Neuroscience

Fundamentals for Rehabilitation

Neuroscience
Fundamentals for Rehabilitation
Third Edition

Laurie Lundy-Ekman, PT, PhD

Professor of Physical Therapy
Pacific University
Hillsboro, Oregon

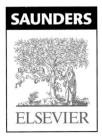

SAUNDERS

ELSEVIER

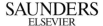

11830 Westline Industrial Drive
St. Louis, Missouri 63146

NEUROSCIENCE: FUNDAMENTALS FOR REHABILITATION, THIRD EDITION
ISBN 13: 978-1-4160-2578-8

Notice

Previous editions copyright © 2002, 1998

Library of Congress Control Number: 2007925845

Publishing Director: Linda Duncan
Editor: Kathryn Falk
Developmental Editor: Andrew Grow
Publishing Services Manager: Pat Joiner-Myers
Senior Project Manager: Karen M. Rehwinkel
Cover Design Direction: Paula Ruckenbrod
Interior Designer: Paula Ruckenbrod

Printed in China

Last digit is the print number: 9 8 7 6 5 4 3 2 1

To my husband Andy and my daughter Lisa

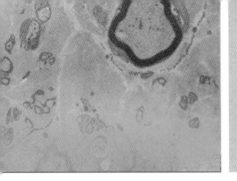

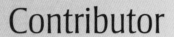

Contributor

Lisa Stehno-Bittel, PT, PhD
Associate Professor
Department of Physical Therapy Education
University of Kansas Medical Center
Kansas City, Kansas

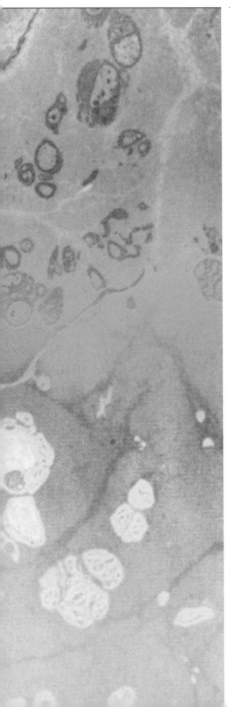

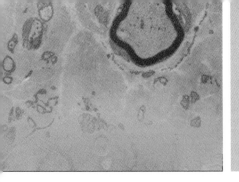

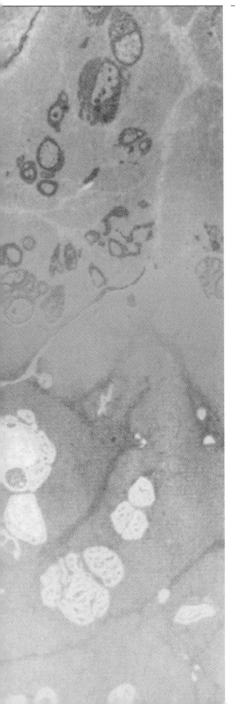

Preface

How do we perceive, feel emotions, move, learn, and remember? And what are the common neural disorders that affect these processes? Neuroscience is the attempt to answer these questions. However, the answers in neuroscience are not static; knowledge progresses rapidly. This third edition of *Neuroscience: Fundamentals for Rehabilitation* reflects updated concepts and recent research. Yet the original purpose of the book remains unaltered: to present carefully selected, clinically important information essential for understanding the neurologic disorders encountered by therapists. Feedback from students, clinicians, and educators indicates that they find the book exceptionally useful both as an introduction to neuroscience and as a reference during clinical practice.

This text is unique in addressing neuroscience issues critical for the practice of physical rehabilitation. Clinical issues including abnormal muscle tone, chronic pain, and control of movement are emphasized, whereas topics often discussed extensively in neuroscience texts, such as the function of neurons in the visual cortex, are omitted.

The text has five sections: Cellular Level, Development, Systems, Regions, and Support Systems. The **Cellular Level** discusses the variety of neural cells, neuron ion channels, membrane potentials, synapses, and mechanisms of learning/memory (Chapters 2-4). **Development** covers embryology of the nervous system and developmental disorders (Chapter 5). Three systems comprise the **Systems** section: somatosensory, autonomic, and motor (Chapters 6-10). The somatosensory system transmits information from the skin and the musculoskeletal system to the brain. The autonomic system conveys information between the brain and smooth muscles, viscera, and glands. The motor system transmits information from the brain to the skeletal muscles. Disorders that affect these three systems are presented. **Regions** covers the peripheral nervous system, spinal region, brainstem and cerebellar region, and the cerebrum (Chapters 11-17). The final section, **Support Systems**, discusses the blood supply and the cerebrospinal fluid system (Chapter 18).

This organization provides the student the opportunity to learn how neural cells operate first, and then apply that knowledge while developing an understanding of systems neuroscience. In learning systems neuroscience, the student develops familiarity with landmarks throughout the nervous system that are revisited in the regions section. The final chapter integrates much of the information from previous chapters in the discussion of the effects of strokes. Thus the text is structured so that subsequent chapters build on the information in earlier chapters, and earlier information is developed more fully and applied to new clinical disorders later in the text. This structure provides a framework for neurologic examination and evaluation: first the systems involved are identified, and then the region(s) implicated are identified.

In addition to the five sections of the book, an **Atlas** of photographs of normal sections of the human brain, with labeled line drawings on the pages facing each photograph, is located at the front of the book and two **Appendices** covering neurochemicals are located at the back of the book.

Distinctive features of this text include:

- Personal stories written by people with neurologic disorders; these stories give the information immediacy and a connection with reality that is sometimes missing from textbook presentations
- Clinical notes containing case examples to challenge students to apply the information to clinical practice
- Disease profiles that provide a quick summary of the features of common neurologic disorders: pathology, etiology, signs and symptoms, region affected, demographics, and prognosis
- Brief introductions to clinical examination techniques

Topics that are new or extensively revised in this edition include:

- Neurotransmitters and neuromodulators
- Neuroplasticity
- Developmental coordination disorder
- Mechanisms of neuropathic pain
- The pain matrix
- Migraine
- Red flags for headache, low back pain, and spinal region disorders
- Golgi tendon organ function
- Stepping pattern generators
- Spasticity
- Effects of anxiety on motor behavior
- Role of movement in the health of peripheral nerves
- Movement of the spinal cord within the vertebral canal
- Evaluation of the dizzy patient
- Effects of behavior on immune function
- Autism spectrum disorders
- Dementia with Lewy bodies
- Locked-in syndrome
- Minimally conscious state

Learning Aids

- **Chapter Outlines, Introductions, and Summaries** clarify the organization of each chapter and reinforce important topics.
- **Terms in bold** highlight important terminology. These terms are defined when first used and are also collected as a glossary at the end of the book.
- **Clinical Notes** are opportunities for the students to test their ability to apply neuroscience information to a specific case. Answers to the Clinical Notes are available at the back of the book.
- **Review Questions** focus student attention on significant topics. Answers to the review questions are available at the back of the book.
- **References** are provided as guides into the research literature.
- Hundreds of original **full-color illustrations** complement content.

Supplementary Learning Resources

Online learning resources to complement this textbook are available at the Elsevier Evolve website (*http://evolve.elsevier.com/Lundy/*). At this website, students will find a workbook, content updates, author contact information, and WebLinks to facilitate further exploration. The workbook provides multiple choice and short-answer questions, matching exercises, drawings to label, and terms to define for each chapter. Correct answers are available online for all of the exercises except the term definitions. Term definitions are available in the glossary of this textbook. In addition to the student resources, instructors using this textbook have access to an online course management system and an image collection of the textbook illustrations. The course management system provides tools for online discussion, a calendar, uploading and downloading of documents, and quiz capability. The images can be downloaded for use in presentations.

The CD contains approximately 40 animations depicting a variety of neurologic disorders and anatomic characteristics. The animations include synaptic activity, action potentials, neural development, muscle spindle, Golgi tendon organ, somatosensory pathways, dermatomes, myotomes, actin-myosin bonds, titin, motor pathways, cauda equina lesion, and the pupillary reflex.

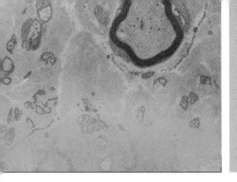

Acknowledgments

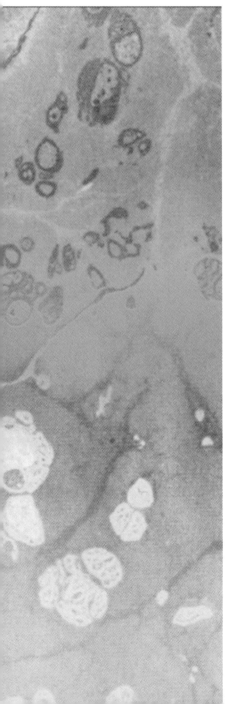

This edition has been significantly improved by the contributions of several key people. Lisa Ekman, content editor, made extensive suggestions for improving the readability and organization of the entire text. Lisa Stehno-Bittel updated and revised Chapters 2, 3, and 4. Erin Jobst provided suggestions for revisions to Chapter 7. Andrew Grow, Developmental Editor, was consistently helpful and encouraging throughout the process. My husband Andy and my daughter Lisa have been patient, good humored, and supportive during the writing of this book.

Students who provided guidance on previous editions include Christopher Boor, Nancy Heinley, Mike Hmura, and Susan Hendrickson. Clinicians and faculty who reviewed previous manuscripts include Anne Burleigh-Jacobs, Renate Powell, Mike Studer, Robert Rosenow, and Daiva Banaitis.

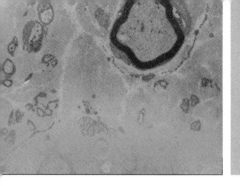

Contents

4 Neuroplasticity   71

5 Development of the Nervous System   85

6 Somatosensory System   105

9 The Motor System: Motor Neurons 187

10 Basal Ganglia, Cerebellum, and Movement 243

**18 Support Systems: Blood Supply and
     Cerebrospinal Fluid System   485**

Neuroscience

Fundamentals for Rehabilitation

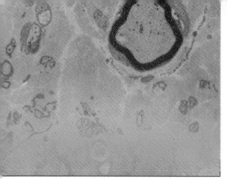

Atlas

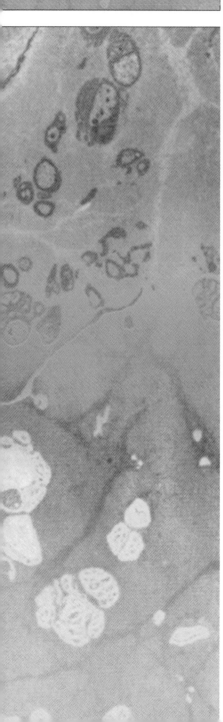

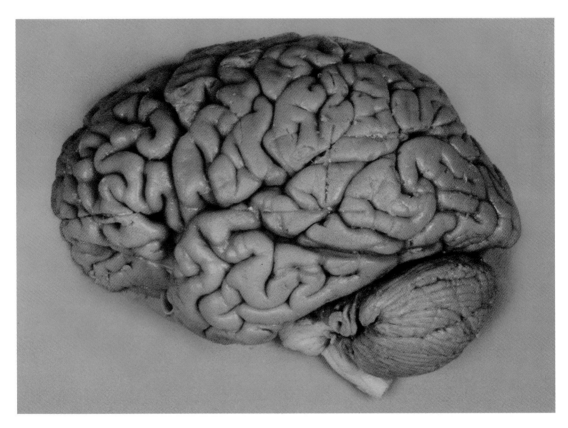

FIGURE A1

Lateral view of the brain. Anterior is to the left. Dotted lines indicate boundaries between areas that are not separated by the sulci. The orbital gyri are part of the frontal lobe. (Photograph courtesy Dr. John W. Sundsten, Department of Biological Structure, University of Washington.)

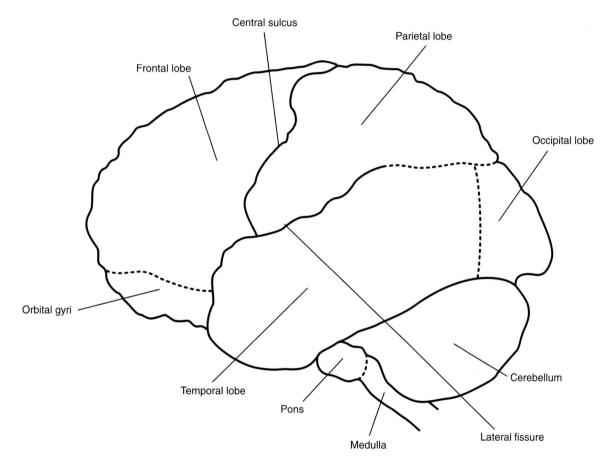

Central sulcus

Parietal lobe

Frontal lobe

Occipital lobe

Orbital gyri

Cerebellum

Temporal lobe

Pons

Lateral fissure

Medulla

FIGURE A1

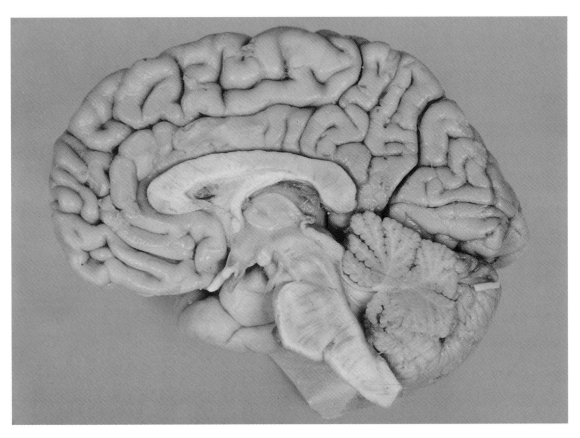

FIGURE A2
Midsaggital view of the brain. Anterior is to the left. (Photograph courtesy Dr. John W. Sundsten, Department of Biological Structure, University of Washington.)

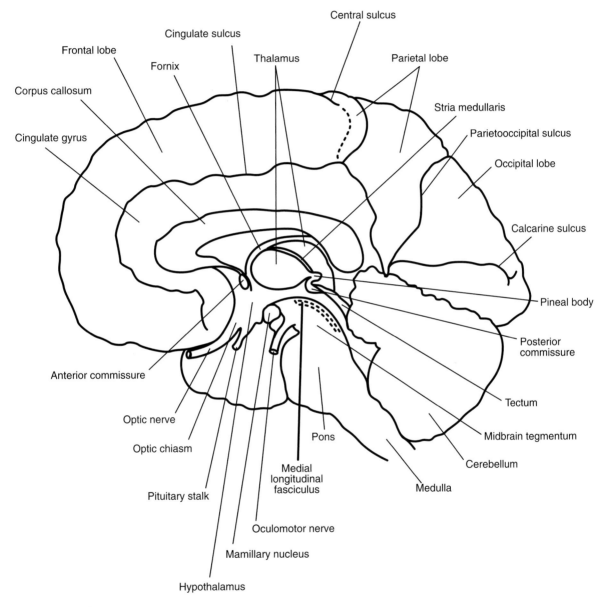

Central sulcus

Cingulate sulcus

Frontal lobe

Fornix

Thalamus

Parietal lobe

Corpus callosum

Stria medullaris

Cingulate gyrus

Parietooccipital sulcus

Occipital lobe

Calcarine sulcus

Pineal body

Posterior commissure

Anterior commissure

Tectum

Optic nerve

Midbrain tegmentum

Optic chiasm

Pons

Cerebellum

Pituitary stalk

Medial longitudinal fasciculus

Medulla

Oculomotor nerve

Mamillary nucleus

Hypothalamus

FIGURE A2

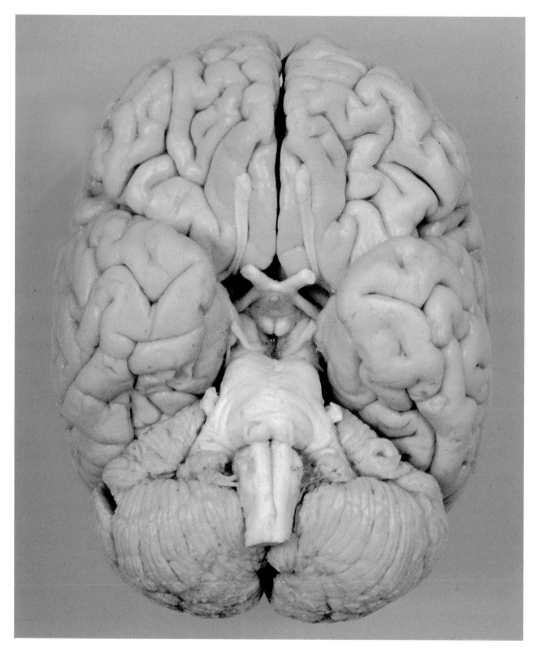

FIGURE A3
Inferior view of the brain. Anterior is at the top. The inset shows the medulla and some of the cranial nerves associated with the medulla. (Photograph courtesy Dr. John W. Sundsten, Department of Biological Structure, University of Washington.)

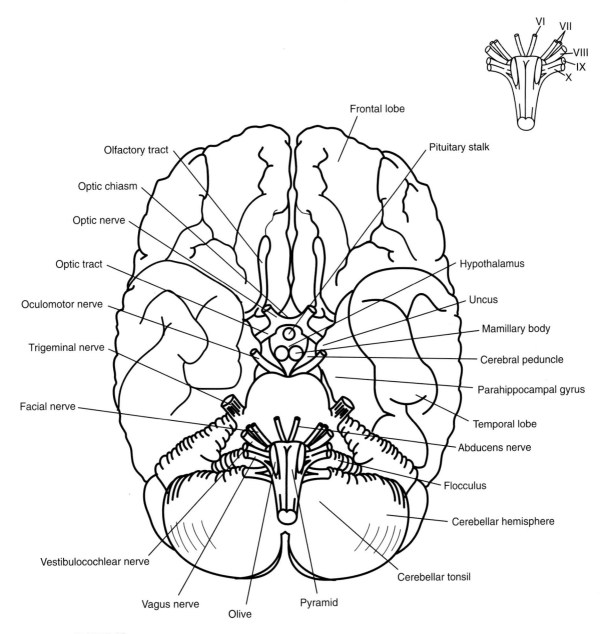

Olfactory tract

Optic chiasm

Optic nerve

Optic tract

Oculomotor nerve

Trigeminal nerve

Facial nerve

Vestibulocochlear nerve

Vagus nerve

Olive

Pyramid

Frontal lobe

Pituitary stalk

Hypothalamus

Uncus

Mamillary body

Cerebral peduncle

Parahippocampal gyrus

Temporal lobe

Abducens nerve

Flocculus

Cerebellar hemisphere

Cerebellar tonsil

VI VII VIII IX X

FIGURE A3

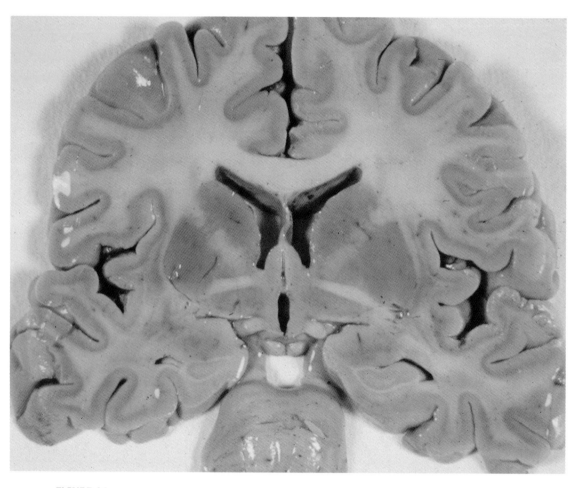

FIGURE A4
Oblique coronal section. See inset of a midsagittal section for the angle of the section. (Photograph courtesy Dr. John W. Sundsten, Department of Biological Structure, University of Washington.)

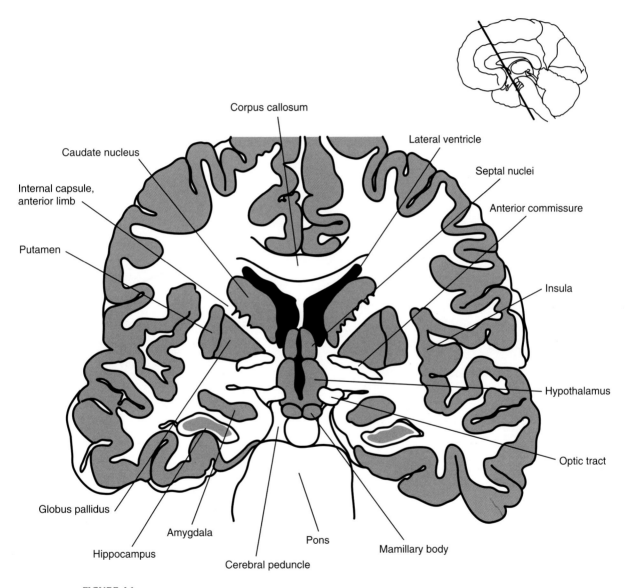

Corpus callosum

Lateral ventricle

Septal nuclei

Caudate nucleus

Anterior commissure

Internal capsule,
anterior limb

Putamen

Insula

Hypothalamus

Optic tract

Globus pallidus

Amygdala

Pons

Mamillary body

Hippocampus

Cerebral peduncle

FIGURE A4

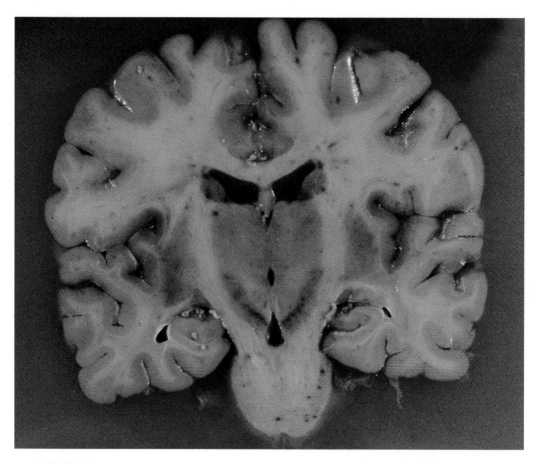

FIGURE A5

Coronal section, through putamen and globus pallidus. Note the direct continuation of the internal capsule into the cerebral penduncle. (Photograph courtesy Dr. John W. Sundsten, Department of Biological Structure, University of Washington.)

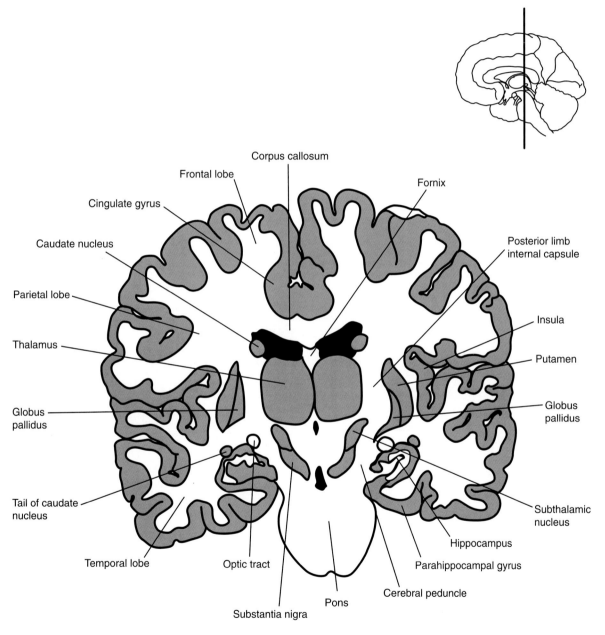

Corpus callosum

Frontal lobe

Cingulate gyrus

Caudate nucleus

Parietal lobe

Thalamus

Globus pallidus

Tail of caudate nucleus

Temporal lobe

Optic tract

Substantia nigra

Pons

Fornix

Posterior limb internal capsule

Insula

Putamen

Globus pallidus

Subthalamic nucleus

Hippocampus

Parahippocampal gyrus

Cerebral peduncle

FIGURE A5

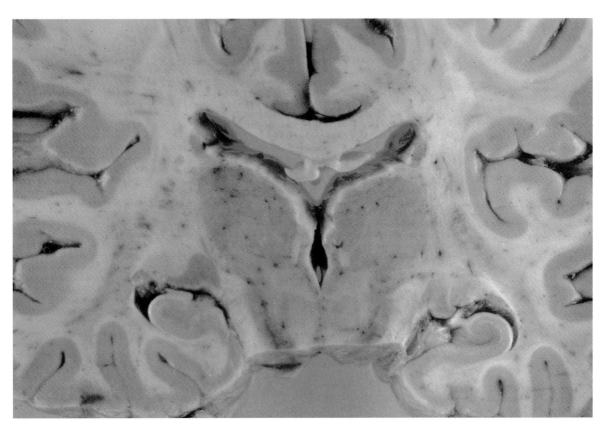

FIGURE A6
Coronal section, through posterior thalamus. (Photograph courtesy Dr. Jeannette Townsend, University of Utah.)

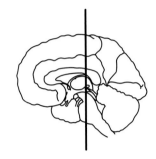

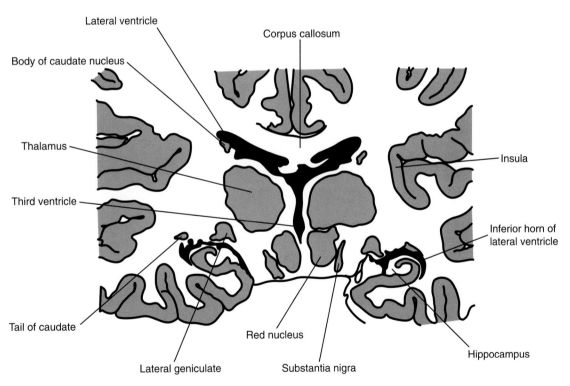

Lateral ventricle

Corpus callosum

Body of caudate nucleus

Thalamus

Insula

Third ventricle

Inferior horn of
lateral ventricle

Tail of caudate

Red nucleus

Hippocampus

Lateral geniculate

Substantia nigra

FIGURE A6

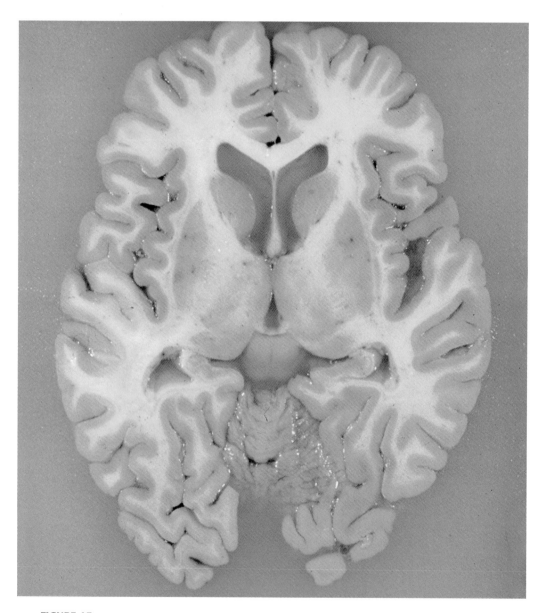

FIGURE A7

Horizontal section. Anterior is at the top. (Photograph courtesy Dr. John W. Sundsten, Department of Biological Structure, University of Washington.)

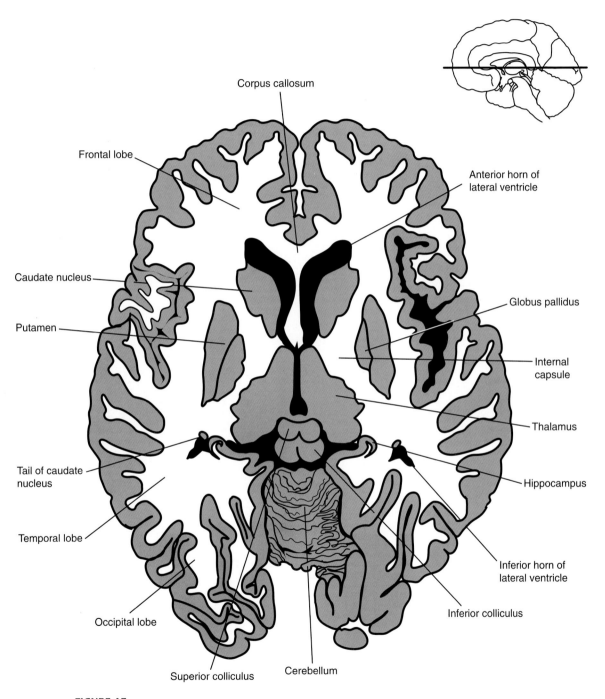

Corpus callosum

Frontal lobe

Anterior horn of
lateral ventricle

Caudate nucleus

Globus pallidus

Putamen

Internal
capsule

Thalamus

Tail of caudate
nucleus

Hippocampus

Temporal lobe

Inferior horn of
lateral ventricle

Occipital lobe

Inferior colliculus

Superior colliculus

Cerebellum

FIGURE A7

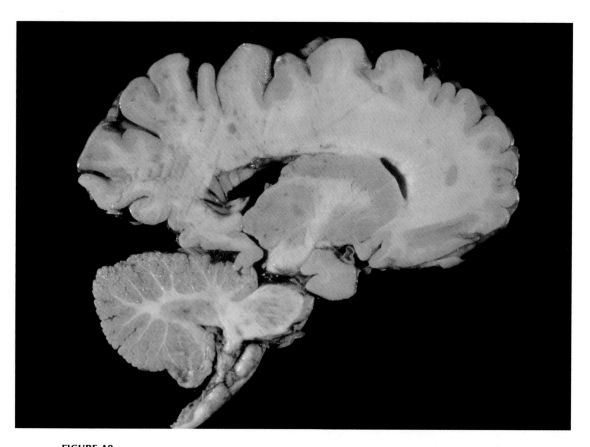

FIGURE A8

Sagittal section, lateral to the midline. Anterior is to the right. In the inset, the cerebellum has been removed to clearly show the location of the section. The section includes the cerebellum. (Photograph courtesy Dr. Jeannette Townsend, University of Utah.)

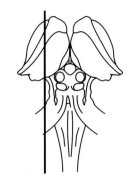

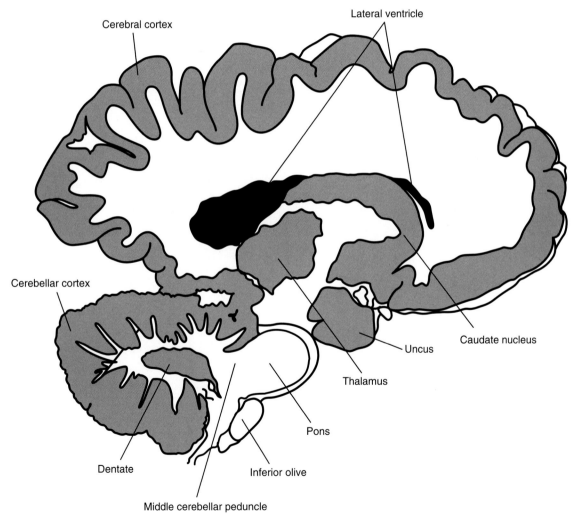

Cerebral cortex

Lateral ventricle

Cerebellar cortex

Caudate nucleus

Uncus

Thalamus

Dentate

Pons

Inferior olive

Middle cerebellar peduncle

FIGURE A8

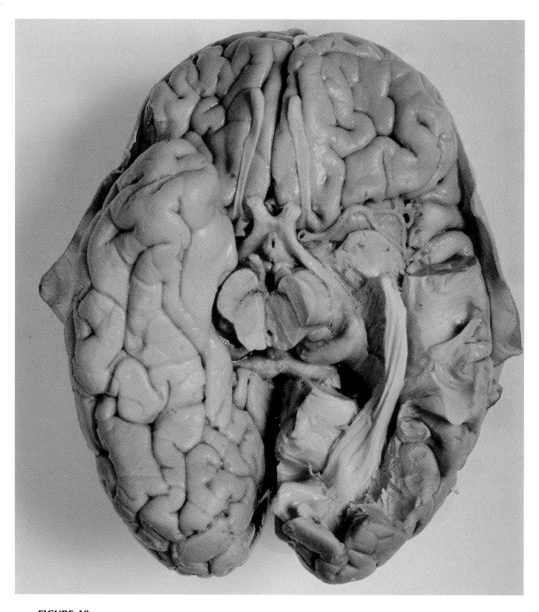

FIGURE A9

Inferior view of the brain. Anterior is at the top. The pons, medulla, and cerebellum have been removed. The temporal and occipital lobes have been partially removed to reveal the visual radiation. (Photograph courtesy Dr. John W. Sundsten, Department of Biological Structure, University of Washington.)

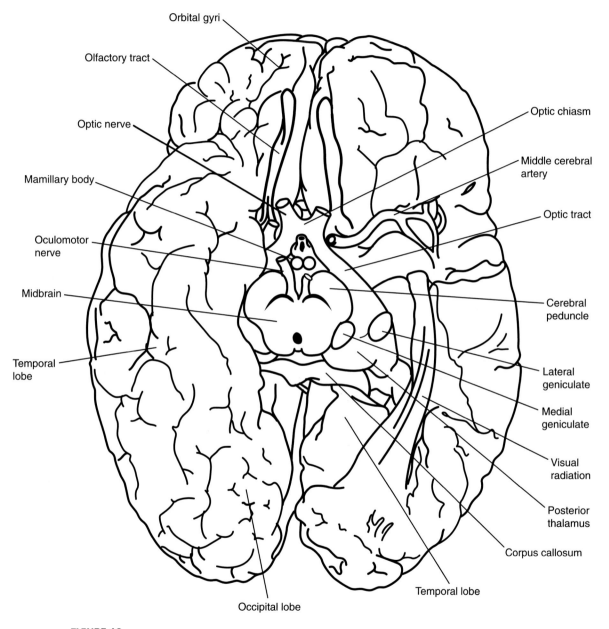

Orbital gyri

Olfactory tract

Optic nerve

Mamillary body

Oculomotor
nerve

Midbrain

Temporal
lobe

Optic chiasm

Middle cerebral
artery

Optic tract

Cerebral
peduncle

Lateral
geniculate

Medial
geniculate

Visual
radiation

Posterior
thalamus

Corpus callosum

Temporal lobe

Occipital lobe

FIGURE A9

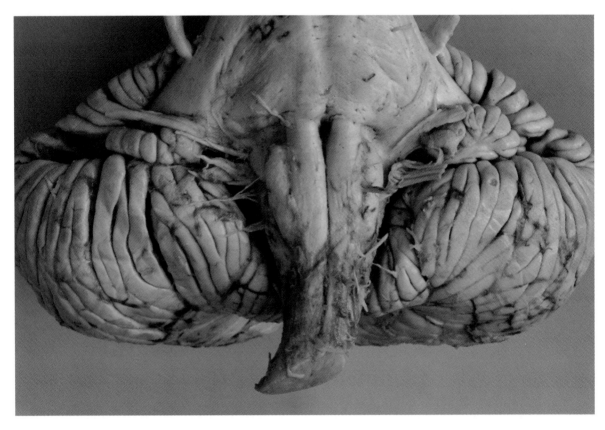

FIGURE A10

Anterior view of the pons, medulla, and cerebellum. On the specimen, only a fragment of the hypoglossal nerve is intact. In the illustration, the initial section of the hypoglossal nerve has been added on the right.

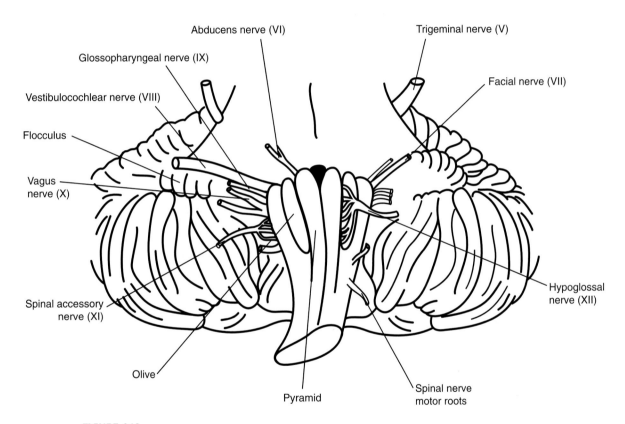

Abducens nerve (VI)

Trigeminal nerve (V)

Glossopharyngeal nerve (IX)

Facial nerve (VII)

Vestibulocochlear nerve (VIII)

Flocculus

Vagus
nerve (X)

Hypoglossal
nerve (XII)

Spinal accessory
nerve (XI)

Olive

Pyramid

Spinal nerve
motor roots

FIGURE A10

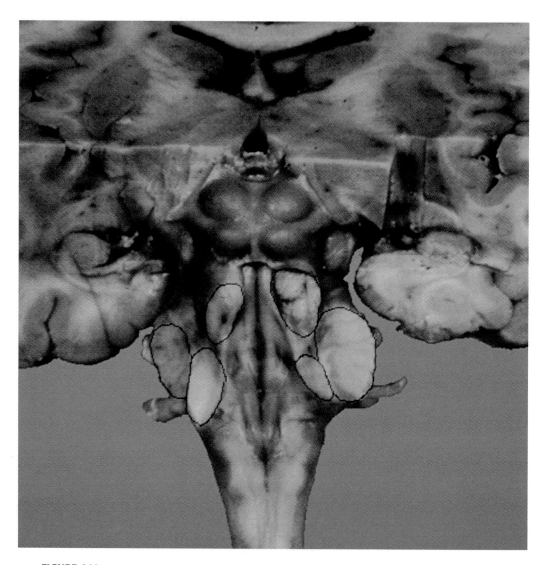

FIGURE A11

Posterior view of the brainstem and cerebral hemispheres. The cerebellum has been removed. The cerebral hemispheres have been sectioned in the horizontal plane and also in the coronal plane through the temporal lobe. The red line indicates the intersection of the planes of section. Above the line is the horizontal section of the cerebrum. See inset of a midsagittal section for the angles of the sections. (Photograph courtesy Dr. John W. Sundsten, Department of Biological Structure, University of Washington.)

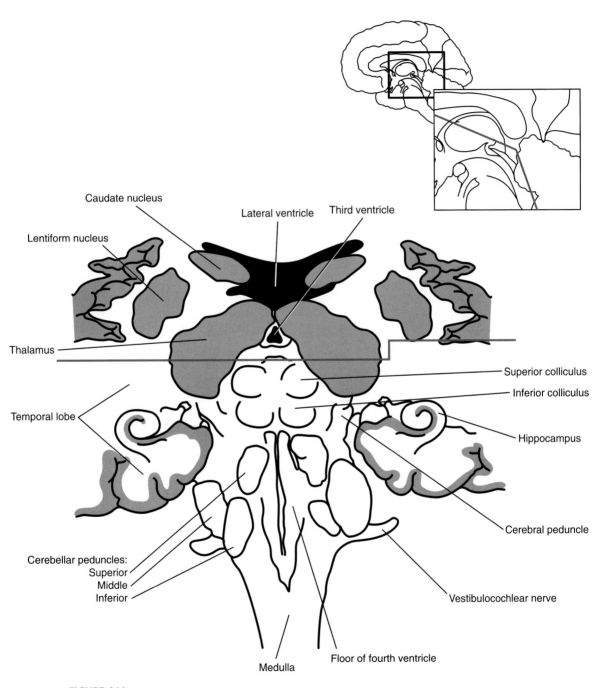

Caudate nucleus

Lentiform nucleus

Lateral ventricle

Third ventricle

Thalamus

Superior colliculus

Inferior colliculus

Temporal lobe

Hippocampus

Cerebral peduncle

Cerebellar peduncles:
Superior
Middle
Inferior

Vestibulocochlear nerve

Medulla

Floor of fourth ventricle

FIGURE A11

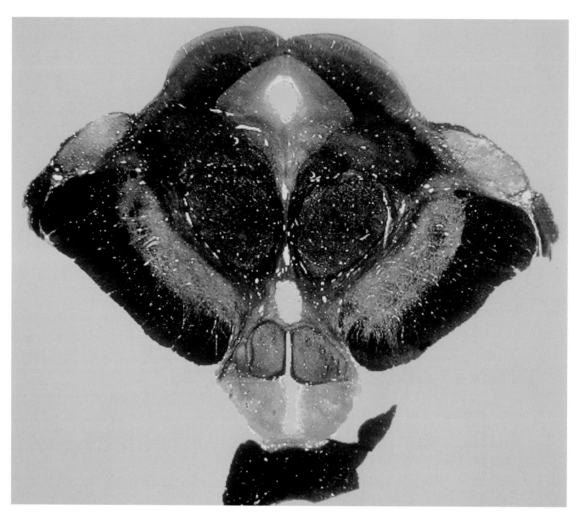

FIGURE A12

Horizontal section of the upper midbrain. Posterior is at the top. The myelin has been stained to appear black instead of light in color. At the bottom of the section, below the dotted line, are structures that are not part of the midbrain: the optic chiasm and the hypothalamus with its mamillary nuclei. In the outline drawing, the shading reflects the natural (unstained) appearance of the tissue, with the gray matter dark and the white matter light. (Photograph courtesy Dr. John W. Sundsten, Department of Biological Structure, University of Washington.)

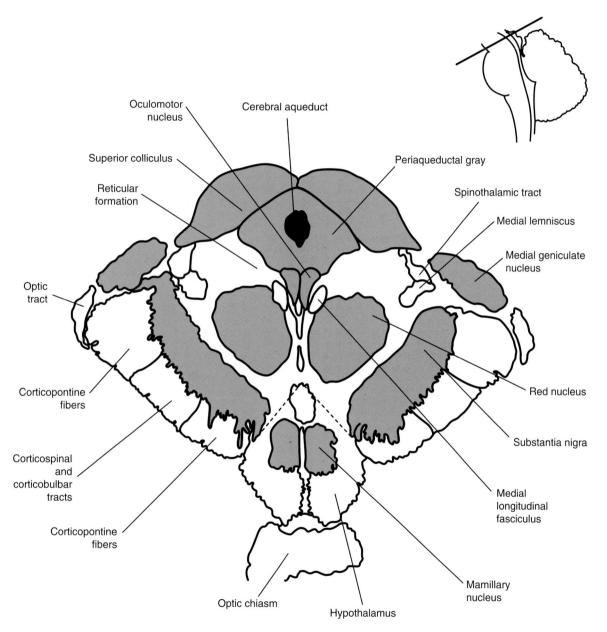

Oculomotor
nucleus

Cerebral aqueduct

Periaqueductal gray

Superior colliculus

Spinothalamic tract

Reticular
formation

Medial lemniscus

Medial geniculate
nucleus

Optic
tract

Red nucleus

Corticopontine
fibers

Substantia nigra

Corticospinal
and
corticobulbar
tracts

Medial
longitudinal
fasciculus

Corticopontine
fibers

Optic chiasm

Hypothalamus

Mamillary
nucleus

FIGURE A12

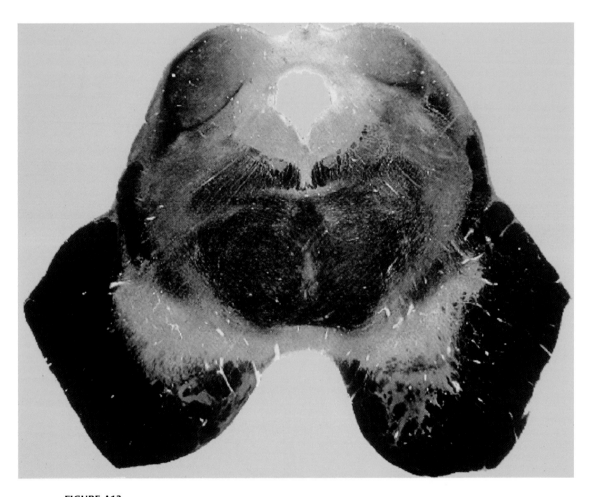

FIGURE A13

Horizontal section of the lower midbrain. Posterior is at the top. The myelin has been stained to appear black instead of light in color. In the outline drawing, the shading reflects the natural (unstained) appearance of the tissue, with the gray matter dark and the white matter light. (Photograph courtesy Dr. John W. Sundsten, Department of Biological Structure, University of Washington.)

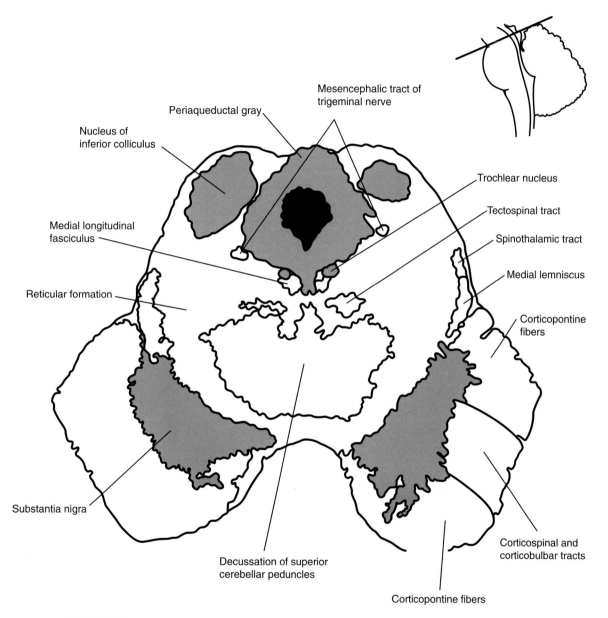

Mesencephalic tract of
trigeminal nerve

Periaqueductal gray

Nucleus of
inferior colliculus

Trochlear nucleus

Tectospinal tract

Spinothalamic tract

Medial longitudinal
fasciculus

Medial lemniscus

Corticopontine
fibers

Reticular formation

Substantia nigra

Decussation of superior
cerebellar peduncles

Corticospinal and
corticobulbar tracts

Corticopontine fibers

FIGURE A13

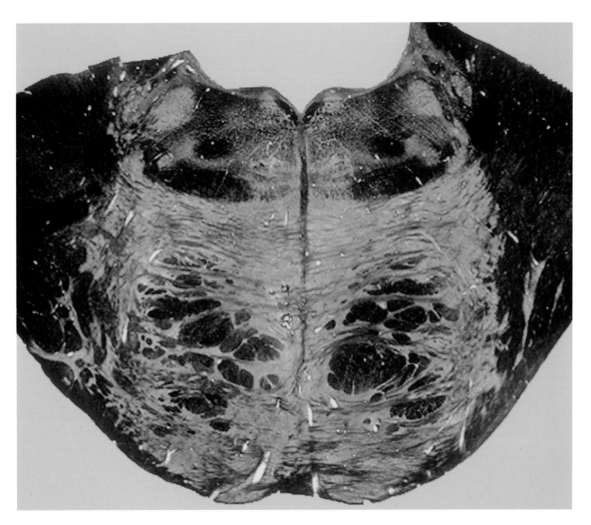

FIGURE A14

Mid-pons. Posterior is at the top. The myelin has been stained to appear black instead of light in color. In the outline drawing, the shading reflects the natural (unstained) appearance of the tissue, with the gray matter dark and the white matter light. (Photograph courtesy Dr. John W. Sundsten, Department of Biological Structure, University Washington.)

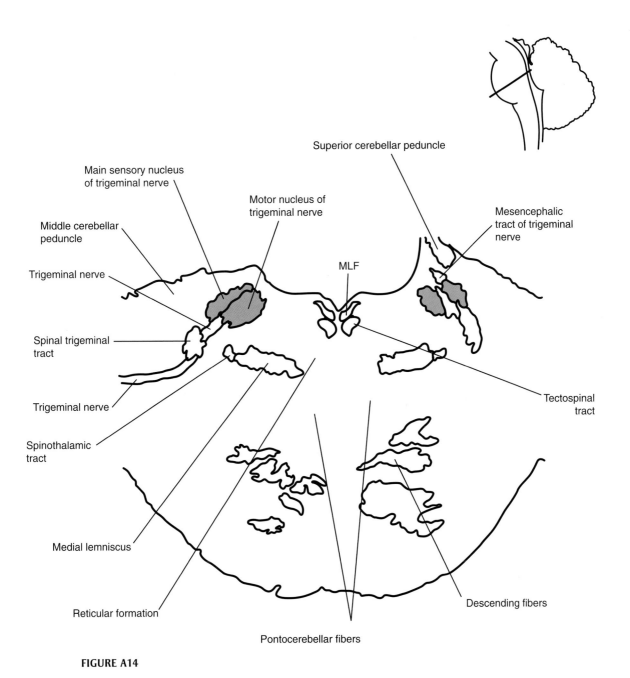

Superior cerebellar peduncle

Main sensory nucleus
of trigeminal nerve

Motor nucleus of
trigeminal nerve

Mesencephalic
tract of trigeminal
nerve

Middle cerebellar
peduncle

Trigeminal nerve

MLF

Spinal trigeminal
tract

Trigeminal nerve

Tectospinal
tract

Spinothalamic
tract

Medial lemniscus

Descending fibers

Reticular formation

Pontocerebellar fibers

FIGURE A14

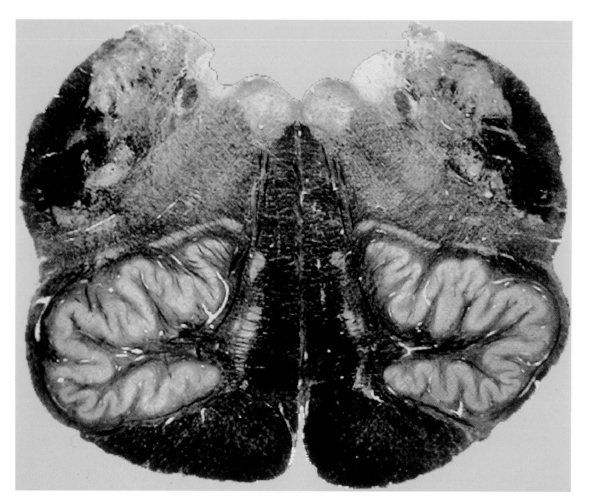

FIGURE A15

Upper medulla. Posterior is at the top. The myelin has been stained to appear black instead of light in color. In the outline drawing, the shading reflects the natural (unstained) appearance of the tissue, with the gray matter dark and the white matter light. (Photograph courtesy Dr. John W. Sundsten, Department of Biological Structure, University Washington.)

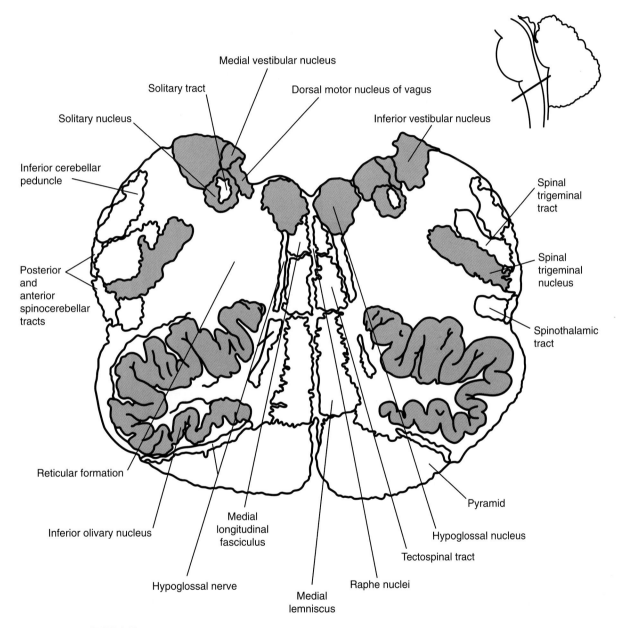

Medial vestibular nucleus

Solitary tract

Solitary nucleus

Dorsal motor nucleus of vagus

Inferior vestibular nucleus

Inferior cerebellar peduncle

Spinal trigeminal tract

Spinal trigeminal nucleus

Posterior and anterior spinocerebellar tracts

Spinothalamic tract

Reticular formation

Pyramid

Inferior olivary nucleus

Medial longitudinal fasciculus

Hypoglossal nucleus

Tectospinal tract

Hypoglossal nerve

Raphe nuclei

Medial lemniscus

FIGURE A15

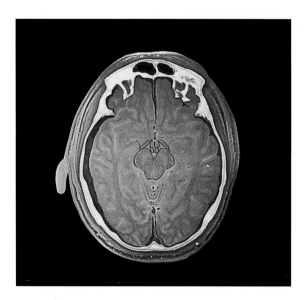

FIGURE A16
Contrast-enhanced CAT (computerized axial tomography) scan of a normal brain. Horizontal section. (From Bo WJ, et al. [1990]. Basic atlas of sectional anatomy with correlated imaging. [2nd ed.]. Philadelphia: Saunders.)

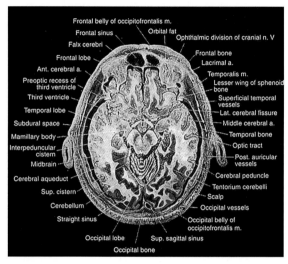

Frontal belly of occipitofrontalis m.
Frontal sinus
Orbital fat
Ophthalmic division of cranial n. V
Falx cerebri
Frontal lobe
Frontal bone
Ant. cerebral a.
Lacrimal a.
Preoptic recess of third ventricle
Temporalis m.
Lesser wing of sphenoid bone
Third ventricle
Superficial temporal vessels
Temporal lobe
Lat. cerebral fissure
Subdural space
Middle cerebral a.
Mamillary body
Temporal bone
Interpeduncular cistern
Optic tract
Midbrain
Post. auricular vessels
Cerebral peduncle
Cerebral aqueduct
Tentorium cerebelli
Sup. cistern
Scalp
Cerebellum
Occipital vessels
Straight sinus
Occipital belly of occipitofrontalis m.
Occipital lobe
Sup. sagittal sinus
Occipital bone

FIGURE A17
Photograph of brain section imaged in A16. (From Bo WJ, et al. [1990]. Basic atlas of sectional anatomy with correlated imaging. [2nd ed.]. Philadelphia: Saunders.)

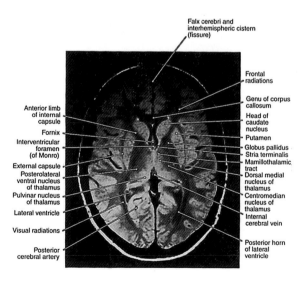

Falx cerebri and interhemispheric cistern (fissure)

Anterior limb of internal capsule
Fornix
Interventricular foramen (of Monro)
External capsule
Posterolateral ventral nucleus of thalamus
Pulvinar nucleus of thalamus
Lateral ventricle
Visual radiations
Posterior cerebral artery

Frontal radiations
Genu of corpus callosum
Head of caudate nucleus
Putamen
Globus pallidus
Stria terminalis
Mamillothalamic tract
Dorsal medial nucleus of thalamus
Centromedian nucleus of thalamus
Internal cerebral vein
Posterior horn of lateral ventricle

FIGURE A18
MRI (magnetic resonance imaging) of a normal brain. Horizontal section. (From Pomeranz SJ [1989]. Craniospinal magnetic resonance imaging. Philadelphia: Saunders.)

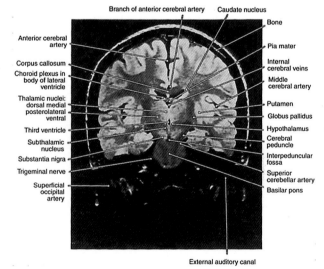

Branch of anterior cerebral artery
Caudate nucleus
Bone
Anterior cerebral artery
Pia mater
Corpus callosum
Internal cerebral veins
Choroid plexus in body of lateral ventricle
Middle cerebral artery
Thalamic nuclei: dorsal medial posterolateral ventral
Putamen
Third ventricle
Globus pallidus
Subthalamic nucleus
Hypothalamus
Substantia nigra
Cerebral peduncle
Trigeminal nerve
Interpeduncular fossa
Superficial occipital artery
Superior cerebellar artery
Basilar pons
External auditory canal

FIGURE A19
MRI (magnetic resonance imaging) of a normal brain. Coronal section. (From Pomeranz SJ [1989]. Craniospinal magnetic resonance imaging. Philadelphia: Saunders.)

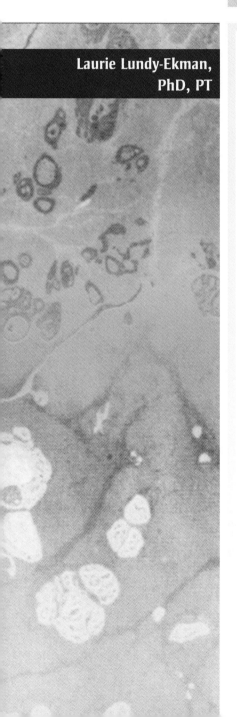

1

Introduction to Neuroscience

Laurie Lundy-Ekman, PhD, PT

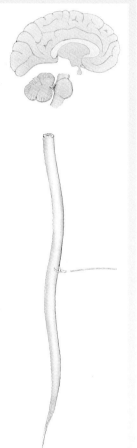

Many people live with functional limitations related to nervous system damage or disease. People who have experienced brain damage, spinal cord injury, birth defects, and neurologic diseases must cope with the effects. Tasks as seemingly simple as sitting, standing, walking, getting dressed, and remembering a name may become incredible challenges. Physical and occupational therapy play a crucial role in helping people regain the ability to function as independently as possible. The design of physical and occupational therapy treatments and the management of each individual case are dependent on an understanding of the nervous system and continued research.

WHAT IS NEUROSCIENCE?

The quest to understand the nervous system is called **neuroscience**. Neuroscience is a relatively new science concerned with the development, chemistry, structure, function, and pathology of the nervous system. Rigorous scientific research on neural function has a relatively short history, beginning in the late 1800s. At that time, physiologists Fritsch and Hitzig reported that electrical stimulation of specific areas of an animal's cerebral cortex elicited movement, and physicians Broca and Wernicke separately confirmed, by autopsy, localized brain damage in people who had language deficits after stroke. About the same time, Hughlings Jackson proposed that multiple brain areas are essential for complex functions such as perception, action, and language.

About 1890, Cajal, a neuroanatomist, established that each nerve cell (neuron) is a distinct, individual cell, not directly continuous with other nerve cells. Sherrington, a physiologist studying involuntary reactions that occur in response to stimuli, proposed that nerve cells were linked by specialized connections he named synapses. The next major advances in understanding the nervous system did not occur until the 1950s, when both the electron microscope and the microelectrode were developed. The electron microscope allows visualization of cellular organelles, and the microelectrode can record the activity of a single nerve cell.

Beginning in the 1970s, new imaging techniques were developed that create clear images of the living spinal cord and brain, unobscured by the surrounding skull and vertebrae. These imaging techniques provide physiologic and pathologic information never before available. Computerized axial tomography (CAT), positron emission tomography (PET), and magnetic resonance imaging (MRI) all use computerized analysis to create an image of the nervous system (Figure 1-1). In a CAT scan, a series of x-rays are analyzed by a computer to generate an image of the density of various areas in the nervous system. PET scans require injecting a radioactive substance into the bloodstream, then using a special camera to record signals emitted by radioactive decay. The amount of radioactive decay in an area is proportional to the local blood flow, so the computer-generated image is an indirect indicator of nerve cell activity. MRI uses a magnetic field to align naturally occurring protons in the body, and then a radio frequency pulse temporarily disrupts the alignment. The signal emitted as the nuclei return to their original position is detected, and these signals are converted into images of the nervous system. MRI can produce excellent three-dimensional images of nervous system tissues and provide information about activity-related changes in blood flow.

In 1985, the development of transcranial magnetic stimulation (TMS) enabled researchers to stimulate brain activity without opening the skull. An electric current in a coil near the scalp generates a magnetic field that passes through the skull. The magnetic field induces an electric current in a small area of the brain (Figure 1-2). The electric current activates local neurons. For example, if a specific part of the motor cortex is stimulated, the hand moves without the intent of the person receiving the stimulation. TMS is usually painless. After TMS, the stimulated brain area is temporarily inactive. Thus TMS allows researchers to investigate the effects of stimulating a part of the brain and, in addition, to study the effects of briefly inactivating part of the brain without damaging the area or using invasive techniques.

All of these techniques used historically to examine neural function are still used today, though with many refinements. Current approaches to understanding the nervous system include multiple levels of analysis:
- Molecular
- Cellular
- Systems
- Behavioral
- Cognitive

Analysis of the Nervous System

Molecular neuroscience investigates the chemistry and physics involved in neural function. Studies of the ionic exchanges required for a nerve cell to conduct information from one part of the nervous system to another and the chemical transfer of information between nerve cells are molecular-level neuroscience. Reduced to their most fundamental level, sensation, moving, understanding, planning, relating, speaking, and most other human functions depend on chemical and electrical changes in nervous system cells.

Cellular neuroscience considers distinctions between different types of cells in the nervous system and how each cell type functions. Inquiries into how an individual neuron processes and conveys information, how information is transferred among neurons, and the roles of non-neural cells in the nervous system are cellular-level questions.

Systems neuroscience investigates groups of neurons that perform a common function. Systems-level analysis studies the connections, or circuitry, of the nervous system. Examples are the proprioceptive system, which conveys position and movement information from the

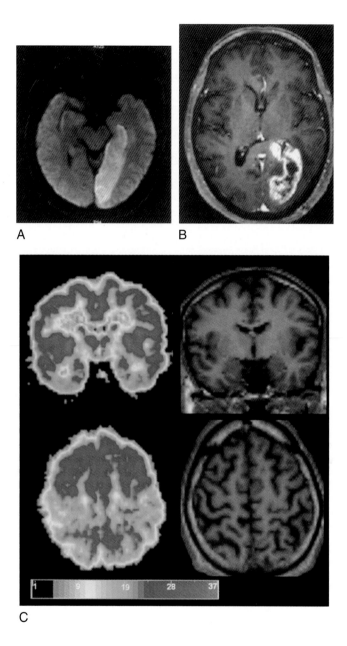

A

B

C

FIGURE 1-1

Computerized imaging of the brain. **A, CAT** (x-ray computed axial tomography). CAT brain scans are typically used to investigate suspected strokes or increased intracranial pressure. In this horizontal section, the whitest area indicates infarction. **B, MRI** (magnetic resonance imaging). MRI produces the best resolution of various soft tissues. In this horizontal section, the whitest area indicates a tumor. **C, PET** (positron emission computed tomography). PET scans are used to assess blood flow, oxygen or glucose metabolism, or receptor location. Often PET scans include a color scale. Compare the PET scans on the left to the MRI scans on the right. The top scans are coronal sections and the bottom scans are horizontal sections. The colors on the PET scans indicate the number of opioid receptors (when activated, decrease the emotional response to pain) in a given area; the highest concentration is indicated in violet. (**A** *from Shetty SK, Lev MH. CT perfusion in acute stroke. 2005. Neuroimaging Clin North Am. 15(3):481-501, ix. Review. P 492.* **B** *from Chenevert TL, Sundgren PC, Ross BD. Diffusion imaging: insight to cell status and cytoarchitecture 2006. Neuroimaging Clin North Am. 16(4):619-632, viii-x. p 492.* **C** *from Hammers A, Lingford-Hughes A. 2006 Opioid imaging. Neuroimaging Clin North Am. 16(4):529-552, vii. P 536.)*

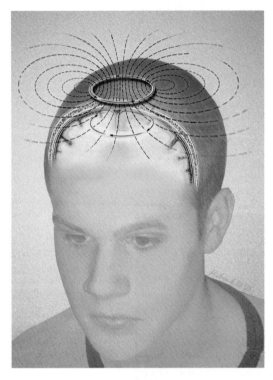

FIGURE 1-2
During transcranial magnetic stimulation, an electromagnetic coil is held against a person's scalp. The coil emits magnetic pulses that pass though the skull and induce an electric current in the brain. This electric current alters the activity of neurons. *(Illustration courtesy L. Kibiuk/Society for Neuroscience.)*

musculoskeletal system to the central nervous system, and the motor system, which controls movement.

Behavioral neuroscience looks at the interaction among systems that influence behavior. For example, studies of postural control investigate the relative influence of visual, vestibular, and proprioceptive sensations on balance under different conditions.

Cognitive neuroscience covers the fields of thinking, learning, and memory. Studies of planning, using language, and the differences between memory for specific events and memory for performing motor skills are examples of cognitive-level analysis.

What Do We Learn from These Studies?

From a multitude of investigations at all levels of analysis in neuroscience, we have begun to be able to answer questions such as the following:

- How do ions influence nerve cell function?
- How does a nerve cell convey information from one location in the nervous system to another?
- How is language formed and understood?
- How does information about a hot stove encountered by a fingertip reach conscious awareness?
- How are the abilities to stand and walk developed and controlled?
- How can modern medicine contribute to the recovery of neural function?
- How can physical and occupational therapy assist a patient in regaining maximal independence after neurologic injury?

The answers to these questions are explored in this text. The purpose of this text is to present the information that is essential for understanding the neurologic disorders encountered by therapists. Therapists who specialize in neurologic rehabilitation typically treat clients with brain and spinal cord disorders. However, clients with neurologic disorders are not confined to neurologic rehabilitation; therapists specializing in orthopedics frequently treat clients with chronic neck or low back pain, nerve compression syndromes, and other nervous system problems. Regardless of area of specialty, a thorough knowledge of basic neuroscience is important for every therapist.

ORGANIZATION OF THIS BOOK

The information in this text is presented in six parts:

 I. *Cellular level:* Structure and functions of the cells in the nervous system
 II. *Development:* How the nervous system forms
 III. *Somatic and autonomic systems:* Groups of neurons that perform a common function
 IV. *Regions:* Areas of the nervous system
 V. *Support systems:* Blood supply and cerebrospinal fluid systems
 VI. *Appendices:* Intracellular messengers; Neurotransmitters and Neuromodulators

Cellular Level

Cells in the nervous system are neurons and glia. A **neuron** is the functional unit of the nervous system, consisting of a nerve cell body and the processes that extend outward from the cell body: dendrites and the axon.

- Neurons that convey information into the central nervous system are afferent.
- Neurons that transmit information from the central nervous system to peripheral structures are efferent.

- Neurons that connect only with other neurons are interneurons.

Glia are non-neuronal cells that provide services for the neurons. Some specialized glial cells form myelin sheaths, the coverings that surround and insulate axons in the nervous system and aid in the transmission of electrical signals. Other types of glia nourish, support, and protect neurons.

Development of the Human Nervous System

The development of the human nervous system in utero and through infancy is considered in this section. Common developmental disorders are also described.

Somatic and Autonomic Systems

The nervous system is composed of many smaller systems, each with distinct functions. Many systems are discussed in the context of an appropriate region of the nervous system; for example, the cognitive system is discussed in the chapter on the cerebrum. However, three systems extend through all regions of the nervous system: the somatosensory, autonomic, and somatic motor systems. The somatosensory system conveys information from the skin and musculoskeletal system to areas of the brain. The autonomic system provides bidirectional communication between the brain and smooth muscle, cardiac muscle, and gland cells. The somatic motor system transmits information from the brain to skeletal muscles. Because much of the nervous system is devoted to somatosensory, autonomic, and motor functions, being familiar with these three systems gives meaning to many of the terms encountered in studying the regions of the nervous system.

Regions of the Nervous System

The nervous system can be divided into four regions: peripheral, spinal, brainstem and cerebellar, and cerebral regions (Figure 1-3).

Peripheral Nervous System

The peripheral nervous system consists of all parts of the nervous system that are not encased in the vertebral column or skull. Peripheral nerves, including the median, ulnar, sciatic, and cranial nerves, are groups of axons.

Spinal Region

The spinal region includes all parts of the nervous system encased in the vertebral column. In addition to the spinal cord, axons attached to the cord are within the spinal region until the axons exit the intervertebral foramen.

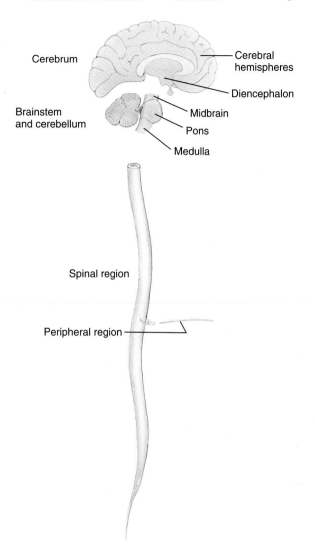

FIGURE 1-3
Lateral view of the regions of the nervous system. Regions are listed on the left, and subdivisions are listed on the right.

Brainstem and Cerebellar Region

The brainstem connects the spinal cord with the cerebral region. The major divisions of the brainstem are the medulla, pons, and midbrain (see Figure 1-3). Although the cranial nerve receptors and axons are part of the peripheral nervous system, because most cranial nerves are functionally and structurally closely related to the brainstem, the cranial nerves are discussed with the brainstem region in this text. Connected to the posterior brainstem is the cerebellum.

Cerebral Region

The most massive part of the brain is the cerebrum, consisting of the diencephalon and cerebral hemispheres (see Figure 1-3). The diencephalon, in the center of the cerebrum, is almost completely surrounded by the cerebral hemispheres. The thalamus and hypothalamus are major structures of the diencephalon. Cerebral hemispheres consist of the cerebral cortex, axons connecting the cortex with other parts of the nervous system, and deep nuclei.

Support Systems

The cerebrospinal fluid and vascular systems provide essential support to the nervous system. Cerebrospinal fluid fills the ventricles, four continuous cavities within the brain, and then circulates on the surface of the central nervous system. Membranous coverings of the central nervous system, the meninges, are part of the cerebrospinal fluid system. The blood supply of the brain is delivered by the internal carotid and vertebral arteries.

Appendices

Appendix A covers intracellular messengers. **Appendix B** lists the actions of the most common neurotransmitters and neuromodulators and neurologic conditions associated with abnormal levels of these chemicals.

INTRODUCTION TO NEUROANATOMY

A general knowledge of basic neuroanatomy is required before proceeding in this text. As noted earlier, the nervous system is divided into four regions: peripheral, spinal, brainstem and cerebellar, and cerebral regions. The peripheral nervous system consists of all nervous system structures not encased in bone. The central nervous system, encased in the vertebral column and skull, includes the spinal cord, brainstem and cerebellar, and cerebral regions.

Parts of the nervous system are also classified according to the type of non-neural structures they innervate. Thus, the somatic nervous system connects with cutaneous and musculoskeletal structures, the autonomic nervous system connects with viscera, and the special sensory systems connect with visual, auditory, vestibular, olfactory, and gustatory (taste) structures.

Terms used to describe locations in the nervous system are listed in Table 1-1.

Planes are imaginary lines through the nervous system (Figure 1-4). There are three planes:
- Sagittal
- Horizontal
- Coronal

A sagittal plane divides a structure into right and left portions. A midsagittal plane divides a structure into right and left halves, while a parallel cut produces parasagittal sections. A horizontal plane cuts across a structure at right angles to the long axis of the structure, creating a horizontal, or cross, section. A coronal plane divides a structure into anterior and posterior portions. The plane of an actual cut is used to name the cut surface; for example, a cut through the brain along the coronal plane is called a *coronal section.*

Cellular Level Neuroanatomy

Differences in cellular constituents produce an obvious feature, the difference between gray and white matter, in sections of the central nervous system (Figure 1-5). White matter is composed of axons, projections of nerve cells that usually convey information away from the cell body, and myelin, an insulating layer of cells that wraps around the axons. Areas with a large proportion of myelin appear white because of the high fat content of myelin. A bundle of myelinated axons that travel together in the central nervous system is called a *tract, lemniscus, fasciculus, column, peduncle,* or *capsule.*

Table 1-1   TERMS USED TO DESCRIBE LOCATIONS IN THE NERVOUS SYSTEM

Term	Definition	Antonym	Definition of Antonym
Superior	Above another part	Inferior	Below another part
Rostral	Toward the head	Caudal	Toward the tail or coccyx
Anterior or ventral	Toward the front	Posterior or dorsal	Toward the back
Medial	Toward the midline	Lateral	Farther from the midline
Proximal	Nearest the point of origin	Distal	Farther from the point of origin
Ipsilateral	On the same side of the body	Contralateral	On the opposite side of the body

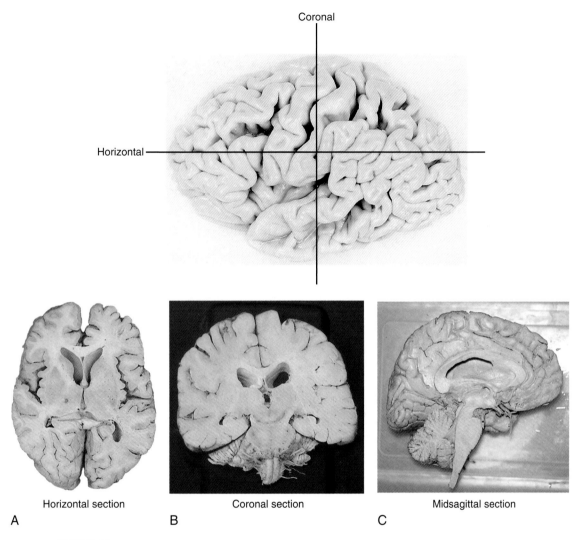

Coronal

Horizontal

Horizontal section

A

Coronal section

B

Midsagittal section

C

FIGURE 1-4
Planes and sections of the brain. *(Lateral view courtesy Dr. Melvin J. Ball.)*

Areas of the central nervous system that appear gray contain primarily neuron cell bodies. These areas are called *gray matter.* Groups of cell bodies in the peripheral nervous system are called *ganglia.* In the central nervous system, groups of cell bodies are most frequently called *nuclei,* although gray matter on the surface of the brain is called *cortex.*

The axons in white matter convey information among parts of the nervous system. Information is integrated in gray matter.

Peripheral Nervous System

Within a peripheral nerve are afferent and efferent axons. Afferent axons carry information from peripheral receptors toward the central nervous system. For example, an afferent axon transmits information to the central nervous system when the hand touches an object. Efferent axons carry information away from the central nervous system; for example, efferent axons carry motor commands from the central nervous system to skeletal muscles

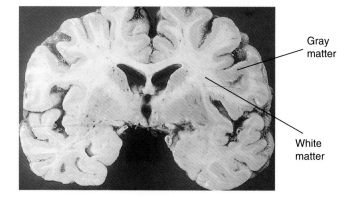

FIGURE 1-5

A coronal section of the cerebrum, revealing white and gray matter. White matter is composed of axons surrounded by large quantities of myelin. Gray matter is mainly composed of neuron cell bodies. (*Courtesy Jeanette Townsend.*)

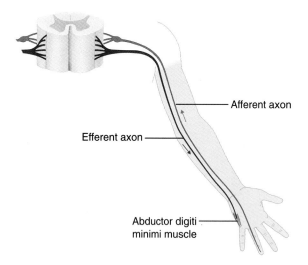

FIGURE 1-6

Afferent and efferent axons in the upper limb. A single segment of the spinal cord is illustrated. The arrows illustrate the direction of information in relation to the central nervous system. By convention, neurons in sensory pathways are often colored blue and neurons in motor pathways are usually colored red.

(Figure 1-6). Peripheral components of the somatic nervous system include axons, sensory nerve endings, and glial cells. In the autonomic nervous system, entire neurons, sensory endings, synapses, ganglia, and glia are found in the periphery.

These components enable peripheral nerves to convey information from sensory receptors into the central nervous system, and also to transmit signals from the central nervous system to skeletal and smooth muscle and glands.

Spinal Region

Within the vertebral column, the spinal cord extends from the foramen magnum (the opening at the inferoposterior aspect of the skull) to the level of the first lumbar vertebra. Distally, the spinal cord ends in the conus medullaris. The spinal cord has 31 segments, with a pair of spinal nerves arising from each segment.

Each spinal nerve is connected to the cord by a dorsal root and a ventral root (Figure 1-7). An enlargement of the dorsal root, the dorsal root ganglion, contains the cell bodies of sensory neurons. Cell bodies of neurons forming the ventral root are located within the spinal cord. The union of the dorsal and ventral roots forms the spinal nerve. The spinal nerve exits the vertebral column via openings between vertebrae, then divides into dorsal and ventral rami that communicate with the periphery. The rami communicantes conduct signals between the spinal cord and the sympathetic ganglia.

Cross-sections of the spinal cord reveal centrally located gray matter forming a shape similar to the letter *H* surrounded by white matter (Figure 1-8). Each side of the gray matter is subdivided into ventral, lateral, and dorsal horns. These horns contain cell bodies of motor neurons, interneurons, and the endings of sensory neurons. The gray matter commissure connects the lateral areas of gray matter. The white matter is divided into three areas (funiculi):

- Anterior column
- Lateral column
- Dorsal column

The meninges, connective tissue surrounding the spinal cord and brain, are discussed later in this chapter.

The spinal cord has two main functions:

- To convey information between the neurons connected to peripheral structures and the brain
- To process information

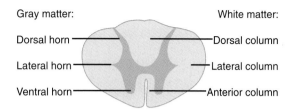

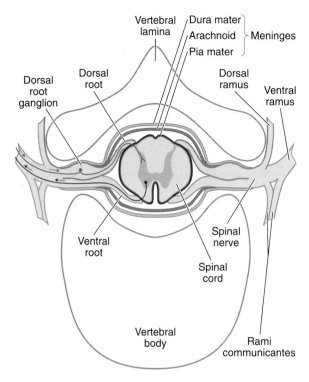

FIGURE 1-7

Spinal region: horizontal section, including vertebra, spinal cord and roots, the spinal nerve, and rami. Afferent and efferent neurons are illustrated on the left side. The spinal nerve is formed of axons from the dorsal and ventral roots. The bifurcation of the spinal nerve into dorsal and ventral rami marks the transition from the spinal region to the peripheral region.

FIGURE 1-8

Cross-section of the spinal cord. The central gray matter is divided into horns and a commissure. The white matter is divided into columns.

The cord conveys somatosensory information to the brain and also conveys signals from the brain to neurons that directly control movement. An example of spinal cord processing of information is the reflexive movement of a limb away from a painful stimulus. Within the cord are the necessary circuits to orchestrate the movement.

Brainstem and Cerebellar Region

Many fiber tracts carrying motor and sensory information travel through the brainstem, while other fiber tracts begin or end within the brainstem. In addition, the brainstem contains important groups of neurons that control equilibrium (sensations of head movement, orienting to vertical, postural adjustments), cardiovascular activity, respiration, and other functions. External features of the brainstem are illustrated in Figure 1-9.

The parts of the brainstem are the medulla, pons, and midbrain.

Medulla

The medulla is continuous with the spinal cord. Features of the anterior surface of the medulla are the olive, the pyramid, and the roots of four cranial nerves. The olive is an oval bump on the superior anterolateral surface of the medulla. The pyramids are axons projecting from the cerebral cortex to the spinal cord. As these fibers cross the midline, they form the pyramidal decussation.

Pons

Superior to the medulla is the pons. The junction of the medulla and pons is marked by a transverse line. The ventral part of the pons forms a large bulge anteriorly, containing fiber tracts and interspersed nuclei. Four cranial nerves attach to the pons.

Midbrain

The superior section of the brainstem is the midbrain. The anterior portion of the midbrain is formed by two cerebral peduncles consisting of fibers that descend from the cerebral cortex. Dorsally, the tectum of the midbrain consists of four small rounded bodies, two superior colliculi and two inferior colliculi. The colliculi are important for orientation to auditory and visual stimuli. Two cranial nerves arise from the midbrain.

The brainstem conveys information between the cerebrum and the spinal cord, integrates information, and regulates vital functions (i.e., respiration, heart rate, and temperature).

Cranial Nerves

Twelve pairs of cranial nerves emerge from the surface of the brain (Figure 1-10). Each cranial nerve is designated by a name and by a Roman numeral. The numbering is

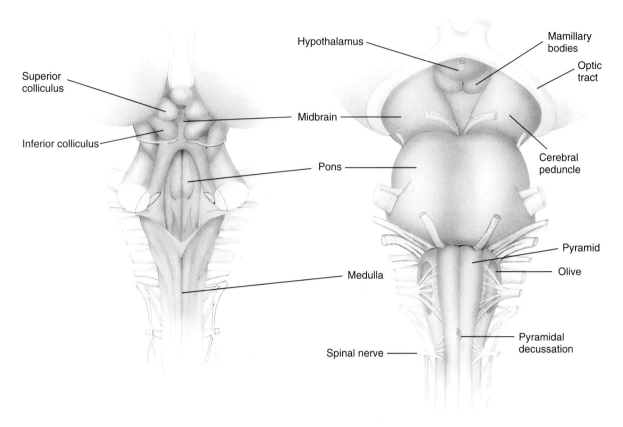

FIGURE 1-9
Brainstem: posterior and anterior views.

according to the site of attachment to the brain, from anterior to posterior. Most cranial nerves innervate structures in the head, face, and neck. The exception is the vagus nerve, which innervates thoracic and abdominal viscera in addition to structures in the head and neck.

Some cranial nerves are purely sensory. The purely sensory cranial nerves are the olfactory (I), optic (II), and vestibulocochlear (VIII) nerves. Other cranial nerves are principally motor but also contain some sensory fibers that respond to muscle and tendon movement. These include the oculomotor (III), trochlear (IV), abducens (VI), accessory (XI), and hypoglossal (XII). The remaining cranial nerves are mixed nerves, containing both motor and sensory fibers. Table 1-2 lists the cranial nerves and their functions.

Cerebellum

The cerebellum consists of two large cerebellar hemispheres and a midline vermis (Figure 1-11). Vermis

means "worm," a fitting description for the appearance of the cerebellar midline. Internally, the cerebellar hemispheres are composed of the cerebellar cortex on the surface, underlying white matter, and centrally located deep nuclei. The cerebellum connects to the posterior brainstem by large bundles of fibers called *peduncles*. The superior, middle, and inferior peduncles join the midbrain, pons, and medulla with the cerebellum. The cerebellum's function is to coordinate movements.

Cerebrum

Diencephalon

The diencephalon consists of four structures (Figure 1-12):
- Thalamus
- Hypothalamus

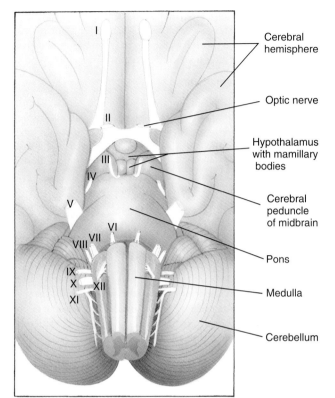

Cerebral hemisphere

Optic nerve

Hypothalamus with mamillary bodies

Cerebral peduncle of midbrain

Pons

Medulla

Cerebellum

FIGURE 1-10

Inferior surface of the brain showing attachments of cranial nerves, except the attachment of cranial nerve IV. Cranial nerve IV attaches to the posterior brainstem (see Figure 1-9).

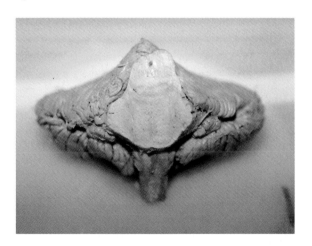

FIGURE 1-11

Anterior view of the cerebellum and brainstem. The midbrain and pons have been partially dissected to show the fiber tracts.

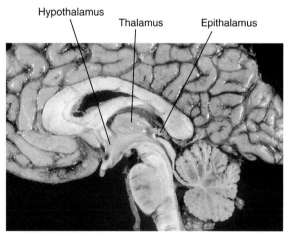

Hypothalamus

Thalamus

Epithalamus

FIGURE 1-12

The parts of the diencephalon that are visible in a midsagittal section are the thalamus, hypothalamus, and epithalamus. The subthalamus is lateral to the plane of section. (*Courtesy Jeanette Townsend.*)

Table 1-2   CRANIAL NERVES

Number	Name	Function
I	Olfactory	Smell
II	Optic	Vision
III	Oculomotor	Moves eyes up, down, medially; raises upper eyelid; constricts pupil
IV	Trochlear	Moves eye medially and down
V	Trigeminal	Facial sensation, chewing, sensation from temporomandibular joint
VI	Abducens	Abducts eye
VII	Facial	Facial expression, closes eyes, tears, salivation, and taste
VIII	Vestibulocochlear	Sensation of head position relative to gravity and head movement; hearing
IX	Glossopharyngeal	Swallowing, salivation, and taste
X	Vagus	Regulates viscera, swallowing, speech, and taste
XI	Accessory	Elevates shoulders, turns head
XII	Hypoglossal	Moves tongue

- Epithalamus
- Subthalamus

The thalamus is a large, egg-shaped collection of nuclei in the center of the cerebrum. The other three structures are named for their anatomic relationship to the thalamus: the hypothalamus is inferior to the thalamus, the epithalamus is located posterosuperior to the thalamus, and the subthalamus is inferolateral to the thalamus. The epithalamus consists primarily of the pineal gland.

Thalamic nuclei relay information to the cerebral cortex, process emotional and some memory information, integrate different types of sensation (i.e., touch and visual information), or regulate consciousness, arousal, and attention. The hypothalamus maintains body temperature, metabolic rate, and the chemical composition of tissues and fluids within an optimal functional range. The hypothalamus also regulates eating, reproductive, and defensive behaviors, expression of emotions, growth,

and the function of reproductive organs. The pineal gland influences the secretion of other endocrine glands, including the pituitary and adrenal glands. The subthalamus is part of a neural circuit controlling movement.

Cerebral Hemispheres

The longitudinal fissure divides the two cerebral hemispheres. The surfaces of the cerebral hemispheres are marked by rounded elevations called *gyri* (singular: gyrus) and grooves called *sulci* (singular: sulcus). Each cerebral hemisphere is subdivided into six lobes (Figure 1-13):

- Frontal
- Parietal
- Temporal
- Occipital
- Limbic
- Insular

The first four lobes are named for the overlying bones of the skull. The limbic lobe is on the medial aspect of the cerebral hemisphere. The insula is a section of the hemisphere buried within the lateral sulcus, revealed by separating the temporal and frontal lobes.

The distinctions among the lobes are clearly marked in only a few cases; the remainder are approximate. Clear distinctions include the following:

- The boundary between the frontal lobe and the parietal lobe, marked by the central sulcus
- The boundary between the parietal lobe and the occipital lobe, clearly marked only on the medial hemisphere by the parieto-occipital sulcus
- The division of the temporal lobe and the frontal lobe, marked by the lateral sulcus.
- The limbic lobe, on the medial surface of the hemisphere, bounded by the cingulate sulcus and by the margin of the parahippocampal gyrus

The entire surface of the cerebral hemispheres is composed of gray matter, called the *cerebral cortex*. The cerebral cortex processes sensory, motor, and memory information and is the site for reasoning, language, nonverbal communication, intelligence, and personality. Deep to the cortex is white matter, composed of axons connecting the cerebral cortex with central nervous system areas. Several collections of these fibers are of particular interest: the commissures and the internal capsule. The commissures are bundles of axons that convey information between the cortices of the left and right cerebral hemispheres. The corpus callosum is a huge commissure that connects most areas of the cerebral cortex. The much smaller anterior commissure connects the temporal lobe cerebral cortices. The internal capsule

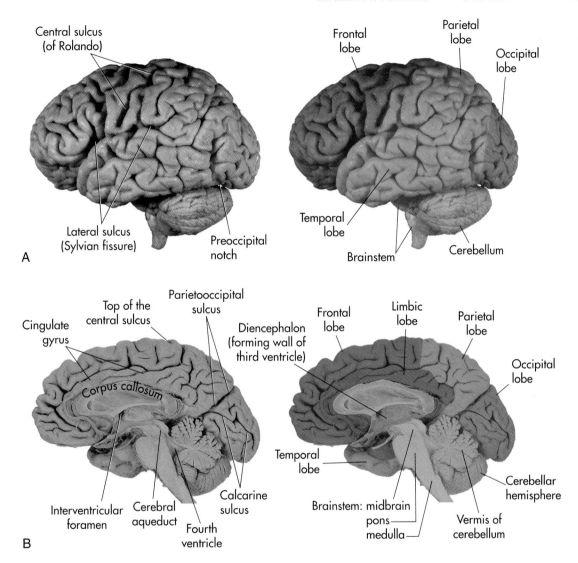

FIGURE 1-13
Major regions and landmarks of the brain in lateral (**A**) and midsagittal (**B**) views. *(Modified from Nolte J. {1999}. The human brain: An introduction to its functional anatomy, ed 4, St Louis: Mosby.)*

consists of axons projecting from the cerebral cortex to subcortical structures and from subcortical structures to the cerebral cortex. The internal capsule is subdivided into anterior and posterior limbs, with a genu (bend) between them (Figure 1-14, *A*).

Within the white matter of the hemispheres are additional areas of gray matter, the most prominent being the basal ganglia. The basal ganglia nuclei in the cerebral hemispheres are the caudate, putamen, and globus pallidus (Figure 1-14). The putamen and globus pallidus together are called the *lenticular nucleus*. The caudate and putamen together are called the *corpus striatum*. Two additional nuclei, the subthalamic (in the diencephalon) and the substantia nigra (in the midbrain) are also part of the basal ganglia neural circuit. The basal ganglia circuit helps to control movement.

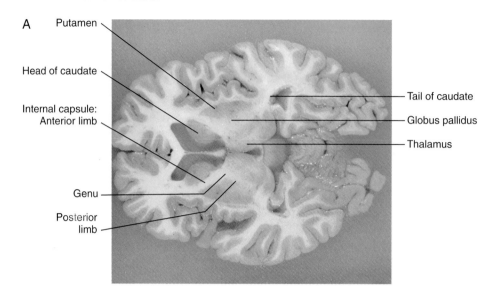

A

Putamen

Head of caudate

Internal capsule:
Anterior limb

Tail of caudate

Globus pallidus

Thalamus

Genu

Posterior
limb

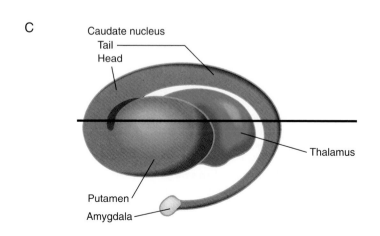

B

Caudate

Putamen

Globus pallidus

Thalamus

FIGURE 1-14
Basal ganglia, thalamus,
and internal capsule.
A, Horizontal section of
the cerebrum. Anterior is
to the left. The internal
capsule is the white
matter bordered by the
head of the caudate and
the thalamus medially
and by the lenticular
nucleus (putamen and
globus pallidus) laterally.
B, Horizontal section of
the cerebrum. Anterior is
to the left. The location
of the basal ganglia
and thalamus within
the white matter of the
cerebral hemispheres is
illustrated. The basal
ganglia are shown in
three dimensions on the
right side of the brain.
C, View from the side
of the left caudate,
putamen, thalamus,
and amygdala. The line
indicates the level of the
section in **B.**

C

Caudate nucleus
Tail
Head

Thalamus

Putamen

Amygdala

Another functional group of structures within the cerebrum is the limbic system, located in the diencephalon and cerebral hemispheres. The limbic system includes parts of the hypothalamus, thalamus, and cerebral cortex; several deep cerebral nuclei, the most prominent being the amygdala; and the hippocampus, a region of the temporal lobe (Figure 1-15). The limbic system is involved with emotions and the processing of some types of memory.

Support Systems

Cerebrospinal Fluid System

Cerebrospinal fluid, a modified filtrate of plasma, circulates from cavities inside the brain to the surface of the central nervous system and is reabsorbed into the venous blood system. The cavities inside the brain are the four ventricles: paired lateral ventricles in the cerebral hemispheres; the third ventricle, a midline slit in the diencephalon; and the fourth ventricle, located posterior to the pons and medulla and anterior to the cerebellum (Figure 1-16). The ventricular system continues through the medulla and spinal cord as the central canal and ends blindly in the caudal spinal cord. Within the ventricles, cerebrospinal fluid is secreted by the choroid plexus. The lateral ventricles are connected to the third ventricle by the interventricular foramina. The third and fourth ventricles are connected by the cerebral aqueduct. Cerebrospinal fluid leaves the fourth ventricle through the lateral foramina and the medial foramen to circulate around the central nervous system.

The meninges, membranous coverings of the brain and spinal cord, are also part of the cerebrospinal fluid system. From outmost to inmost, the meninges are the dura, arachnoid, and pia. Only the first two can be observed in gross specimens; the pia is a very delicate membrane adherent to the surface of the central nervous system. The arachnoid, also a delicate membrane, is named for its resemblance to a spider's web. The dura, named for its toughness, has two projections that separate parts of the brain: the falx cerebri separates the cerebral hemispheres, and the tentorium cerebelli separates the posterior cerebral hemispheres from the cerebellum (Figure 1-17). Within these dural projections are spaces called *dural sinuses,* which return cerebrospinal fluid and venous blood to the jugular veins. The cerebrospinal fluid system regulates the contents of the extracellular fluid and also provides buoyancy to the central nervous system by suspending the brain and spinal cord within fluid and membranous coverings.

Vascular Supply

This section is presented regionally, beginning with blood supply to peripheral nerves, then spinal cord, followed by vasculature of the brain.

VASCULAR ANATOMY

Peripheral nerves are accompanied by blood vessels. Branches from the blood vessels pierce the epineurium surrounding the peripheral nerves. Arterioles and venules travel parallel to fascicles of neurons (Figure 1-18) to provide ionic exchange and nourishment.

Blood is supplied to the spinal cord by three spinal arteries running vertically along the cord: one is in the anterior midline and two are posterior, on either side of midline but medial to the dorsal roots (Figure 1-19). The anterior spinal artery supplies the anterior two-thirds of the cord. The posterior spinal arteries supply the posterior third of the cord. The spinal arteries receive blood via the vertebral and medullary arteries. The medullary arteries are branches of vertebral, cervical, thoracic, and lumbar arteries. There are seven to ten medullary arteries. The vertebral arteries that supply blood to the upper spinal cord enter the skull through the foramen magnum to supply part of the brain.

Two pairs of arteries supply blood to the brain (Figure 1-20):
* Two internal carotid arteries
* Two vertebral arteries

The internal carotid arteries provide blood to most of the cerebrum, while the vertebral arteries provide blood to the occipital and inferior temporal lobes and to the brainstem region. The paired internal carotid arteries supply the anterior, superior, and lateral cerebral hemispheres. The paired vertebral arteries supply the brainstem, cerebellum, and posteroinferior cerebrum. The arterial branches discussed in the following sections are only the major arteries. Each artery has many branches, an elaborate capillary bed, and multiple arteriovenous junctions.

Vascular Supply to the Brainstem and Cerebellum

The brainstem and cerebellum are supplied by branches of the vertebral arteries and branches of the basilar artery (Figure 1-21). The basilar artery is formed by the union of the vertebral arteries. Each **vertebral artery** has three main branches: the anterior and posterior spinal arteries and the posterior inferior cerebellar artery. The medulla

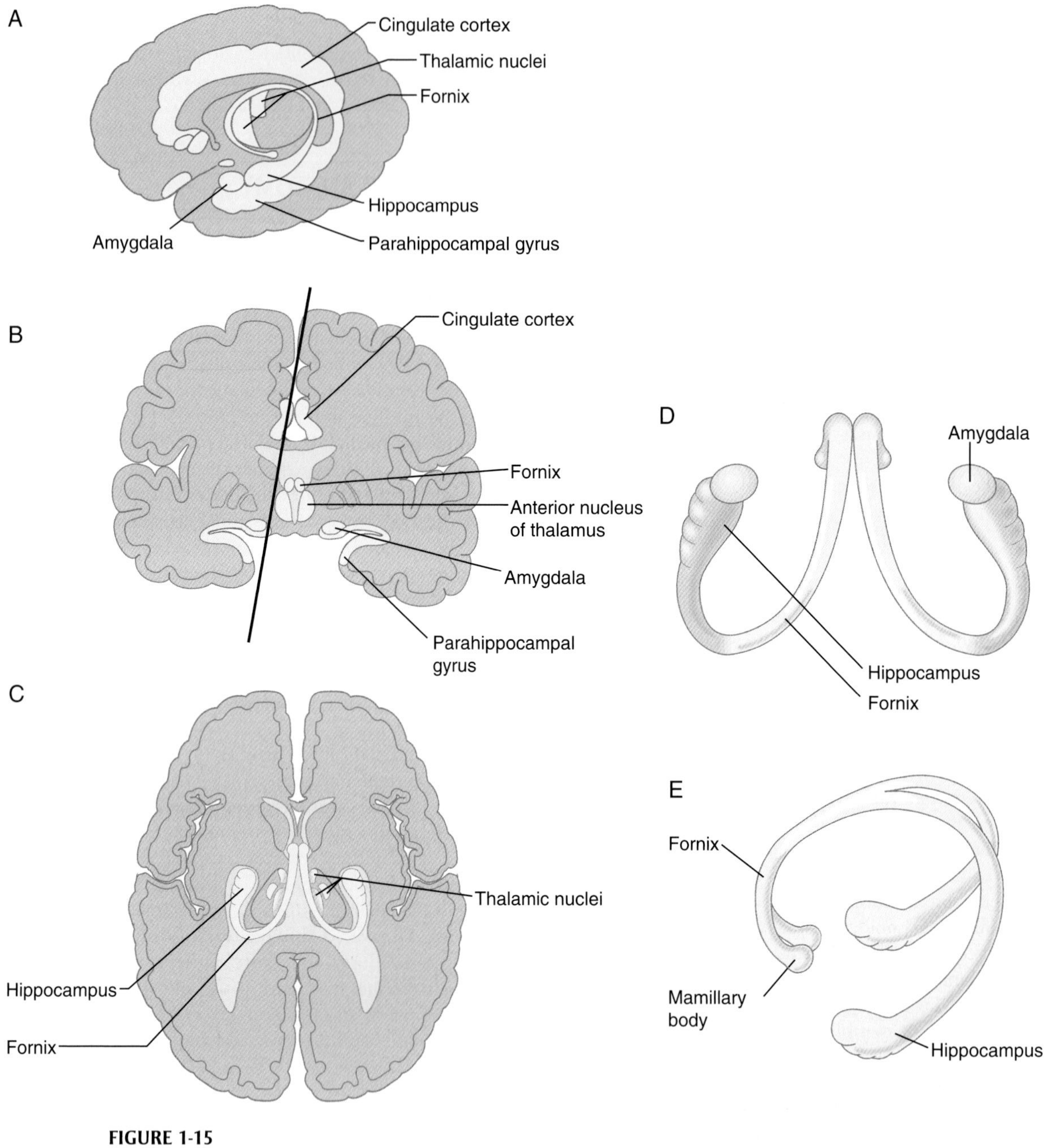

FIGURE 1-15

Limbic system. The structures in light pink are parts of the limbic system. **A,** View of the limbic structures on the right side of the brain. Anterior is to the left. The plane of the section is at approximately the angle indicated in part **B. B,** Coronal section of the brain. The blue area is a fluid-filled space in the brain, part of the ventricle system (see Figure 1-16). **C,** Horizontal section. Anterior is at the top. View is from above showing the hippocampus and fornix in three dimensions. The hippocampus is below the plane of the section, and the fornix is above the plane of the section. The amygdala is within the white matter and thus is not visible in this section. **D,** The hippocampus, fornix, and amygdala from above. Anterior is at the top. **E,** The mamillary body, fornix, and hippocampus. View is from above and laterally. Anterior is toward the left.

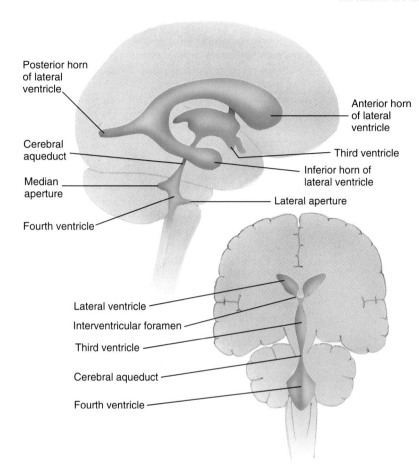

FIGURE 1-16

The four ventricles: two lateral ventricles, the third ventricle, and the fourth ventricle. Each lateral ventricle is within a cerebral hemisphere. The third ventricle is between the left and right thalamus, and the fourth ventricle is posterior to the pons and medulla and anterior to the cerebellum.

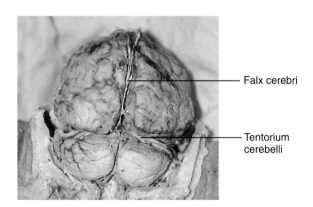

FIGURE 1-17

The dura mater covering the posterior brain has been removed to reveal the dural projections: the falx cerebri and the tentorium cerebelli.

receives blood from all three branches of the vertebral arteries. The posterior inferior cerebellar artery also supplies the inferior cerebellum.

Near the pontomedullary junction, the vertebral arteries join to form the **basilar artery.** The basilar artery and its branches (anterior inferior cerebellar, superior cerebellar) supply the pons and most of the cerebellum. At the junction of the pons and midbrain, the basilar artery divides to become the **posterior cerebral arteries.** The posterior cerebral artery is the primary blood supply to the midbrain.

Vascular Supply to Cerebral Hemispheres

Internal Carotid and Posterior Cerebral Arteries

The cerebrum is entirely supplied by the internal carotid and posterior cerebral arteries. The internal carotid

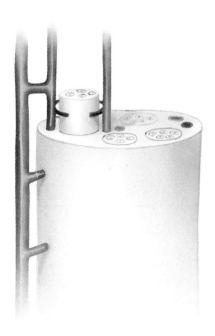

FIGURE 1-18
Blood supply to a group of axons within a peripheral nerve.

arteries enter the skull through the temporal bones; small branches from each internal carotid become posterior communicating arteries that join the internal carotid with the posterior cerebral artery. Near the optic chiasm, the internal carotid divides into anterior and middle cerebral arteries (see following sections). Together, the posterior cerebral arteries and branches of the internal carotid arteries form the circle of Willis to supply the cerebrum.

Circle of Willis

The circle of Willis is an anastomotic ring of nine arteries, supplying all of the blood to the cerebral hemispheres (see Figure 1-20). Six large arteries anastomose via three small communicating arteries. The large arteries are the anterior cerebral artery (a branch of the internal carotid), the internal carotid, and the posterior cerebral (branches of the basilar). The anterior communicating artery (unpaired) joins the anterior cerebral arteries together, and the posterior communicating artery links the internal carotid with the posterior cerebral artery.

Cerebral Arteries

Each of the three major cerebral arteries (anterior, middle, posterior) has both cortical branches (supplying the cortex and outer white matter) and deep branches (to central gray matter and adjacent white matter).

From its origin, the **anterior cerebral artery** moves medially and anteriorly, into the longitudinal fissure.

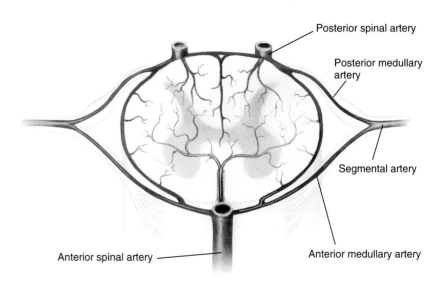

Posterior spinal artery

Posterior medullary artery

Segmental artery

Anterior medullary artery

Anterior spinal artery

FIGURE 1-19
Blood supply of the spinal cord.

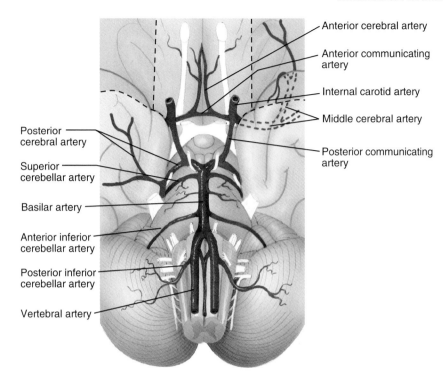

Anterior cerebral artery

Anterior communicating artery

Internal carotid artery

Middle cerebral artery

Posterior communicating artery

Posterior cerebral artery

Superior cerebellar artery

Basilar artery

Anterior inferior cerebellar artery

Posterior inferior cerebellar artery

Vertebral artery

FIGURE 1-20
Arterial supply of the brain. The posterior circulation, supplied by the vertebral arteries, is labeled on the left. The anterior circulation, supplied by the internal carotid arteries, is labeled on the right. The area supplied by the posterior cerebral artery is indicated in yellow; the middle cerebral artery territory is blue, and the anterior cerebral artery territory is green. The watershed area, supplied by small anastomoses at the ends of the large cerebral arteries, is indicated by dotted black lines.

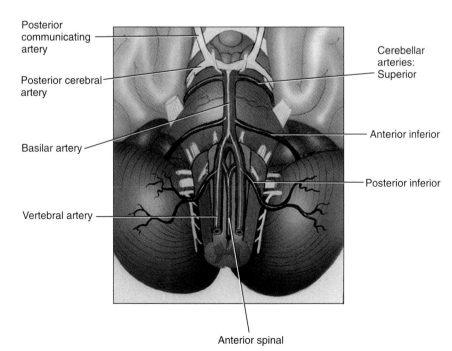

Posterior communicating artery

Posterior cerebral artery

Basilar artery

Vertebral artery

Cerebellar arteries:
Superior

Anterior inferior

Posterior inferior

Anterior spinal

FIGURE 1-21
Blood supply of the brainstem and cerebellum. Each artery is color coded to match the territory it supplies.

The artery sweeps up and back above the corpus callosum, its branches supplying the medial surface of the frontal and parietal lobes (Figure 1-22). The **middle cerebral artery** supplies the internal capsule, globus pallidus, putamen, and caudate, then passes through the lateral sulcus. The branches of the middle cerebral artery fan out to supply most of the lateral hemisphere. The **posterior cerebral artery** wraps around and supplies the midbrain and then supplies the occipital lobe and parts of the medial and inferior temporal lobes. The major cerebral arteries connect at their beginning (via the circle of Willis) and at their ends (watershed area [see Figure 1-22]). The **watershed area** is an area of marginal blood flow on the surface of the lateral hemispheres, where small anastomoses link the ends of the cerebral arteries.

> The anterior cerebral artery supplies the anterosuperior parts of the medial cerebral hemisphere. The middle cerebral artery supplies most of the lateral cerebral hemisphere, caudate, and parts of the putamen and internal capsule. The posterior cerebral artery supplies the midbrain, occipital lobe, and parts of the medial and inferior temporal lobe.

In addition to the branches of major cerebral arteries supplying deep structures, two other arteries supply only deep structures: the **anterior and posterior choroidal arteries.** The anterior choroidal (a branch of the internal carotid) supplies choroid plexus in the lateral ventricles, and parts of the visual pathway (optic tract and optic radiations; see Chapter 15), putamen, thalamus,

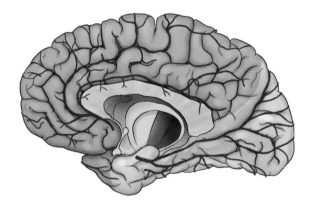

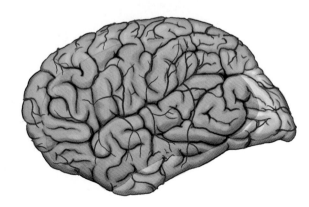

FIGURE 1-22
The large cerebral arteries: anterior, middle, and posterior. The area supplied by the anterior cerebral artery is green, the area supplied by the middle cerebral artery is pink, and the area supplied by the posterior cerebral artery is yellow.

internal capsule, and hippocampus. The posterior choroidal (a branch of the posterior cerebral artery) supplies the choroid plexus of the third ventricle and parts of the thalamus and hippocampus (Figure 1-23). Figure 1-24 illustrates the arterial supply of cerebrum in coronal section.

In contrast to other parts of the body that have major veins corresponding to the major arteries, venous blood from the cerebrum drains into dural (venous) sinuses. Dural sinuses are canals between layers of dura mater. In turn, the dural sinuses drain into the jugular veins. The vascular system provides oxygen, ionic exchange, and nourishment for the cells of the nervous system. Table 1-3 reviews the arterial supply of the central nervous system.

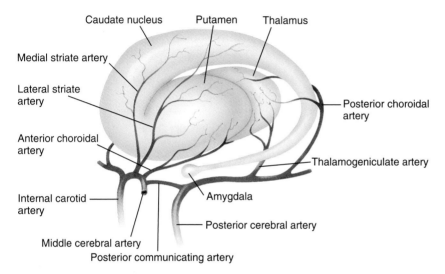

FIGURE 1-23
Branches of the internal carotid artery supply parts of the caudate and putamen. The supply to the putamen is via the anterior choroidal artery. The posterior choroidal artery, a branch of the posterior cerebral artery, supplies the choroids plexus of the third ventricle and parts of the thalamus and hippocampus.

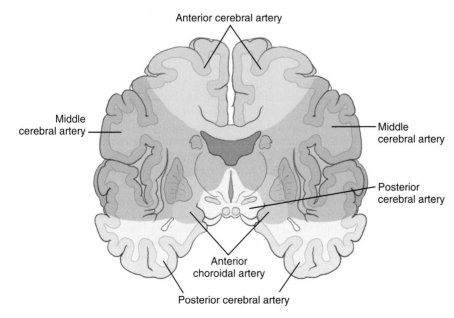

FIGURE 1-24
Coronal section illustrating the arterial supply of the cerebrum.

Table 1-3 ARTERIAL SUPPLY OF THE CENTRAL NERVOUS SYSTEM

Artery	Area Supplied
Vertebral Artery Branches	
Anterior and posterior spinal arteries	Spinal cord and medulla
Posterior inferior cerebellar artery	Medulla and cerebellum
Basilar Artery Branches	
Anterior inferior cerebellar and superior cerebellar artery	Pons and cerebellum
Posterior cerebral artery Branch: Posterior choroidal	Midbrain, occipital lobe, and inferomedial temporal lobe
	Choroid plexus of third ventricle; parts of thalamus and hypothalamus
Internal Carotid Branches	
Anterior choroidal	Choroid plexus in lateral ventricles, parts of the visual pathway (optic tract and optic radiations), parts of the putamen, thalamus, internal capsule, and hippocampus
Anterior cerebral artery	Medial frontal and parietal lobes
Middle cerebral artery	Globus pallidus, putamen, most of lateral hemisphere, part of internal capsule and caudate

INCIDENCE AND PREVALENCE OF DISORDERS

Incidence is the proportion of a population that develops a **new** case of the disorder within a defined time period. Incidence is typically reported per 100,000 people. For example, when I asked 40 adults who had a new cavity in the past year, only one new case was reported, indicating an incidence of 2500 per 100,000. **Prevalence** is the current proportion of the population with the condition, including both old and new cases. The prevalence rate is typically reported per 1000 people. The prevalence of dental cavities in the same group of people was 39/40, indicating a prevalence of 975 per 1000.

Migraine headache has a low incidence and a high prevalence, because prevalence is the cumulative sum of past year incidence rates. The incidence of migraine is 1,000/100,000 people per year (1% of the population develops a new case during a given year; Gilmour and Wilkins, 2001). The migraine prevalence for women is 33,000/100,000 and for men is 13,000/100,000; 33% for women and 13% for men; (Hankey and Wardlaw, 2002). In contrast, the motor neuron disease called *amyotrophic lateral sclerosis (ALS)* is fatal. Only 50% of people with ALS survive more than 36 months after the onset of the first symptom (Evans et al., 2000). The annual incidence of ALS is 2/100,000, and the prevalence is 5/100,000 (Hankey and Wardlaw, 2002). Figure 1-25 indicates the incidence of selected neurologic disorders. Because the incidence in the general population is unknown, spinal bifida and complex regional pain syndrome were not included in Figure 1-25. Spina bifida occurs 50 times per 100,000 live births (Northrup et al. 2000) and complex regional pain syndrome occurs following 1%-5% of traumatic injuries (Reddy, 2002).

CLINICAL APPLICATION OF LEARNING NEUROSCIENCE

For therapists, the main purpose in studying the nervous system is to understand the effects of nervous system lesions. A **lesion** is an area of damage or dysfunction. Signs and symptoms following a lesion of the nervous system depend on the location of the lesion. For example, complete destruction of a specific area of cerebral cortex severely interferes with hand function. The cause of the damage could be blood supply interruption, a tumor, or local inflammation, but regardless of the cause, damage to that area of the cerebral cortex compromises the dexterity of the hand. Depending on their distribution in the nervous system, lesions can be categorized as follows:

- Focal: limited to a single location
- Multifocal: limited to several, nonsymmetrical locations
- Diffuse: affecting bilaterally symmetrical structures but does not cross the midline as a single lesion

A tumor in the spinal cord is an example of a focal lesion. A tumor that has metastasized to several locations is multifocal. Alzheimer's disease, a memory and cognitive disorder, is diffuse because it affects cerebral structures bilaterally but does not cross the midline as a single lesion.

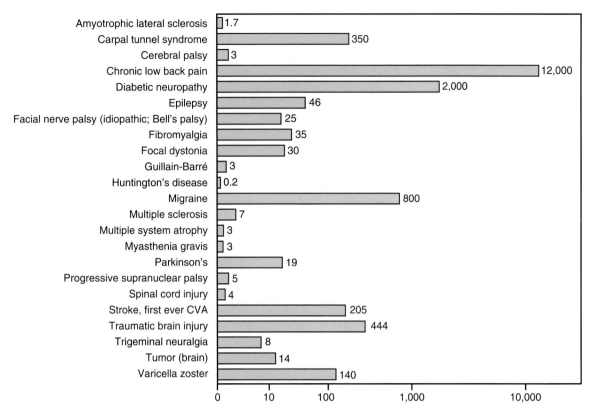

FIGURE 1-25
Incidence of selected neurologic disorders per 100,000 population in one year. *(Data from Andersson 1999, Bower et al. 1997, Diabetes Control and Complications Trial Research Group 1993, Gallagher et al. 2004, Hankey and Wardlaw 2002, Jackson et al. 2004, Jager et al. 2000, Kokmen et al. 1994, Lyngberg et al. 2005, MacDonald et al. 2000, Nordstrom et al. 1998, Nutt et al. 1988, Schrag et al. 1999, and Sorenson et al. 2003.)*

> Regardless of the cause of nervous system dysfunction, the resulting signs and symptoms depend on the site and size of the lesion(s).

Neurologic Evaluation

The neurologic evaluation has two parts:
- History
- Examination

The purpose of the neurologic evaluation is to determine the probable etiology of the neurologic problems so that appropriate care can be provided. The etiologies that affect the nervous system include the following:
- Trauma
- Vascular disorders
- Inflammation
- Degenerative disorders
- Neoplasms
- Immunologic disorders
- Toxic or metabolic disorders

History

A history is essentially a structured interview to determine the symptoms that lead the person to seek physical or occupational therapy. Knowing the typical speed of onset and the expected pattern of progression for each category of pathology is critical for recognizing when a specific client's signs and symptoms necessitate referral to a medical practitioner.

The speed of onset and pattern of progression provide important clues to the etiology, or cause, of nervous

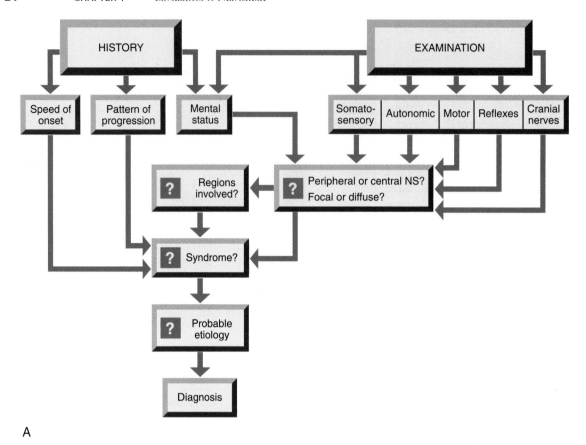

FIGURE 1-26
Flowcharts illustrating the process of neurologic evaluation. **A,** The generalized process. A"?" indicates a
question that can be answered by analyzing the information that flows into that box.

system dysfunction. Speed of onset is classified as
follows:
- Acute, indicating minutes or hours to maximal signs
  and symptoms
- Subacute, progressing to maximal signs and symptoms over a few days
- Chronic, gradual worsening of signs and symptoms
  continuing for weeks or years

Acute onset usually indicates a vascular problem,
subacute onset frequently indicates an inflammatory
process, and chronic onset often suggests either a tumor
or degenerative disease. In cases of trauma, the etiology
is usually obvious, and in cases of immune, toxic, or
metabolic disorders, the speed of onset varies according
to the specific cause. The pattern of progression can be
stable, improving, worsening, or fluctuating.

While discussing the person's history, the therapist
can often obtain adequate information about the person's
mental status:
- Is the person awake?
- Is the person aware?
- Is the person able to respond appropriately to
  questions?

Examination

Specific tests are performed to assess the function of the
sensory, autonomic, and motor systems. These tests are
described in subsequent chapters. If indicated, additional
tests that assess function within specific regions of the
nervous system may be performed.

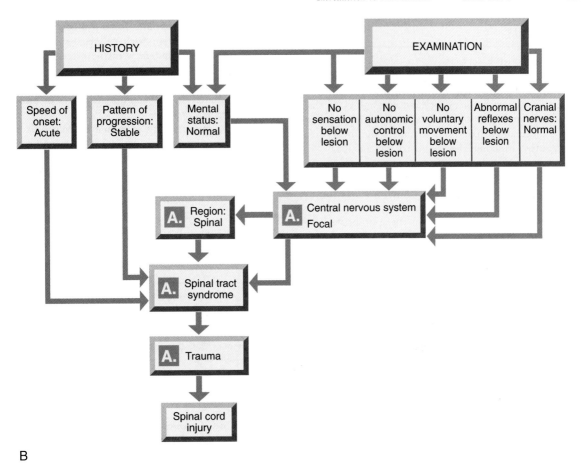

B

FIGURE 1-26, cont'd

B, Application of the neurologic evaluation process. The findings on the history and examination are indicated, as are the subsequent steps to reach a diagnosis. "**A.**" indicates an answer to a question in **A.** In this case, the diagnosis is spinal cord injury.

Diagnosis

By synthesizing the information from the history and the examination, the therapist begins to answer the following questions:
- Is the lesion in the peripheral or central nervous system?
- Are the signs symmetrical on the right and left sides of the body?
- Is the lesion focal, multifocal, or diffuse?
- Does the pattern of signs and symptoms indicate a syndrome?

- What region or regions of the nervous system are involved?
- What is the probable etiology?
- What is the diagnosis?

Figure 1-26 shows, in the form of flowcharts, how information is integrated to reach a diagnosis. In many cases, the therapist is able to reach a diagnosis. In other cases the therapist may not be able to answer several of the diagnostic questions, or the diagnosis may be beyond the scope of physical therapy practice. In such cases, the person must be referred to the appropriate medical practitioner.

SUMMARY

To understand the nervous system, each level of analysis is essential. As noted by Joaquin Fuster (1994), a brain researcher and psychiatrist, "the problem with the molecular approach to higher neurophysiology is that it proceeds at the wrong (i.e., impractical) level of discourse and analysis (like trying to understand the written message by studying the chemistry of the ink)." To extend Fuster's analogy, if there is a problem with the ink, then studying the ink's chemistry is appropriate. If there is a problem at the molecular level, with the supply of particular ions or molecules required by the nervous system, then the molecular level is the appropriate level of analysis. However, a molecular-level approach to understanding language is not practical; a cognitive-level analysis is appropriate. Some dysfunctions in the nervous system interfere with cellular-level processes, other dysfunctions interfere with the processing of one type of information, and still others interfere with all functions processed in a specific area. To understand each type of dysfunction, the appropriate levels of analysis must be applied.

Scientific investigations at each level of analysis have revealed many details of neural function. These details have promoted an improved understanding of function and provided new insight into the treatment of neurologic disorders. Continued neuroscience research and continued development of new treatment regimens can only bring us closer to a full understanding of nervous system function in health, disease, and recovery.

References

Andersson GB (1999). Epidemiological features of chronic low-back pain. Lancet, 354(9178), 581-585.

Bower JH, Maraganore DM, et al. (1997). Incidence of progressive supranuclear palsy and multiple system atrophy in Olmsted County, Minnesota, 1976 to 1990. Neurology, 49(5), 1284-1288.

Diabetes Control and Complications Trial Research Group (1993). The effect of intensive treatment of diabetes on the development and progression of long-term complications in insulin-dependent diabetes mellitus. New England Journal of Medicine, 329, 977-986.

Evans RW, Baskin DS, et al. (2000). Prognosis of neurological disorders. New York, Oxford University Press.

Fuster JM (1994). Brain systems have a way of reconciling "opposite" views of neural processing; the motor system is no exception. In Cordo P, Harnad S, (Eds). Movement control (p. 139). Cambridge, England: Cambridge University Press.

Gallagher AM, Thomas JM, et al. (2004). Incidence of fatigue symptoms and diagnoses presenting in UK primary care from 1990 to 2001. Journal of the Royal Society of Medicine, 97(12), 571-575.

Gilmour H, Wilkins K (2001). Migraine. Health Reports, 12(2), 23-40.

Hankey GJ, Wardlaw JM (2002). Clinical neurology (pp. 95, 534). New York, Demos Medical Publishing.

Jackson AB, Dijkers M, et al. (2004). A demographic profile of new traumatic spinal cord injuries: Change and stability over 30 years. Archives of Physical Medicine and Rehabilitation, 85(11), 1740-1748.

Jager TE, Weiss HB, et al. (2000). Traumatic brain injuries evaluated in U.S. emergency departments, 1992-1994. Academic Emergency Medicine, 7(2), 134-140.

Kokmen E, Ozekmekci FS, et al. (1994). Incidence and prevalence of Huntington's disease in Olmsted County, Minnesota (1950 through 1989). Archives of Neurology, 51(7), 696-698.

Lyngberg AC, Rasmussen BK, et al. (2005). Incidence of primary headache: A Danish epidemiologic follow-up study. American Journal of Epidemiology, 161(11), 1066-1073.

MacDonald BK, Cockerell OC, et al. (2000). The incidence and lifetime prevalence of neurological disorders in a prospective community-based study in the UK (see comments). Brain, 123(Pt 4), 665-676.

Nordstrom DL, DeStefano F, et al. (1998). Incidence of diagnosed carpal tunnel syndrome in a general population. Epidemiology, 9(3), 342-345.

Northrup H, Volcik KA (2000). Spina bifida and other neural tube defects. Current Problems in Pediatrics, 30(10), 313-332.

Nutt JG, Muenter MD, et al. (1988). Epidemiology of focal and generalized dystonia in Rochester, Minnesota. Movement Disorders, 3(3), 188-194.

Reddy RV (2002). Complex regional pain syndrome. In Biller J, (Ed). Practical neurology, ed 2, Philadelphia, Lippincott Williams & Wilkins, 687-697.

Schrag A, Ben-Shlomo Y, et al. (1999). Prevalence of progressive supranuclear palsy and multiple system atrophy: A cross-sectional study. Lancet, 354(9192), 1771-1775.

Sorenson EJ, Stalker AP, et al. (2002). Amyotrophic lateral sclerosis in Olmsted County, Minnesota, 1925 to 1998. Neurology, 59(2), 280-282.

Volpe JJ (2001). Neurology of the newborn. Philadelphia, Saunders.

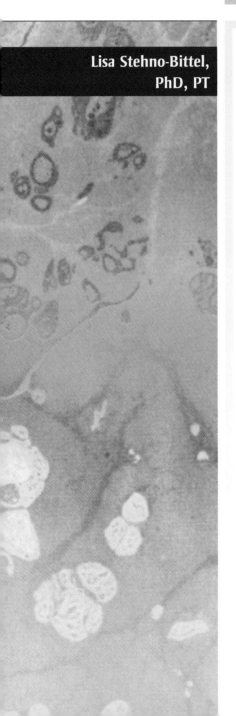

2 Physical and Electrical Properties of Cells in the Nervous System

Lisa Stehno-Bittel, PhD, PT

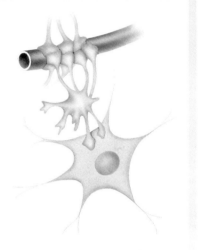

I am a 37-year-old female college professor and physical therapist living with multiple sclerosis (MS). Prior to teaching, I was a full-time physical therapist for 6 years, working with neurologically impaired adults in rehabilitation settings. I began teaching physical therapy when I was 29 years old.

When I was 28 years old, I experienced early symptoms of MS. My right arm felt numb for about 3 days. A few weeks after the numbness subsided, I experienced a right foot drop. This progressed over 24 hours, and I was seen in an emergency room. Initial tests included a lumbar puncture and myelogram, evoked potentials, and a CT scan, all of which produced normal results. I continued to have mildly slurred speech and weakness on my right side. These symptoms resolved in about 10 days. I underwent an MRI, which confirmed the diagnosis of MS secondary to the discovery of a lesion in the cortex. About 6 weeks later, I suffered rapid-onset (about 2 hours) symptoms of left-sided weakness, inability to swallow, unclear speech, and sensory deficits on the left side. I experienced Lhermitte's sign* and had (and continue to have) a perfect midline cut (up to but not including the face) in which the right side of my body feels as if it is on fire, every minute of every day.

In the 9 years that I have had MS, I have experienced nine attacks (although none in the past 27 months). Each attack has been different. I have had two that were purely sensory involving both lower limbs, two that were purely autonomic in which I vomited for hours, and one that was a visual field cut only. The others had elements of sensory, motor, visual, and vestibular problems. I have not experienced any bowel or bladder dysfunction.

I have had nearly full return of function following every attack, with the only remaining symptoms being persistent sensory hypersensitivity on my right side (greater in the limbs than in the trunk), mild visual disturbances including hypersensitivity to light and diminished night-driving ability, impaired vibratory sensation, and minor balance deficits. None of the unresolved symptoms has changed my life in a major way. I am active and have only made some minor

---

Lhermitte's sign: abrupt electric-like shocks traveling down the spine upon flexion of the head.

accommodative changes. I do not suffer from increased levels of fatigue or have difficulty with heat, unlike many people with MS. I consider my condition to be fairly static. I maintain my fitness with aerobic and anaerobic activities.

I have not had any type of therapy except as a participant in research studies. As a regular participant in research studies in the Portland, Oregon, area, I have been involved in a cell-cloning study and a study using the drug Betaseron. I am currently midway through a 2-year study of Avonex, an interferon treatment. Before the Avonex study, I would typically have one attack per year, including during the 2-year period of the Betaseron study, in which I received a placebo. I have not had an attack in 27 months. Part of that time I received Betaseron treatments via subcutaneous injections, and part incorporates the period since I initiated the Avonex interferon study protocol of weekly intramuscular injections. Because the course of MS is unpredictable and the Avonex study is incomplete, conclusions cannot be drawn regarding the effectiveness of the treatment. I also attribute my continued health to other practices, including diet, exercise, stress management, and purpose in my life. I believe all these factors play positive roles in maintaining health and preventing or minimizing the disease state.

—*Lori Avedisian*

INTRODUCTION

With an average 21 billion cerebral cortical neurons and 150,000 kilometers of myelinated nerve fibers (Pakkenberg et al., 2003) controlling sensation, movement, autonomic, and mental processes, the human nervous system is incredibly complex. This vast network of cells constantly develops new interactions and modifies output based on input to the system. The functions of the human body require chemical and electrical interactions among neural cells. Sensory information from peripheral receptors is conveyed to the spinal cord and brain, where it is analyzed as perception of the environment. On the basis of this sensory information, a motor command may be issued for the coordinated movement of muscles. Chemical and electrical interactions within the brain are also responsible for memory of experiences and movements.

This chapter, which will introduce the basic physical, electrical, and chemical properties of the nervous system, is divided into three sections: The first covers **neurons** (nerve cells), the second describes **glia** (cells that support neurons), and the third covers **stem cells** (precursors to neurons and glial cells).

STRUCTURE OF NEURONS

Neurons receive information, process it, and generate output. They have the same basic components as all animal cells. The organelles of a neuron include a nucleus, Golgi bodies, mitochondria, lysosomes, and endoplasmic reticulum. The nucleus, Golgi apparatus, and rough endoplasmic reticulum are restricted to the **soma,** or cell body, of the neuron. Other organelles, such as the mitochondria and smooth endoplasmic reticulum, are distributed throughout the neuron. A plasma membrane surrounds the cell, separating the extracellular environment from its contents. Table 2-1 lists information about each organelle.

Neurons are easily identified under a microscope because of their unique shape. Long protein strands called microtubules, microfilaments, and neurofilaments make up the cell's cytoskeleton and are responsible for maintaining the unique neuronal shape. Because neurons secrete neurotransmitter substances to communicate, they must produce a large quantity and variety of proteins, which are synthesized at the soma. The mechanism that transports proteins to other sites in the cell will be discussed later in this chapter.

Components of Neurons

A typical neuron has four components (Figure 2-1):

Table 2-1   FUNCTION OF CELLULAR ORGANELLES

Organelle	Function
Nucleus	Control center, contains the neuron's genetic material, directs the metabolic activity of the neuron
Mitochondria	Convert nutrients into an energy source the neuron can use; i.e., synthesize adenosine triphosphate
Endoplasmic reticulum	Rough endoplasmic reticulum (called Nissl substance in neurons): synthesizes and transports proteins Smooth endoplasmic reticulum: synthesizes and transports lipids
Ribosomes	Protein synthesis: free ribosomes (not attached to endoplasmic reticulum) synthesize proteins for the neuron's own use; ribosomes attached to rough endoplasmic reticulum synthesize neurotransmitters
Golgi apparatus	Packages neurotransmitter

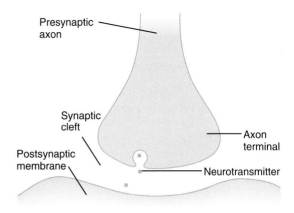

FIGURE 2-2

A synapse, the site of communication between neurons or between a neuron and a muscle or gland. The components of a synapse are the axon terminal of the presynaptic neuron, the synaptic cleft, and the postsynaptic membrane.

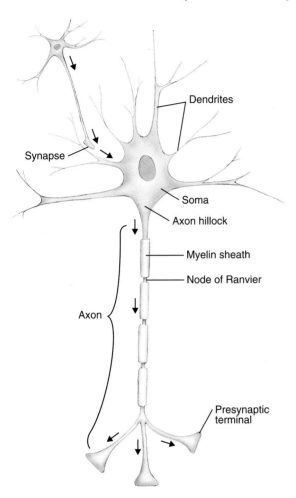

FIGURE 2-1

Parts of a neuron: the cell body (soma), the input units (dendrites), and the output unit (axon) with its presynaptic terminals. The axon hillock and nodes of Ranvier contribute to electrical signaling within the neuron. Also shown is a synapse, where a presynaptic terminal of one neuron communicates with a dendrite of a postsynaptic neuron. Arrows indicate the direction of information transfer.

- Dendrites
- Axon
- Presynaptic terminals
- Soma

Dendrites, branchlike extensions that serve as the main input sites for the cell, project from the soma. They are specialized to receive information from other

cells. Another process extending from the soma is the **axon,** reaching from the cell body to target cells. As dendrites are neuronal input sites, the axon is the output unit of the cell, specialized to send information to other neurons, muscle cells, or glands. Most neurons have a single axon that arises from a specialized region of the cell, called the **axon hillock.** Axons vary in length. The shortest axons are less than 1 mm in length (Purves et al., 2001), whereas axons that transmit motor information from the spinal cord to the foot may be up to 1 meter long. Axons end in **presynaptic terminals,** or fingerlike projections that are the transmitting elements of the neuron. Neurons transmit information about their activity via the release of chemicals called **neurotransmitters** from the presynaptic terminals into the **synaptic cleft.** The synaptic cleft is the space between neurons, and serves as the site for interneuronal communication (Figure 2-2). Communication across the synaptic cleft will be described fully in Chapter 3. Briefly, the presynaptic neuron releases a neurotransmitter into the synaptic cleft, the neurotransmitter diffuses from one side of the cleft to the other, and then the neurotransmitter binds to receptors on the postsynaptic neuron, muscle cell, or gland.

> The basic functions of a neuron are reception, integration, transmission, and transfer of information.

As stated earlier, most of the neurotransmitters used for neuronal signaling are produced in the **soma** of the cell. Thus, the cell must have a mechanism for transporting neurotransmitters and other substances from the soma to the presynaptic terminal at the end of the axon. This process is called **axoplasmic transport** (Figure 2-3). When material travels from the soma along the axon toward the presynaptic terminal, the process is called **anterograde transport.** Some substances must be transported from the synapse back to the soma, which is known as **retrograde transport.** Axonal transport can occur at a wide variety of speeds and appears to slow with the aging process (Frolkis and Tanin, 1999).

> Neurons are electrically active cells with structural and functional specializations of dendrites, axons, and synaptic terminals. Cellular organelles within neurons make and transport neurotransmitters for cell-to-cell interaction.

Types of Neurons

Although the four general components of the neuron remain the same—dendrites, axon, presynaptic terminal, and soma—the organization of these parts varies with the type of neuron. Vertebrate neurons are classified into two groups:

- Bipolar
- Multipolar

Bipolar Cells

This classification is based on the number of processes that directly arise from the cell body (Figure 2-4, *A*). Bipolar cells have two primary processes that extend from the cell body:

- Dendritic root
- Axon

The dendritic root divides into multiple dendritic branches, and the axon projects to form its presynaptic terminals. The retinal bipolar cell in the eye is an example of this type of cell.

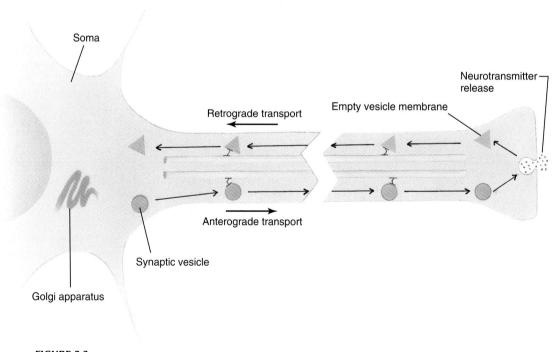

FIGURE 2-3

Axoplasmic transport. Substances required by the axon are delivered from the soma via anterograde transport. Retrograde transport moves substances from the axon to the soma. The proteins that "walk" the vesicles along the microtubules are shown in red.

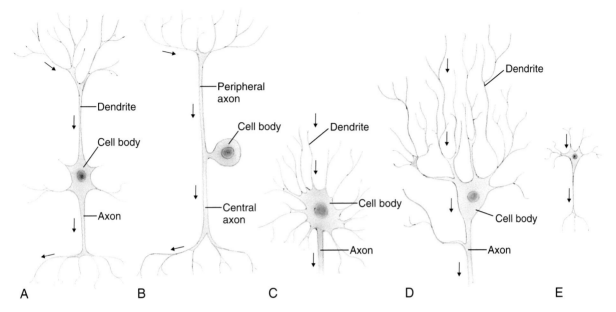

FIGURE 2-4
Morphology of neurons. Cells are not drawn to the same scale. Arrows indicate the direction of information flow. **A,** Bipolar cell of the retina. **B,** Pseudounipolar cell, a neuron that transmits information from the periphery into the central nervous system. These cells are unique in having two axons: a peripheral axon that conducts signals from the periphery to the cell body, and a central axon that conducts signals into the spinal cord. **C,** Multipolar cell. Multipolar cells have many dendrites and a single axon. The cell represented transmits information from the spinal cord to skeletal muscle. **D,** Multipolar cell typical of cerebellum. **E,** Interneuron. This type of cell is distributed throughout the central nervous system.

Pseudounipolar cells, a subclass of bipolar cells, appear to have a single projection from the cell body that divides into two axonal roots. Pseudounipolar cells have two axons and no true dendrites. The most common pseudounipolar cells are sensory neurons, which bring information from the body into the spinal cord (Figure 2-4, *B*). The peripheral axon conducts sensory information from the periphery to the cell body, while the central axon conducts information from the cell body to the spinal cord.

Multipolar Cells

Multipolar cells have multiple dendrites arising from many regions of the cell body and a single axon. They are the most common cells in the vertebrate nervous system, with a variety of different shapes and dendritic organizations. Multipolar cells are specialized to receive and accommodate huge amounts of synaptic input to their dendrites. An example of a multipolar cell is the spinal motor neuron, which projects from the spinal cord to innervate skeletal muscle fibers. A typical spinal motor

cell receives approximately 8,000 synaptic contacts on its dendrites and 2,000 contacts on the cell body itself. Multipolar cells in the cerebellum, called Purkinje cells, receive as many as 150,000 contacts on their expansive dendritic trees.

TRANSMISSION OF INFORMATION BY NEURONS

Neurons function by undergoing rapid changes in electrical potential across the cell membrane. An electrical potential across a membrane exists when the distribution of ions creates a difference in electrical charge on each side of the cell membrane. Four types of membrane channels allow ions to flow across the membrane:
- Leak
- Modality-gated
- Ligand-gated
- Voltage-gated

Membrane Channels

All channels serve as openings through the membrane. Without these openings, the membrane is impermeable to charged molecules. When the channels are open, ions including Na^+, K^+, Cl^-, and Ca^{2+} diffuse through the openings. **Leak channels** allow diffusion of a small number of ions through the membrane at a slow continuous rate. The other channels are termed *gated* because they open in response to a stimulus and close when the stimulus is removed.

Modality-gated channels, specific to sensory neurons, open in response to mechanical forces (i.e., stretch, touch, and pressure), temperature changes, or chemicals. **Ligand-gated channels** open in response to a neurotransmitter binding to the surface of a channel receptor on a postsynaptic cell membrane. When open, the channels allow the flow of electrically charged ions between the extracellular and intracellular environments of the cell, resulting in the generation of local potentials. **Voltage-gated channels** open in response to changes in electrical potential across the cell membrane (Figure 2-5). The shape of these proteins in the membrane depends on the membrane's electrical potential. Changes in membrane potential produce a structural change of the channel that causes the channel to either open or close. Voltage-gated channels open almost instantaneously, and close as quickly. They are ultimately responsible for the electrical signals that are the basis of information transfer in the nervous system. Voltage-gated channels are important in the release of neurotransmitters (see Chapter 3) and the formation of action potentials, as will be discussed later in this chapter.

Electrical Potentials

A rapid change in electrical charge across the cell membrane transmits information along the length of an axon and elicits release of chemical transmitters to other neurons or to the electrically excitable membrane of a muscle. The difference in electrical charge, carried by ions, is referred to as the membrane's *electrical potential*. Three types of electrical potentials in neurons are essential for transmission of information:

- Resting membrane potential
- Local potential
- Action potential

Resting Membrane Potential

The membrane potential is the difference in electrical charge (also called *voltage*) across the cell membrane, and is essential to the function of neurons. When the

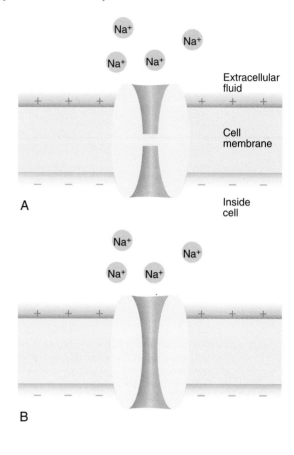

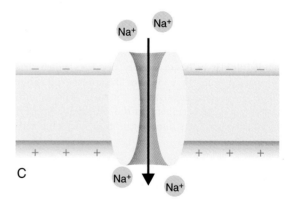

FIGURE 2-5
A sodium ion channel. Ion channels are proteins that span the cell membrane. **A,** When the ion channel is closed, ions cannot pass through the channel. **B,** Application of voltage to the cell membrane causes the channel to change configuration. **C,** This allows ions to pass through the gate. Because the concentration of Na^+ is greater outside the neuron than inside, opening the Na^+ channels produces an influx of Na^+ into the neuron.

neuron is not transmitting information, the value of the electrical potential across the membrane is called the **resting membrane potential.** The resting membrane potential is a steady-state condition with no net flow of ions across the membrane. Although some individual ions may continually move across the membrane through leak channels, when the cell is at its resting membrane potential there is no net change in the total distribution of ions across the two sides.

Without the ability of the membrane to maintain electrical charges on opposite sides, there would be no neuronal signaling. The cell membrane serves as a capacitor, separating the electrical charges on either side of the plasma membrane. An unequal distribution of ionic charge across the membrane is essential for neurons to be excitable. Two forces act on ions to determine their distribution across the plasma membrane: the **concentration gradient** and the **electrical gradient.**

In a simplified example, consider what happens if only sodium chloride (NaCl) ions are outside the cell and the membrane channels allow only Na^+ to pass through, as illustrated in Figure 2-6. When the channels are closed, no ions move across the membrane (Figure 2-6, *A*), and the membrane potential is constant. When the channels open, Na^+ flows from the region of high Na^+ concentration to low Na^+ concentration, in this case from outside to inside the cell (Figure 2-6, *B*). Only a certain amount of Na^+ enters the cell, because an electrical force (electrical gradient) across the membrane is produced as Na^+ ions move into the cell. Because only Na^+ passes through the membrane, Cl^- remains outside with its negative charge (Figure 2-6, *C*). The negative charge attracts Na^+ out of the cell, and an electrical-chemical equilibrium is achieved. Once Na^+ equilibrium is achieved, even if Na^+ channels remain open, there is no net movement of Na^+ ions across the membrane.

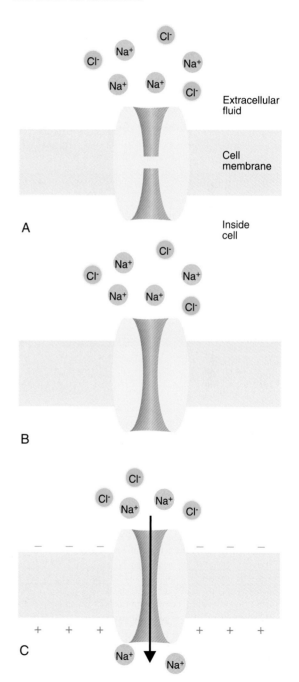

FIGURE 2-6

A simple electrochemical gradient. **A,** NaCl is only present outside the cell. A closed Na^+ channel in the membrane does not allow ions to move through the membrane. **B,** The Na^+ channel opens. **C,** Na^+ flows into the cell, but Cl^- is trapped outside, leaving the unbalanced negative charges on the outside of the membrane. Only a certain number of sodium ions can flow through the open channel before the negative charge of the Cl^- attracts the Na^+ back out of the cell. The distribution of electrical charge is symbolized by the negative signs lining the outside of the cell membrane and the positive signs along the inside of the cell membrane. At this point, the ions are in *electrochemical equilibrium.* Electrochemical equilibrium is reached when there is no net movement of ions across the membrane. The difference in electrical charge inside versus outside the cell produces a resting membrane potential. Note that in neurons, establishing the resting membrane potential involves other ions in addition to the two illustrated in this simplified example.

These opposing chemical and electrical forces control the movement of ions. Equilibrium of the distribution of a specific ion is reached when there is no net movement of that ion across the membrane. Individual ions continue to diffuse through the membrane, but equal quantities of the ion enter and leave the cell.

In the example, Na^+ and Cl^- were specified as the only ions existing outside the cell initially. The cell creates an ionic gradient with ion pumps that use energy in the form of adenosine triphosphate (ATP) to actively move ions against their electro-chemical gradient. Most important to the resting membrane potential is the Na^+-K^+ pump, which carries two K^+ ions into the cell and three Na^+ ions out of the cell with each cycle. Thus, as long as the cell has ATP, an unequal distribution of K^+ and Na^+ will exist across the membrane.

In neurons, the proper electrochemical gradient and resulting membrane resting potential are maintained by:
- The Na^+-K^+ pump
- Negatively charged molecules (anions) trapped inside the neuron, because they are too large to diffuse through the channels

- The passive diffusion of ions through leak channels in the cell membrane.

The membrane potential is defined as the difference in the voltage in the cytoplasm minus the voltage in the extracellular environment. Typically, the resting membrane potential of a neuron is measured at approximately −70 mV, indicating that the inside of the neuron contains more negative charges than the outside (Figure 2-7).

> The unequal distribution of ions creates an electrical charge across the neuron's membrane known as the *membrane potential*. The distribution of a specific ion depends on (1) the concentration gradient of the ion and (2) the electrical forces acting on the ion.

Changes From Resting Membrane Potential. Resting membrane potential is significant because it prepares the membrane for changes in electrical potential. Sudden changes in membrane potential result from the flow of

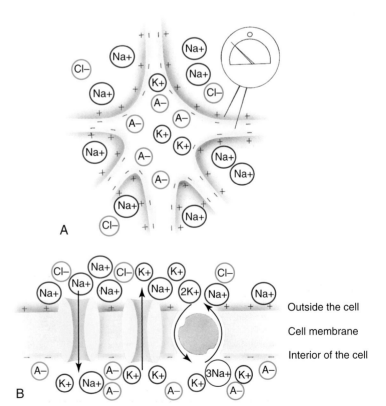

FIGURE 2-7

Resting membrane potential. **A,** Resting membrane potential is measured by comparing the electrical difference between the inside and the outside of the cell membrane. At rest, the inside of the cell membrane is approximately 70 mV more negative than the outside of the cell membrane. A-, anion. **B,** The resting membrane potential is maintained via passive diffusion of ions across the cell membrane and via active transport of Na^+ and K^+ by Na^+-K^+ pumps. The concentrations of Na^+ and Cl^- are kept higher on the outside compared to the inside of the cell, while the concentration of K^+ is kept higher on the inside compared to the outside of the cell. High concentrations of unneutralized negative charged molecules (anions) inside the cell also contribute to the negative resting membrane potential.

Outside the cell

Cell membrane

Interior of the cell

electrically charged ions through gated channels spanning the cell membrane (see Figure 2-5). The cell is **depolarized** when the membrane potential becomes less negative than the resting potential. Depolarization increases the likelihood that the neuron will generate a transmittable electrical signal, and is considered excitatory. Conversely, when the cell is hyperpolarized, the membrane potential becomes more negative than the resting potential. Hyperpolarization decreases the neuron's ability to generate an electrical signal, and is considered inhibitory.

These sudden, brief changes last only milliseconds. Gradual and longer-lasting changes in membrane potential are referred to as **modulation.** Modulation involves small changes in the membrane's electrical potential that alter the flow of ions across a cell membrane.

> Alteration in membrane potential occurs when ion channels open to selectively allow the passage of specific ions.

Local Potentials and Action Potentials

The initial change in membrane potential is called a local potential because it spreads only a short distance along the membrane. Action potentials are much larger changes in electrical potential. An action potential involves a brief, large depolarization that can be repeatedly regenerated along the length of an axon. Because it can be regenerated, an action potential actively spreads long distances to transmit information down the axon to the presynaptic chemical release sites of the presynaptic terminal. Electrical potentials within each neuron conduct information in a predictable and consistent direction. Conduction originates with local potentials at the receiving sites of the neuron: in sensory neurons, the receiving sites are the sensory receptors; in motor and interneurons, the receiving sites are on the postsynaptic membrane. If the change in local potential results in sufficient depolarization of the cell membrane, then an action potential will be generated and actively spread along the length of the cell axon. The sufficient level of depolarization for generation of an action potential is called the threshold level. Only when the electrical potential exceeds the threshold level is an action potential generated.

Figure 2-8 illustrates the events that transmit sensory information along an axon, starting with a local potential change and developing into an action potential. This sequence is as follows:
1. Deformation of a peripheral pressure receptor
2. Change in local membrane potential of the sensory ending
3. Development of an action potential in the sensory axon
4. Release of transmitter from the sensory neuron presynaptic terminal
5. Binding of transmitter to the ligand-gated channel on the postsynaptic cell membrane
6. Activation of synaptic potential in the postsynaptic membrane

The specific features of local and action potentials are summarized in Table 2-2 and are discussed in the following sections.

Local Potentials. Local potentials are categorized as either **receptor potentials** or **synaptic potentials,** depending on whether they are generated at a peripheral receptor of a sensory neuron or at a postsynaptic membrane. Generation of these local potentials is dependent on the characteristics of gated ion channels within the cell membrane. Peripheral receptors have modality-gated channels, while postsynaptic membranes have ligand-gated channels.

Local receptor potentials are generated when the peripheral receptors of a sensory neuron are stretched, compressed, deformed, or exposed to thermal or

Table 2-2   FEATURES OF LOCAL AND ACTION POTENTIALS

Characteristic	Local Potential	Action Potential
Amplitude	Small, graded	Large, all-or-none
Effect on membrane	Either depolarizing or hyperpolarizing	Depolarizing
Propagation	Passive	Active and passive
Ion channels responsible for the change in membrane potential	Sensory neuron end-receptor: modality-gated channel Postsynaptic membrane: ligand-gated channel	Voltage-gated channels

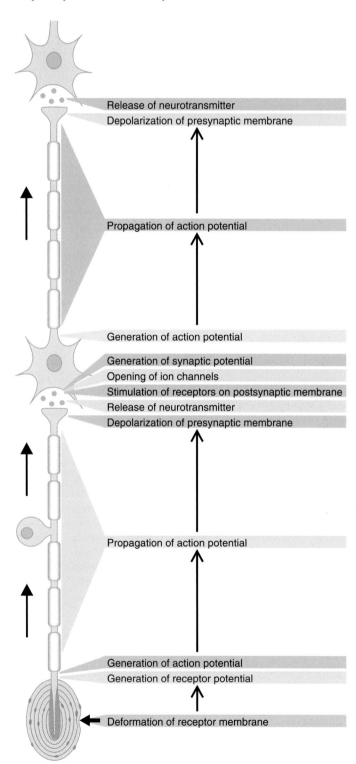

FIGURE 2-8

Sequence of events following stimulation of a sensory receptor. The flow of information via the interaction among receptor potentials, action potentials, and synaptic potentials is shown. A receptor potential is generated by mechanical change (pressure) of the end-receptor. An action potential propagates along the axon of the sensory neuron from the periphery to the spinal cord. Release of chemical transmitters at the synapse with the second neuron generates a synaptic potential in the second neuron. If sufficient stimuli are received by the second neuron, an action potential is generated in this neuron. The action potential propagates along the axon. When the action potential reaches the axon terminal, a chemical transmitter is released from the terminal. The transmitter then binds to receptors on the membrane of the third neuron, and opening of membrane channels generates synaptic potentials.

chemical agents. These changes in protein structure of the membrane cause modality-gated ion channels to open, encoding the sensory information into a flow of ionic current. For example, stretching a muscle opens ion channels in the membrane of sensory receptors embedded in the muscle. Opening of the channels results in ionic flow and generation of receptor potentials that are graded in both amplitude and duration. If the stimulus is larger or longer-lasting, the resulting receptor potential will also be larger or longer-lasting. Most receptor potentials are depolarizing (and therefore excitatory). However, sensory stimulation can also cause a receptor potential that is hyperpolarizing (and therefore inhibitory). A receptor potential is purely localized to the receptive surface of the sensory neuron and can only spread passively a very short distance along the axon. Within one millimeter of travel, the receptor potential is only one-third its original amplitude.

Local synaptic potentials are generated in motor neurons and interneurons when they are stimulated by input from other neurons. When a presynaptic neuron releases its neurotransmitter, the chemical travels across the synaptic cleft and interacts with chemical receptor sites on the membrane of the postsynaptic cell (see Figure 2-8). Binding of the neurotransmitter to receptors on the postsynaptic cell opens ligand-gated ion channels, locally changing the resting membrane potential of the cell. The action of the neurotransmitter on the membrane channel determines whether the synaptic potential will be depolarizing (excitatory) or hyperpolarizing (inhibitory). Similar to receptor potentials, synaptic potentials can only spread passively and are graded in both amplitude and duration: if the neurotransmitter is available in larger amounts for a longer time, the resulting synaptic potential will also be larger and longer-lasting.

Because local potentials can only spread passively along their receptors or synaptic membranes, they generally travel only 1 to 2 mm. In addition, the amplitude decreases with the distance traveled. The strength of the local potentials can be increased and multiple potentials integrated via the processes of temporal summation and spatial summation (Figure 2-9). **Temporal summation** is the combined effect of a series of small potential changes that occur within milliseconds of each other. **Spatial summation** is the process by which either receptor or synaptic potentials generated in different regions of the neuron are added together. Via summation, a sufficient number of potentials occurring within a short period of time cause significant changes in the membrane potential and either promote or inhibit the generation of an action potential.

> Neurons undergo rapid changes in the electrical potential of the membrane to conduct electrical signals. Receptor and synaptic potentials are graded in amplitude and duration and conduct local electrical information in the neuron.

Action Potentials. Because receptor and synaptic potentials only spread passively over short distances, another cellular mechanism, the action potential, is essential for rapid movement of information over long distances. An **action potential** is a large depolarizing signal that is actively propagated along an axon by the repeated generation of a signal. Because they are actively propagated, action potentials transmit information over longer distances than receptor or synaptic potentials. The meaning of the signal is determined not by the signal itself but by the neural pathway along which it is conducted. Unlike local input signals, which vary in amplitude, the action potential is **all-or-none.** This means that every time even minimally sufficient stimuli are provided, an action potential will be produced. Stronger stimuli produce action potentials of the same voltage and duration as minimally sufficient stimuli do. The initiation or firing of an action potential is similar to the striking of a key on a computer keyboard. Regardless of whether the key is struck gently and slowly or rapidly and hard, the letter will be inscribed when the sufficient amount of pressure is achieved. The shape of the letter is not influenced by how hard the key is pressed.

In neurons the generation of action potentials involves a sudden influx of Na^+ through voltage-gated channels. Although voltage-gated Na^+ channels are generally absent in the region of the receptor terminal and the synaptic membrane, there is a dense distribution of these channels within approximately 1 mm of the input regions. In sensory neurons, the region closest to the receptor with a high density of Na^+ channels is called the *trigger zone.* In interneurons and motor neurons, the region closest to the synapse with a high density of Na^+ channels is called the *axon hillock.* The receptor or synaptic potentials that have passively traveled a short distance toward the trigger zone or axon hillock are both spatially and temporally summated. If the summation of local potentials depolarizes the membrane beyond a voltage threshold level, then the opening of many voltage-dependent Na^+ channels generates an action potential. If the summation does not result in depolarization exceeding the threshold, then there will be no action potential.

The stimulus intensity that is just sufficient to produce an action potential is called the **threshold stimulus**

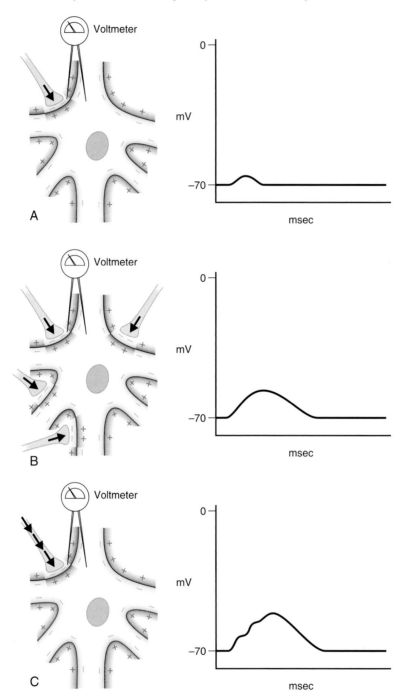

FIGURE 2-9
Integration of local signals. **A,** A single weak input to a cell results in only a slight depolarization of the membrane. **B,** Spatial summation of several different inputs results in a significant depolarization of the membrane. **C,** Temporal summation of several inputs in rapid succession results in significant depolarization of the membrane.

intensity. Typically, a 15-mV depolarization (a change in membrane potential from −70 mV to −55 mV) is sufficient to trigger an action potential. When the voltage across the membrane reaches −55 mV, many voltage-dependent Na^+ channels open. Na^+ flows rapidly into the cell, propelled by the high extracellular Na^+ concentration and attracted by the negative electrical charge inside the membrane. When K^+ channels open later, K^+ leaves the cell, repelled by the positive electrical charge inside the membrane (created by the influx of Na^+) and by the K^+ concentration gradient. The membrane becomes temporarily more polarized than when at rest. This process is called *hyperpolarization.* The resting membrane potential is restored by the diffusion of ions through leak channels. Figure 2-10 illustrates the change in membrane potential during an action potential. The peak occurs at about 35 mV, and then the potential quickly drops back toward the resting membrane potential.

In summary, an action potential is produced by a sequence of three events:

1. A rapid depolarization due to opening of the voltage-gated Na^+ channels
2. A decrease in Na^+ conduction due to closing of the channels
3. A rapid repolarization due to opening of voltage-gated K^+ channels

Owing to continued efflux of K^+, repolarization is followed by a period of hyperpolarization, during which the membrane potential is even more negative than during resting. When the membrane is hyperpolarized, it is more difficult to initiate a subsequent action potential. During this time the membrane is said to be **refractory**. The characteristics of the ion channels define the refractory period. Some channels become inactivated immediately after opening for an action potential and require a specific amount of time before they can be activated again for a subsequent action potential. The refractory period can be divided into two distinct states:

* Absolute refractory period
* Relative refractory period

During the **absolute refractory period,** the membrane is unresponsive to stimuli. This state occurs because the Na^+ channels responsible for the upstroke of the action potential cannot be reopened for a specific period of time following their closure. The **relative refractory period** occurs during the later part of the action potential (Figure 2-11). During this period the membrane potential is returning toward its resting level and may even be hyperpolarized. A stimulus may activate the Na^+ channels at this time, but it must be stronger than normal. The refractory period promotes

forward propagation of the action potential while preventing its backward flow. If there were no refractory period, the passive flow of ions associated with an action potential could spread both forward and backward along the length of the axon. Although the flow of K^+ out of the cell restores the resting membrane potential, the resting levels of ion concentration must be restored over time by the Na^+-K^+ pump actively moving Na^+ out of the neuron and K^+ into the neuron.

Action potentials are an all-or-none electrical response to the local depolarization of a membrane. Depolarization of the membrane to the threshold level depends on opening of voltage-gated Na^+ channels. Repolarization depends on the opening of the K^+ channels.

Propagation of Action Potentials. Once an action potential has been generated, the change in electrical potential spreads passively along the axon to the adjacent region of the membrane. When depolarization of the adjacent, inactive region reaches threshold, another action potential is generated. This process, the passive spread of depolarization to adjacent membrane and the generation of new action potentials, is repeated along the entire length of the axon (Figure 2-12). This process is analogous to lighting a trail of gunpowder: once the trail has been lit, the heat generated ignites the adjacent gunpowder and the process propagates down the trail. The propagation of an action potential is dependent on both passive properties of the axon and active opening of ion channels distributed along the length of the axon.

Some axons are specialized for faster action potential propagation. These faster-conducting axons have two structural adaptations that improve their passive properties:

* Increased diameter of the axon
* Myelination

The effect of these adaptations on propagation of an electrical signal along an axon is similar to the flow of water through a hose. A wider hose will allow more water through in less time. Similarly, a larger diameter axon will allow more current flow, with less time required to change the electrical charge of the adjacent membrane. Wrapping a leaky hose with tape will prevent water from leaking through the wall of the hose, ensuring that most of the water will travel to the end of the hose. Similarly, myelination prevents the leakage of current across the axon membrane.

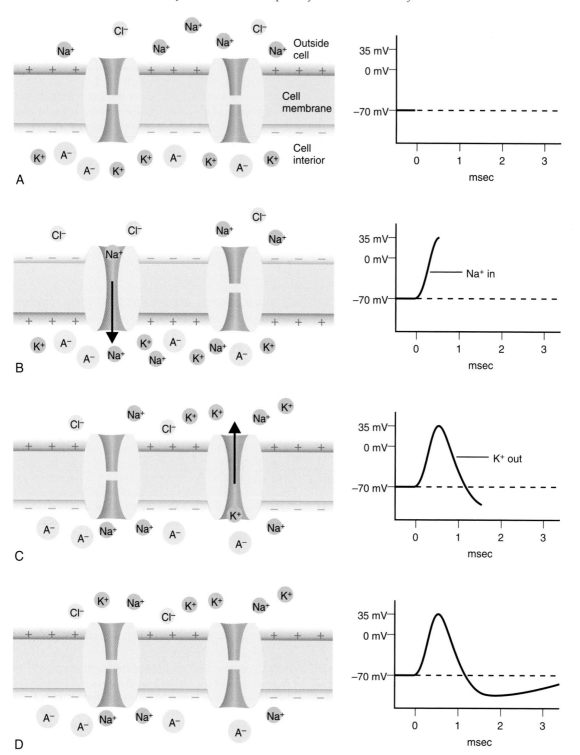

FIGURE 2-10   *See legend on opposite page.*

FIGURE 2-10
Action potential. **A,** In this example, the resting membrane
potential of the cell is −70 mV and membrane channels
are closed. **B,** Initiation of the action potential begins with
opening of voltage-sensitive Na⁺ channels and a rapid influx of
Na⁺, causing the cell membrane to become less negative (i.e.,
depolarized). **C,** Closing of the Na⁺ channels and opening of
K⁺ channels then causes a reversal of membrane potential.
D, Ultimately, a brief hyperpolarization of the membrane
results in the potential becoming more negative than the resting
potential. Later, the cell membrane returns to resting potential
after the closure of the membrane channels via the action of the
Na⁺-K⁺ pump *(not shown).*

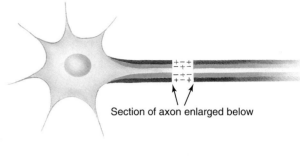

Section of axon enlarged below

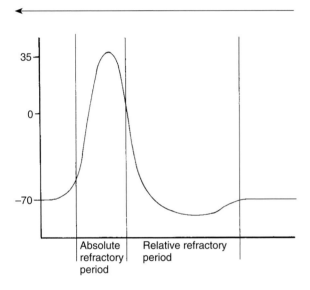

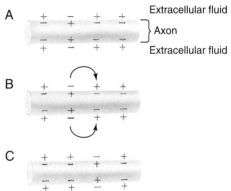

Extracellular fluid
} Axon
Extracellular fluid

FIGURE 2-12
Propagation of action potential. **A,** A depolarizing current
passively spreads down the axon, causing the interior of the
axon to become more positive than when the membrane is
resting. **B,** In the adjacent membrane, when the depolarizing
current reaches threshold level, Na⁺ channels open, causing
rapid depolarization of the membrane. **C,** An action potential is
generated, and the depolarizing current continues to propagate
down the axon.

FIGURE 2-11
Refractory periods. During and immediately following the action
potential are two refractory periods. The absolute refractory
period corresponds to the time the firing level is reached until
repolarization (reversal of potential) is one-third complete. The
relative refractory period corresponds to the time immediately
following the absolute refractory period until the membrane
potential returns to the resting level.

Myelination is the presence of a sheath of proteins and
fats surrounding an axon. Myelin provides insulation,
preventing current flow across the axonal membrane.
If ions were allowed to run down their electrochemical gradient during propagation of the action
potential, the amplitude of the potential would dissipate as the impulse traveled down the axon. Similarly,
when a hose has leaky walls, the flow diminishes as
distance from the faucet increases. In an axon, to keep
the amplitude of the action potential above threshold,

the uneven distribution of ions must be maintained (the
membrane potential cannot be allowed to return to the
resting potential). When there is a greater separation
of charges across the axon membrane, as provided by
myelin, fewer positive ions must be deposited along the
inner membrane to depolarize the membrane to a threshold level; therefore, current flow for a shorter period
of time can result in membrane depolarization over a
greater distance.

Myelination increases the speed of action potential
propagation and the distance a current can passively
spread. Thicker myelin leads to faster conduction and
greater chances for action potential propagation. Myelinated axons have small patches of that lack myelin, called
nodes of Ranvier. The nodes are specialized for active
propagation of an action potential by allowing ion flow

across the membrane. Nodes of Ranvier are distributed every 1 to 2 mm along the axon and contain high densities of Na^+ channels and K^+ channels. An action potential spreads rapidly along a myelinated region, then slows when crossing the high-capacitance, unmyelinated region of the node of Ranvier. The high capacitance at the node stores charge, preparing to produce an action potential. As a node becomes depolarized, voltage-gated Na^+ channels open, generating a new action potential and the spread of ionic current along the axon to the next node (Figure 2-13). Consequently, as the action potential propagates down a myelinated axon, it appears to quickly jump from node to node. This is called **saltatory conduction.** Because Na^+ channels remain open only a brief time, the generation of a refractory period again plays a critical role in the forward propagation of the action potential, by preventing the backward flow of electrical potential. Propagation of the action potential in a myelinated axon requires that a new action potential be generated at each node of Ranvier and passed on down the axon. In this manner, the action potential maintains its size and shape as it travels along the axon.

> Action potentials are propagated down the length of an axon via both passive and active membrane properties.

DIRECTION OF INFORMATION FLOW IN NEURONS

Normally, information within a neuron is only transferred in one direction. Depending on its role in the direction of information transfer, a neuron falls into one of three functional groups:
- Afferent neurons
- Efferent neurons
- Interneurons

Afferent neurons carry sensory information from the outer body toward the central nervous system. **Efferent neurons** relay commands from the central nervous system to smooth and skeletal muscles. **Interneurons,** the largest class of neurons, act throughout the nervous system, processing information locally or conveying information short distances. For example, interneurons in the spinal cord control the activity of local reflex circuits within the spinal cord.

The terms *afferent* and *efferent* can also refer to the direction of information conveyed by a particular group of neurons within the central nervous system. For example, when thalamocortical neurons convey information from the thalamus to the cerebral cortex, this information is efferent from the thalamus and afferent to the cerebral cortex. Neuronal pathways within the central nervous

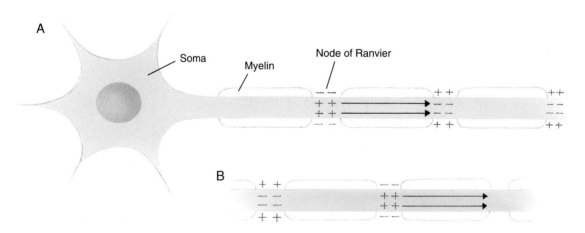

FIGURE 2-13
Saltatory conduction, or the process by which an action potential appears to jump from node to node down an axon. **A,** A depolarizing potential spreads rapidly along the myelinated regions of the axon, then slows when crossing the unmyelinated node of Ranvier. **B,** When an action potential is generated at a node of Ranvier, the depolarizing potential again spreads quickly across myelinated regions, appearing to jump from node to node.

system are commonly named by combining the name of efferent (i.e., site of origin) and afferent (i.e., site of termination) regions. For example, corticospinal neurons originate in the cerebral cortex and terminate in the spinal cord.

INTERACTIONS BETWEEN NEURONS

The specificity and diversity of function within the nervous system can be attributed to neuronal convergence and neuronal divergence. **Convergence** is the process by which multiple inputs from a variety of cells terminate on a single neuron. **Divergence** is the process whereby a single neuronal axon may have many branches that terminate on a multitude of cells. Via temporal and spatial summation, a sufficient number of convergent inputs occurring within a short period of time causes significant changes in the membrane potential and either promotes or inhibits the generation of an action potential.

Through the processes of convergence and divergence (Figure 2-14), a single stimulus may produce a substantial response. An example of convergence is the neural input to sensory association areas in the cerebral cortex, where information from hearing, vision, and touch is integrated. An example of divergence is the signaling of information from a pinprick. The pinprick activates end-receptors of a sensory neuron that transmits infor-

mation about tissue damage. The message is conveyed to multiple neurons in the spinal cord, eliciting a motor response that moves the body part away from the stimulus. Other neurons relay information that leads to conscious awareness of pain.

> Divergent and convergent synaptic connections contribute to the distribution of information throughout the nervous system.

GLIA: SUPPORTING CELLS

Glial cells form a critical support network for neurons. In early research, glia was thought to be a substance similar to glue, responsible for determining the shape of the nervous system: The term *glia* is derived from the Greek word for glue. Electron microscopy revealed glia as more complex, composed of cells. More recently, studies have shown that glial cells do more than provide the structure for the nervous system; they actually transmit information (Parpura and Haydon, 2000). Further, glial cells may be actively involved in the pathogenesis of a number of ailments, including the cognitive and memory disorder Alzheimer's disease (Schubert et al., 1998) and the disorders associated with multiple sclerosis.

Types of Glia

Glial cells are categorized by size and function. Large glial cells are called **macroglia** and small glial cells are **microglia.**

Macroglial Cells

Macroglial cells are classified into three groups:
- Astrocytes
- Oligodendrocytes
- Schwann cells

Astrocytes are star-shaped macroglial cells found throughout the central nervous system. For years these cells were thought to provide support for neurons, which were considered the only signaling cells. However, over the past twenty years understanding of the role of astrocytes has changed dramatically. Of the glial cells, astrocytes are thought to have the most direct role in cell signaling (Araque et al., 1999).

Astrocytes can be stimulated by signals from adjacent neurons or by mechanical changes (changes in shape or pressure). Stimulated astrocytes spread waves of Ca^{++} to neighboring astrocytes. These calcium waves can be

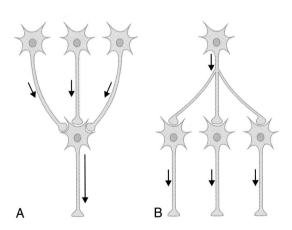

FIGURE 2-14
Convergence and divergence. **A,** Convergent input to interneurons and motor neurons in the spinal cord includes afferent input from the musculoskeletal system and input from the brain. **B,** Divergent output includes the activation of several neurons by single inputs. Only a few of the actual connections are shown.

regulated by neuronal activity (Cornell-Bell et al., 1990; Rouach et al., 2000). Spontaneous calcium waves can also arise from astrocytes without input from other astrocytes or neurons.

Communication between neurons and astrocytes travels in both directions. As noted above, neurons can stimulate astrocytes. Stimulation of astrocytes can increase or decrease communication between neurons (Araque et al., 1999). Stimulated astrocytes can release glutamate, a neurotransmitter (Parpura and Haydon, 2000; Vesce et al., 1999). Even though astrocytes release neurotransmitters, they do not have synaptic contacts and do not generate action potentials. Instead, astrocytes use an elaborate signaling pathway, with calcium diffusing through openings (called *gap junctions*) from one cell to the next (Figure 2-15). Signaling in gap junctions is bidirectional, because calcium can diffuse through them in either direction.

Astrocytes also serve important functions in the maintenance of normal neuronal signaling (Walz, 2000). They act as scavengers, taking up extra K^+ ions in the extracellular environment, removing chemical transmitters from the synaptic cleft between neurons, and cleaning up other debris in the extracellular space. Astrocytes have end-feet connect neurons and blood capillaries (Figure 2-16), providing a nutritive function for neurons. They are components of the blood-brain barrier, which will be discussed in Chapter 18. Finally, astrocytes are thought to play an important role in early central nervous system development by providing a pathway for migrating neurons. This same pathway may be important during recovery from an injury.

Oligodendrocytes and Schwann cells form a protective covering called the *myelin sheath,* which insulates the axon. The macroglia use lipids and proteins to create this covering. Neurons of the central nervous system are myelinated by oligodendrocytes, while neurons of the peripheral nervous system are myelinated by Schwann cells. Schwann cells are considered the only supporting cells of the peripheral nervous system, and must provide for the peripheral nervous system all of the functions performed by other classes of glial cells in the central nervous system. When peripheral nerves are inflamed, Schwann cells act as phagocytes, cells that ingest and destroy bacteria and other cells. Myelin is an effective insulator for neurons, shielding them from the extracellular

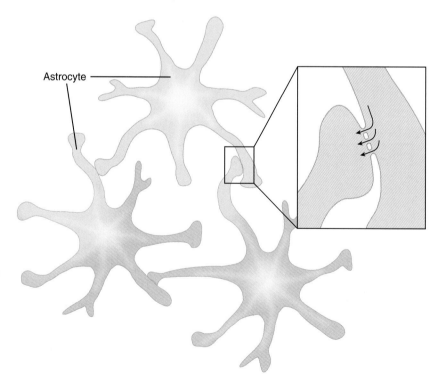

Astrocyte

FIGURE 2-15

Communication between astrocytes. The green color indicates the presence of Ca⁻. The upper astrocyte has been stimulated, producing a wave of Ca⁻ ions passing through the gap junctions from the stimulated cell to the unstimulated cell. The insert shows a magnification of the gap junction.

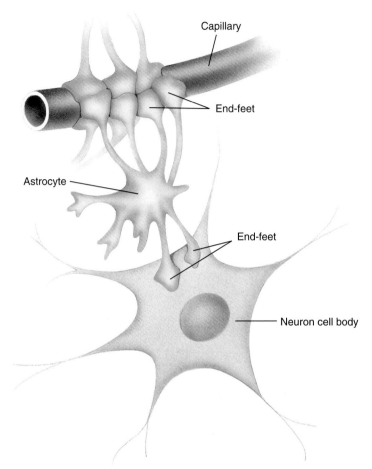

Capillary

End-feet

Astrocyte

End-feet

Neuron cell body

FIGURE 2-16
Astrocyte end-feet. Astrocytes form a
connection between neurons and capillaries,
providing nutrition.

environment. Oligodendrocytes in the central nervous system envelop several axons from different neurons. In the peripheral nervous system, a Schwann cell may wrap around one axon or several axons (Figure 2-17). An axon is considered **myelinated** when the sheath wraps completely around the axon, usually several times. If the myelin sheath only partially covers the axon, the neuron is classified as **unmyelinated**, even though the term *partially myelinated* would be more accurate.

Microglial Cells

Microglial cells normally function as phagocytes. Microglia act as the central nervous system's immune system and clean the neural environment. They are activated during nervous system development and following injury, infection, or disease. During normal develop-

ment of the nervous system, many neurons that don't make strong synaptic contacts die. As neural cells die, whether as part of normal development or from a pathologic process, the dying cells secrete proteins that attract microglia into the nervous system. The microglia clean up and remove debris from the dying cells. Recently, abnormal activation of microglia has been identified in various disease states including Parkinson's disease (a movement disorder), Alzheimer's disease, amyotrophic lateral sclerosis (a movement disorder), and stroke (Tzeng et al., 2005).

In diseases associated with aging, including Alzheimer's disease, microglia may become activated and stimulate neighboring astrocytes. The result can be a loss of the physiologic buffering function of both the microglia and the astrocytes, and the release of toxic compounds

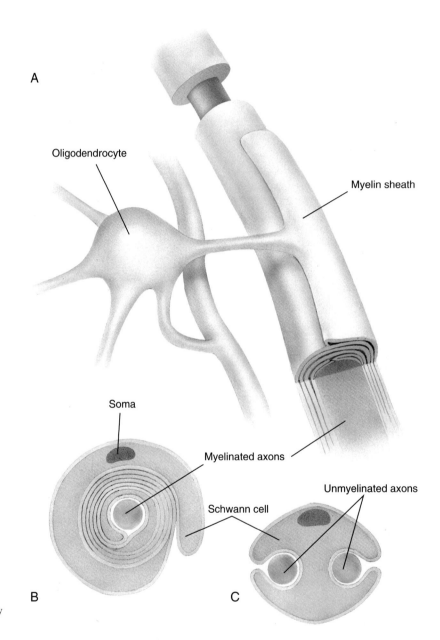

FIGURE 2-17
Myelination. **A,** Oligodendrocytes
provide myelin sheaths in the
central nervous system. **B** and **C,**
Schwann cells provide insulation to
peripheral axons. Myelinated axons
are completely enveloped by Schwann
cells. Unmyelinated axons are partially
surrounded.

into the neuronal environment (Schubert et al., 2000).
Also, human immunodeficiency virus (HIV), associated
with acquired immunodeficiency syndrome (AIDS), can
activate microglia and stimulate a cascade of cellular
breakdown. Clearly, there is a delicate balance between

the normal, protective roles of microglia and the more
recently identified destructive roles. As researchers continue to investigate the intricate functions of glial cells,
the roles of these cells in health and disease of the nervous
system are increasingly appreciated.

> Oligodendrocytes and Schwann cells contribute to the myelination of neurons throughout the nervous system. Astrocytes and microglia contribute to the nutritive and cleanup functions throughout the central nervous system. Astrocytes also exchange signals with other astrocytes and neurons.

Myelin: Clinical Application

Myelin is critical to the conduction of information in the nervous system. As an action potential travels along an axon from a myelinated region to an area where myelin has been damaged, the resistance to the electrical signal increases. The propagation of the electrical current slows and may eventually stop before it reaches the next site of conduction. Why some neurons have myelinated axons and others are unmyelinated is still a mystery, but clues are starting to come into place. First, there appears to be a size requirement, as short axons are not myelinated. In addition, diffusible nerve growth factor appears to regulate the myelination process (Sherman and Brophy, 2005).

Considerable advances have been made recently using cell implantation to enhance neuronal regeneration in demyelinating diseases and following nerve trauma. For example, in animals, Schwann cell implants result in significant regeneration of axons across a spinal cord transection (Xu et al., 1999). This regeneration is often associated with improved motor function, and has great potential as a medical intervention for people with spinal cord injuries.

Peripheral Nervous System Demyelination

Peripheral neuropathy is any pathologic change involving peripheral nerves. Peripheral neuropathies often involve destruction of the myelin surrounding the largest, most myelinated sensory and motor fibers, resulting in disrupted proprioception (awareness of limb position) and weakness. Autoimmune disorders, metabolic abnormalities, viruses, trauma, and toxic chemicals can cause peripheral demyelination.

Guillain-Barré syndrome involves acute inflammation and demyelination of peripheral sensory and motor fibers. The person's immune system generates antibodies that attack Schwann cells. Guillain-Barré syndrome often occurs 2 to 3 weeks after a mild infection. In severe cases, segmental demyelination is so extreme that axons within the myelin sheath degenerate, resulting in greater residual disorders than in people whose axons remain intact (Figure 2-18).

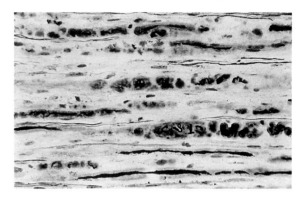

FIGURE 2-18

A nerve biopsy showing peripheral demyelination and axon degeneration that occurs in severe Guillain-Barré syndrome. *(Courtesy Dr. Melvin J. Ball.)*

Signs and symptoms of the syndrome include decreased sensation and motor paralysis. Cranial nerves of the face may be affected, causing difficulty with chewing, swallowing, speaking, and facial expressions. Pain is prominent in some cases. Patients most often report deep aching pain or hypersensitivity to touch. Typically, signs and symptoms have rapid onset followed by a plateau and then gradual recovery. In most cases a person affected by Guillain-Barré syndrome will experience complete recovery. In severe cases, the nerves of the autonomic nervous system and the respiratory system become affected, causing changes in cardiac and respiratory function. Ten percent of people with Guillain-Barré syndrome die of cardiac or respiratory failure. (See Box 2-1 on Guillain-Barré syndrome.)

Medical treatment may include **plasmapheresis** and **intravenous immunoglobulin therapy.** Plasmapheresis is the process of filtering the blood plasma to remove the circulating antibodies responsible for attacking the Schwann cells. **Intravenous immunoglobulin therapy** neutralizes specific antibodies and decreases inflammation (Kuwabara, 2004). Occupational therapy is directed at activities of daily living, including self-care. Physical therapy initially entails stretching and range-of-motion exercises during the acute phase of the disorder. In the recovery phase, physical therapy is directed toward strengthening and the return of functional mobility. When voluntary movement is present, exercise should be gentle to avoid overwork damage in partially denervated muscles (Zelig et al., 1988).

BOX 2-1   GUILLIAN-BARRÉ SYNDROME

Pathology
Demyelination

Etiology
Probably autoimmune

Speed of Onset
Acute, subacute, or chronic

Signs and Symptoms
Weakness is greater than sensory loss; may have pain or hypersensitivity to touch

Consciousness
Normal

Cognition, Language, and Memory
Normal

Sensory
Abnormal sensations (tingling, burning); pain

Autonomic
Blood pressure fluctuation, irregular cardiac rhythms

Motor
Paresis or paralysis; may include respiratory muscles

Cranial Nerves
Motor cranial nerves most affected (eye and facial movements, chewing, swallowing)

Region Affected
Peripheral nervous system

Demographics
Affects all ages, no gender preference

Incidence
1.3 per 100,000 people per year (Kuwabara, 2004)

Lifetime Prevalence
0.2 per 1000 (MacDonald et al., 2000)

Prognosis
Progressively worse for 2-3 weeks, then gradual improvement; 10% mortality rate (Kuwabara, 2004)
Complete functional recovery occurs in 75% of patients

Destruction of Schwann cells impedes conduction of electrical signals along sensory and motor pathways of the peripheral nervous system.

Central Nervous System Demyelination

Central nervous system demyelination involves damage to the myelin sheaths in the brain and spinal cord. Multiple sclerosis (MS) occurs when the immune system

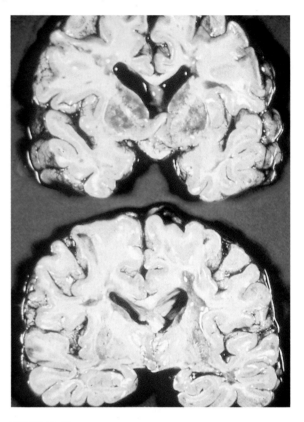

FIGURE 2-19
A coronal section of the cerebrum showing central demyelination. The abnormal areas in the white matter are plaques characteristic of multiple sclerosis. *(Courtesy Dr. Melvin J. Ball.)*

produces antibodies that attack oligodendrocytes (Tzakos et al., 2005). The destruction of the oligodendrocytes in MS produces patches of demyelination, called **plaques,** in the white matter of the central nervous system (Figure 2-19). Similar to demyelination of peripheral neurons, demyelination of central nervous system neurons causes slowed or blocked transmission of signals (Martino et al., 2000).

Signs and symptoms of MS include weakness, lack of coordination, impaired vision, double vision, impaired sensation, and slurred speech (Kaufman et al., 2000; Vleugels et al., 2000). In addition, there may be disruption of memory and emotions. Diagnosis is difficult because MS usually manifests with one sign that may completely resolve. For example, a person might report blindness in one eye, caused by edema or inflammation in the optic tract, and then not experience any signs for months. Neurologic signs that completely resolve, including this temporary blindness, disappear when the swelling and inflammation subside. Diagnosis has improved with the use of imaging techniques and other tests. Demyelination and axonal transection produce relatively permanent impairments (Trapp, 1998).

MS onset most commonly occurs between the ages of 20 and 40 years, and women are three times more frequently affected than men. MS progresses, although some people experience periods of remission.

Physical and occupational therapists work to maintain or improve function where possible. Patients are encouraged to avoid high temperatures and excessive exertion, since increases in body temperature are believed to interfere with the activity of membrane proteins in axons, further disabling action potential conduction. (See Box 2-2 on multiple sclerosis.) Fortunately, medical treatment includes a variety of new drugs that are making major improvements in patients' quality of life (Polman and Uitdehaag, 2000).

Destruction of oligodendrocytes impedes conduction of electrical signals along pathways of the central nervous system.

NEURAL STEM CELLS

The nervous system, unlike many other tissues, has a limited ability to repair itself following injury. Mature neurons cannot reproduce. However, in the past decade, neural stem cells have been discovered in both developing and adult brains. These cells are immature and undifferentiated, the precursors to both neurons and glial cells. Through maturation and differentiation, stem cells can give rise to different types of cells in the central nervous system (Lynch and Portis, 2000). Growth factors have been shown to have an effect on stem cell proliferation (Gage, 2000). Experimentally, adult neural cells can be derived from these primitive cells. The characteristics of neural stem cells include the ability to:
- Self-renew
- Differentiate into most types of neurons and glial cells
- Populate developing and degenerating regions of the central nervous system

The role of neural stem cells in the mature brain is not clear. However, there is a great deal of excitement concerning the possible role of stem cells in brain cell implants. In particular, preliminary stem cell transplantations have been completed in patients with the motor

---

BOX 2-2   MULTIPLE SCLEROSIS

Pathology
Demyelination

Etiology
Probably autoimmune

Speed of Onset
Can be acute, subacute, or chronic

Time Course
Exacerbations and remissions

Signs and Symptoms
  Consciousness
  Normal
  Cognition, Language, and Memory
  Infrequently affects thinking and/or memory
  Sensory
  Tingling, numbness, pins and needles
  Autonomic
  Bladder disorders, sexual impotence in men, genital anesthesia in women
  Motor
  Weakness, incoordination, reflex changes
  Cranial Nerves
  Partial blindness in one eye, double vision, dim vision, eye movement disorders

Region Affected
Central nervous system

Demographics
Typical age at onset is 20-40 years; affects 3 times as many women as men
  Incidence
  7 per 100,000 people per year (MacDonald et al., 2000)
  Lifetime Prevalence
  2 per 1000 (MacDonald et al., 2000)

Prognosis
Variable course; very rarely fatal; most people with MS live a normal life span

---

neuron disease amyotrophic lateral sclerosis, which is significant because currently there is no effective treatment for this disease (Silani and Corbo, 2004). Neurons survive and proliferate after implantation only if they are immature, like stem cells (Bjorklund and Lindvall, 2000). The ability of stem cells to differentiate in the brain and make connections with existing neurons has been verified. This ability is greatest in the young, even fetal, brain, but it can also occur in adult animal brains. One barrier to the use of neuronal stem cells as therapeutic tools will be the difficulty in obtaining them from the brain.

SUMMARY

All nervous system activity relies on the complex physical and electrical properties of cells. Diverse, adaptable, and versatile, these cells affect both normal and abnormal activity. Although physical and occupational therapists work with patients' entire bodies, the basis for rehabilitation lies on the cellular level. A thorough understanding of the roles of these cells—and their contributions to movement, activity, and disease—allows a therapist to more effectively treat patients.

CLINICAL NOTES

Case 1

I.D., a 19-year-old man, suffered severe flu symptoms, requiring him to stay home from work for 2 days. Four days after his return to work, I.D. noted tingling and numbness in his fingers. By the end of the day, he noticed his hand movements were clumsy. The following day I.D. returned to work. Midday he was unable to stand and could not use his hands. At the hospital, nerve conduction studies for both motor and sensory pathways were conducted. (To test peripheral sensory nerve pathways, an electrical stimulus is given to the skin on a distal point over a nerve and recorded with surface electrodes at a more proximal point over the same nerve. The time required for transmitting the signal between the two points indicates the conduction velocity. Peripheral motor conduction studies are similar, except the electrical stimulus is given proximally over the nerve and recorded from the skin over an associated muscle.) The studies for I.D. indicated that peripheral sensory and motor conduction times were significantly prolonged bilaterally.

   I.D. had suffered peripheral nerve demyelination, presumably due to an autoimmune response to some form of viral infection. With the loss of myelin, nerve conduction was severely impaired. I.D. had sensory loss and muscular weakness that significantly impaired his ability to move. Following medical treatment, he was referred to physical therapy for range-of-motion exercises, strengthening exercises, and functional mobility training.

Questions

1. The disease was confirmed to involve the peripheral nervous system. Did the loss of myelin involve oligodendrocytes or Schwann cells?
2. How does a loss of myelin along peripheral sensory fibers affect the propagation of action potentials in the affected axons?
3. Would the loss of myelin in sensory neuron fibers impair the generation of local receptor potentials or the propagation of action potentials?

Case 2

J.R. is a 27-year-old woman with MS who was admitted to the hospital twice in the past year with complaints of bilateral lower-extremity weakness and blurred vision. Upon examination, she exhibited about 30% of normal muscle strength in the left lower extremity and about 50% of normal strength in the right lower extremity. She exhibited mild left foot drop during the swing phase of gait and slight knee hyperextension during the stance phase. At the hospital, visual evoked potentials were evaluated to assess nerve conduction velocity along the visual tracts. Evoked potentials are extracted from an electroencephalogram (EEG) recorded during repetitive presentation of a flash of light. The time from the stimulus to the appearance of the potential on the EEG indicates the central conduction time. For J.R., decreased visual sensory conduction times were determined. J.R. was referred to physical therapy for strengthening exercises and gait training with an ankle-foot orthosis. The physician's orders specified low-repetition exercises and avoidance of physical overexertion.

Questions

1. Delayed conduction times for the evoked potentials suggest a problem with sensory conduction within the central nervous system. What nervous system abnormality can explain the delayed sensory nerve conduction times?
2. What mechanism related to generation of the action potential may be directly impaired by increases in body temperature associated with overexertion?

REVIEW QUESTIONS

1. Do dendritic projections function as input units or output units for a neuron?
2. Name one example of a pseudounipolar cell. Why is it called pseudounipolar?
3. What is the specialized function of multipolar cells?
4. What are the three major ions that contribute to the electrical potential of a cell membrane in its resting state?
5. Define the terms *depolarization* and *hyperpolarization* with respect to resting membrane potential.
6. If a membrane channel opens when it is bound by a neurotransmitter, what type of membrane channel is it?
7. What does the term *graded* mean with respect to the generation of local receptor and synaptic potentials?
8. How is the resting membrane potential maintained?
9. Why is the hyperpolarization of a neuronal membrane considered inhibitory?
10. Peripheral receptors have what types of ion channels?
11. List two types of local potential summation that can result in depolarization of a membrane to the threshold level.
12. The generation of an action potential requires the influx of what ion? Is the influx mediated by a voltage-gated channel?
13. Do large-diameter or small-diameter axons promote faster conduction velocity of an action potential?
14. What are the unique features of the nodes of Ranvier that promote generation of an action potential?
15. Names of tracts in the central nervous system identify the origin and termination of the tract. Where does the spinothalamic tract originate? Where does this tract terminate?
16. Are networks composed of interneuronal convergence and divergence found throughout the central nervous system or only in the spinal cord?
17. List two ways in which glial cells differ from nerve cells.
18. What are the four functions of astrocytes in the mature nervous system?
19. To what critical function do both oligodendrocytes and Schwann cells contribute in the nervous system?
20. What are the differences between oligodendrocytes and Schwann cells?
21. Compare and contrast Guillain-Barré syndrome and multiple sclerosis.

References

Araque A, Sanzgiri RP, et al. (1999). Astrocyte-induced modulation of synaptic transmission. Canadian Journal of Physiology and Pharmacology, 77, 699-706.

Bjorklund A, Lindvall O (2000). Cell replacement therapies for central nervous system disorders. Nature Neuroscience, 3(6), 537-544.

Cornell-Bell AH, Finkbeiner SM, et al. (1990). Glutamate induces calcium waves in cultured astrocytes: Long range glial signaling. Science, 247, 470-473.

Frolkis VV, Tanin SA (1999). Peculiarities of axonal transport of steroid hormones (hydrocortisone, testosterone) in spinal root fibres of adult and old rats. Neuroscience, 92(4), 1399-1404.

Gage FH (2000). Mammalian neural stem cells. Science, 287, 1433-1438.

Kaufman M, Moyer D, et al. (2000). The significant change for the Timed 25-Foot Walk in the Multiple Sclerosis Functional Composite. Multiple Sclerosis, 6(4), 286-290.

Kuwabara S (2004). Guillain-Barré syndrome: Epidemiology, pathophysiology and management. Drugs, 64(6), 597-610.

Lynch WP, Portis JL (2000). Neural stem cells as tools for understanding retroviral neuropathogenesis. Virology, 271, 227-233.

MacDonald BK, Cockerell OC, et al. (2000). The incidence and lifetime prevalence of neurological disorders in a prospective community-based study in the UK (see comments). Brain, 123(4), 665-676.

Martino G, Furlan R, et al. (2000). Cytokines and immunity in multiple sclerosis: The dual signal hypothesis. Journal of Neuroimmunology, 109(1), 3-9.

Pakkenberg B, Pelvig D, et al. (2003). Aging and the human neocortex. Experimental Gerontology, 38(1-2), 95-99.

Parpura V, Haydon PG (2000). Physiological astrocytic calcium levels stimulate glutamate release to modulate adjacent neurons. Proceedings of the National Academy of Sciences of the United States of America, 97(15), 8629-8634.

Polman CH, Uitdehaag BM (2000). Drug treatment of multiple sclerosis. British Medical Journal, 321, 490-494.

Purves D, Augustine GJ, et al. (2001). Neural signaling. Neuroscience, ed 2, Sunderland, MA: Sinauer Associates.

Rouach N, Glowinski J, et al. (2000). Activity-dependent neuronal control of gap-junctional communication in astrocytes. Journal of Cell Biology, 149, 1513-1526.

Schubert P, Morino T, et al. (2000). Cascading glia reactions: A common pathomechanism and its differentiated control by cyclic nucleotide signaling. Annals of the New York Academy of Sciences, 903, 24-33.

Schubert P, Ogata T, et al. (1998). Pathological immuno-reactions of glial cells in Alzheimer's disease and possible sites of interference. Journal of Neurological Transmission (Supplement), 54, 167-174.

Sherman DL, Brophy PJ (2005). Mechanisms of axon ensheathment and myelin growth. Nature Reviews. Neuroscience, 6, 683-690.

Silani V, Corbo M (2004). Cell-replacement therapy with stem cells in neurodegenerative diseases. Current Neurovascular Research, 1(3), 283-289.

Trapp BD, Peterson J, et al. (1998). Axonal transection in the lesions of multiple sclerosis. New England Journal of Medicine, 338(5), 278-285.

Tzakos AG, Troganis A, et al. (2005). Structure and function of the myelin proteins: Current status and perspectives in relation to multiple sclerosis. Current Medicinal Chemistry, 12(13), 1569-1587.

Tzeng SF, Hsiao HY, et al. (2005). Prostaglandins and cyclooxygenases in glial cells during brain inflammation. Current Drug Targets. Inflammation and Allergy, 4(3), 335-340.

Vesce S, Bezzi P, et al. (1999). The highly integrated dialogue between neurons and astrocytes in brain function. Science Progress, 82, 251-270.

Vleugels L, Lafosse C, et al. (2000). Visuoperceptual impairment in multiple sclerosis patients diagnosed with neuropsychological tasks. Multiple Sclerosis, 6(4), 241-254.

Walz W (2000). Role of astrocytes in the clearance of excess extracellular potassium. Neurochemistry International, 36, 291-300.

Xu XM, Zhang SX, et al. (1999). Regrowth of axons into the distal spinal cord through a Schwann-cell-seeded mini-channel implanted into hemisected adult rat spinal cord. European Journal of Neuroscience, 11, 1723-1740.

Zelig G, Ohry A, et al. (1988). The rehabilitation of patients with severe Guillain-Barré syndrome. Paraplegia, 26(4), 250-254.

3 Synapses and Synaptic Transmission

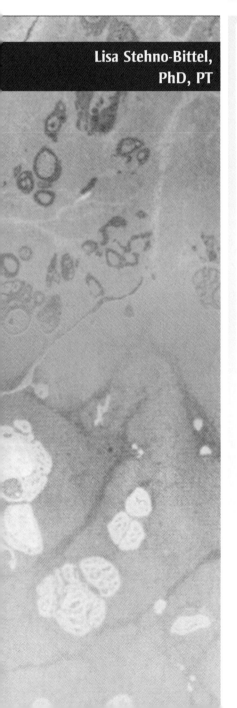

**Lisa Stehno-Bittel,
PhD, PT**

When I was young, I found the story of mutiny on the Bounty fascinating. I thought *mutiny* sounded like a word I should have in my vocabulary. Little did I know I would one day use the word in the context of my own body. Today my immune system wages a mutiny of sorts: I have myasthenia gravis (MG).

My disease first became apparent a year ago, when I was a 28-year-old college student completing the prerequisites for a graduate program in physical therapy. My vision started behaving strangely. I experienced dizziness and disorientation when I tried to scan from one point to another. It was as though one eye couldn't keep up with the other. I visited my ophthalmologist, who suggested everything from a brain tumor to multiple sclerosis. After a battery of tests, including an MRI, all of his theories had been eliminated. Fortunately I was then referred to a neuroophthalmologist, who knew what I had before he even examined me. He gave me a Tensilon test, which was positive, and officially diagnosed MG, which is a disease that affects muscle receptors, interfering with muscle contraction.

My life has changed significantly over the last year. I am lucky, however, because the disease only affects my eyes at this point. I experience double vision much of the time, and I have difficulty keeping my eyelids open. I have learned that I depended on my eyes in ways I had never realized. I most notice the absence of depth perception, caused by weakness of the muscles that should normally align my eyes.

After quick deterioration at the onset of the disease, my condition stabilized. I take a medication called pyridostigmine bromide (Mestinon), which controls my symptoms to some degree for short periods of time. I also underwent a thymectomy last summer because studies have shown that, for largely unknown reasons, removal of the thymus gland can result in dramatic improvement in patients with MG. These improvements can take up to a year to manifest themselves. I have noticed modest improvements in my condition since the surgery. I have received no physical therapy for my disease because at this point it affects only the oculomotor (eye movement control) portion of my vision.

—*David Hughes*

INTRODUCTION

Neural communication takes place at synapses. Diseases and disorders that interfere with synaptic communication can disrupt any aspect of neural function, from thinking to nerve-muscle signaling to the regulation of mood. Most drugs that affect the central nervous system act at the synapse. This chapter discusses how synapses function, including the roles of neurotransmitters and neuromodulators, synaptic receptors, and neurotransmitter agonists and antagonists. This chapter also covers some of the diseases and disorders caused by synaptic failure.

Structure of the Synapse

At a synapse, a neuron and a postsynaptic cell communicate. The postsynaptic cell can be a gland, a muscle cell, or another neuron. A synapse comprises a presynaptic terminal, a postsynaptic terminal, and the synaptic cleft (Figure 3-1). The **presynaptic terminal,** located at the end of the axon, is a projection specialized for the release

of chemicals. The membrane region of the receiving cell is the **postsynaptic terminal.** The space between the two terminals is called the **synaptic cleft.** The presynaptic terminal contains vesicles (small membrane-bound packets) of chemicals called **neurotransmitters.** Neurotransmitters transmit information across the cleft. The postsynaptic membrane contains **receptors,** with specialized molecules designed to bind specific neurotransmitters.

Events at the Synapse

The following steps summarize synaptic communication. This sequence is also shown in Figure 3-2.

1. An action potential (a brief pulse of electrical current that travels along the axon) arrives at the presynaptic terminal.
2. The membrane of the presynaptic terminal depolarizes, opening voltage-gated Calcium (Ca^{++}) channels.
3. Influx of Ca^{++} into the neuron terminal, combined with the liberation of Ca^{++} from intracellular stores, triggers the movement of synaptic vesicles, which contain neurotransmitters, toward a release site in the membrane (Zucker, 1993).
4. Synaptic vesicles fuse with the membrane, releasing neurotransmitter into the cleft.
5. Neurotransmitter diffuses across the synaptic cleft.
6. Neurotransmitter that contacts a receptor on the postsynaptic membrane binds to that receptor.
7. The receptor changes shape. The changed configuration of the receptor either:
   • Opens an ion channel associated with the membrane receptor, or
   • Activates intracellular messengers associated with the membrane receptor.

Synaptic contact between neurons can occur on the cell body (axosomatic), the dendrites (axodendritic), or the axon (axoaxonic) of the postsynaptic neuron (Figure 3-3). A single neuron can have multiple synaptic inputs in each region as described in Chapter 2 under "Interactions Between Neurons."

The total number of action potentials reaching the terminal directly influences the amount of neurotransmitter released. Strong excitatory stimuli to the presynaptic cell lead to a greater number of action potentials reaching the presynaptic terminal. Also, the duration of the stimulus to the presynaptic cell influences the series of subsequent action potentials: When the presynaptic cell is stimulated for more time, the series of action potentials is also longer.

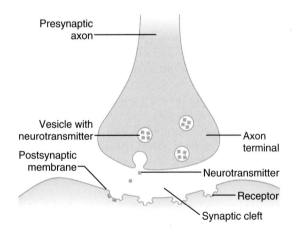

FIGURE 3-1

Synapse. An axon terminal from one neuron communicating via neurotransmitter with any region of membrane on another neuron, muscle cell, or gland forms a synapse.

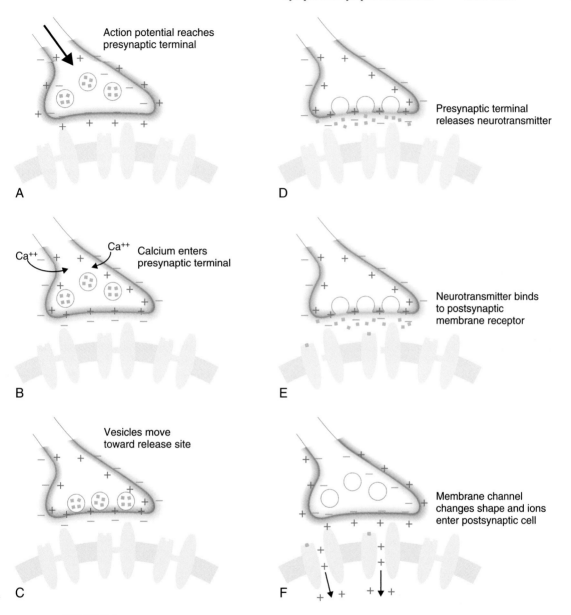

FIGURE 3-2
Series of events at an active chemical synapse. **A,** The action potential reaches the axon terminal. **B,** The change in electrical potential causes the opening of voltage-dependent Ca^{++} channels and the influx of Ca^{++}. **C,** Elevated levels of Ca^{++} then promote the movement of synaptic vesicles to the membrane. **D,** The synaptic vesicles bind with the membrane, then release neurotransmitter into the synaptic cleft. **E,** Neurotransmitter diffuses across the synaptic cleft and activates a membrane receptor. **F,** In this case, the receptor is associated with an ion channel that opens when the receptor site is bound by neurotransmitter, allowing positively charged ions to enter the postsynaptic cell.

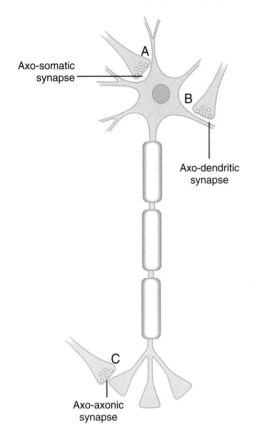

Axo-somatic synapse

Axo-dendritic synapse

Axo-axonic synapse

FIGURE 3-3

Types of synapses. **A,** Axosomatic connection between the axon of a presynaptic neuron and the cell body or soma of a postsynaptic neuron. **B,** Axodendritic connection between the axon of a presynaptic neuron and a dendrite of a postsynaptic neuron. **C,** Axoaxonic connection between the axon of a presynaptic neuron and the axon of a postsynaptic neuron.

An increase in either the strength or the duration of a stimulus to the presynaptic cell results in the release of greater quantities of neurotransmitter.

ELECTRICAL POTENTIALS AT SYNAPSES

Some of the neurotransmitters released into the synaptic cleft bind with receptors on the postsynaptic membrane. The chemical stimulation of these receptors can result in the opening of membrane ion channels. If the synapse is neuromuscular, axosomatic, or axodendritic, the flux of ions in the postsynaptic membrane generates a local

postsynaptic potential. Axoaxonic activity produces presynaptic effects.

Postsynaptic Potentials

Postsynaptic potentials are local changes in ion concentration across the postsynaptic membrane. When a neurotransmitter binds to a receptor that opens ion channels on the postsynaptic membrane, the effect may be local depolarization or hyperpolarization. A local depolarization is an **excitatory postsynaptic potential** (EPSP). A local hyperpolarization is an **inhibitory postsynaptic potential** (IPSP).

Excitatory Postsynaptic Potential

An EPSP occurs when neurotransmitters bind to postsynaptic membrane receptors that open ion channels, allowing a local, instantaneous flow of Na^+ or Ca^{++} into the neuron. The flux of positively charged ions into the cell causes the postsynaptic cell membrane to become depolarized (less negative), creating an EPSP (Figure 3-4). Summation of EPSPs can lead to generation of an action potential (see Chapter 2).

Excitatory postsynaptic potentials are common throughout both the central and peripheral nervous systems. For example, activation of synapses between a neuron and a muscle cell at the neuromuscular junction results in EPSPs that lead to excitation of the muscle. The action of the neurotransmitter acetylcholine is always excitatory to the muscle cell. Binding of acetylcholine opens membrane channels that allow Na^+ influx into the muscle cell, initiating a series of events leading to mechanical contraction the muscle cell. Every action potential in a lower motor neuron (a neuron that innervates muscle) elicits a contraction of the muscle cell because lower motor neurons release sufficient amounts of transmitter to bind to and activate the many receptors on a muscle cell membrane.

Inhibitory Postsynaptic Potential

An IPSP is a local hyperpolarization of the postsynaptic membrane, which decreases the possibility of an action potential. In contrast to the EPSP, an IPSP involves a local flow of Cl^- and/or K^+ in response to a neurotransmitter binding to postsynaptic membrane receptors (Figure 3-5). The postsynaptic ion channels open, allowing Cl^- into the cell or K^+ out of the cell. This causes the local postsynaptic cell membrane to become hyperpolarized (more negative). Hyperpolarization can inhibit the generation of an action potential in the postsynaptic cell. If excitatory postsynaptic potentials coincide with inhibitory postsynaptic potentials,

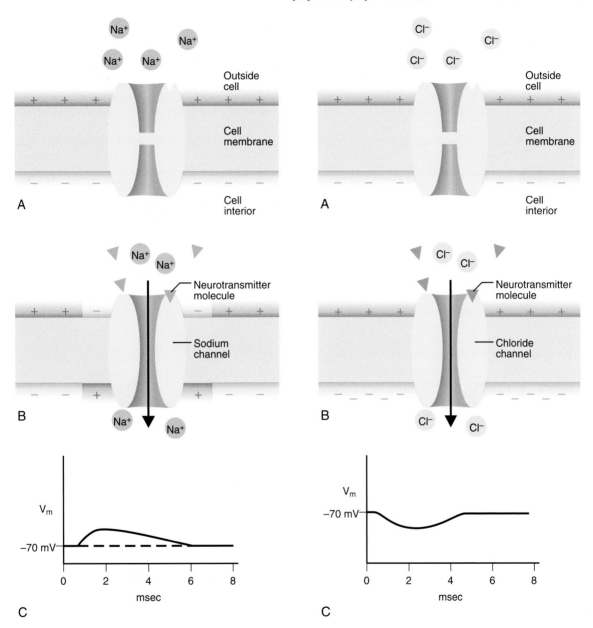

FIGURE 3-4

Excitatory postsynaptic potential. **A,** The resting membrane, with Na^+ channels closed. **B,** Neurotransmitter released into the synaptic cleft binds with membrane receptors that stimulate the opening of ligand-gated Na^+ channels. A resulting influx of Na^+ depolarizes the membrane and causes excitation of the neuron. **C,** The resulting postsynaptic membrane potential is more positive than the resting membrane potential.

FIGURE 3-5

Inhibitory postsynaptic potential. **A,** The resting membrane, with Cl^- channels closed. **B,** Neurotransmitter released into the synaptic cleft binds with membrane receptors, which stimulates the opening of ligand-gated Cl^- channels. A resulting influx of Cl^- hyperpolarizes the membrane and thereby causes inhibition of the neuron. **C,** The resulting postsynaptic membrane potential is more negative than the resting membrane potential.

summation determines whether an action potential will be generated. If the preponderance of input to a neuron is inhibitory, an action potential is not generated in the postsynaptic neuron. Only if sufficient depolarization occurs to reach threshold is an action potential generated in the postsynaptic cell.

> At the postsynaptic membrane, changes in membrane potential can be either excitatory or inhibitory to the neuron.

Presynaptic Facilitation and Inhibition

Activity at a synapse can be influenced by **presynaptic facilitation,** which allows more neurotransmitter to be released, or **presynaptic inhibition,** which allows less (Figure 3-6). Presynaptic facilitation intensifies signals that are interpreted as pain. Presynaptic inhibition can diminish the same signals. For example, concentrating on a painful shoulder can increase the level of activation of brain areas associated with the pain experience, while distraction can lessen the brain activity. Presynaptic effects occur when the amount of neurotransmitter released by a neuron is influenced by previous activity in an axoaxonic synapse. Neurotransmitter released from

the axon terminal of one neuron binding with receptors on the axon terminal of a second neuron alters the membrane potential of the second terminal. For example, activity at axoaxonic synapses between axons descending from the brain and axons of somatosensory neurons can facilitate or inhibit signals interpreted as painful. This presynaptic effect intensifies or relieves the perception of pain.

Presynaptic facilitation occurs when a presynaptic axon releases neurotransmitter that slightly depolarizes the axon terminal of a second neuron. This causes a small Ca^{++} influx into the second neuron's postsynaptic terminal. Because of this small Ca^{++} influx, the duration of an action potential in the second neuron increases. The prolonged action potential allows more Ca^{++} than normal to enter the second neuron's postsynaptic terminal. The increased Ca^{++} concentration causes more vesicles of neu-

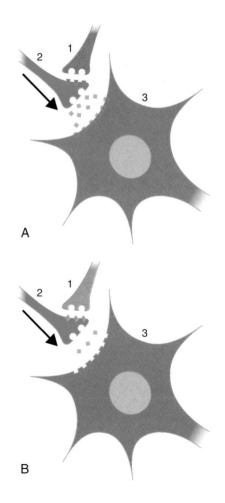

FIGURE 3-6

Presynaptic facilitation and presynaptic inhibition. In both panels, the interneuron is labeled *1,* the presynaptic neuron is labeled *2,* and the postsynaptic neuron is labeled *3.* In **A,** the interneuron (*1*) has just been fired, releasing neurotransmitter that is bound to receptors on the axon terminal of the presynaptic neuron (*2*). The binding of the neurotransmitter will facilitate the release of neurotransmitter by the presynaptic neuron (*2*). Thus, when an action potential (*indicated by the arrow*) reaches the axon terminal of the presynaptic neuron, more Ca^{++} enters the presynaptic terminal and more transmitter than normal is released by the presynaptic neuron. The result is increased stimulation of the postsynaptic neuron (*3*) owing to the increased release of neurotransmitter. **B,** The opposite effect. The interneuron (*1*) has released a neurotransmitter that is bound to the axon terminal of the presynaptic neuron (*2*). The binding of this transmitter will inhibit the release of neurotransmitter by the presynaptic neuron. Thus, when an action potential reaches the axon terminal of the presynaptic neuron, less Ca^{++} than normal enters the terminal and less neurotransmitter is released by the presynaptic neuron. The result is decreased stimulation of the postsynaptic cell membrane (*3*), owing to the decreased release of neurotransmitter into the synaptic cleft between the presynaptic neuron and postsynaptic neuron.

rotransmitter than usual to move to the cell membrane and release transmitter into the synapse. Accordingly, the facilitated neuron releases more neurotransmitter to its target postsynaptic cell (Figure 3-6, *A*).

Presynaptic inhibition occurs when an axon releases neurotransmitter that slightly hyperpolarizes the axonal region of a second neuron. When an action potential occurs in the second neuron, the duration of the action potential is decreased in the axon terminal of the second neuron due to the local inhibition of the axon terminal membrane. As a result of the decreased duration of the action potential, Ca^{++} influx is reduced. Accordingly, the inhibited neuron releases less neurotransmitter onto its target postsynaptic cell (Figure 3-6, *B*).

> The release of neurotransmitters from an axon terminal can be either facilitated or inhibited by the chemical action at an axoaxonic synapse.

NEUROTRANSMITTERS AND NEUROMODULATORS

Neurotransmitters and neuromodulators are chemicals critical to health and disease in the nervous system. Most drugs administered to patients with diseases of the nervous system either mimic the action of a neurotransmitter or neuromodulator, or block the ability of the neurotransmitter or neuromodulator to interact with its receptor.

Neurotransmitters may excite or inhibit the postsynaptic neuron, depending on the molecule released and the receptors present on the postsynaptic membrane. Neurotransmitters affect the postsynaptic neuron either directly, by activating ion channels, or indirectly, by activating proteins inside the postsynaptic neuron. Neurotransmitters that act directly are classified as fast-acting, because they have actions that are extremely short-lived: less than 1/1000 of a second. Neurotransmitters that act indirectly are classified as slow-acting, because their transmission requires 1/10 of a second to minutes. Slow-acting neurotransmitters regulate fast synaptic transmission by controlling the amount of neurotransmitter released from presynaptic terminals. They can also influence the actions of fast-acting neurotransmitters on the postsynaptic membrane (Greengard, 2001).

Neuromodulators alter neural function by acting at a distance away from the synaptic cleft (Figure 3-7). Neuromodulators are released into the extracellular

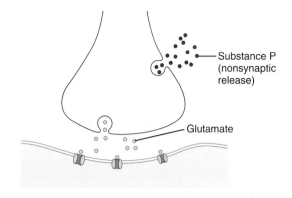

FIGURE 3-7
Cotransmission of neurotransmitter and neuromodulator. In this example, the transmitter is glutamate and the modulator is Substance P. This combination is released by the axons of neurons that convey information perceived as pain. Depolarization of the presynaptic terminal membrane initiates events that culminate in the simultaneous release of neuromodulator (Substance P) into the extracellular space (nonsynaptic release) and neurotransmitter (glutamate) into the synaptic cleft.

fluid and modulate the activity of many neurons. Their effects manifest more slowly and usually last longer than those of neurotransmitters. In general, neuromodulators require seconds before their cellular effects are observed, and these effects last from minutes to days. While neuromodulators are not released directly into the synaptic cleft, they often act in conjunction with neurotransmitters. The same molecule can act as a neurotransmitter or a neuromodulator, depending on whether the molecule is released only at specific synapses or is released into the extracellular space. For example, Substance P, a short-chain polypeptide discussed later in this chapter, acts as a neurotransmitter between certain neurons in the spinal cord, but as a neuromodulator in the hypothalamus.

Chemical synaptic transmission requires several steps. The neurotransmitter must be synthesized, stored, and released, then interact with the post-synaptic receptor, and finally be removed from the synaptic cleft. Until recently, neuroscientists believed each neuron used only one chemical substance for transmission. For example, a cholinergic neuron would only use acetylcholine as a neurotransmitter. However, not only does a neuron contain more than one neurotransmitter ready for release, but researchers have found evidence that neurons may release multiple transmitters simultaneously (Jonas et al., 1998). This finding greatly complicates the

**Table 3-1 COMMON NEUROTRANSMITTERS/
NEUROMODULATORS**

Type	Transmitter/Modulator
Cholinergic	Acetylcholine (ACh)
Amino acid	γAminobutyric acid (GABA)
	Glutamate (Glu)
	Glycine (Gly)
	Aspartate
Amine	Dopamine (DA)
	Histamine
	Norepinephrine (NE)
	Serotonin (5-HT)
Peptide	Endorphins
	Enkephalins
	Substance P
Other	Nitric oxide

classification of neurons and synapses. Researchers identify new compounds as putative neurotransmitters on a continual basis. The chemicals that most commonly function as neurotransmitters and neuromodulators are listed in Table 3-1. This chapter focuses on the neurotransmitters and neuromodulators that have been characterized extensively.

SPECIFIC NEUROTRANSMITTERS AND NEUROMODULATORS

Acetylcholine

Acetylcholine (ACh) is the major conveyor of information in the peripheral nervous system. All neurons that synapse with skeletal muscle fibers (lower motor neurons) use ACh to elicit fast-acting effects on muscle membranes. ACh also has slow-acting effects in the peripheral nervous system that regulate heart rate and other autonomic functions. In the central nervous system, slow action and neuromodulation by ACh is involved in the control of movement and selection of objects of attention (Pepeu and Giovannini, 2004; Aston-Jones and Cohen, 2005).

Amino Acids

Amino acid transmitters—glutamate, aspartate, glycine, and gamma aminobutyric acid (GABA)—are typically fast-acting. Glutamate and aspartate have powerful excitatory effects on neurons in virtually every region

of the brain. **Glutamate,** the principal fast excitatory transmitter of the central nervous system (Meldrum, 2000), elicits neural changes that occur with learning and development. However, glutamate may also contribute to neuron death following central nervous system damage. Chapter 4 discusses the destructive role of glutamate.

Glycine and GABA are inhibitory transmitters. **Glycine** inhibits postsynaptic membranes, primarily in the brainstem and spinal cord. **GABA** is the major inhibitory neurotransmitter in the central nervous system, particularly at interneurons within the spinal cord. Inhibitory effects produced by GABA and glycine prevent excessive neural activity. Low levels of these transmitters can cause neural overactivity, leading to seizures.

> The most prevalent fast-acting neurotransmitters are glutamate and GABA.

Amines

Amines are distributed widely throughout the nervous system. Members of this family include dopamine, norepinephrine, serotonin, and histamine. Dopamine, norepinephrine, and serotonin are produced by neurons in the brain stem that project throughout the cerebral cortex and other gray matter areas. In the central nervous system, amines act as both slow-acting neurotransmitters and as neuromodulators (Aston-Jones and Cohen, 2005; Vizi, 2000).

Dopamine affects motor activity, cognition, and behavior. Signaling pathways that use dopamine have been implicated in the pathophysiology of schizophrenia (a disorder of thinking) and Parkinson's disease (a disorder of movement). Dopamine is associated with feelings of pleasure and reward, and thus motivates certain behaviors. These feelings of reward affect behaviors as important as eating, and as destructive as addiction. Cocaine and amphetamines directly affect dopamine signaling by interfering with dopamine **reuptake** into the presynaptic neuron. Impeding dopamine reuptake prolongs dopamine activity, allowing it to continue to bind and activate receptors repeatedly. Cocaine produces euphoria and stereotyped behaviors including pacing and nail biting by interfering with the reuptake protein. Amphetamines energize users by increasing the release of dopamine and blocking dopamine reuptake.

Norepinephrine is used by the autonomic nervous system, the thalamus, and the hypothalamus. It plays a vital role in active surveillance by increasing attention to sensory information. The highest levels of norepinephrine are associated with vigilance (for example, when driving on a crowded freeway), and the lowest levels occur during sleep. Norepinephrine is also essential in producing the "fight-or-flight" reaction to stress. Overactivity of the norepinephrine system produces fear and, in extreme cases, panic, by acting on cortical and limbic regions. Excessive levels of norepinephrine can produce **panic disorder,** the abrupt onset of intense terror, a sense of loss of personal identity, and the perception that familiar things are strange or unreal, combined with signs of increased sympathetic nervous system activity.

Serotonin levels affect mood and perception of pain. Low levels of serotonin are associated with depression and suicidal behavior. The antidepressant Prozac (fluoxetine) is a selective blocker of serotonin reuptake. By blocking serotonin reuptake, the drug ensures that serotonin will remain in the synapses longer, providing more opportunity for serotonin to bind with receptors. There are at least 14 different subtypes of serotonin receptors. This diversity gives the system several ways of responding to the same neurotransmitter.

Although it is often referred to as an amine modulator, histamine is chemically a distant relative to the other compounds in this category. As a neurotransmitter, histamine is concentrated in the hypothalamus, an area of the brain known for regulating hormonal function, and increases arousal (Goutagny et al., 2004).

> Dopamine, norepinephrine, serotonin, and histamine function as slow-acting neurotransmitters and neuromodulators.

Peptides

Neuroactive peptides can affect neuronal signaling by acting as traditional hormones, neurotransmitters, or neuromodulators. Peptides in the central nervous system may act as single neurotransmitters within the synaptic junction, but most researchers believe they work in conjunction with other neurotransmitters and neuromodulators within the same synapse. One of the most common neuropeptides is **Substance P.** When tissue is injured, Substance P stimulates nerve endings at the site of injury and within the spinal cord to intensify the neural signals perceived as pain. Substance P acts as a neurotransmitter in this case, carrying information from the periphery to the spinal cord and brain. Substance P has also been strongly implicated as a neuromodulator in the pathophysiology of pain syndromes that involve perception of normally innocuous stimuli as painful.

Calcitonin gene-related peptide frequently acts as a neuromodulator. By activating second messengers (described later in this chapter) in the post-synaptic cell, calcitonin gene-related peptide phosphorylates the ACh receptor, resulting in a decreased likelihood that ACh will activate its own receptor when bound. This is a classical example of a neuromodulator affecting the synaptic transmission by a neurotransmitter. The neuromodulator effects of calcitonin gene-related peptide also appear to be involved in long-term neural changes in response to pain stimuli (Ren et al., 2005).

Another group of neuro-active peptides is called the **endogenous opioid peptides,** because they bind the same receptors that the drug opium binds. This group includes endorphins, enkephalins, and dynorphins. Opioids inhibit neurons in the central nervous system that are involved in the perception of pain.

Nitric Oxide

Some diffusible agents have neuromodulator effects. For example, nitric oxide, a known regulator of the vascular system, is also active in the brain. **Nitric oxide** appears to be involved in persistent changes in the postsynaptic response to repeated stimuli and in cell death of neurons. These processes, called *long-term potentiation* and *excitotoxicity,* respectively, are explained in Chapter 4.

SYNAPTIC RECEPTORS

Once a neurotransmitter is released into the synaptic cleft, it must bind to a receptor on the postsynaptic membrane to have an effect. The receptors on the postsynaptic neuron are typically named according to the neurotransmitter/neuromodulator to which they bind. For example, the receptors that bind GABA are called GABA receptors. As stated previously, there are typically several types of receptors that will bind the same neurotransmitter. Thus, the effect of a neurotransmitter is not based on the chemical itself, but on the type of receptor to which it binds.

Receptors produce either direct or indirect actions. Neurotransmitter receptors act directly as ion channels when the receptor and ion channel comprise a single functional unit. Receptors act indirectly by using intracellular activity to activate ion channels or cause other changes within the postsynaptic neuron. Examples of receptors in each of these categories are provided below.

Postsynaptic receptors use three mechanisms to transduce signals. When activated, receptors produce fast or slow responses, by

- Directly opening ion channels (fast synaptic transmission),
- Indirectly opening ion channels (slow synaptic transmission), or
- Activating a cascade of intracellular events (slow synaptic transmission).

Direct Activation of Ion Channels: Ligand-Gated Channels

Ligand-gated ion channels consist of proteins that function both as receptors for the neurotransmitter and as ion channels. The gates of these channels open in response to a specific chemical ligand binding to the receptor surface (see Figures 3-4 and 3-5). Neurotransmitters and hormones are endogenous ligands, because they are produced within the organism. Drugs, because they are produced outside the organism, are exogenous ligands.

Typically if a neurotransmitter is not bound to the receptor of a ligand-gated channel, the gate is closed, and no ions pass through. However, if neurotransmitter is bound to the receptor, the gate opens, and specific ions are allowed to flow through the gate according to their electrochemical gradients. Electrochemical gradients are affected by the distribution of electrical charge and the concentration gradient of the specific ion (see Chapter 2).

In the resting state, a ligand-gated channel is closed, not allowing any ions to flow through. When a specific neurotransmitter approaches the channel and binds to the receptor, the gate opens, and ions diffuse down their electrochemical gradient across the neuron's membrane. Even inhibitory neurotransmitters act by opening ion channels. When GABA binds to certain receptors, channels selective for Cl^- open. Chloride diffuses down its electrochemical gradient and into the cell, carrying the negative charge. Although the ion channel may be open for only a few milliseconds, enough ions cross the membrane to make substantial changes in the local membrane potential. The additional negative charge entering the cell hyperpolarizes the membrane, making it less likely to reach threshold and fire an action potential. Thus some ligand-gated ion channels inhibit neuronal activation.

In general, ion channels will open and close rapidly as long as the neurotransmitter is present in the synaptic cleft. Some ligand-gated channels have shut-off mechanisms that inactivate the channel after a certain

period of time, even when the ligand is still present in the extracellular fluid. All other receptors become inactivated when the neurotransmitter is removed from the synaptic cleft, either by degradation or by reuptake of the neurotransmitter back into the presynaptic axon terminal.

> Rapid and brief opening of membrane channels occurs when a neurotransmitter binds to the receptor site of the membrane channel.

Indirect Activation of Ion Channels

Ion channels can also be opened indirectly, causing reactions slower than those of direct activation. Guanine nucleotide binding proteins (G-proteins) indirectly open ion channels by acting as cytoplasmic shuttles, moving between the receptor and target effector proteins on the internal surface of the cell membrane.

When the receptor is activated by a neurotransmitter, the following sequence takes place (Figure 3-8), (Casey and Gilman, 1988; Lamb and Pugh, 1992):

1. The receptor protein changes shape.
2. The G-protein becomes activated (via replacement of guanosine diphosphate by guanosine triphosphate).
3. The active subunits of G-proteins, α and $\beta\gamma$, break free from the receptor to act as cytoplasmic signaling shuttles.
4. The subunits bind to a membrane ion channel.
5. The ion channel changes shape and opens.
6. The subunits become deactivated and reassociate with the receptor.

When the membrane receptor is not activated, the $\alpha\beta\gamma$ complex is bound to the receptor.

> When a neurotransmitter binds to an extracellular membrane receptor with an associated intracellular G-protein, activation of the G-protein elicits cellular events that develop slowly and last longer than the effects of ligand-gated channels. The G-protein can also cause persistent opening of membrane channels.

Cascade of Intracellular Events: Second-Messenger Systems

G-protein second-messenger systems are responsible for some of the most profound and long-lasting changes in

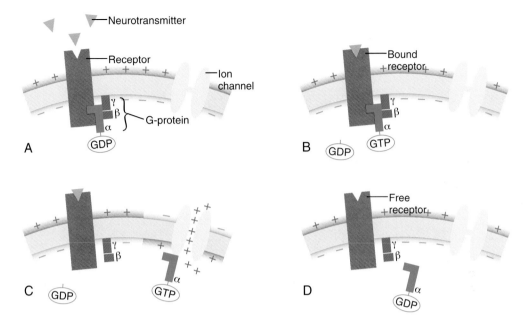

FIGURE 3-8

G-protein–gated ion channel. **A,** In the nonstimulated state, the $\alpha\beta\gamma$ G-protein complex is associated with a membrane receptor. **B,** Neurotransmitter binds to the membrane receptor, causing a conformational change and activation of the G-protein. The α chain detaches from the membrane receptor. **C,** The α-guanosine triphosphate (GTP) complex binds to a membrane-spanning G-protein channel. A conformational change in the protein channel causes the channel to open, and ions flow into the cell. **D,** The α chain is inactivated and released from the protein channel. The channel closes, and the α chain returns to its host membrane receptor to bind with the $\beta\gamma$ chain. (*GDP:* Guanosine diphosphate.)

the nervous system. Via their second-messenger pathways, G-proteins affect long-acting systems that regulate mood, pain perception, movement, motivation, and cognition.

By activating intracellular target proteins, initiating a cascade of intracellular events, the G-proteins can:

- Activate genes, causing the cell to manufacture different neurotransmitters or other specific cellular products,
- Open membrane ion channels, or
- Modulate calcium concentrations inside the cell. Internal stores of Ca^{++} liberated in response to second-messenger systems regulate metabolism and other cellular processes. In this case, Ca^{++} acts as a third messenger.

In second-messenger systems, the neurotransmitter is the first messenger, delivering the message to the receptor but remaining outside the cell. The second messenger, produced inside the cell, conveys the message

and activates responses inside the cell. This can alter a variety of cellular functions. A second-messenger system is similar to a fire department's response to an emergency: The first messenger (neurotransmitter) is analogous to a caller reporting a fire. A receptor conveys relevant information, as an emergency dispatcher does. Second messengers are analogous to firefighters, activating responses within the cell itself.

Some of the same neurotransmitters that act on ligand-gated and G-protein–mediated ion channel receptors can also act on receptors that work through second messenger systems. Figure 3-9 shows the difference between neurotransmitter binding to ligand-gated channels and neurotransmitter binding to G-protein–mediated receptors.

When a G-protein activates an intracellular target protein, the target protein generates a second messenger, which either modulates a membrane channel or affects enzyme activity. Via the G-protein pathway, a single neurotransmitter molecule may elicit a cascade

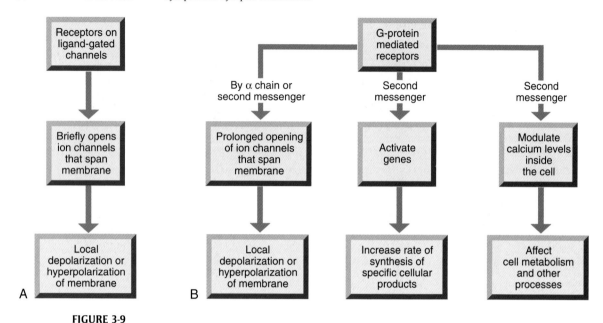

FIGURE 3-9
The effects of neurotransmitter binding to a receptor. **A,** The effects of neurotransmitter binding to a ligand-gated channel. **B,** The effects of G-protein–mediated receptors.

of cellular responses through the indirect activation of the second messenger (Figure 3-10). For example, one second-messenger system produces prostaglandins, substances that regulate vasodilation and increase inflammation. Aspirin and other nonsteroidal anti-inflammatory drugs reduce pain and inflammation by inhibiting one of the enzymes in this G-protein–initiated cascade. Appendix A describes several common second messengers.

The receptor tyrosine kinase is another class of receptors that act through second messengers. Most frequently, these receptors are involved in cell growth, cellular movement, and cell death (Manning et al., 2002). Dysfunction of specific receptor tyrosine kinases, or their agonists, has been implicated in multiple sclerosis (Sobel, 2005), schizophrenia (Kwon et al., 2005), and sensory neuropathies (Mutoh et al., 2005).

The G-Protein Pathway Amplifies the Signal

One activated receptor can stimulate a number of G-proteins (Figure 3-11). Each subunit of the G-protein can carry a different signal to the second messengers. Each of the second messengers may activate a number of other downstream molecules. Figure 3-12 illustrates the series of events in a G-protein second-messenger system.

SPECIFIC RECEPTORS

Acetylcholine Receptors

Receptors that bind ACh fall into two categories: nicotinic and muscarinic. These receptors are distinguished by their ability to bind certain drugs. Nicotine, derived from tobacco, selectively activates the nicotinic receptors. Muscarine, a poison derived from mushrooms, activates only the muscarinic receptors. Fast-acting nicotinic receptors directly open ion channels, allowing a rapid increase in intracellular Na^+ and Ca^{++}, resulting in local depolarization. **Nicotinic receptors** are found at the neuromuscular junction, autonomic ganglia, and in some areas of the central nervous system. The nicotinic receptors of the brain have been implicated in a number of functions, including neuronal development, memory, and learning. Nonsynaptic nicotinic receptors are prevalent in the hippocampus and sensory cortex (Dani and Bertrand, 2007; Jones et al., 1999), and are implicated in the cognitive disorder Alzheimer's disease (Kem, 2000). Nicotine addiction is discussed in Chapter 17.

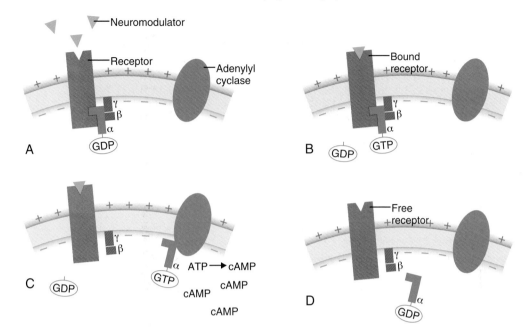

FIGURE 3-10

G-protein acting on a second-messenger system. **A** and **B,** The cellular events are the same as in Figure 3-7, **A** and **B. C,** The α-guanosine triphosphate (GTP) complex binds to a membrane-spanning G-protein enzyme called adenylyl cyclase. A conformational change in the protein enzyme causes the enzyme to produce adenosine triphosphate (ATP), which is converted to cyclic adenosine monophosphate (cAMP). The cAMP acts as a second messenger, activating a variety of cellular proteins including kinases and protein channels. **D,** The α chain is inactivated and released from the protein enzyme. The enzyme is inactivated, and the α chain returns to its host membrane receptor to bind with the βγ chain. (*GDP:* Guanosine diphosphate.)

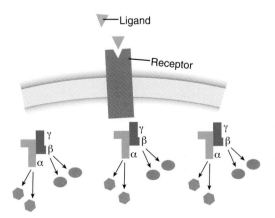

FIGURE 3-11

G-protein action. A neurotransmitter (a type of ligand) binds to one receptor, activating it. The receptor sequentially binds three G-protein molecules. The G-protein molecules dissociate from the receptor and split into α and βγ subunits. The α and βγ subunits of the G-protein molecules each transmit the signal to multiple effector molecules. Thus the signal generated by the binding of a neurotransmitter with a receptor is diversified and amplified.

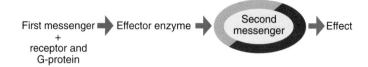

FIGURE 3-12

G-protein–mediated second-messenger system. These systems involve: (1) binding of a neurotransmitter to a G-protein–associated membrane receptor, (2) activation of an effector enzyme, (3) increased levels of a second messenger, and (4) a cellular and physiologic event. An example of a cellular event is increased production of prostaglandins, resulting in the physiologic events of vasodilation, increased inflammation, and increased signals in neurons that signal tissue damage. Different second-messenger systems can produce changes in cellular metabolism.

Muscarinic receptors are G-protein receptors. Their activation produces a slow, prolonged response that is either excitatory or inhibitory. Muscarinic receptors are found mainly on autonomic effector cells in the heart and some regions of the brain. Thus, the actions of ACh on muscarinic receptors contribute to the regulation of cardiac muscle, smooth muscle, and glandular activity (see Chapter 8). There are many subtypes of muscarinic receptors, which are distributed throughout the nervous system.

Glutamate Receptors

Glutamate receptors either directly open ion channels or activate G-protein pathways. Glutamate receptors that couple to G-proteins are called *metabotropic glutamate receptors* (Meldrum, 2000). The ligand-gated ion channels that bind glutamate are called AMPA (alpha-amino-3-hydroxy-5-methyl-4-isoxazolepropionic acid), kainate, or NMDA (*N*-methyl-D-aspartate) receptors. Activation of AMPA and kainate receptors causes fast depolarization of the postsynaptic neuron (Lees, 2000). The NMDA receptor is unique, because to open the ion channel, glutamate must be bound to the receptor and, simultaneously, the membrane must depolarize. Thus the NMDA receptor is both voltage and ligand-gated. Activation of an NMDA receptor causes the associated channel to open and close very slowly. The channel is permeable to Na^+, Ca^{++}, and K^+. The resulting prolonged ionic changes inside the postsynaptic neuron produce long-term potentiation (LTP), a prolonged increase in the size of the postsynaptic response to a given stimulus (Trist, 2000). LTP, important in development and learning, is described further in Chapter 4.

In contrast to these positive roles for NMDA receptors, abnormal activity of these receptors is associated with numerous disorders. The level of glutamate in the local environment of the NMDA receptors must, therefore, be finely regulated because exposure of neurons to high concentrations of glutamate for only a few minutes can lead to neuronal cell death (see Chapter 4) (Meldrum, 2000). Overactivity of NMDA receptors may cause epileptic seizures. The illicit drug phencyclidine ("angel dust") binds to the NMDA receptor and blocks the flow of ions. Changes in glutamate transmission are associated with a number of central nervous system pathologies, including chronic pain, depression, Parkinson's disease, schizophrenia, and the neuronal injury associated with acute stroke (Meador-Woodruff and Healy, 2000; Trist, 2000).

GABA Receptors

As previously discussed, GABA is the most common fast-acting inhibitory neurotransmitter. GABA binds to two types of receptors, referred to as GABA$_A$ and GABA$_B$.

GABA$_A$ receptors are ligand-gated Cl^- channels that open when GABA binds to the receptor, producing hyperpolarization of the postsynaptic membrane. GABA$_A$ receptors are found in nearly every neuron. Barbiturate drugs mimic the action of GABA and bind to the GABA$_A$ subtype. Barbiturates are used pharmacologically for sedation, to decrease anxiety, and as anticonvulsants for treating seizures. In addition, they provide a feeling of euphoria, all of which can be explained by the drugs' ability to activate GABA$_A$ receptors.

GABA also activates slow-acting responses. GABA$_B$ receptors are linked to ion channels via second-messenger systems. Baclofen, a muscle relaxant used to treat excessive muscle contraction, increases the presynaptic release of GABA that activates the GABA$_B$ receptors in the spinal cord. Baclofen is often used to treat excessive muscle contractions in chronic spinal cord injury.

Amine Receptors

Dopamine activates at least five subtypes of receptors. These receptors all use second messenger systems to suppress the activity of Ca^{++} channels. Dopamine affects motor activity, motivation, and cognition. Drugs that act on dopamine receptors alter movement, motivation, and thinking.

Norepinephrine receptors are G-protein–mediated receptors with two major subtypes, called α and β. Activation of α norepinephrine receptors causes relaxation of intestinal smooth muscle. Some β receptors are found in the heart and increase the force and rate of heart contraction. Drugs called β-blockers decrease blood pressure by occupying the binding site but not activating the norepinephrine receptor. In the brain, activation of norepinephrine receptors can produce either excitatory or inhibitory responses.

Serotonin receptors also come in multiple forms and are coupled to different signaling pathways. Some are G-protein receptors, and others are ligand-gated channels opening Na^+ and K^+ channels. A multitude of brain functions are regulated by serotonin receptors, including sleep, cognition, perception (including pain), motor activity, and mood. LSD, a hallucinogenic drug, activates one set of serotonin receptors.

RECEPTOR REGULATION

Receptors may be regulated by:
- Receptor internalization or
- Receptor inactivation.

Overstimulation of postsynaptic receptors can cause a decrease in the number of receptors at the surface. The activated receptors are *internalized* when part of the postsynaptic membrane folds into the cell, creating a receptor-containing vesicle that buds off into the cytoplasm. These "used" receptors may be recycled back to the membrane, ready for subsequent activation, or they may be degraded by the cell and replaced with newly formed receptor molecules.

Inactivation leaves the total number of receptors at the membrane constant but switches some off, so that the number of functional receptors decreases. An example of this mechanism is the β-adrenergic receptor, which binds norepinephrine. Following receptor activation, an intracellular kinase phosphorylates the receptor. Phosphorylation blocks the ability of subsequent norepinephrine molecules to activate the receptor. Only when the receptor has been dephosphorylated can it be activated by a ligand.

> Neurotransmitters and neuromodulators are the chemicals released from an axon terminal. Their effects depend on the type of receptor they bind with. Neurotransmitter effects are local, limited to the postsynaptic membrane. Neuromodulators are released into the extracellular fluid and affect the function of many neurons.

NEUROTRANSMITTER AGONISTS AND ANTAGONISTS

Drugs that affect the nervous system usually bind with receptors or prevent the release of neurotransmitters or neuromodulators. If a drug binds to the receptor and mimics the effects of naturally occurring neurotransmitters, the drug called an **agonist**. If, on the other hand, a drug prevents the release of neurotransmitters or binds to the receptor and impedes the effects of a naturally occurring transmitter, the drug is called an **antagonist**. Because nicotine binds to certain ACh receptors and elicits the same effects as the neurotransmitter would, nicotine is an ACh agonist.

Botulinum toxin A (Botox) is a neurotransmitter antagonist used to improve the functional abilities of people with movement abnormalities caused by central nervous system disorders. Botulinum toxin A is naturally produced by a family of bacteria and, when ingested, causes widespread paralysis by inhibiting the release of ACh at the neuromuscular junction (Borg-Stein and Stein, 1993). When small doses of botulinum toxin A are therapeutically injected directly into an overactive muscle, the local effect is muscle paralysis (Cromwell and Paquette, 1996). This paralysis lasts for up to 12 weeks (Borg-Stein and Stein, 1993) and can result in improved range of motion, resting limb position, and functional movements.

DISORDERS OF SYNAPTIC FUNCTION

Diseases that affect the neuromuscular junction and ion channels in the central nervous system interfere with synaptic function.

Diseases Affecting the Neuromuscular Junction

Signaling between efferent nerve terminals and muscle cells can be disrupted by disease. For example, in Lambert-Eaton syndrome, antibodies destroy voltage-gated Ca^{++}

channels in the presynaptic terminal (Rowland, 1991). The blockage of Ca^{++} influx into the terminal results in decreased release of neurotransmitter and decreased excitation of the muscle, causing muscle weakness. Lambert-Eaton syndrome typically occurs in people with small cell cancers of the lung.

Another disease that affects synaptic transmission at the neuromuscular junction is **myasthenia gravis.** In this autoimmune disease, antibodies attack and destroy nicotinic receptors on muscle cells. Normal amounts of ACh are released into the cleft, but have few receptors to bind. In myasthenia gravis, repetitive use of the muscle leads to increased weakness. Muscles that contract frequently—eye and eyelid muscles, for instance—become weak, causing drooping of the eyelids and misalignment of the eyes. Other commonly affected muscles control facial expression, swallowing, proximal limb movements, and respiration. Proximal limb weakness typically causes difficulty reaching overhead, climbing stairs, and rising from a chair. Drugs that inhibit the breakdown of ACh usually improve function because they increase the amount of time ACh is available to bind with remaining receptors. The autoimmune assault on ACh receptors can be countered with:

- Removal of the thymus gland, an immune organ that functions abnormally in myasthenia gravis, contributing to the damage of ACh receptors,
- Immunosuppressive drugs, or
- Plasmapheresis (the process of removing blood from the body, centrifuging the blood to separate plasma from cells, then returning the blood cells and replacing the plasma with a plasma substitute).

These treatments produce a relatively good prognosis in myasthenia gravis; the survival rate is better than 90%. Onset in women typically occurs between the ages of 20 and 30 years, while in men onset most commonly occurs between the ages of 60 and 70 years. Occasionally, remissions occur in the course of the disease, but stabilization and progression are more frequent outcomes (Box 3-1).

Diseases affecting the neuromuscular junction generally impede the transmission of a signal by decreasing the release of neurotransmitter at the synapse or preventing the transmitter from activating the postsynaptic membrane receptor.

Channelopathy

Channelopathy is a disease that involves dysfunction of ion channels (Margari et al., 2005). For example, genetic

---

BOX 3-1   MYASTHENIA GRAVIS

Pathology
Decreased number of muscle membrane acetylcholine receptors

Etiology
Autoimmune

Speed of Onset
Chronic

Signs and Symptoms
Usually affects eye movements or eyelids first
Consciousness
Normal
Cognition, Language, and Memory
Normal
Sensory
Normal
Autonomic
Normal
Motor
Fluctuating weakness; weakness increases with muscle use
Cranial Nerves
Cranial nerves are normal; however, skeletal muscles innervated by cranial nerves show fluctuating weakness (because the disorder affects the muscle membrane receptors)

Region Affected
Peripheral

Demographics
Can occur at any age; women more often affected than men
Incidence
3 per 100,000 people per year (MacDonald et al., 2000)
Lifetime Prevalence
0.4 per 1000 (MacDonald et al., 2000)

Prognosis
Stable or slowly progressive; with medical treatment, >90% survival rate

---

mutations in both voltage-gated and ligand-gated ion channels are implicated in several inherited neurologic disorders, especially in diseases that disrupt skeletal muscle coordination (Graves and Hanna, 2005). Several studies of families with inherited disorders of voluntary movement have linked the hyperexcitability of ion channels in the brain and muscle to abnormal movements, epilepsy, and migraines (Guerrini, 2001).

SUMMARY

Scientific understanding of synaptic transmission has changed dramatically over the past 15 years. Researchers have discovered that multiple neurotransmitters may be released simultaneously from a single presynaptic terminal, found new categories of molecules that act as synap-

tic neurotransmitters, and begun to comprehend the role of neuromodulators. The complexity of events at the synaptic cleft leaves researchers much to discover. Because most drugs that act on the central nervous system act at the synapse, both past and future research in this field are critical to understanding health and disease.

CLINICAL NOTES

Case 1

M.J., a 54-year-old woman, suffers from small cell cancer of the lung and exhibits generalized, progressive muscle weakness. Medical evaluation determines that M.J.'s weakness is related to a neuromuscular junction disorder consistent with Lambert-Eaton syndrome. In this syndrome, the voltage-gated Ca^{++} channels in the axon terminals at the synapse between the motor neuron and muscle are disrupted. Plasmapheresis—the process of removing blood from the body, centrifuging the blood to separate the plasma from the cells, then returning the blood cells and replacing the plasma with a plasma substitute—effectively reduces M.J.'s weakness. The benefit from plasmapheresis supports the hypothesis that the disease involves circulating antibodies to the Ca^{++} channels in the motor axon terminals, because the circulating antibodies are removed with the plasma.

Questions

1. The neurotransmitter released at the synaptic junction between the motor axon and the muscle is ACh. Why would destruction of the Ca^{++} channels in the axon terminal disrupt the release of ACh from the axon terminal?
2. Would physical therapy be beneficial for increasing M.J.'s strength if the antibodies to the Ca^{++} channel continue to circulate?

Case 2

S.B., a 12-year-old girl, has significant gait abnormalities resulting from cerebral palsy. She walks on her toes and exhibits a scissor gait, with her legs strongly adducted with each step. S.B. has shown no significant improvements in gait with standard physical therapy exercise, gait training, or range-of-motion exercise. Her physicians now want to inject a small amount of botulinum toxin into the gastrocnemius and adductor magnus muscles of both legs in an effort to reduce involuntary muscle activity and improve gait.

Questions

1. By what mechanism could the injection of botulinum toxin reduce involuntary muscle activity?
2. At the neuromuscular junction, ACh acts via a ligand-gated receptor. Is the action of ACh on the nicotinic, ligand-gated receptor the same as its action on the muscarinic, G-protein–mediated receptor?

REVIEW QUESTIONS

1. What is the difference between postsynaptic inhibition and presynaptic inhibition?
   Which one results in a decreased release of neurotransmitter?
2. The release of neurotransmitter from synaptic vesicles is dependent on the influx of what ion into the presynaptic terminal?
3. What is an EPSP?
4. Does direct activation of a membrane ion channel by a neurotransmitter or indirect activation via second-

messenger systems result in faster generation of a synaptic potential?
5. How long do the effects of neurotransmitter binding persist? How long do the effects of neuromodulator binding persist?
6. How does binding of a neurotransmitter to the receptor of a ligand-gated ion channel cause the channel to open?
7. How do G-proteins contribute to a cascade of cellular events?

8. Is the effect of a neurotransmitter determined by the transmitter itself or by the type of receptor?

9. When glutamate binds to a ligand-gated receptor, what happens?

10. Which neurotransmitter has effects on both motor activity and on the ability to think?

11. What are the actions of Substance P?

12. What is the role of endogenous opioid peptides?

13. What transmitter and which type of receptors are essential for long-term potentiation?

14. Is the number of receptors on a neuron's cell membrane constant throughout the life of the neuron?

References

Aston-Jones G, Cohen JD (2005). An integrative theory of locus coeruleus-norepinephrine function: adaptive gain and optimal performance. Annual Review of Neuroscience, 28, 403-450.

Borg-Stein J, Stein J (1993). Pharmacology of botulinum toxin and implications for use in disorders of muscle tone. Journal of Head Trauma and Rehabilitation, 8, 103-106.

Casey PJ, Gilman AG (1988). G-protein involvement in receptor-effector coupling. Journal of Biological Chemistry, 263, 2577-2580.

Cromwell SJ, Paquette VL (1996). The effect of botulinum toxin A on the function of a person with poststroke quadriplegia. Physical Therapy, 76(4), 395-402.

Dani JA, Bertrand D (2007). Nicotinic acetylcholine receptors and nicotinic cholinergic mechanisms of the central nervous system, 47, 699-729.

Goutagny R, Verret L, et al. (2004). Posterior hypothalamus and regulation of vigilance states. Archives Italiennes de Biologie, 142(4), 487-500.

Graves TD, Hanna MG (2005). Neurological channelopathies. Postgraduate Medical Journal, 81(951), 20-32.

Greengard P (2001). The neurobiology of slow synaptic transmission. Science, 294(5544), 1024-1030.

Guerrini R (2001). Idiopathic epilepsy and paroxysmal dyskinesia. Epilepsia 42, 36-41.

Jonas P, Bischofberger J, et al. (1998). Corelease of two fast neurotransmitters at a central synapse. Science, 281, 419-424.

Jones S, Sudweeks S, et al. (1999). Nicotinic receptors in the brain: Correlating physiology with function. Trends in Neuroscience, 22, 555-561.

Kem WR (2000). The brain alpha 7 nicotinic receptor may be an important therapeutic target for the treatment of Alzheimer's disease. Behavioural Brain Research, 113, 169-181.

Kwon OB, Longart M, et al. (2005). Neuregulin-1 reverses long-term potentiation at CA1 hippocampal synapses.

Lamb TD, Pugh EN Jr. (1992). G-protein cascades: Gain and kinetics. Trends in Neurosciences, 15(8), 291-298.

Lees GJ (2000). Pharmacology of AMPA/kainite receptor ligands and their therapeutic potential in neurological and psychiatric disorders. Drugs, 59, 33-78.

MacDonald BK, et al. (2000). The incidence and lifetime prevalence of neurological disorders in a prospective community-based study in the UK (see comments). Brain, 123(4), 665-676.

Manning G, Whyte DB, et al. (2002). The protein kinase complement of the human genome. Science, 298, 1912-1934.

Margari L, Presicci A, et al. (2005). Channelopathy: Hypothesis of a common pathophysiologic mechanism in different forms of paroxysmal dyskinesia. Pediatric Neurology, 32(4), 229-235.

Meador-Woodruff JH, Healy DJ (2000). Glutamate receptor expression in schizophrenic brain. Brain Research: Brain Research Reviews, 31, 288-294.

Meldrum BS (2000). Glutamate as a neurotransmitter in the brain: Review of physiology and pathology. Journal of Nutrition, 130, 1007S-1015S.

Mutoh T, Tachi M, et al. (2005). Impairment of the Trk-neurotrophin receptor by the serum of a patient with subacute sensory neuropathy. Archives of Neurology, 62(10), 1612-1615.

Pepeu G, Giovannini MG (2004). Changes in acetylcholine extracellular levels during cognitive processes. Learning & Memory, 11(1), 21-27.

Ren K, Novikova SI, et al. (2005). Neonatal local noxious insult affects gene expression in the spinal dorsal horn of adult rats. Molecular Pain, 1, 27.

Rowland LP (1991). Diseases of chemical transmission at the nerve-muscle synapse: Myasthenia gravis. In ER Kandel, JH Schwartz, TM Jessell (Eds.), Principles of neural science, ed 3, pp 235-243. New York: Elsevier.

Sobel RA (2005). Ephrin A receptors and ligands in lesions and normal-appearing white matter in multiple sclerosis. Brain Pathology, 15(1), 35-45.

Trist DG (2000). Excitatory amino acid agonists and antagonists: Pharmacology and therapeutic applications. Pharmaceutica Acta Helvetiae, 74, 221-229.

Vizi, ES (2000). Role of high-affinity receptors and membrane transporters in nonsynaptic communication and drug action in the central nervous system, 52(1), 63-90.

Zucker RS (1993). Calcium and transmitter release. Journal Physiology (Paris), 87(1), 25-36.

4

Neuroplasticity

Lisa Stehno-Bittel, PhD, PT

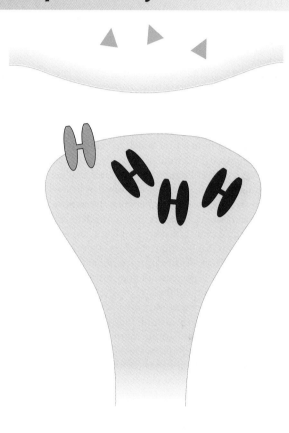

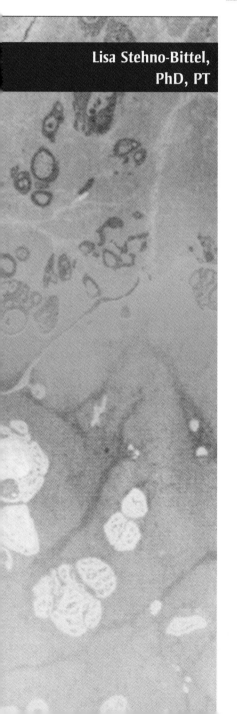

INTRODUCTION

Our experiences and our states of health or disease continuously create and break neuronal connections. **Neuroplasticity** is the ability of neurons to change their function, chemical profile (amount and types of neurotransmitters produced), or structure (Woolf and Salter, 2000). It is essential for recovery from damage to the central nervous system. By definition, neuroplasticity lasts more than a few seconds and is not periodic.

Researchers have demonstrated neuroplasticity by studying animals raised in environments with toys and challenging obstacles. These animals develop more dendritic branching and more synapses per neuron, and have higher gene expression for certain protein products in the brain, than animals without stimulation (Johansson, 2000).

Neuroplasticity is a general term used to encompass the following mechanisms:

- Habituation
- Learning and memory
- Cellular recovery after injury

HABITUATION

Habituation, one of the simplest forms of neuroplasticity, is a decrease in response to a repeated, benign stimulus. In studies of animal posture and locomotion performed in the late 1800s, the pioneering neuroscientist Charles Sherrington observed that certain reflexive behaviors, such as withdrawing a limb from a mildly painful stimulus, ceased after several repetitions of the same stimulus. Sherrington proposed that the decreased responsiveness resulted from a functional decrease in the synaptic effectiveness of the stimulated pathways to the motor neuron (reviewed in French, 1970). Later studies confirmed that habituation of the withdrawal reflex is due to a decrease in synaptic activity between the sensory neurons and interneurons. The cellular mechanisms responsible for habituation are not completely understood. However, with habituation there is a decrease in the release of excitatory neurotransmitters, including glutamate, and perhaps a decrease in free intracellular Ca^{++}. Generally, after many seconds of rest, the effects of habituation are no longer present, and a reflex can be elicited in response to sensory stimuli. However, with prolonged repetition of stimulation, more permanent, structural changes occur: the number of synaptic connections decreases. For example, people with tinnitus (ringing in the ear) can use hearing aids to habituate to the ringing over a prolonged period of time (Folmer and Carroll, 2006).

In occupational and physical therapy, the term *habituation* is applied to techniques and exercises intended to decrease the neural response to a stimulus. For example, some children are extremely reactive to stimulation on their skin. Therapists treat this abnormal sensitivity, called tactile defensiveness, by gently stimulating the child's skin, then gradually increasing the intensity of stimulation. This is intended to achieve habituation to the tactile stimulation. In people with specific types of vestibular disorders, movements that induce dizziness and nausea are repeatedly performed, again with the purpose of achieving habituation to the movements.

> Short-term changes in neurotransmitter release and postsynaptic receptor sensitivity can result in a decreased response to specific, repetitive stimuli.

LEARNING AND MEMORY: LONG-TERM POTENTIATION

Unlike the short-term, reversible effects of habituation, learning and memory involve persistent, longlasting changes in the strength of synaptic connections (Wiersma-Meems et al., 2005). Neuroimaging techniques reveal that during the initial phases of motor learning, large and diffuse regions of the brain show synaptic activity. With repetition of a task, there is a reduction in the number of active regions in the brain. Eventually, when a motor task has been learned, only small, distinct regions of the brain show increased activity during performance of the task (Floyer-Lea and Matthews, 2005). For example, learning to play a musical instrument requires numerous brain regions. As skill increases, fewer areas are activated. Eventually, playing the instrument requires only a few small, specific regions (Meister et al., 2005).

Long-term memory requires the synthesis of new proteins and the growth of new synaptic connections. With repetition of a specific stimulus, the synthesis and activation of proteins alter the neuron's excitability and promote the growth of new synaptic connections, especially at dendritic spines (Johansson, 2004). **Long-term potentiation** (LTP), a cellular mechanism for the formation of memory, has been intensively studied in the hippocampus (Perez-Otano and Ehlers, 2005). The hippocampus, in the temporal lobe, is essential for processing memories that can be easily verbalized. For example, the hippocampus is important in remembering names, but not in remembering how to perform motor acts like riding a bicycle. Long-term potentiation also occurs in motor and somatosensory cortex, cerebellum, and visual cortex, contributing to motor, somatosensory, and visual learning (Llansola et al., 2005; Perez-Otano and Ehlers, 2005).

Long-term potentiation is essential to neural recovery following an injury or insult. Additionally, LTP may have harmful consequences; it may contribute to the development of chronic pain syndromes, including low back pain (see Chapter 7).

Improved memory is related to an increase in synaptic activity and metabolic changes that enhance the efficiency of cell firing. With repetition of a specific stimulus, the synthesis and activation of new proteins can alter the neuron's excitability and promote or inhibit the growth of synaptic connections.

The mechanism responsible for long-term potentiation is the conversion of silent synapses to active synapses.

Silent synapses lack functional glutamate alpha-amino-3-hydroxy-5-methyl-4-isoxazolepropionic acid (AMPA) receptors. Because these synapses lack functional AMPA receptors, they are inactive under normal conditions. Silent synapses can be converted to active synapses via long-term potentiation. A set of mobile AMPA receptors cycles between the cytoplasm and the synaptic membrane (Luscher et al., 2000), providing the mechanism for sudden activation of silent synapses.

The morphology, or shape, of the postsynaptic membrane also changes with long-term potentiation (Fischer et al., 1998; Luscher et al., 2000). Figure 4-1 illustrates one proposed mechanism for morphologic changes in the synapse following stimulation (Luscher et al., 2000). The

budlike shape on the postsynaptic membrane is a dendritic spine, a preferential site for synapse formation. The morphologic remodeling of the synaptic membrane and the functional changes in synaptic strength are probably related. First Ca^{++} enters the postsynaptic cell through channels associated with NMDA (*N*-methyl-D-aspartate) glutamate receptors, resulting in phosphorylation of AMPA receptors and insertion of AMPA receptors into the membrane (Luscher et al., 2000). Subsequently the postsynaptic membrane remodels, generating a new dendritic spine. For a neuron to structurally change, there must be genetic alterations in the cell during the learning process. Calcium is a predominant regulator of gene activity, important because the nucleus itself

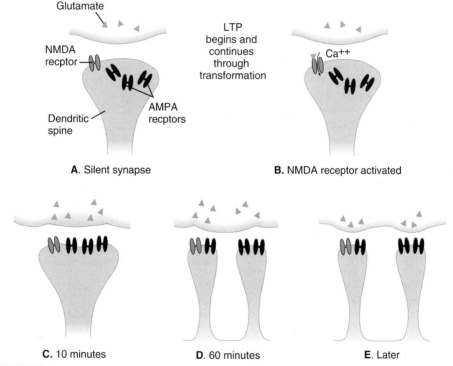

FIGURE 4-1

Structural changes in a synapse induced by long-term potentiation. **A,** The NMDA receptor crosses the membrane allowing cations to pass through either direction. The receptor binds glutamate. The budlike shape of the postsynaptic membrane represents a dendritic spine. Dendritic spines are protrusions on dendrites that are preferential sites of synapses. This is a silent synapse, with AMPA receptors located in the cytoplasm, not in the cell membrane. **B,** Then, long-term potentiation is initiated by the activity of NMDA receptors. **C,** In response to increased Ca^{++} from NMDA receptor activity, AMPA receptors are inserted into the cell membrane. **D,** With continued stimulation, the postsynaptic membrane generates a new dendritic spine. **E,** Finally, structural changes occur in the presynaptic cell, producing a new synapse. *(Modified from Luscher C, Nicoll RA, et al. (2000). Synaptic plasticity and dynamic modulation of the postsynaptic membrane. Nature Neuroscience, 3(6), 547.)*

contains Ca^{++} ion channels (Stehno-Bittel et al., 1995), which may regulate transport across the nuclear membrane (Stehno-Bittel, 1995). This localization of calcium to the nucleus can "turn on" particular genes important in neuronal function (Bading et al., 1993). Thus, changes in calcium within the cell are likely to be one of the signals leading to altered gene regulation during the learning process (Bading, 1999).

Clinically, magnetic stimulation can improve motor memory. Transcranial magnetic stimulation of the motor cortex enhances the duration of motor memory (Butefisch et al., 2004). Magnetic stimulation of afferent pathways induces long-term potentiation, producing an increase in the amplitude of excitatory postsynaptic potentials (EPSPs) of an associated neuron. The EPSP facilitation (i.e., long-term potentiation) can last up to several days.

Finally, non-neuronal cells also play a critical role in brain plasticity. Astrocytes change rapidly in response to changes in stimulation patterns. In rats raised in enriched environments, contact between astrocytes and neurons is greater than in rats raised in standard cages (Jones and Greenough, 1996). This suggests that nonsynaptic transmission of information is important in neuroplasticity.

> Long-term changes, including the synthesis of new proteins and growth of new synaptic connections, result in a maintained response and memory of specific, repetitive stimuli.

CELLULAR RECOVERY FROM INJURY

Injuries that damage or sever axons cause degeneration, but may not result in cell death. Some neurons have the ability to regenerate the axon. In contrast to injury to the axon, injuries that destroy the cell body of a neuron invariably lead to death of the cell. When a neuron dies, the nervous system promotes recovery by altering specific synapses, functionally reorganizing the central nervous system, and changing neurotransmitter release in response to neural activity. These processes are described in more detail below.

Axonal Injury

Axon severance injuries typically occur in the peripheral nervous system where the axons extend a long distance and are not protected by the vertebral column or skull. Axons may be severed by injuries from sharp objects (knives, machinery) or by extreme stretch that pulls the

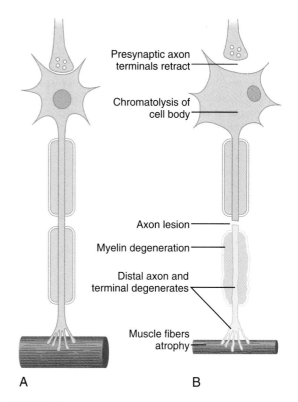

FIGURE 4-2

Wallerian degeneration. **A,** Normal connections before an axon is severed. **B,** Degeneration following severance of an axon. Degeneration following axonal injury involves several changes: (1) the axon terminal degenerates, (2) myelin breaks down and forms debris, and (3) the cell body undergoes metabolic changes. Subsequently, (4) presynaptic terminals retract from the dying cell body, and (5) postsynaptic cells degenerate. In this illustration the postsynaptic cell is a muscle cell.

axon apart. When an axon is severed, the part connected to the cell body is referred to as the proximal segment, and the part isolated from the cell body is called the distal segment. Immediately after injury, the cytoplasm leaks out of the cut ends, and the segments retract away from each other. Once isolated from the cell body, the distal segment of the axon undergoes a process called **wallerian degeneration** (Figure 4-2). When the distal segment of an axon degenerates, the myelin sheath pulls away from that segment. The axon swells and breaks into shorter segments. The terminals rapidly degenerate, and their loss is followed by death of the entire distal segment. Glial cells scavenge the area, cleaning up debris from the degeneration. In addition to axonal degeneration, the associated cell body undergoes degenerative changes called **central chromatolysis,** which occasionally leads to cell death. If a postsynaptic cell loses most of its synaptic inputs due to damage of the presynaptic neurons, the postsynaptic cell degenerates and may die.

The regrowth of damaged axons is called **sprouting.** Sprouting takes two forms: collateral and regenerative (Figure 4-3). Collateral sprouting occurs when dendrites of neighboring neurons reinnervate a denervated target. Collateral sprouting occurs when a denervated target is reinnervated by branches of intact axons of neighboring neurons. Regenerative sprouting occurs when an axon and its target cell (a neuron, muscle, or gland) have been damaged. The injured axon sends out side sprouts to a new target. Functional regeneration of axons occurs most frequently in the peripheral nervous system,

partly because the production of nerve growth factor (NGF) by Schwann cells contributes to the recovery of peripheral axons. Recovery is slow, with approximately 1 mm of growth per day, or about 1 inch of recovery per month.

Peripheral axon sprouting can cause problems when an inappropriate target is innervated. For example, after peripheral nerve injury, motor axons may innervate different muscles than they previously did, resulting in unintended movements when the neurons fire (Freidenberg and Hermann, 2004). These unintended movements, called **synkinesis,** are usually short-lived, as the affected individual relearns muscle control. Similarly, in the sensory systems, innervation of sensory receptors by axons that previously innervated a different type of sensory receptor can cause confusion of sensory modalities.

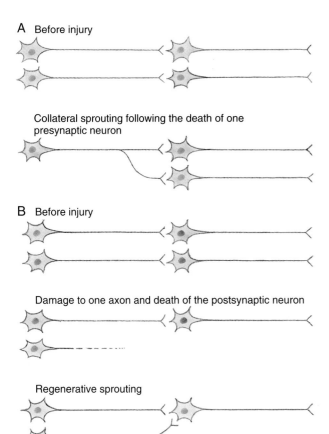

A Before injury

Collateral sprouting following the death of one presynaptic neuron

B Before injury

Damage to one axon and death of the postsynaptic neuron

Regenerative sprouting

FIGURE 4-3

Axonal sprouting. The new growth of axons following injury involves two types of sprouting—collateral sprouting **(A),** in which a denervated neuron attracts side sprouts from nearby undamaged axons, and regenerative sprouting **(B),** in which the injured axon issues side sprouts to form new synapses with undamaged neurons.

Damaged axons of peripheral neurons can recover from injury, and targets deprived of input from damaged axons can attract new inputs to maintain nervous system function.

Functional axon regeneration does not occur in central nervous system axons. Development of glial scars and the absence of nerve growth factor prevent axonal regeneration in the brain and spinal cord. Glial scars, formed by astrocytes and microglia, physically block axonal regeneration, and also may release growth-inhibiting factors such as neurite outgrowth inhibitor (Nogo) (Chen et al., 2002). Nogo is expressed in oligodendrocytes, but not in Schwann cells (He and Koprivica, 2004). The exact role of Nogo in halting recovery after injury is unclear. When researchers eliminated both copies of the active Nogo gene in a group of rodents, the results were mixed: some animals demonstrated improvement in CNS recovery, while others showed no effect (He and Koprivica, 2004). Drugs currently in development block the effects of Nogo and other growth inhibitors—and could be useful in CNS recovery—by targeting inhibitory proteins, blocking receptor-binding sites, or inhibiting the second-messenger signaling cascade (Kastin and Pan, 2005).

Synaptic Changes

Following central nervous system injury, the body uses several mechanisms to overcome damage. Synaptic mechanisms include recovery of synaptic effectiveness, denervation hypersensitivity, synaptic hypereffectiveness, and unmasking of silent synapses (Figure 4-4). After injury, local edema may compress a presynaptic neuron's cell body or axon, producing focal ischemia and interfering with microvascular function (del Zoppo and Mabuchi, 2003). The reduced blood flow interferes with neural function, including synthesis and transport of neurotransmitters, causing some synapses to become inactive. Once edema has resolved, relief of pressure on the presynaptic neuron restores normal cellular function, allowing synthesis and transport of neurotransmitters, which causes **synaptic effectiveness** to return. **Denervation hypersensitivity** occurs when presynaptic axon terminals are destroyed and new receptor sites develop on the postsynaptic membrane in response to transmitter released from other nearby axons (Obata et al., 2004). **Synaptic hypereffectiveness** occurs when only some branches of a presynaptic axon are destroyed. The remaining axon branches receive all of the neurotransmitter that would normally be shared among the

terminals, resulting in larger than normal amounts of transmitter being released onto postsynaptic receptors. Another synaptic change is **unmasking (disinhibition) of silent synapses.** In the normal nervous system, many synapses seem to be unused unless injury to other pathways results in their activation (Poncer, 2003).

Researchers are just beginning to identify the mechanisms responsible for these changes. Many of the same mechanisms responsible for brain plasticity during learning are involved in the recovery period following brain injury. These include NMDA receptor activity and changes in the levels of Ca^{++} ions and of the neurotransmitter Substance P (Zipfel et al., 2000). Transmission by nitric oxide, the diffusible neuromodulator discussed in Chapter 3, has also been implicated in modulation of synaptic function (Kara and Friedlander, 1998).

Functional Reorganization of the Cerebral Cortex

In the adult brain, cortical areas routinely adjust the way they process information. They also retain the ability to develop new functions. Changes at individual synapses reorganize the brain, which can have significant functional consequences. Researchers map functional areas of the cerebral cortex by recording neuron activity in response to sensory stimulation or during active muscle contractions. Cortical representation areas, called cortical maps, can be modified by sensory input, experience, and learning, and brain injury. If a person regularly performs a skilled motor task, the cortical representation of that area will be enlarged. For example, string instrument players have an enlarged area representing fingers of the left hand, while their right hands have only an average finger map (Elbert et al., 1995).

Magnetic resonance imaging (MRI) of the cortex indicates reassignment of neuron function in adults. In people with upper limb amputations, much of the cortical area that would normally be devoted to the missing hand becomes reorganized for representation of the face (Lotze et al., 2001). The face representation expands to occupy the adjacent cortical area that no longer receives input from the hand.

Reorganization of representations in the cortex has also been demonstrated by researchers who ask amputees to report where they feel referred sensations (Lotze et al., 2001). Referred sensations are sensations felt in one place in response to a stimulus applied in another place. For example, when researchers touch the chin of a person who lacks a fifth finger, the amputee reports a tingling sensation in that missing finger. A consistent, precise relationship between the stimulated points and

A   Edema

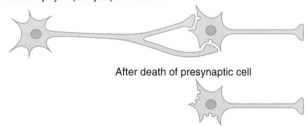

B   Before injury to presynaptic neuron

After death of presynaptic cell

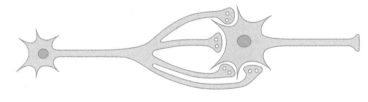

C   Before injury to presynaptic cell

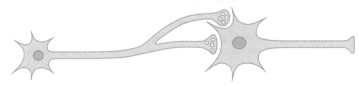

After loss of some presynaptic terminals

FIGURE 4-4

Synaptic changes following injury. **A,** Recovery of synaptic effectiveness occurs with the reduction in local edema that interfered with action potential conduction. **B,** Denervation hypersensitivity occurs after destruction of presynaptic neurons deprives postsynaptic neurons of an adequate supply of neurotransmitter. The postsynaptic neurons develop new receptors at the remaining terminals. **C,** Synaptic hypereffectiveness occurs after some presynaptic terminals are lost. Neurotransmitter accumulates in the undamaged axon terminals, resulting in excessive release of transmitter at the remaining terminals.

the location of phantom sensation has been reported (Lotze et al., 2001).

Less drastic changes than amputation may elicit brain reorganization. Functional magnetic resonance imaging (fMRI) shows significant brain reorganization in patients who develop hand paresis following surgery for brain tumors (Reinges et al., 2005). Figure 4-5 shows changes in the fMRI before and after surgery. Preoperatively, the motor cortex on the right side of the image *(A)* was the

major area activated, but after resection of the tumor, the same task was accomplished with activation in multiple areas of the brain including the ipsilateral side *(B)*.

Brain reorganization has also been demonstrated in people with deafness or blindness. People with congenital deafness have enhanced peripheral vision to moving stimuli, compared to hearing subjects (Bavelier et al., 2000), and people with blindness use a visual area of the cortex when reading Braille (Pascual-Leone et al.,

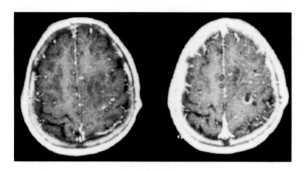

FIGURE 4-5

A functional magnetic resonance image (fMRI) illustrates changes in brain activity during finger and thumb movement before and after surgery to remove a brain tumor. **A,** Prior to surgery, hand movement was normal and the primary motor area of the cerebral cortex was most active during the movements. **B,** After surgery, the hand was paretic and activity in the primary motor area of the cerebral cortex decreased. However, activity in other motor areas of the cerebral cortex increased post surgery. *(From Reinges MH, Krings T, et al. (2005). Prospective demonstration of short-term motor plasticity following acquired central paresis, Neuroimage, 24(4), 1252, Figure 3.)*

2005). Functional reorganization after nerve injury is probably also a factor in some chronic pain syndromes, in which pain persists despite the apparent healing of the precipitating injury. This type of plasticity is discussed in Chapter 7.

Although nervous system plasticity research is in its infancy, researchers are beginning to explain mechanisms of learning and recovery from injury. Plasticity allows for recovery from nervous system injury; however, active movement is crucial for optimizing motor recovery.

> Cortical areas routinely adjust to changes in sensory input and develop new functions dependent on required motor output.

Activity-Related Changes in Neurotransmitter Release

Neuronal activity regulates neurotransmitter production and release. Repeated stimulation of somatosensory pathways can cause increases in inhibitory neurotransmitters, decreasing the sensory cortex response to overstimulation. Understimulation can have the opposite effect, causing the cortex to be more responsive to weak sensory inputs. Improved understanding of cellular mechanisms involved in plasticity may lead to improved clinical

rehabilitation of peripheral and central nervous system disorders in both children and adults.

One potentially beneficial treatment of neurochemical disorders uses genetic manipulation to influence neuroplasticity. Researchers are designing procedures to genetically modify existing neurons so the neurons can make and secrete chemicals that are deficient in the brain. Laboratory studies have shown that transfer of a gene for nerve growth factor into neurons that secrete the neurotransmitter dopamine can protect those neurons from degenerative changes (Sun et al., 2005). Furthermore, increased levels of nerve growth factor and other neurotropic factors may protect neurons by promoting neuron survival, resistance to injury, and plasticity (Sun et al., 2005).

METABOLIC EFFECTS OF BRAIN INJURY

When the brain suffers a stroke or traumatic injury, neurons deprived of oxygen for a prolonged period die and do not regenerate. This damage is not always limited to directly affected neurons. **Excitotoxicity** (cell death caused by overexcitation of neurons) may add more damage. Oxygen-deprived neurons release large quantities of glutamate, an excitatory neurotransmitter, from their axon terminals (Zipfel et al., 1999). Excessive glutamate kills postsynaptic neurons that receive particularly high concentrations. Glutamate at normal concentrations is crucial for central nervous system function; however, at excessive concentrations glutamate is toxic to neurons.

The processes involved in excitotoxicity are diagrammed in Figure 4-6. First, glutamate binds persistently to the NMDA-type glutamate receptor in the cell membrane (Waxman and Lynch, 2005). Stimulation of this receptor results in an influx of Ca^{++} into the cell, and indirectly facilitates the release of internal Ca^{++} stores. With the increase in Ca^{++} inside the cell, more K^+ diffuses out of the cell, requiring increased glycolysis to provide energy for the Na^+-K^+ pump to actively transport K^+ into the cell. Together, the increased glycolysis and the increased Ca^{++} lead to several destructive consequences for neurons:

- Increased glycolysis liberates excessive amounts of lactic acid, lowering the intracellular pH and resulting in acidosis that can break down the cell membrane.
- High intracellular Ca^{++} levels activate Ca^{++}-dependent digestive enzymes called *proteases*. These activated proteases break down cellular proteins.

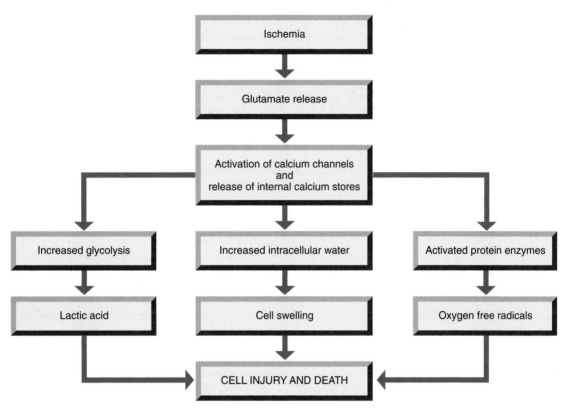

FIGURE 4-6
Schematic process of excitotoxicity. Following an initial ischemic insult, excessive intracellular calcium concentrations result in three pathways of cellular destruction: increased glycolysis, increased intracellular water, and activated protein enzymes.

- Ca^{++} activates protein enzymes that liberate arachidonic acid, producing substances that cause cell inflammation and produce oxygen free radicals. Oxygen free radicals are charged oxygen particles detrimental to mitochondrial functions of the cell.
- An influx of water associated with the ionic influx causes cell edema.

Ultimately, these cellular events lead to cell death and potential propagation of neural damage if the dying cell releases glutamate and overexcites its surrounding cells. Excitotoxicity contributes to the neuronal damage in cerebrovascular accident (stroke), traumatic brain injury, and neural degenerative diseases. Glutamate receptors and some Ca^{++} channels have also been implicated in the neuronal disruption associated with acquired immunodeficiency syndrome (AIDS). The future pharmaceutical treatment of stroke, head injury, and neural degenerative diseases may be directed toward blocking the NMDA type of glutamate receptor and thus preventing the cascade of cell death related to excitotoxicity. However, blocking these receptors may kill cells on the peripheral region of the ischemia due to low Ca^{++} levels (Zipfel et al., 1999). The toxic effects of Ca^{++} at both low and high concentrations mean that researchers are challenged to find successful pharmacologic interventions.

In addition to the possible pharmaceutical blocking of NMDA-type glutamate receptors for management of an ischemic insult to the brain, other treatments may be directed specifically toward blocking the effects of Ca^{++} and free radicals. In animals, when oxygen and blood glucose levels are diminished by an occlusion of blood flow to the brain, levels of the intracellular messenger inositol trisphosphate (IP_3) are increased. This increase stimulates the release of Ca^{++} from intracellular storage sites and promotes a variety of cellular activities. With high cellular activity in the absence of adequate glucose, there is an increase in lactose, free radicals, and other metabolic end products that poison the cell. Also, when IP_3 is broken down by the cell, its by-product, diacylglycerol, breaks down into free fatty acid metabolites that can be poisonous to the cell. Future pharmaceutical treatment of stroke and traumatic brain injury may also be directed toward blocking the IP_3 pathway or administering drugs that act as scavengers for oxygen free radicals. These treatments could potentially prevent the cascade of cell death related to the production of fatty acid metabolites.

> In response to ischemia, cells can die either directly from lack of oxygen or indirectly from the cascade of events resulting from increased stimulation of glutamate receptors.

EFFECTS OF REHABILITATION ON PLASTICITY

Following brain injury, both the intensity of rehabilitation and the amount of time between the injury and initiation of rehabilitation influence the recovery of neuronal function. Prolonged lack of active movement following cortical injury may lead to subsequent loss of function in adjacent, undamaged regions of the brain. However, retraining movements prevent subsequent damage in adjacent areas of cortex (Nudo et al., 1996). Using monkeys, researchers mimicked a stroke by damaging a small part of the motor cortex associated with hand movement control. When retraining of hand movements was initiated 5 days following the original injury, researchers found no loss of function in undamaged adjacent cortical regions. In some cases, neural reorganization took place, and the hand representation of the cortex extended into regions of the cortex formerly occupied by shoulder and elbow representations (Nudo et al., 1996). Because functional reorganization coincided with the recovery of fine finger movements, some researchers believe rehabilitation has a direct effect on the integrity and reorganization of adjacent, undamaged regions of motor cortex.

Conclusive evidence indicates that early rehabilitation is key to improved recovery (Teasell et al., 2005). Biernaskie et al. (2004) produced small lesions in the sensorimotor cortices of rats, and then initiated enriched rehabilitation 5 days or 30 days post stroke. The enriched rehabilitation consisted of housing four to six rats in a cage with a variety of objects designed to encourage (not force) coordinated use of the impaired forelimb. After receiving 5 weeks of treatment, rats whose rehabilitation began 5 days post lesion retrieved more than twice as many food pellets using the impaired forelimb as the rats who also received 5 weeks of treatment but whose rehabilitation began 30 days post lesion. Delay reduces the impact of therapy.

The type of therapy offered is also important to the ultimate success of treatment. Task-specific practice is essential for motor learning (Bayona et al., 2005). Transcranial magnetic stimulation and functional magnetic imaging show that task-specific training, as opposed to traditional stroke rehabilitation, produces long-lasting cortical reorganization in the brain areas activated (Classen et al., 1998).

Constraint-induced movement is one type of task-specific training used in people with chronic dysfunction resulting from a stroke. In this technique, use of the unaffected upper limb is constrained by a sling. The patient then practices functional movements with the affected upper extremity. Selected patients (only 20%-25% of patients have enough hand movement to qualify for the therapy; Wolf et al., 2005) experience small improvements in upper limb movement (Mark and Taub, 2004).

However, excessively vigorous rehabilitation of motor function too soon after the injury can be counterproductive. Constraint-induced movement of an impaired limb immediately after an experimental lesion of the sensorimotor cortex in adult rats has been shown to dramatically increase neuronal injury and result in long-lasting deficits in limb placement, decreased response to sensory stimulation, and defective use of the limb for postural support (Kozlowski et al., 1996). Furthermore, the cortices of these animals showed large increases in the volume of the lesions, and an absence of dendritic growth or sprouting. These results suggest that immediate, intense, constraint-induced movement of an impaired limb may expand brain injury. Preliminary data indicate that excitotoxicity, caused by use-dependent increases in cortical activity, is a possible explanation for the increase in lesion size (Kozlowski et al., 1996). These harmful effects only occur with extreme overuse of the impaired extremity immediately after the lesion. If rats have lesions induced in the sensorimotor cortex and are able to freely use both forelimbs after the surgery, dendritic complexity increases in the cortex that controls the impaired extremity and no increase in cortical damage occurs (Schallert et al., 2003). Rehabilitation training initiated 3 to 5 days after a lesion does not increase lesion size or worsen behavioral outcomes (Biernaskie et al., 2004).

SUMMARY

In the last 20 years, researchers have made remarkable progress in understanding the nervous system's ability to heal and adapt following injury. Neuroplasticity, which enables people to recover from neural injuries, is an essential concept for those designing therapeutic interventions. An understanding of this key concept is essential to physical and occupational therapists, as well as those designing pharmacologic treatments. Therapists can optimize recovery by initiating therapy early, avoiding vigorous use or overuse of impaired extremities during the first few days post central nervous system injury, and practicing specific tasks to elicit beneficial adaptive neuroplasticity.

CLINICAL NOTES

Case 1

BG, a 37-year-old woman, suffered a compound fracture of her right distal radius and ulna following a fall while ice-skating. Internal fixation of the fracture was required, and BG was restricted to very limited use of her dominant right arm and hand. Postoperatively, BG reported decreased sensation in the fourth and fifth fingers of her right hand. Due to the severity of the fracture, some of the ulnar nerve fibers had been damaged. Six weeks after injury, BG was referred to therapy for range-of-motion exercises of the right wrist and hand and low-resistance exercise. Grip strength in the right hand was two-thirds that in the left hand. During therapy, BG reported "burning sensations" and "pins and needles" in the digits of her right hand.

Questions

1. Is it possible for damaged or severed ulnar nerve axons to recover after injury?
2. Should the therapist anticipate the abnormal sensory sensations to diminish over the course of a few months?

Case 2

KS, a 52-year-old man, experienced some right-sided weakness and then collapsed while working on his farm. Several hours passed before KS was found. He was transported to the local hospital, where doctors determined he had suffered a stroke. The stroke resulted from sudden blockage of an artery, preventing blood flow to a region of the brain. KS experienced a right facial droop, inability to move his right arm and leg, and decreased sensation on the right side of the body. KS required maximal assistance for all mobility, and was referred to occupational and physical therapy.

Questions

1. Was the brain damage associated with the stroke most likely confined only to the cells that were deprived of oxygen due to decreased blood flow?
2. If excitotoxicity was in part responsible for the severity of the stroke, which principal excitatory neurotransmitter would be involved?

REVIEW QUESTIONS

1. Define neuroplasticity.
2. When therapists repeatedly provoke unwanted reactions in people with tactile defensiveness, what is the intent?
3. What is the mechanism of long-term potentiation?
4. Define wallerian degeneration.
5. What are some consequences of axonal sprouts innervating inappropriate targets?
6. Can adult mammals' cortical motor and sensory maps change?
7. Define the term *excitotoxicity*.

8. Name one end product of glycolysis that contributes to cell death.
9. Identify two mechanisms by which excessive levels of intracellular calcium promote cell death.
10. Can some of the brain damage associated with strokes, traumatic injury, and degenerative diseases potentially be reduced with the administration of pharmaceutical agents?
11. What are the effects of constraint-induced movement following a stroke?

References

Bading H (1999). Nuclear calcium-activated gene expression: Possible roles in neuronal plasticity and epileptogenesis. Epilepsy Research, 36(2), 225-231.

Bading H, Ginty DD, et al. (1993). Regulation of gene expression in hippocampal neurons by distinct calcium pathways. Science, 260, 181-186.

Bavelier D, Tomann A, et al. (2000). Visual attention to the periphery is enhanced in congenitally deaf individuals. Journal of Neuroscience, 20(17), RC93.

Bayona NA, Bitensky J, et al. (2005). The role of task-specific training in rehabilitation therapies. Topics in Stroke Rehabilitation, 12(3), 58-65.

Biernaskie J, Chernenko G, et al. (2004). Efficacy of rehabilitative experience declines with time after focal ischemic brain injury. Journal of Neuroscience, 24(5), 1245-1254.

Butefisch CM, Khurana V, et al. (2004). Enhancing encoding of a motor memory in the primary motor cortex by cortical stimulation. Journal of Neurophysiology, 91(5), 2110-2116.

Chen ZJ, Negra M, et al. (2002). Oligodendrocyte precursor cells: Reactive cells that inhibit axon growth and regeneration. Journal of Neurocytology, 31(6-7), 481-495.

Classen J, Liepert J, et al. (1998). Rapid plasticity of human cortical movement representation induced by practice. Journal of Neurophysiology, 79(2), 1117-1123.

del Zoppo GJ, Mabuchi T (2003). Cerebral microvessel responses to focal ischemia. J Journal of Cerebral Blood Flow and Metabolism, 23(8), 879-894.

Elbert T, Pantev C, et al. (1995). Increased cortical representation of the fingers of the left hand in string players. Science, 270, 305-307.

Fischer M, Kaech S, et al. (1998). Rapid actin-based plasticity in dendritic spines. Neuron, 20, 847-854.

Floyer-Lea A, Matthews PM (2005). Distinguishable brain activation networks for short- and long-term motor skill learning. Journal of Neurophysiology, 94(1), 512-518.

Folmer RL, Carroll JR (2006). Long-term effectiveness of ear-level devices for tinnitus. Otolaryngology—Head and Neck Surgery, 134(1), 132-137.

Freidenberg SM, Hermann RC (2004). The breathing hand: Obstetric brachial plexopathy reinnervation from thoracic roots? Journal of Neurology, Neurosurgery, and Psychiatry, 75(1), 158-160.

French RD (1970). Some concepts of nerve structure and function in Britain, 1875-1885: Background to Sir Charles Sherrington and the synapse concept. Medical History, 14(2), 154-165.

He Z, and Koprivica V (2004). The Nogo signaling pathways for regeneration block. Annual Review of Neuroscience, 27, 341-368.

Johansson BB (2000). Brain plasticity and stroke rehabilitation. Stroke, 31, 223-230.

Johansson BB (2004). Brain plasticity in health and disease. The Keio Journal of Medicine, 53(4), 231-246.

Jones TA, Greenough WT (1996). Ultrastructural evidence for increased contact between astrocytes and synapses in rats reared in a complex environment. Neurobiology of Learning and Memory, 65, 48-56.

Kara P, Friedlander MJ (1998). Dynamic modulation of cerebral cortex synaptic function by nitric oxide. Progress in Brain Research, 118, 183-198.

Kastin AJ, Pan W (2005). Targeting neurite growth inhibitors to induce CNS regeneration. Current Pharmaceutical Design, 11(10), 1247-1253.

Kozlowski DA, James DC, et al. (1996). Use-dependent exaggeration of neuronal injury after unilateral sensorimotor cortex lesions. Journal of Neuroscience, 16(15), 4776-4786.

Llansola M, Sanchez-Perez A, et al. (2005). Modulation of NMDA receptors in the cerebellum. 1. Properties of the NMDA receptor that modulate its function. Cerebellum, 4(3), 154-161.

Lotze M, Flor H, et al. (2001). Phantom movements and pain. An fMRI study in upper limb amputees. Brain, 124(11), 2268-2277.

Luscher C, Nicoll RA, et al. (2000). Synaptic plasticity and dynamic modulation of the postsynaptic membrane. Nature Neuroscience, 3(6), 545-550.

Mark VW, Taub E (2004). Constraint-induced movement therapy for chronic stroke hemiparesis and other disabilities. Restorative Neurology and Neuroscience, 22(3-5), 317-336.

Meister I, Krings T, et al. (2005). Effects of long-term practice and task complexity in musicians and nonmusicians performing simple and complex motor tasks: Implications for cortical motor organization. Human Brain Mapping, 25(3), 345-352.

Nudo RJ, Wise BM, et al. (1996). Neural substrates for the effects of rehabilitative training on motor recovery after ischemic infarct. Science, 272, 1791-1794.

Obata K, Yamanaka H, et al. (2004). Contribution of degeneration of motor and sensory fibers to pain behavior and the changes in neurotrophic factors in rat dorsal root ganglion. Experimental Neurology, 188(1), 149-160.

Pascual-Leone A, Amedi A, et al. (2005). The plastic human brain cortex. Annual Review of Neuroscience, 28, 377-401.

Perez-Otano I, Ehlers MD (2005). Homeostatic plasticity and NMDA receptor trafficking. Trends in Neurosciences, 28(5), 229-238.

Poncer JC (2003). Hippocampal long term potentiation: Silent synapses and beyond. Journal de Physiologie (Paris), 97(4-6), 415-422.

Reinges MH, Krings T, et al. (2005). Prospective demonstration of short-term motor plasticity following acquired central paresis. Neuroimage, 24(4), 1248-1255.

Schallert T, Fleming SM, et al. (2003). Should the injured and intact hemispheres be treated differently during the early phases of physical restorative therapy in experimental stroke or parkinsonism? Physical Medicine and Rehabilitation Clinics of North America, 14(1 Suppl), S27-S46.

Stehno-Bittel L, Luckhoff A, et al. (1995). Calcium release from the nucleus by InsP3 receptor channels. Neuron, 14, 163-167.

Stehno-Bittel L (1995). Calcium signalling in normal and abnormal brain function. Neurology Report, 19(2), 12-17.

Sun M, Kong L, et al. (2005). Comparison of the capability of GDNF, BDNF, or both, to protect nigrostriatal neurons in a rat model of Parkinson's disease. Brain Research, 1052(2), 119-129.

Teasell R, Bitensky J, et al. (2005). The role of timing and intensity of rehabilitation therapies. Topics in Stroke Rehabilitation, 12(3), 228-237.

Waxman EA, Lynch DR (2005). N-methyl-D-aspartate receptor subtypes: Multiple roles in excitotoxicity and neurological disease. Neuroscientist, 11(1), 37-49.

Wiersma-Meems R, Van Minnen J, et al. (2005). Synapse formation and plasticity: The roles of local protein synthesis. Neuroscientist, 11(3), 228-237.

Wolf SL, Thompson PA, et al. (2005). The EXCITE trial: Attributes of the Wolf Motor Function Test in patients with subacute stroke. Journal of Neurologic Rehabilitation, 19(3), 194-205.

Woolf CJ, Salter MW (2000). Neuronal plasticity: Increasing the gain in pain. Science, 288, 1765-1768.

Zipfel GJ, Babcock DJ, et al. (2000). Neuronal apoptosis after CNS injury: The roles of glutamate and calcium (In Process Citation). Journal of Neurotrauma, 17(10), 857-869.

Zipfel G J, Lee J-M, et al. (1999). Reducing calcium overload in the ischemic brain. New England Journal of Medicine, 341, 1543-1544.

5 Development of the Nervous System

Laurie Lundy-Ekman, PhD, PT

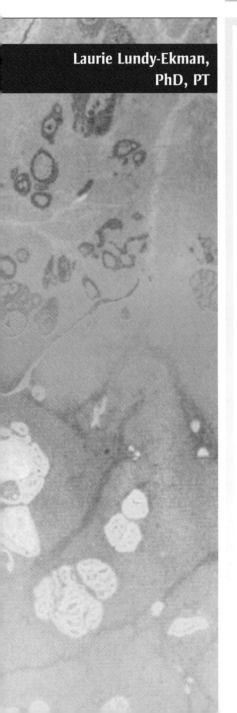

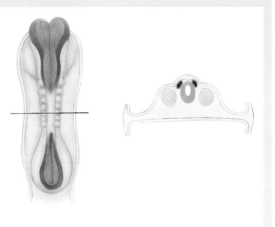

I am a 22-year-old student. Next year I will complete my master's degree in physical therapy, and I plan to specialize in pediatrics. Helping children with neurologic deficits is very important to me, as I was diagnosed with cerebral palsy at 2 years of age. At that time, a friend asked my parents if they would let me be seen by a pediatric specialist because the friend noticed that I was still crawling while all the children I was playing with were walking. I had no other signs of delayed development, verbally, cognitively, or socially, but motorically I was far behind my peers. Unlike the pediatricians that I had seen previously, who said that I would outgrow my motoric delay, this specialist confirmed what my parents had suspected. A diagnosis of mild spastic diplegic cerebral palsy* was made, and my parents searched for things they could do to encourage my development.

I have yet to understand why my doctors did not tell my parents about physical therapy. Fortunately, I started school 3 years later, and my physical education teacher took an interest. To the best of his abilities, he used his skills as an educator and read extensively over the next 6 years to provide opportunities for me to develop motor skills. My first formal therapy session came in eighth grade, when I was referred by the school to an occupational therapist for an evaluation and to develop a physical education program that I could do independently. That visit sparked my interest in rehabilitation, shaping my choice of career.

As I mentioned, my cerebral palsy is mild. My cognitive skills are not affected, and my upper limb coordination is near normal. One physician's record states that there was some involvement of my left upper limb, but I do not notice any problems except when my reflexes are tested. I am inclined to think that any decrease in upper limb coordination is due to lack of challenges at a younger age, but I cannot confirm this suspicion. The most significant physical impact cerebral palsy has had on my life is on my gait pattern and recreational activities.

---

*Bilateral excessive muscle stiffness with weakness, usually affecting the lower limbs.

As a child, motor dysfunction was more a daily problem than it is now because I could not keep up with my friends. I still struggle at times. Most recently, I struggled with learning to perform dependent-patient transfers in physical therapy school. Personally, I think that the greatest impact cerebral palsy has had on my life is a psychological one. There are still some things I would like to learn to do, but failing with motor activities as a child has influenced what I am willing to try now. On the other hand, that is why I am becoming a physical therapist: I want children and adults to know that physical limitations do not have to prevent them from enjoying life as much as anyone else.

—*Heidi Boring*

INTRODUCTION

From a single fertilized cell, an entire human being can develop. How is the exquisitely complex nervous system generated during development? Genetic and environmental influences act on cells throughout the developmental process, stimulating cell growth, migration, differentiation, and even cell death and axonal retraction to create the mature nervous system. Some of these processes are completed in utero, while others continue during the first several years after birth. Understanding the beginnings of the nervous system is vital for comprehending developmental disorders and helpful in understanding the anatomy of the adult nervous system.

DEVELOPMENTAL STAGES IN UTERO

Humans in utero undergo three developmental stages:
- Preembryonic
- Embryonic
- Fetal

Preembryonic Stage

The preembryonic stage lasts from conception to 2 weeks. Fertilization of the ovum usually occurs in the uterine tube. The fertilized ovum, a single cell, begins cell division as it moves down the uterine tube and into the cavity of the uterus (Figure 5-1). By repeated cell division, a solid sphere of cells is formed. Next, a cavity opens in the sphere of cells. At this stage of development, the sphere is called a *blastocyst*. The outer layer of the blastocyst will become the fetal contribution to the placenta, and the inner cell mass will become the

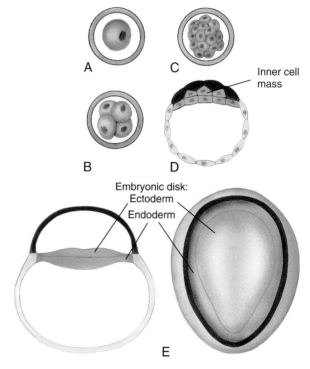

FIGURE 5-1

A, Fertilized ovum, a single cell. **B,** Four-cell stage. **C,** Solid sphere of cells. **D,** Hollow sphere of cells. The inner cell mass will become the embryonic disk. **E,** The two-layered embryonic disk, shown in cross section *(left)* and from above *(right)*. The upper layer of the disk is the ectoderm, and the lower layer is the endoderm.

embryo. The blastocyst implants into the endometrium of the uterus. During implantation, the inner cell mass develops into the embryonic disk, consisting of two cell layers: ectoderm and endoderm. Soon, a third cell layer, mesoderm, forms between the other two layers.

Embryonic Stage

During the embryonic stage, from the second to the end of the eighth week, the organs are formed (Figure 5-2). The ectoderm develops into sensory organs, epidermis, and the nervous system. The mesoderm develops into dermis, muscles, skeleton, and the excretory and circulatory systems. The endoderm differentiates to become the gut, liver, pancreas, and respiratory system.

Fetal Stage

The fetal stage lasts from the end of the eighth week until birth. The nervous system develops more fully

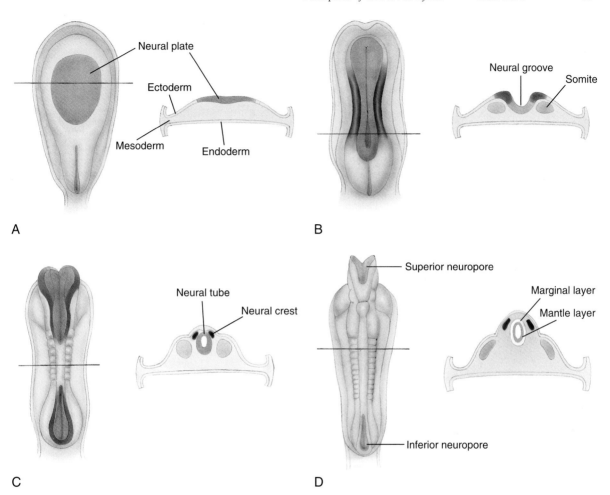

FIGURE 5-2
Cross sections through the embryo are shown on the right. On the left, the view is from above the embryo.
A, Day 16 (Compare with Figure 5-1, **E.**) **B,** The midline section of the neural plate moves toward the interior of the embryo, creating the neural groove (day 18). **C,** The folds of the neural plate meet, forming the neural tube. The neural crest separates from the tube and from the remaining ectoderm (day 21). **D,** The open ends of the neural tube are neuropores. The neural tube differentiates into an inner mantle layer and an outer marginal layer.

and myelination (insulation of axons by fatty tissue) begins.

The nervous system develops from ectoderm, the outer cell layer of the embryo.

FORMATION OF THE NERVOUS SYSTEM

Formation of the nervous system occurs during the embryonic stage and has two phases. First, tissue that will become the nervous system coalesces to form a tube running along the back of the embryo. When the ends of the tube close, the second phase, brain formation, commences.

Neural Tube Formation (Days 18 to 26)

The nervous system begins as a longitudinal thickening of the ectoderm, called the **neural plate** (see Figure 5-2, *A*). The plate forms on the surface of the embryo, extending from the head to the tail region, in contact with amniotic fluid. The edges of the plate fold to create the **neural groove,** and the folds grow toward each other (see Figure 5-2, *B*). When the folds touch (day 21), the neural tube is formed (see Figure 5-2, *C*). The neural tube closes first in the future cervical region. Next, the groove rapidly zips closed rostrally and caudally, leaving open ends called neuropores (see Figure 5-2, *D*). Cells adjacent to the neural tube separate from the tube and the remaining ectoderm to form the **neural crest.** When the crest has developed, the neural tube and the neural crest move inside the embryo. The overlying ectoderm (destined to become the epidermal layer of skin) closes over the tube and neural crest. The superior neuropore closes by day 27, and the inferior neuropore closes about 3 days later.

By day 26, the tube differentiates into two concentric rings (see Figure 5-2, *D*). The **mantle layer** (inner wall) contains cell bodies and will become gray matter. The **marginal layer** (outer wall) contains processes of cells, whose bodies are located in the mantle layer. The marginal layer develops into white matter, consisting of axons and glial cells.

> The brain and spinal cord develop entirely from the neural tube.

Relationship of Neural Tube to Other Developing Structures

As the neural tube closes, the adjacent mesoderm divides into spherical cell clusters called **somites** (see Figure 5-2, *B*). Developing somites cause bulges to appear on the surface of the embryo (Figure 5-3). The somites first appear in the future occipital region, and new somites are added caudally. The anteromedial part of a somite, the **sclerotome,** becomes the vertebrae and the skull. The posteromedial part of the somite, the **myotome,** becomes skeletal muscle. The lateral part of the somite, the **dermatome,** becomes dermis (Figure 5-4).

As the cells of the mantle layer proliferate in the neural tube, grooves form on each side of the tube, separating the tube into ventral and dorsal sections (see Figure 5-4). The ventral section is the **motor plate** (also called *basal plate*). Axons from cell bodies located in the motor plate grow out from the tube to innervate the myotome region of the somite. As development continues, this association leads to the formation of a **myotome:** a group of muscles derived from one somite and innervated by a single spinal nerve. Thus, myotome has two meanings:

FIGURE 5-3

Photographs of embryos early in the fourth week. In **A,** the embryo is essentially straight, whereas the embryo in **B** is slightly curved. In **A,** the neural groove is deep and is open throughout its entire extent. In **B,** the neural tube has formed between the two rows of somites but is widely open at the rostral and caudal neuropores. The neural tube is the primordium of the central nervous system (brain and spinal cord). *(Courtesy Professor Hideo Nishimura.)*

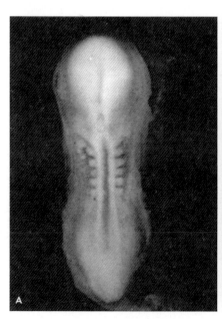
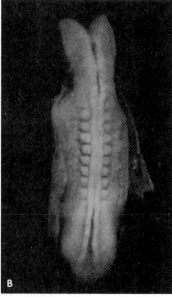

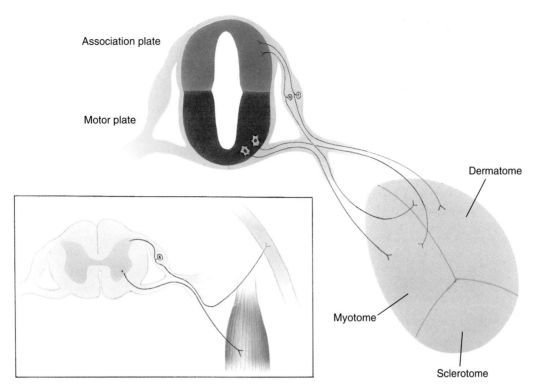

FIGURE 5-4
The neurons connecting the neural tube with the somite are shown. The mantle layer of the neural tube has differentiated into a motor plate (ventral) and an association plate (dorsal). The inset illustrates the same structures in maturity. The following changes have occurred: part of the neural plate → spinal cord, motor plate → ventral horn, association plate → dorsal horn, myotome → skeletal muscle, and dermatome → dermis.

(1) an embryologic section of the somite and (2) after the embryonic stage, a group of muscles innervated by a segmental spinal nerve. Neurons whose cell bodies are in the basal plate become motor neurons, which innervate skeletal muscle, and interneurons. In the mature spinal cord, the gray matter derived from the basal plate is called the *ventral horn.*

The dorsal section of the neural tube is the **association plate** (also called *alar plate*). In the spinal cord, these neurons proliferate and form interneurons and projection neurons. In the mature spinal cord, the gray matter derived from the association plate is called the *dorsal horn* (see Figure 5-4).

Neurons in the dorsal region of the neural tube process sensory information. Neurons with cell bodies in the ventral region innervate skeletal muscle.

The **neural crest** separates into two columns, one on each side of the neural tube. The columns break up into segments that correspond to the dermal areas of the somites. Neural crest cells form peripheral sensory neurons, myelin cells, autonomic neurons, and endocrine organs (adrenal medulla and pancreatic islets). The cells that become peripheral sensory neurons grow two processes; one connects to the spinal cord, and the other innervates the region of the somite that will become dermis. Like the term *myotome,* **dermatome** has two meanings: (1) the area of the somite that will become dermis, and (2) after the embryonic stage, the dermis innervated by a single spinal nerve. The peripheral sensory neurons, also known as primary sensory neurons, convey information from sensory receptors to the association plate. The cell bodies of the peripheral sensory neurons are outside the spinal cord, in the dorsal root ganglion.

> The peripheral nervous system, with the exception of motor neuron axons, develops from the neural crest.

Until the third fetal month, spinal cord segments are adjacent to corresponding vertebrae, and the roots of spinal nerves project laterally from the cord. As the fetus matures, the spinal column grows faster than the cord. As a result, the adult spinal cord ends at the L1-L2 vertebral level. Caudal to the thoracic levels, roots of the spinal nerves travel inferiorly to reach the intervertebral foramina (Figure 5-5). The collection of lumbosacral nerve roots that extend inferior to the end of the spinal cord is the cauda equina (named for resemblance to a horse's tail; Figure 5-6). Disorders of the cauda equina are discussed in Chapter 12. The filum terminale is a continuation of the dura, pia, and glia connecting the end of the spinal cord with the coccyx. The end of the spinal cord is the conus medullaris.

Brain Formation (Begins Day 28)

When the superior neuropore closes, the future brain region of the neural tube expands to form three enlargements (Figure 5-7): the **hindbrain** (rhomben-cephalon), **midbrain** (mesencephalon), and **forebrain** (prosencephalon). Soon two additional enlargements appear, providing the brain with five distinct regions. The enlargements, like their precursor neural tube, are hollow. In the mature nervous system, the fluid-filled cavities are called *ventricles.*

The hindbrain divides into two sections; the lower section becomes the **myelencephalon,** and the upper section becomes the **metencephalon.** These later differentiate to become the medulla, pons, and cerebellum. In the upper hindbrain, the central canal expands to form the fourth ventricle. The pons and upper medulla are anterior to the fourth ventricle, and the cerebellum is posterior. In the cerebellum, the mantle layer gives rise to both deep nuclei and the cortex. To become the cortex, the mantle layer cell bodies migrate through the white matter to the outside.

The **midbrain** enlargement retains its name, midbrain, throughout development. The central canal becomes the cerebral aqueduct in the midbrain, connecting the third and fourth ventricles.

The posterior region of the forebrain stays in the midline to become the **diencephalon.** The major structures are the **thalamus** and the **hypothalamus.** The midline cavity forms the third ventricle.

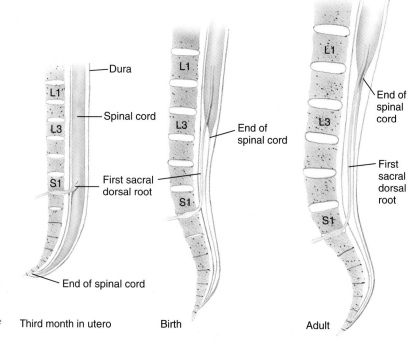

FIGURE 5-5

After the third month in utero, the rate of growth of the vertebral column exceeds that of the spinal cord. The passage of the nerve roots through specific intervertebral foramina is established early in development, so the lower nerve roots elongate within the vertebral canal to reach their passage. For simplicity, only the first sacral nerve root is illustrated.

Dura

Spinal cord

First sacral dorsal root

End of spinal cord

Third month in utero

L1

L3

S1

End of spinal cord

Birth

L1

L3

S1

End of spinal cord

First sacral dorsal root

Adult

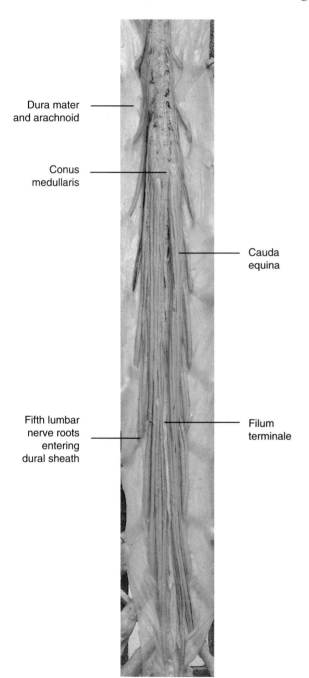

FIGURE 5-6

Dorsal surface of the lower end of the spinal cord and the cauda equina. Because the spinal cord does not grow as long as the vertebral column, the lumbosacral nerve roots extend below the end of the spinal cord, forming the cauda equina. *(From Abrahams PH, Marks SC, et al. (2003). McMinn's color atlas of human anatomy, ed 5, p 109, Philadelphia: Mosby.)*

The anterior part of the forebrain becomes the **telencephalon.** The central cavity enlarges to form the lateral ventricles (Figure 5-8). The telencephalon becomes the **cerebral hemispheres;** the hemispheres expand so extensively that they envelop the diencephalon. The cerebral hemispheres consist of deep nuclei, including the basal ganglia (groups of cell bodies); white matter (containing axons); and the cortex (layers of cell bodies on the surface of the hemispheres). As the hemispheres expand ventrolaterally to form the temporal lobe, they attain a *C* shape. As a result of this growth pattern, certain internal structures, including the caudate nucleus (part of the basal ganglia) and lateral ventricles, also become *C* shaped (Figure 5-9).

Continued Development During Fetal Stage

Lateral areas of the hemispheres do not grow as much as the other areas, with the result that a section of cortex becomes covered by other regions. The covered region is the **insula** (see Atlas A-4), and the edges of the folds that cover the insula meet to form the lateral sulcus. In the mature brain, if the lateral sulcus is pulled open, the insula is revealed. The surfaces of the cerebral and cerebellar hemispheres begin to fold, creating sulci, grooves into the surface, and gyri, elevations of the surface. Table 5-1 summarizes normal brain development.

CELLULAR-LEVEL DEVELOPMENT

The progressive developmental processes of cell proliferation, migration, and growth, extension of axons to target cells, formation of synapses, and myelination of axons are balanced by the regressive processes that extensively remodel the nervous system during development.

Epithelial cells that line the neural tube divide to produce neurons and glia. The neurons migrate to their final location by one of two mechanisms: (1) sending a slender process to the brain surface and then hoisting themselves along the process or (2) climbing along radial glia (long cells that stretch from the center of the brain to the surface) (Chotard and Salecker, 2004). The neurons differentiate appropriately after migrating to their final location. The function of each neuron—visual, auditory, motor, and so on—is not genetically determined. Instead, function depends on the area of the brain where the neuron migrates. Daughter cells of a specific mother cell may assume totally different functions, depending on the location of migration (Gotz, 2003).

How do neurons in one region of the nervous system find the correct target cells in another region? For

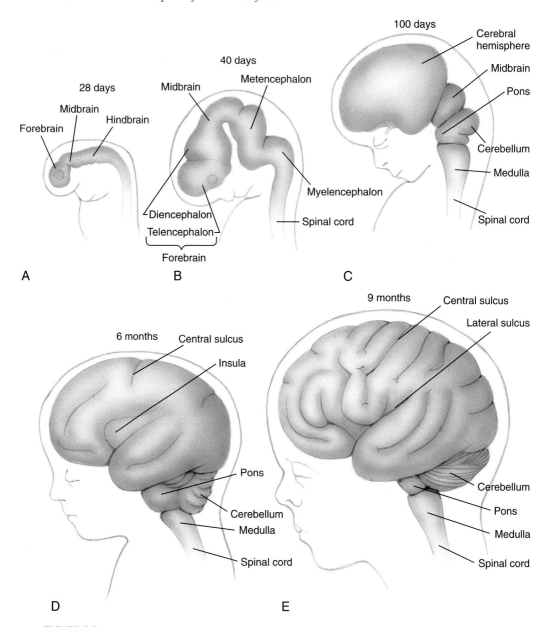

FIGURE 5-7

Brain formation. **A,** Three-enlargement stage. **B,** Five-enlargement stage. **C,** Telencephalon has grown so extensively that the diencephalon is completely covered in a lateral view. **D,** The insula is being covered by continued growth of adjacent areas of the cerebral hemisphere. **E,** Folding of the surface of the cerebral and cerebellar hemispheres continues.

example, how do neurons in the cortex direct their axons down through the brain to synapse with specific neurons in the spinal cord? A process emerges from the neuron cell body. The forward end of the process expands to form a **growth cone** that samples the environment,

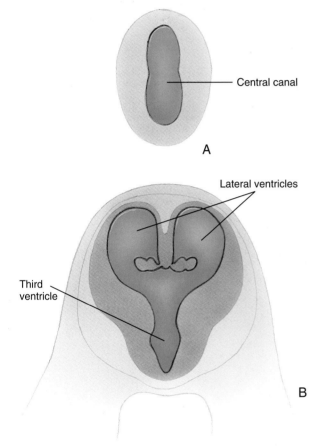

FIGURE 5-8
Formation of ventricles. **A,** Central canal in neural tube. **B,** Coronal section of developing telencephalon.

contacting other cells and chemical cues. The growth cone recoils from some chemicals it encounters and advances into other regions where the chemical attractors are specifically compatible with the growth cone characteristics.

When the growth cone contacts its target cell, synaptic vesicles soon form, and microtubules that formerly ended at the apex of the growth cone project to the presynaptic membrane. With repeated release of neurotransmitter, the adjacent postsynaptic membrane develops a concentration of receptor sites. In early development, many neurons develop that do not survive. **Neuronal death** claims as many as half of the neurons formed during the development of some brain regions. The neurons that die are probably ones that failed to establish the optimal connections with their target cells or were too inactive to maintain their connection. Thus, development is partially dependent on activity. Some neurons that survive retract their axons from certain target cells while leaving other connections intact. For example, in the mature nervous system, a muscle fiber is innervated by only one axon. During development, several axons may innervate a single muscle cell. This polyneuronal innervation is eliminated during development (Martin, 2005). These two regressive processes, neuronal death and **axon retraction,** sculpt the developing nervous system.

Neuronal connections also sculpt the developing musculature. Experiments that change motor neuron connections to a muscle fiber demonstrate that muscle fiber type (fast or slow twitch) is dependent on innervation. **Fast twitch muscle** is converted to slow twitch if innervated by a slow motor neuron, and **slow twitch muscle** can be converted to fast twitch if innervated by a fast motor neuron (Pette, 2001).

Before neurons with long axons become fully functional, their axons must be insulated by a **myelin sheath,** composed of lipid and protein. The process of acquiring a myelin sheath is **myelination.** The process begins in the fourth fetal month; most sheaths are completed by the end of the third year of life. The process occurs at

Table 5-1		SUMMARY OF NORMAL BRAIN DEVELOPMENT		
Hindbrain	→	Metencephalon	→	Pons, upper medulla, cerebellum, fourth ventricle
		Myelencephalon	→	Lower medulla
Midbrain	→	Midbrain	→	Midbrain, cerebral aqueduct
Forebrain	→	Diencephalon	→	Thalamus, hypothalamus, third ventricle
		Telencephalon	→	Cerebral hemispheres, including basal ganglia, cerebral cortex, lateral ventricles

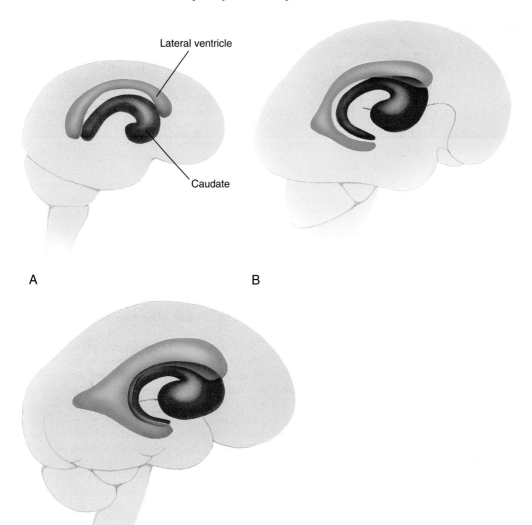

FIGURE 5-9
The growth pattern of the cerebral hemispheres results in a *C* shape of some of the internal structures. The changing shapes of the caudate nucleus and lateral ventricle are shown.

different rates in each system. For instance, the motor roots of the spinal cord are myelinated at about 1 month of age, but tracts sending information from the cortex to activate motor neurons are not completely myelinated, and therefore not fully functional, until a child is approximately 2 years old. Thus, if neurons that project from cerebral cortex to motor neurons were damaged perinatally, motor deficits might not be observed until the child was older. For example, if some of the cortical neurons controlling lower limb movements were damaged at birth, the deficit might not be recognized until the child is more than a year old and has difficulty standing and walking. This is an example of **growing into deficit**: nervous system damage that occurred earlier is not evident until the systems damaged would normally have become functional.

DEVELOPMENTAL DISORDERS: IN UTERO AND PERINATAL DAMAGE OF THE NERVOUS SYSTEM

The central nervous system is most susceptible to major malformations between day 14 and week 20, as the fundamental structures of the central nervous system are forming. After this period, growth and remodeling continue; however, insults cause functional disturbances and/or minor malformations.

Neural Tube Defects

Anencephaly, formation of a rudimentary brainstem without cerebral and cerebellar hemispheres, occurs when the cranial end of the tube remains open and the forebrain does not develop. The skull does not form over the incomplete brain, leaving the malformed brainstem and meninges exposed. Anencephaly can be detected by maternal blood tests, amniotic fluid tests, and ultrasound imaging. The causes include chromosomal abnormalities, maternal nutritional deficiencies, and maternal hyperthermia. Most fetuses with this condition die before birth, and almost none survive more than a week after birth.

Arnold-Chiari malformation is a developmental deformity of the hindbrain. There are two types of Arnold-Chiari malformation. Arnold-Chiari type I is not associated with defects of the lower neural tube and consists of herniation of the cerebellar tonsils through the foramen magnum into the vertebral canal. Both the medulla and pons are small and deformed. Often, people with the Arnold-Chiari I malformation have no symptoms. If symptoms do occur, they begin during adolescence or early adulthood. The most frequent complaints are severe head and neck pain, usually suboccipital. The headaches may be induced by coughing, sneezing, or straining. The deformity may be associated with restriction of cerebrospinal fluid flow, producing hydrocephalus (see Chapter 18). Hydrocephalus is an excessive volume of cerebrospinal fluid (CSF). The pressure exerted by the CSF may interfere with the function of adjacent structures, causing sensory and motor disorders. The malformation of lower cranial nerves and of the cerebellum may result in problems with tongue and facial weakness, decreased hearing, dizziness, weakness of lateral eye movements, and problems with coordination of movement. Visual disturbances include double vision, floaters or flashing lights, loss of vision from part of the visual field, blurred vision, and discomfort in response to light (Milhorat et al., 1999). If the deficits are stable,

no medical treatment is indicated. If the deficits are progressing, surgical removal of the bone immediately surrounding the malformation may be indicated. Abnormalities of the upper cervical cord may cause loss of pain and temperature sensation on the shoulders and lateral upper limbs (see Chapter 12). See Milhorat et al., 1999 for clinical and MRI findings in a large group of people with symptomatic Arnold-Chiari type I.

In Arnold-Chiari type II (Figure 5-10), the signs are present in infancy. Type II consists of malformation of the brainstem and cerebellum leading to extension of the medulla and cerebellum through the foramen magnum. Type II often produces progressive hydrocephalus (blockage of flow of cerebrospinal fluid; see Chapter 18), paralysis of the sternocleidomastoid muscles, deafness, bilateral weakness of lateral eye movements, and facial weakness (Box 5-1). Arnold-Chiari type II is almost always associated with another disorder, the incomplete closure of the neural tube, called meningomyelocele (see below).

Spina bifida is the neural tube defect that results when the inferior neuropore does not close (Figure 5-11). Developing vertebrae do not close around an incomplete neural tube, resulting in a bony defect at the distal end of the tube. Maternal nutritional deficits (eating less than 400 μg of folic acid per day during early pregnancy) are associated with higher incidence of the disorder. The severity of the defect varies; if neural tissue does not

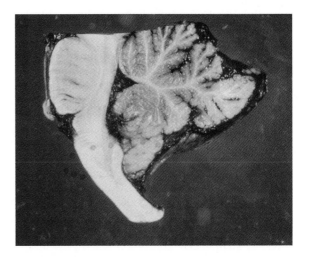

FIGURE 5-10
The Arnold-Chiari malformation consists of malformation of the pons, medulla, and inferior cerebellum. The green dots indicate the level of the foramen magnum. The medulla and inferior cerebellum protrude into the foramen magnum.

BOX 5-1 ARNOLD-CHIARI MALFORMATION

Pathology
Developmental abnormality
Etiology
Unknown
Speed of Onset
Unknown
Signs and Symptoms
Consciousness
Normal
Cognition, Language, and Memory
Normal
Sensory
Headache, usually suboccipital, initiated by or exacerbated by coughing, straining, and sneezing; may have loss of pain and temperature sensation on shoulders and lateral upper limbs if upper central spinal cord is abnormal
Autonomic
Vomiting secondary to hydrocephalus
Motor
Uncoordinated movements; paresis; impaired fine-motor coordination of hands

Cranial Nerves
Vertigo (sensation of spinning); deafness; tongue, facial muscle, and lateral eye movement weakness; difficulty swallowing
Vision
Temporary visual disturbances
Region Affected
Upper spinal cord, brainstem, and cerebellum
Demographics
Prevalence
Only affects developing nervous system
2.4 per 1,000 (Speer et al., 2000)
Incidence
Unknown. In a series of 12,226 MRI reports, 1.0% had 3 mm or greater herniation. Of those patients with 5 mm or more of herniation, 31% did not have Arnold-Chiari—related symptoms at the time of the scan (Elster and Chen, 1992)
Prognosis
Defect is stable; symptoms are stable or progressive

protrude through the bony defect (spina bifida occulta), usually spinal cord function is normal. In spina bifida cystic, the meninges and in some cases the spinal cord protrude through the posterior opening in the vertebrae. The three types of spina bifida cystica, in order of increasing severity, are: meningocele, meningomyelocele, and myeloschisis. **Meningocele** is protrusion of the meninges through the bony defect. In some cases, meningocele may be asymptomatic. In other cases, spinal cord function may be impaired. In **meningomyelocele,** neural tissue with the meninges protrudes outside the body. Meningomyelocele always results in abnormal growth of the spinal cord and some degree of lower-extremity dysfunction; often, bowel and bladder control is impaired (Figure 5-12). No consensus exists on proper medical management of meningomyelocele. **Myeloschisis** is the most severe defect, consisting of a malformed spinal cord open to the surface of the body, which occurs when the neural folds fail to close (Box 5-2).

Tethered Spinal Cord

During development, rarely the end of the spinal cord adheres to the one of the lower vertebra, thus tethering the spinal cord to the bone. As the person grows, the resulting traction on the inferior spinal cord causes: dermatomal and myotomal deficits in the lower limbs, pain the saddle region (part of the body that would contact a horse saddle) and lower limbs, and bowel and bladder dysfunction. Less often, a tethered cord syndrome interferes with movement control signals descending from the brain. If the traction on the spinal cord is mild, signs may only occur when mechanical stress increases and/or the onset of signs may not occur until adolescence or later.

Forebrain Malformation

The prosencephalon normally divides into two cerebral hemispheres. Rarely, this division does not occur, resulting in a single cerebral hemisphere, often associated with facial abnormalities: a single eye (or no eye), a deformed nose, and cleft lip and palate. The defect is called holoprosencephaly. Genetic factors have been implicated in the disorder. The disorder can be identified in utero by genetic tests and by ultrasound.

Exposure to Alcohol or Cocaine in Utero

What are the consequences of maternal substance abuse? Fetal alcohol syndrome (consisting of impairment of the

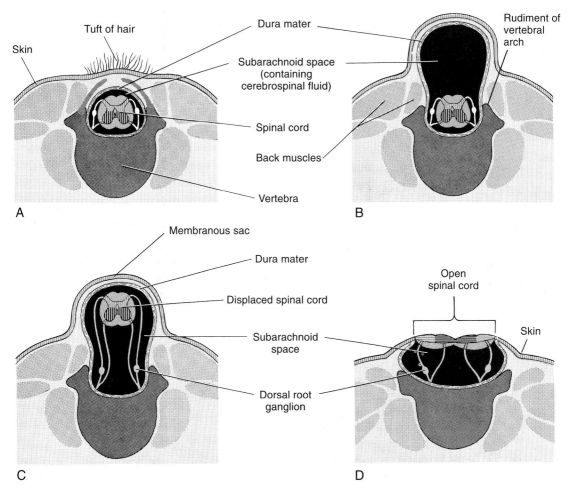

FIGURE 5-11

Various types of spina bifida and the commonly associated malformations of the nervous system. **A,** Spina bifida occulta. About 10% of people have this vertebral defect in L5, S1, or both. Neural function is usually normal. **B,** Spina bifida with meningocele. **C,** Spina bifida with meningomyelocele. **D,** Spina bifida with myeloschisis. The types illustrated in **B** to **D** are often referred to collectively as spina bifida cystica because of the cystlike sac that is associated with them. *(From Moore K L, Persaud, TVN (2003). The developing human, Clinically oriented embryology, p 437. Philadelphia: Saunders.)*

central nervous system, growth deficiencies before and/or after birth, and facial anomalies) and the milder syndrome of alcohol-related birth defects are examples of substance abuse interfering with development during gestation. Both syndromes are due to maternal alcohol intake. Physical characteristics include an abnormally small head, an indistinct philtrum (groove above upper lip), a thin upper lip, and a short vertical space between the open eyelids. Malformation of the cerebellum, cere-

bral nuclei, corpus callosum, neuroglia, and neural tube leads to cognitive, movement, and behavioral problems. Intelligence, memory, language, attention, reaction time, visuospatial abilities, decision making, goal-oriented behavior, fine- and gross-motor skills, and social and adaptive functioning are impaired (Riley and McGee, 2005).

The effects of in utero exposure to cocaine depend on the stage of development. Disturbance of neuronal

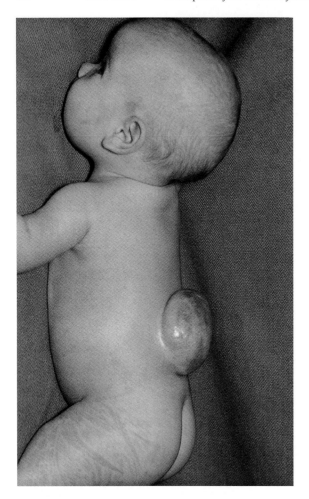

FIGURE 5-12
Meningomyelocele in an infant, resulting in paralysis of the lower limbs. *(From Parkinson D (2003). In Moore KL, Persaud TVN. The developing human: Clinically oriented embryology. Philadelphia: Saunders.)*

BOX 5-2   SPINA BIFIDA CYSTICA

Pathology
  Developmental abnormality
Etiology
  Some cases due to maternal nutritional deficits
Speed of Onset
  Unknown
Signs and Symptoms
  *Signs and symptoms vary, depending on location and
    severity of the malformation*
  Consciousness
  Normal
  Cognition, Language, and Memory
  *Usually normal in meningocele; retardation frequently
    accompanies meningomyelocele and myeloschisis*
  Somatosensation in Lower Limbs
  Meningocele: may be impaired
  Meningomyelocele: impaired or absent
  Myeloschisis: absent
  Autonomic
  *Meningomyelocele/ myeloschisis: lack of bladder and
    bowel control*
  Motor
  *Meningocele and meningomyelocele: paresis of lower
    limbs*
  Myeloschisis: paralysis of the lower limbs
  Cranial Nerves
  Normal
Region Affected
  Inferior spinal cord
Demographics
  Prevalence
  Only affects developing nervous system
  *4 per 10,000 live births (Centers for Disease Control
    and Prevention, 2004)*
Prognosis
  Defect is stable

proliferation is the most frequent consequence of cocaine exposure during neural development, but interference with other neurodevelopmental processes also occurs. Cocaine exposure in utero causes difficulties with attention and impulse control (Frank et al., 2001).

Abnormal Location of Cells

What happens when the process of cell migration goes awry? Cells fail to reach their normal destination. In the cerebral cortex, this results in abnormal gyri, due to abnormal numbers of cells in the cortex, and heterotopia, the displacement of gray matter, commonly into the deep cerebral white matter. Seizures are often associated with heterotopia.

Mental Retardation

Abnormalities of dendritic spines are found in many cases of mental retardation (Halpain et al., 2005, Carlisle and Kennedy, 2005). Dendritic spines are projections from the dendrites, common in cerebral and cerebellar cortex projection neurons, which are the preferential sites of synapses.

Cerebral Palsy

Cerebral palsy is a movement and postural disorder caused by permanent, nonprogressive damage of a developing brain. In premature infants, the brain damage usually occurs postnatally. Cerebral palsy is classified according to the type of motor dysfunction. The most common are as follows:

- Spastic (Figure 5-13)
- Athetoid
- Ataxic
- Mixed

In spastic cerebral palsy, the damaged neurons are adjacent to the ventricles. Muscle shortening in spastic cerebral palsy often results in toe walking and a scissor gait. In scissor gait, one leg swings in front of the other instead of straight forward, producing a crisscross motion of the legs during walking. In athetoid cerebral palsy, the neuronal damage is in the basal ganglia. Athetoid cerebral palsy is characterized by slow, writhing movements of the extremities and/or trunk. In ataxic cerebral palsy, the damage is in the cerebellum. Ataxic cerebral palsy consists of incoordination, weakness, and shaking during voluntary movement. If more than one type of abnormal movement coexist in a person, the disorder is classified as mixed type. Cerebral palsy is also classified according to the area of the body affected: hemiplegia affects both limbs on one side of the body, quadriplegia affects all four limbs equally, and diplegia indicates that the upper limbs are less severely affected than both lower limbs.

According to a consensus statement by the International Cerebral Palsy Task Force, the understanding of the etiology of cerebral palsy has changed with recent scientific advances (Task Force on Neonatal Encephalopathy and Cerebral Palsy, 2003). Traditionally, cerebral palsy was believed to result from difficulties during the birth process. However, epidemiologic studies indicate that most cases of cerebral palsy result from events before the onset of labor, or in the newborn after delivery. The causes of cerebral palsy include abnormal development in utero, metabolic abnormalities, disorders of the immune system, coagulation disorders, infections, trauma, and hypoxia. Only 10 percent of cases involve hypoxia, and even these may have originated before birth rather than during labor or delivery. Further, only 20 percent of cases of spastic quadriplegic cerebral palsy are associated with difficulties during labor or delivery, and athetoid cerebral palsy is infrequently associated with difficult labor or delivery. Hemiplegic cerebral palsy, spastic diplegia, and ataxic cerebral palsy are not associated with difficult labor or delivery (Task Force on Neonatal Encephalopathy and Cerebral Palsy, 2003). Of 52 premature infants whose umbilical cord gases were analyzed, only three had oxygen deprivation (Holcroft 2003). Neuroimaging (Figure 5-14) reveals the variety of pathologies that cause cerebral palsy (Lin, 2003).

Cognitive, somatosensory, visual, auditory, and speech deficits are frequently associated with cerebral palsy. **Growing into deficit** is common in cerebral palsy. Although the nervous system damage is not progressive, new problems appear as the child reaches each age for normal developmental milestones: that is, when the child reaches the age when most children walk, the inability of the child with cerebral palsy to walk independently at the usual age becomes apparent (Box 5-3).

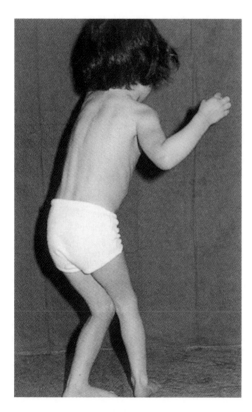

FIGURE 5-13
Child with spastic cerebral palsy. Note the flexion contractures of the right arm and both knees, and internal rotation of the left lower limb. *(From Forbes CD, Jackson WF (1997). Color atlas and text of clinical medicine, 2nd edition. London: Mosby.)*

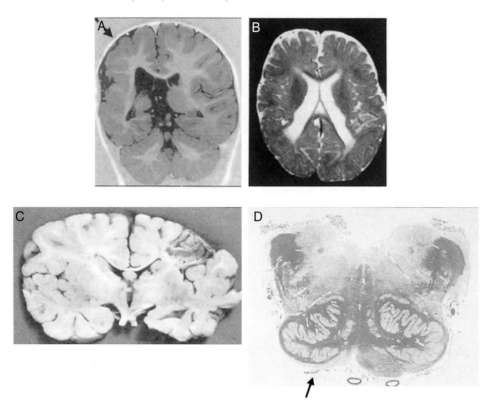

FIGURE 5-14

Neuroimaging of cerebral palsy pathology. A variety of developmental brain abnormalities can cause cerebral palsy. **A,** Patient has hemiplegic cerebral palsy and began walking at the typical age for hemiplegia (18-22 months). The arrow indicates abnormal right hemisphere development, with many small folds of the cerebral cortex. **B,** Horizontal section showing enlarged ventricles secondary to death of the adjacent white matter. The corpus callosum is extremely thin. The clinical presentation is spastic diplegia. (Compare this section with Atlas Figure 17.) **C,** Coronal section through the hemispheres of an 8-month-old infant showing a cortical-subcortical infarct and a small internal capsule. **D,** Transverse section of the medulla from the same infant as **C.** The arrow points to the absence of the medullary pyramid caused by loss of corticospinal tract axons. *(From Lin JP (2003). The cerebral palsies: A physiological approach. Journal of Neurology, Neurosurgery, and Psychiatry, Mar(74), Suppl 1, i27. Reproduced with permission from the BMJ Publishing Group.)*

Even at birth, the infant brain is far from its adult form. Thus, damage during development has different consequences than injury of a fully developed brain.

Developmental Coordination Disorder

Children with normal intellect, without traumatic brain injury or cerebral palsy or other neurologic problems, who lack the motor coordination to perform tasks that most children their age are able to perform, are considered to have developmental coordination disorder (DCD). The condition is usually permanent, continuing into adulthood (Missiuna et al., 2003). These children lag behind their peers in dressing, using utensils, handwriting, and/or athletics. Currently a variety of standards and tests are used to diagnose DCD. Slowed movement time is the single characteristic that reliably differentiates children with DCD from those without the disorder (Missiuna et al, 2003). Hadders-Algra (2003) postulates two forms of DCD, a milder form associated with a moderate risk for learning and behavioral problems and a more severe form that is strongly correlated with attention and learning difficulties.

BOX 5-3 CEREBRAL PALSY

Pathology
Developmental abnormality

Etiology
Abnormal development in utero, metabolic abnormalities, disorders of the immune system, coagulation disorders, infections, trauma, or, rarely, hypoxia. The central nervous system damage occurs before the second birthday.

Speed of Onset
Unknown

Signs and Symptoms
Consciousness
Normal
Cognition, Language, and Memory
Frequently associated with mental retardation and language deficits, although some people with cerebral palsy have above normal intelligence and memory
Sensory
May be normal or impaired
Autonomic
Usually normal

Motor
Spastic type: paresis, muscle shortening, increased muscle resistance to movements
Athetoid type: slow, writhing movements
Ataxic type: incoordination, weakness, shaking during voluntary movements
Cranial Nerves
Not directly affected; however, due to abnormal neural input, the output of motor cranial nerves is impaired

Region Affected
Brain; some abnormalities in spinal cord

Demographics
Only developing nervous system affected

Prevalence
2-3 per 100,000 live births per year (Topp et al., 2001)

Prognosis
The abnormality is stable, but functional limitations may only become obvious as the person grows

---

Autism

Autism indicates a range of abnormal behaviors including impaired social skills. Three disorders comprise the autism spectrum: autistic disorder, Asperger's disorder, and pervasive developmental disorder not otherwise specified. People with autistic disorder engage in repetitive behaviors, have limited interests, appear to lack imagination, and are uninterested in interacting with other people. Some people with autistic disorder are mute, others can speak but do not initiate conversation. People with Asperger's disorder speak and have normal or better intelligence. However, their limited social skills, their narrow range of interests, and their repetitive and frequently obsessive behaviors interfere with school, work, and/or social life. Pervasive developmental disorder not otherwise specified indicates atypical behaviors similar to autism or Asperger's yet not meeting all of the criteria for a diagnosis of autism or Asperger's.

Summary of Developmental Disorders

Major deformities of the nervous system occur before week 20 because the gross structure is developing during this time. After 20 weeks of normal development, damage to the immature nervous system causes minor malformations and/or disorders of function. Table 5-2 summarizes

the processes of development and the consequences of damage during the peak time of each process.

NERVOUS SYSTEM CHANGES DURING INFANCY

Many animal experiments have investigated the consequences of sensory deprivation on the infant nervous system. These experiments indicate that **critical periods** during development are crucial for normal outcomes. Critical periods are the time when neuronal projections compete for synaptic sites; thus, the nervous system optimizes neural connections during the critical period.

One example of changing the functional properties of the nervous system was demonstrated in infant monkeys. Monkeys raised with one eyelid sutured shut from birth to 6 months were permanently unable to use vision from that eye, even after the sutures were removed. Recordings indicated that the retinal cells responded normally to light and the information was relayed correctly to the visual cortex, but the visual cortex did not respond to the information (Hubel and Wiesel, 1977). Occluding vision in one eye in an adult monkey for an equivalent period of time had relatively little effect on vision once

Table 5-2   SUMMARY OF DEVELOPMENTAL PROCESSES AND THE CONSEQUENCES OF INTERFERENCE WITH SPECIFIC DEVELOPMENTAL PROCESSES

Developmental Process	Peak Time of Occurrence	Disorders Secondary to Interference with Developmental Process
Neural tube formation	In utero weeks 3-4	Anencephaly, Arnold-Chiari malformation, spina bifida occulta, meningocele, meningomyelocele, myeloschisis
Formation of brain enlargements	In utero months 2-3	Holoprosencephaly
Cellular proliferation	In utero months 3-4	Fetal alcohol syndrome, cocaine-affected nervous system
Neuronal migration	In utero months 3-5	Heterotopia, seizures
Organization (differentiation, growth of axons and dendrites, synapse formation, selective neuron death, retraction of axons)	In utero month 5 to early childhood	Mental retardation, trisomy 21, cerebral palsy
Myelination	Birth to 3 years after birth	Unknown

visual input was restored. Thus the critical period for tuning the visual cortex is during the first 6 months of development in monkeys.

Critical periods are times when axons are competing for synaptic sites. Normal function of neural systems is dependent on appropriate experience during the critical period.

Changes analogous to the functional disuse in the monkeys explain the decrease in ability to learn a new language after early childhood. At birth, the cerebral cortex hearing areas are sensitive to all speech sounds. By 6 months, nonnative phoneme distinctions (like "r" from "l" in Japanese) have been eliminated from the auditory perceptual map (Kuhl, 2000). Therefore older children and adults have great difficulty hearing, as well as pronouncing, nonnative phonemes. However, in normal 9-month-old American infants, five hours of exposure to Chinese speakers during a 1-month period preserves the ability to distinguish among Mandarin speech sounds (Kuhl et al., 2003). This indicates that critical periods do not end abruptly, however the neuroplasticity is optimal for learning a specific task during a particular critical period. Learning a new language is possible during adulthood, but the adult will probably never sound like a native speaker. During critical periods, experience regulates the competition between inputs, affecting the electrical activity, molecular mechanisms, and inhibitory

action that produce permanent structural changes in the nervous system (Hensch, 2004).

Interruption of development during a critical period may explain some of the differences in outcome between perinatal and adult brain injury. In people with cerebral palsy, damage to fibers descending from the cerebrum to the spinal cord during fetal development or at birth may eliminate some competition for synaptic sites during a critical period, causing persistence of inappropriate connections and abnormal development of spinal motor centers (Eyre et al., 2001). These inappropriate connections and developmental deficits in spinal motor centers, in addition to the deficiency of descending control, result in abnormal movement. The adult with brain damage loses descending control, but because development is complete, inappropriate connections or abnormal spinal motor circuits do not compound the dysfunction.

SUMMARY

During the preembryonic stage, three layers of cells form: ectoderm, mesoderm, and endoderm. During the embryonic stage, the nervous system develops from ectoderm. During the fetal stage, the nervous system continues to develop and myelination of axons begins.

Somites appear during the embryonic stage. Parts of the somite are the myotome, destined to become skeletal muscle, and the dermatome, destined to become dermis. The association of a single spinal nerve with a specific spinal nerve leads to the formation of a myotome: a group of skeletal muscles innervated by a spinal nerve. Similarly the skin innervated by a single spinal nerve is a dermatome.

The inferior part of the neural tube becomes the spinal cord. The superior part of the neural tube differentiates to become the medulla, pons, midbrain, cerebellum, diencephalons, and cerebral hemispheres. During development neural cells multiply, migrate, and grow. Neurons extend their axons to target cells, synapses form, and axons are myelinated. Neuronal death, claiming up to half of the neurons that develop in some

brain regions, and axon retraction prune the developing nervous system. Damage to the developing nervous system may cause deficits that are not recognized until later in development, when the system that was damaged would become functional. This delayed loss of function is called *growing into deficit.*

Malformations of the central nervous system include anencephaly, Arnold-Chiari malformation, spina bifida, and forebrain malformation. Other disorders that occur during development include tethered spinal cord, mental retardation, cerebral palsy, developmental coordination disorder, and autism.

CLINICAL NOTES

Case 1

A 2-year-old boy has no reaction to any stimulation below the level of the umbilicus. He does not voluntarily move his lower limbs, his lower limb muscles are atrophied, and he has no voluntary control of his bladder or bowels. His mother reports that he had surgery on his back 2 days after birth. Above the level of the umbilicus, sensation and movement are within normal limits.

Questions
1. The nervous system deficits affect which of the systems: sensory, autonomic, or motor?
2. The lesion is in what region of the nervous system: the peripheral, spinal, brainstem, or cerebral region?

Case 2

Mary, a 2-year-old girl, is not yet attempting to stand. She has been slower than her peers in developing motor skills. The mother reports that Mary's lower body always felt "stiff as a board" when she was lifted and held. The mother also reports difficulty dressing and changing Mary when Mary is agitated, because the girl's legs strongly adduct. Mary is not yet toilet trained. Even when Mary is calm, her muscles are more stiff than normal. The therapist finds that Mary's somatosensation is intact throughout the body, her upper body has normal strength for her age, and the muscles of her lower limbs are weak.

Questions
1. The nervous system deficits affect which of the systems: sensory, autonomic, or motor?
2. The lesion is in what region of the nervous system?
3. What is the most likely diagnosis?

REVIEW QUESTIONS

1. When do the organs form during development?
2. List the steps in formation of the neural tube.
3. What is a myotome?
4. Describe the changes in the neural tube that lead to formation of the brain.

5. List the progressive processes of cellular-level development.
6. Describe the regressive processes of cellular-level development.
7. Explain the concept of "growing into deficit."

8. Describe the anatomical deficit in each of the following: anencephaly, Arnold-Chiari malformation, and the four types of spina bifida.

9. What are the differences between Arnold-Chiari type I and type II?

10. About half of the cases of severe mental retardation are associated with what developmental defect?

11. What is cerebral palsy? List the major types of cerebral palsy. What causes cerebral palsy?

12. What are critical periods?

References

Carlisle HJ, Kennedy MB (2005). Spine architecture and synaptic plasticity. Trends in Neurosciences, 28(4), 182-187.

Centers for Disease Control and Prevention. (2004). Spina bifida and anencephaly before and after folic acid mandate—United States, 1995-1996 and 1999-2000. Morbidity and Mortality Weekly Report, 53(17), 362-365.

Chotard C, Salecker I (2004). Neurons and glia: Team players in axon guidance. Trends in Neurosciences, 27(11), 655-661.

Elster AD, Chen MUM (1992). Chiari I malformations: Clinical and radiologic reappraisal. Radiology, 183, 347-353.

Eyre JA, Taylor JP, et al. (2001). Evidence of activity-dependent withdrawal of corticospinal projections during human development. Neurology, 57(9), 1543-1554.

Frank DA, Augustyn M, et al. (2001). Growth, development, and behavior in early childhood following prenatal cocaine exposure: A systematic review. Journal of the American Medical Association, 285(12), 1613-1625.

Gotz M (2003). Glial cells generate neurons—master control within CNS regions: Developmental perspectives on neural stem cells. Neuroscientist, 9(5), 379-397.

Hadders-Algra M (2003). Developmental coordination disorder: Is clumsy motor behavior caused by a lesion of the brain at early age? Neural Plasticity, 10(1-2), 39-50.

Halpain S, Spencer K, et al. (2005). Dynamics and pathology of dendritic spines. Progress in Brain Research, 147, 29-37.

Hensch TK (2004). Critical period regulation. Annual Review of Neuroscience, 27, 549-579.

Holcroft CJ, Blakemore, KJ, et al. (2003). Association of prematurity and neonatal infection with neurologic morbidity in very low birth weight infants. Obstetrics and Gynecology, 101(6), 1249-1253.

Hubel DH, Wiesel TN (1977). Ferrier Lecture: Functional architecture of macaque monkey visual cortex. Proceedings of the Royal Society of London, Series B: Biological Sciences, 198, 1-59.

Kuhl PK (2000). A new view of language acquisition. Proceedings of the National Academy of Sciences of the United States of America, 97(22), 11850-11857.

Kuhl PK, Tsao FM, et al. (2003). Foreign-language experience in infancy: Effects of short-term exposure and social interaction on phonetic learning. Proceedings of the National Academy of Sciences of the United States of America, 100(15), 9096-9101.

Lin JP (2003). The cerebral palsies: A physiological approach. Journal of Neurology, Neurosurgery, and Psychiatry, Mar(74), Suppl 1, i23-i29.

Martin JH (2005). The corticospinal system: From development to motor control. Neuroscientist, 11(2), 161-173.

Milhorat TH, Chou MW, et al. (1999). Chiari I malformation redefined: Clinical and radiographic findings for 364 symptomatic patients. Neurosurgery, 44(5), 1005-1017.

Missiuna CA, Rivard L, et al. (2003). Early identification and risk management of children with developmental coordination disorder. Pediatric Physical Therapy, 15: 32-38.

Pette D (2001). Historical Perspectives: Plasticity of mammalian skeletal muscle. Journal of Applied Physiology, 90(3), 1119-1124.

Riley EP, McGee CL (2005). Fetal alcohol spectrum disorders: An overview with emphasis on changes in brain and behavior. Experimental Biology and Medicine (Maywood, NJ), 230(6), 357-365.

Speer MC, George TM, et al. (2000). A genetic hypothesis for Chiari I malformation with or without syringomyelia. Neurosurgery Focus, 8(3), 1-4.

Task Force on Neonatal Encephalopathy and Cerebral Palsy (2003). Neonatal Encephalopathy and Cerebral Palsy: Defining the Pathogenesis and Pathophysiology. American College of Obstetricians and Gynecologists (in collaboration with the American Academy of Pediatrics). Washington, DC.

Topp M, Uldall P, et al. (2001). Cerebral palsy births in eastern Denmark, 1987-90: Implications for neonatal care. Paediatric and Perinatal Epidemiology, 15(3), 271-277.

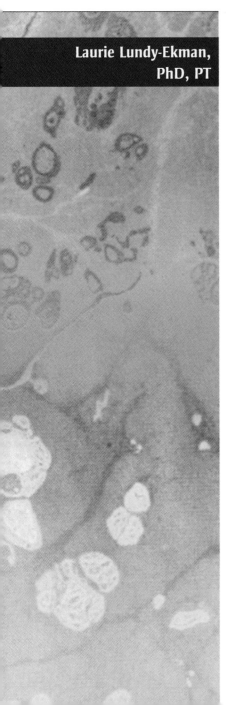

6

Somatosensory System

Laurie Lundy-Ekman, PhD, PT

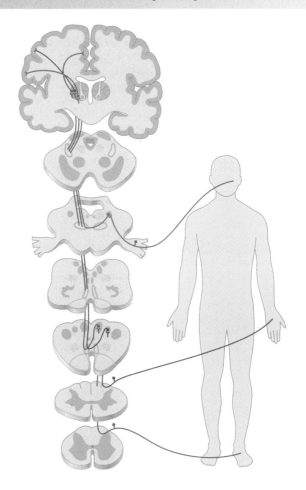

INTRODUCTION

Sensation allows us to investigate the world, move accurately, and avoid or minimize injuries. This chapter discusses somatosensation, the sensory information from the skin and musculoskeletal systems. The special senses of smell, vision, hearing, and equilibrium and the sensations from the viscera are discussed in subsequent chapters.

Sensory information from the skin is called *superficial* or *cutaneous.* Superficial sensory information includes touch, pain, and temperature. Touch sensation includes superficial pressure and vibration. In contrast, sensory information from the musculoskeletal system includes proprioception and pain. Proprioception provides information regarding stretch of muscles, tension on tendons, position of joints, and deep vibration. Proprioception includes both static joint position sense and kinesthetic sense, sensory information about movement.

All pathways that convey somatosensory information share similar anatomic arrangements. Receptors in the periphery encode the mechanical, chemical, or thermal stimulation received into receptor potentials (see Chapter 2). If the receptor potentials exceed the threshold of the trigger zone, an action potential is generated in a peripheral axon. The action potential is conducted along a peripheral axon, to a soma in a dorsal root ganglion, then along the proximal axon into the spinal cord. Within the spinal cord, the information ascends via axons in the white matter to various regions of the brain. The information is transmitted through a series of neurons and synapses.

> Information in the somatosensory system proceeds from the receptor through a series of neurons to the brain.

The diameter of the axons, the degree of axonal myelination, and the number of synapses in the pathway determine how quickly the information is processed. Much somatosensory information is not consciously perceived but is processed at the spinal level in local neural circuits or by the cerebellum to adjust movements and posture. The distinction between sensory information (nerve impulses generated from the original stimuli) and sensation (awareness of stimuli from the senses) should be noted throughout this chapter. Perception, the interpretation of sensation into meaningful forms, occurs in the cerebrum. Perception is an active process of interaction between the brain and the environment. To perceive involves acting on the environment—moving the eyes, moving the head, or touching objects—in addition to interpreting sensation.

PERIPHERAL SOMATOSENSORY NEURONS

Sensory Receptors

Sensory receptors are located at the distal ends of peripheral neurons. Each type of receptor is specialized, responding only to a specific type of stimulus, the adequate stimulus, under normal conditions. Based on the characteristics of the adequate stimulus, somatosensory receptors are classified as follows:

- Mechanoreceptors, responding to mechanical deformation of the receptor by touch, pressure, stretch, or vibration
- Chemoreceptors, responding to substances released by cells, including damaged cells following injury or infection
- Thermoreceptors, responding to heating or cooling

A subset of each type of somatosensory receptors is classified as nociceptors. Nociceptors are preferentially sensitive to stimuli that damage or threaten to damage tissue. Stimulation of nociceptors results in a sensation of pain. For example, when pressure mechanoreceptors are stimulated by stubbing a toe, the sensation experienced is pain rather than pressure. The receptors that encode the pain message are nociceptors, not the lower-threshold pressure receptors that convey information experienced as nonpainful pressure. Information from each of these types of receptors may reach awareness, but much of the information is used to make automatic adjustments and is selectively prevented from reaching consciousness by descending and local inhibitory connections.

Receptors that respond as long as a stimulus is maintained are called **tonic receptors.** For example, some stretch receptors in muscles, the tonic stretch receptors, fire the entire time a muscle is stretched. Receptors that adapt to a constant stimulus and stop responding are called **phasic receptors.** Muscles also contain phasic stretch receptors, which respond only briefly to a quick stretch. Another example of phasic receptors is the brief response of pressure receptors after putting on a wrist watch.

Somatosensory Peripheral Neurons

The cell bodies of most peripheral sensory neurons are located outside the spinal cord in the dorsal root ganglia or outside the brain in cranial nerve ganglia. Peripheral sensory neurons have two axons:

- Distal axons conduct messages from receptor to the cell body.
- Proximal axons project from the cell body into the spinal cord or brainstem.

Some proximal axons that enter the spinal cord extend as far as the medulla before synapsing.

Peripheral axons, also called *afferents,* are classified according to axon diameter. The most commonly used system for classifying peripheral sensory axons designates the axons in order of declining diameter: Ia, Ib, II, or $A\beta$, $A\delta$, C (Figure 6-1). The diameter of an axon is functionally important: larger-diameter axons

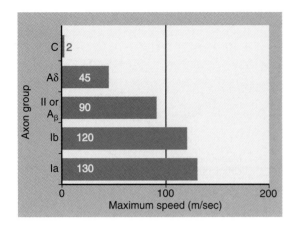

FIGURE 6-1
Conduction velocity of sensory axons.

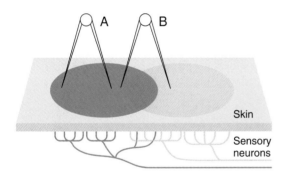

FIGURE 6-2
Receptive fields. The areas of skin innervated by each neuron are indicated on the surface of the skin. **A,** The caliper points touching the skin would be perceived as one point because both points are within the receptive field of one neuron. **B,** The caliper points would be perceived as two points because the points are contacting the receptive field of two neurons.

transmit information faster than smaller-diameter axons. The faster conduction occurs because resistance to current flow is lower in large-diameter axons and because the large-diameter axons are myelinated, allowing saltatory conduction of the action potential (see Chapter 2).

Cutaneous Innervation

The area of skin innervated by a single afferent neuron is called the *receptive field* for that neuron (Figure 6-2). Receptive fields tend to be smaller distally and larger proximally. Distal regions of the body also have a greater

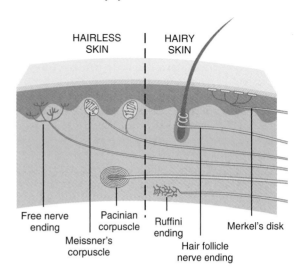

FIGURE 6-3
Cutaneous receptors.

density of receptors than the proximal areas. The combination of smaller receptive fields and greater density of receptors distally enables us to distinguish between two closely applied stimuli on a fingertip, while the same stimuli cannot be distinguished on the trunk.

Sensations from skin include the following:
- Touch
- Pain
- Temperature

Touch information is categorized as fine touch or coarse touch. **Fine touch** includes a variety of receptors (Figure 6-3) and subsensations. The superficial fine touch receptors have small receptive fields, allowing resolution of closely spaced stimuli. The superficial fine touch receptors are Meissner's corpuscles, sensitive to light touch and vibration, and Merkel's disks, sensitive to pressure. Hair follicle receptors, sensitive to displacement of a hair, also have small receptive fields. The subcutaneous fine touch receptors have large receptive fields, providing less localization and discrimination of stimuli. Subcutaneous fine touch receptors are pacinian corpuscles, responsive to touch and vibration, and Ruffini's corpuscles, sensitive to stretch of the skin. All of the fine touch receptors transmit information on $A\beta$ afferents.

Coarse touch is mediated by free endings throughout the skin (see Figure 6-3). These free nerve endings provide information perceived as crudely localized touch or pressure and the sensations of tickle and itch.

Nociceptors are free nerve endings, responsive to stimuli that damage or threaten tissue. Nociceptors provide information perceived as pain. **Thermal receptors,** also free nerve endings, respond to either warmth or cold within the temperature range that does not damage tissue. The information from all of the free nerve endings is conveyed by Aβ and C afferents. Although the various tactile receptors respond to different types of stimuli, natural stimuli typically activate several types of tactile receptors (Vallbo, 1995).

As noted in Chapter 5, the area of skin innervated by axons from cell bodies in a single dorsal root is a dermatome. In the brachial and lumbosacral plexus, sensory axons innervating specific parts of the limbs are separated from other axons arising in the same dorsal root and regrouped to form peripheral nerves. Thus peripheral nerves, such as the median nerve, have a different pattern of innervation than the dermatomes. Dermatomes and the cutaneous distribution of peripheral nerves in the posteromedial upper limb are illustrated in Figure 6-4. Dermatomes and the cutaneous distribution of peripheral nerves throughout the body are illustrated in Figure 6-5.

Although cutaneous receptors are not proprioceptors, the information from cutaneous receptors contributes to our sense of joint position and movement. The contribution of cutaneous receptors is primarily kinesthetic, responding to stretching of or increasing pressure on the skin. However, Ruffini's corpuscles discharge in response to static joint angles.

> Cutaneous receptors respond to touch, pressure, vibration, stretch, noxious stimuli, and temperature.

Musculoskeletal Innervation

Muscle Spindle

The sensory organ in muscle is the **muscle spindle,** consisting of muscle fibers, sensory endings, and motor endings (Figure 6-6). The sensory endings of the spindle respond to stretch, that is, changes in muscle length and the velocity of length change. Quick and tonic stretch of the spindle is registered by type Ia afferents. Tonic stretch of a muscle is monitored by type II afferents. Small efferent fibers to the ends of muscle spindle fibers adjust spindle fiber stretch so the spindle is responsive through the physiologic range of muscle lengths.

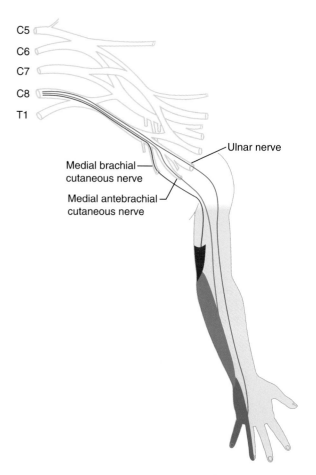

FIGURE 6-4

Cutaneous innervation of the posteromedial upper limb. All of the afferent axons enter the spinal cord through the C8 dorsal root, so the dermatome innervating the posteromedial upper limb is C8. However, three peripheral nerves distribute the axons of sensory neurons to the periphery. Thus, afferents from the posteromedial hand travel in the ulnar nerve, afferents from the posteromedial forearm travel in the medial antebrachial cutaneous nerve, and afferents from the upper posteromedial arm travel in the medial brachial cutaneous nerve. Therefore, a complete lesion of the ulnar nerve superior to the wrist would deprive the area colored blue of sensation, yet the green and red regions would still be innervated. A C8 dorsal root lesion would deprive the entire posteromedial upper limb of sensation.

Intrafusal and Extrafusal Fibers

Muscle spindles are embedded in skeletal muscle. Because the spindle is fusiform (tapered at the ends), the specialized muscle fibers inside the spindle are designated **intrafusal fibers;** the ordinary

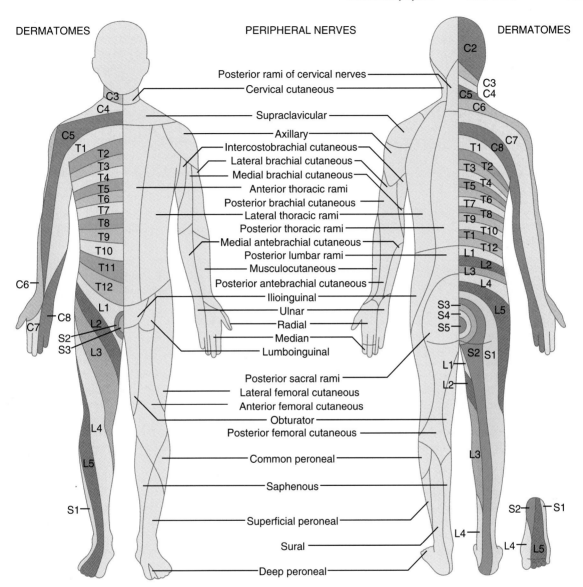

FIGURE 6-5
Dermatomes and cutaneous distribution of peripheral nerves.

skeletal muscle fibers outside the spindle are **extrafusal.** The ends of the intrafusal fibers connect to extrafusal fibers, so stretching the muscle stretches the intrafusal fibers. To serve the dual purposes of providing information about the length and rate of change in length of the muscle, the spindle has two types of muscle fibers, two types of sensory afferents, and two types of efferents.

Intrafusal fibers are contractile only at their ends; the central region cannot contract. The arrangement of nuclei in the central region characterizes the two types of intrafusal fibers:

- **Nuclear bag fibers** have a clump of nuclei in the central region.
- **Nuclear chain fibers** have nuclei arranged single file.

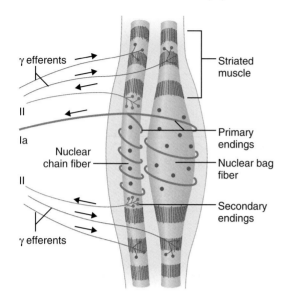

FIGURE 6-6

Simplified illustration of a muscle spindle. The intrafusal muscle fibers are nuclear chain and nuclear bag fibers. Stretch of the central region of intrafusal fibers is sensed by primary and secondary endings. The sensory information is conveyed to the central nervous system by type Ia and type II afferents. Efferent control of intrafusal fibers is via gamma motor neurons.

For spindles to monitor muscle length and rate of change in length, two different sensory endings are required:

- **Primary endings** of type Ia neurons wrap around the central region of each intrafusal fiber.
- **Secondary endings** of type II afferents end mainly on nuclear chain fibers adjacent to the primary endings.

Because of their appearance, primary endings are also known as *annulospiral endings,* and secondary endings are called *flower-spray endings.* The discharge of primary endings is both phasic and tonic. The phasic discharge is maximal during quick stretch and fades quickly, as when a tendon is tapped with a reflex hammer. The tonic discharge is sustained during constant stretch; the rate of firing is proportional to the stretch of spindle fibers. Secondary endings respond only tonically.

If a muscle is passively stretched, the muscle spindles respond to the stretch (Figure 6-7, *A*). If the ends of intrafusal fibers were not contractile, the sensory endings would register change only when the muscle was fully elongated; if the muscle were contracted even slightly, the spindle would be slack, rendering the sensory

endings insensitive to stretch (Figure 6-7, *B*). To maintain sensitivity of the spindle throughout the normal range of muscle lengths, **gamma motor neurons** fire, causing the ends of the intrafusal fibers to contract. Contracting the ends of the intrafusal fibers stretches the central region, thus maintaining sensory activity from the spindle (Figure 6-7, *C*). Gamma efferent control is dual, with **gamma dynamic axons** ending on nuclear bag fibers to adjust the sensitivity of primary afferents and **gamma static axons** innervating both types of intrafusal fibers to tune the sensitivity of both primary and secondary afferents (Taylor et al., 2004).

> Muscle length is signaled by type Ia and II afferents, reflecting stretch of the central region of both types of intrafusal fibers. Spindle sensitivity to changes in length is adjusted by gamma static efferents. Velocity of change in muscle length is signaled only by type Ia afferents, with information mainly from nuclear bag fibers whose sensitivity is adjusted by gamma dynamic efferents.

Golgi Tendon Organs

Tension in tendons is relayed from Golgi tendon organs, encapsulated nerve endings woven among the collagen strands of the tendon near the musculotendinous junction (Figure 6-8, *left*). Golgi tendon organs are sensitive to very slight changes (<1 g) in the tension on a tendon and respond to tension exerted both by active contraction and by passive stretch of muscle (Chalmers, 2004). Information is transmitted from Golgi tendon organs into the spinal cord by type Ib afferents.

Joint Receptors

Joint receptors respond to mechanical deformation of the capsule and ligaments (Figure 6-8, *right*). Ruffini's endings in the joint capsule signal the extremes of joint range and respond more to passive than to active movement. Paciniform corpuscles respond to movement, but not when joint position is constant. Ligament receptors are similar to Golgi tendon organs and signal tension. Free nerve endings are most often stimulated by inflammation. The afferents associated with the joint receptors are as follows:

- Ligament receptors—type Ib
- Ruffini's and paciniform endings—type II
- Free nerve endings—types Aδ and C.

Fully normal proprioception requires muscle spindles, joint receptors, and cutaneous mechanoreceptors.

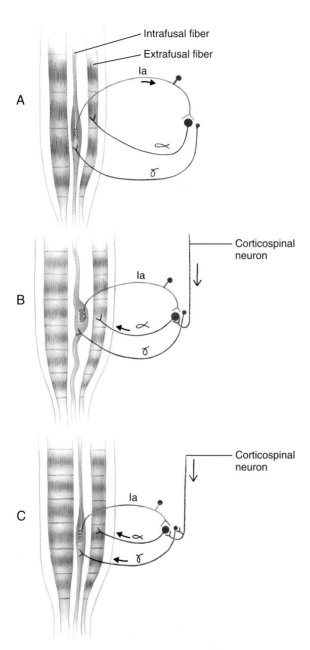

Intrafusal fiber

Extrafusal fiber

Ia

A

B

Corticospinal neuron

Ia

α

γ

C

Corticospinal neuron

Ia

α

γ

FIGURE 6-7

A, During passive stretch, spindles are elongated as the muscle is stretched. This stretch activates the spindle sensory receptors. The arrow indicates action potentials transmitted by the type Ia afferent. **B,** Excitation of the alpha motor neuron via the corticospinal neuron results in contraction of the extrafusal muscle fibers. If the gamma motor neurons do not fire when the alpha motor neurons to the extrafusal muscles fire, the intrafusal central region will be relaxed and the afferent neurons inactive. This does not occur in a normal neuromuscular system. **C,** Normally, during active muscle contraction, alpha and gamma motor neurons are simultaneously active. The firing of gamma motor neurons causes the ends of intrafusal fibers to contract, thus maintaining the stretch on the intrafusal central region and preserving the ability of the sensory endings to indicate stretch.

Muscle spindles respond to quick and to prolonged stretch of the muscle. Tendon organs signal the force generated by muscle contraction or by passive stretch of the tendon. Joint receptors respond to mechanical deformation of joint capsules and ligaments.

Summary: Function of Different-Diameter Axons

Large-diameter afferents transmit information from specialized receptors in muscles, tendons, and joints. Medium-sized afferents transmit information from joint capsules, muscle spindles, and cutaneous touch, stretch, and pressure receptors. The smallest-diameter afferents convey crude touch, nociceptive, and temperature information from both the musculoskeletal system and the skin. Table 6-1 summarizes the axon types, associated receptors, and adequate stimuli for the somatosensory system. Two systems are used to classify somatosensory axons: Roman numerals for proprioceptive axons, and letters for all others.

PATHWAYS TO THE BRAIN

Three types of pathways bring sensory information to the brain (Table 6-2):
- Conscious relay pathways
- Divergent pathways
- Unconscious relay pathways

An important distinction among the types of pathways is the fidelity of information conveyed. Pathways

This redundancy probably reflects the importance of proprioception to the control of movement. People with total hip joint replacements retain good proprioception, despite the loss of joint proprioceptors (Nallegowda et al., 2003).

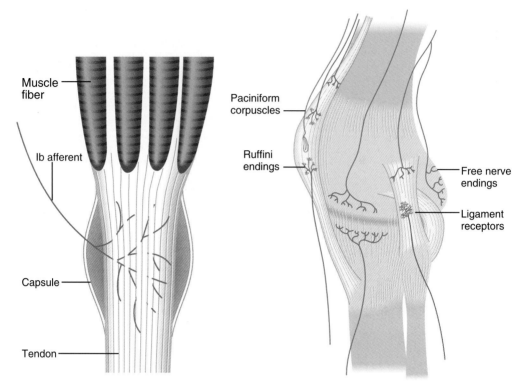

FIGURE 6-8
Left, Golgi tendon organ. *Right,* Joint receptors.

that transmit signals with high fidelity provide accurate details regarding the location of the stimulation. For example, high-fidelity signals from the fingertips allow people to recognize two points separated by as little as 1.6 mm as being distinct points and to identify precisely where on the fingertip the stimulation occurred. The ability to identify the location of stimulation is achieved by the anatomic arrangement of axons in the pathways. In high-fidelity pathways, a somatotopic arrangement of information is created. **Somatotopic** refers to information arranged similarly to the anatomical organization of the body. To create somatotopic arrangement, axons from one part of the body are close to axons carrying signals from adjacent parts of the body and are segregated from axons carrying information from distant parts of the body. For example, axons carrying information from the thumb are near axons carrying information from the index finger and relatively distant from axons carrying information from the toes.

In describing pathways in the nervous system, only the neurons with long axons that connect distant regions of the nervous system are counted. These neurons with long axons are called *projection neurons.* The convention for numbering or naming only the projection neurons omits the small, integrative interneurons interposed between the projection neurons. Thus, a three-neuron pathway means three projection neurons, but a number of interneurons may also be linked in the pathway.

Within the central nervous system, a bundle of axons with the same origin and a common termination is called a **tract.** Somatosensory pathways are often named for the origin and termination of the tract that contains the second neuron in the series. The second neuron in the spinothalamic pathway originates in the spinal cord and terminates in the thalamus. Thus, the second neuron in the pathway travels in the **spinothalamic tract,** and the tract lends its name to the entire pathway. The pathway includes the neuron that brings the information into the

Table 6-1 AXON CLASSIFICATIONS, ASSOCIATED RECEPTORS, AND ADEQUATE STIMULI FOR THE SOMATOSENSORY SYSTEM									
Axon Size*	Proprioception			Cutaneous and Subcutaneous Touch and Pressure			Pain and Temperature		
	Roman Numeral Classification	Receptors	Stimulus	Letter Classification	Receptors	Stimulus	Letter Classification	Receptors	Stimulus
Large myelinated	Ia	Muscle spindles	Muscle stretch	—			—		
	Ib	Golgi tendon organs	Tendon tension	—			—		
		Ligament receptors	Ligament tension						
Medium myelinated	II	Muscle spindles	Muscle stretch	Aβ	Meissner's	Touch, vibration	—		
					Pacinian	Touch, vibration			
		Paciniform & Ruffini's type receptors in joint capsules	Joint movement		Ruffini's	Skin stretch			
					Merkel's	Pressure			
					Hair follicle	Pressure			
Small myelinated							Aδ	Free nerve ending	Tissue damage, temperature, coarse touch
Small unmyelinated							C	Free nerve ending	Tissue damage, temperature, itch, tickle

*The axon correlates with speed of conduction; thus, the large, myelinated fibers conduct fastest and the unmyelinated fibers have the slowest conduction speeds.

Table 6-2   SOMATOSENSORY PATHWAYS

Type	Information Conveyed	Anatomic Name	Termination
Conscious relay	Discriminative touch and conscious proprioception	Dorsal column/medial lemniscus	Primary sensory area cerebral cortex
	Discriminative pain and temperature	Spinothalamic	Primary sensory area cerebral cortex
Divergent	Slow, aching pain	Spinomesencephalic	Midbrain
		Spinoreticular	Reticular formation
		Spinolimbic	Amygdala, basal ganglia, many areas of cerebral cortex
Unconscious relay	Movement-related information	Spinocerebellar	Cerebellum

central nervous system, the neuron in the spinothalamic tract, and the neuron from the thalamus to the cerebral cortex.

The first type of pathways, **conscious relay pathways,** bring information about location and type of stimulation to the cerebral cortex. The information in conscious relay pathways is transmitted with high fidelity, thus providing accurate details regarding the stimulus and its location. Because the information in these pathways allows us to make fine distinctions about stimuli, the term *discriminative* is used to describe the sensations conveyed in conscious relay pathways. Discriminative touch and proprioceptive information ascends ipsilaterally in the posterior spinal cord. Discriminative pain and temperature information crosses the midline soon after entering the cord and then ascends contralaterally.

The second type of pathways, **divergent pathways,** transmit information to many locations in the brainstem and cerebrum and use pathways with varying numbers of neurons. The sensory information is used at both conscious and unconscious levels. Aching pain is a form of sensation that is transmitted via divergent pathways in the central nervous system.

The third type of pathways, **unconscious relay pathways,** bring unconscious proprioceptive and other movement-related information to the cerebellum. This information plays an essential role in automatic adjustments of our movements and posture.

> Conscious relay pathways convey high-fidelity, somatotopically arranged information to the cerebral cortex. Divergent pathways convey information that is not somatotopically organized to many areas of the brain. Unconscious relay pathways convey movement-related information to the cerebellum.

CONSCIOUS RELAY PATHWAYS TO CEREBRAL CORTEX

All four types of somatosensation reach conscious awareness:
- Touch
- Proprioception
- Pain
- Temperature

The pathways involve three projection neurons. The pathways to consciousness travel upward in the spinal cord via two routes:
- Dorsal columns
- Anterolateral tracts

The routes in the spinal cord are composed of white matter, because myelin promotes rapid conduction along the axons. The dorsal columns carry sensory information about discriminative touch and conscious proprioception; discriminative pain and temperature information travels in the anterolateral tracts. To be aware of sensory information, the information must reach the thalamus, where crude awareness is possible (Van der Werf et al., 2002). For discriminative perception, stimuli localized with fine resolution, information must be processed by the cerebral cortex.

If peripheral afferent information is absent, awareness of body parts can be lost. Oliver Sacks, a neurologist, recounts his strange experience of believing that he had lost his leg following severe damage to several nerves in a climbing accident. The complete loss of sensation from his leg led to a lack of awareness of the limb. Although he was not paralyzed, he was unable to voluntarily take a step until his physical therapist moved his leg passively, giving him the concept of how to move the injured leg (Sacks, 1984).

Discriminative Touch and Conscious Proprioception

Discriminative touch includes localization of touch and vibration and the ability to discriminate between two closely spaced points touching the skin. **Conscious proprioception** is the awareness of the movements and relative position of body parts. The integration of touch and proprioceptive information in the cerebral cortex allows identification of an object by touch and pressure information. **Stereognosis** is the ability to use touch and proprioceptive information to identify an object; for example, a key in the hand can be identified without vision. The information conveyed in this pathway is important for recognizing objects by touch, controlling fine movements, and making movements smooth.

The pathway for discriminative touch and conscious proprioception uses a three-neuron relay (Figures 6-9 and 6-10):

- The primary, or first-order, neuron conveys information from the receptors to the medulla.
- The secondary, or second-order, neuron conveys information from the medulla to the thalamus.
- The tertiary, or third-order, neuron conveys information from the thalamus to the cerebral cortex.

Dorsal Column/Medial Lemniscus System

Stimulation of receptors at the distal end of the primary neuron is conveyed to the cell body in the dorsal root ganglion. The primary neuron's proximal axon enters the spinal cord via the dorsal root, then ascends in the ipsilateral dorsal column. Axons from the lower limb occupy the more medial section of the dorsal column, called the **fasciculus gracilis**. Axons from the upper limb occupy the lateral section of the dorsal column, called the **fasciculus cuneatus**. This pattern occurs because nerve fibers entering the dorsal column from higher segments are added laterally to the fibers already in the dorsal column from lower segments.

The axons that ascend in the fasciculus gracilis synapse with second-order neurons in the **nucleus gracilis** of the medulla. The axons in the fasciculus cuneatus synapse with second-order neurons in the **nucleus cuneatus** of the medulla. Thus, in a tall person a primary neuron could be 6 feet long, extending from a toe to the medulla.

Throughout the spinal cord, primary neurons of the discriminative touch/conscious proprioception pathway have many collateral branches entering the gray matter. Some collaterals contribute to motor control, some influence activity in neurons in other sensory systems, and others influence autonomic regulation.

Cell bodies of the second-order neurons are located in the nucleus gracilis or cuneatus. Axons from the second-order neurons cross the midline as the internal arcuate fibers, then ascend to the thalamus as the **medial lemniscus**. The second-order neurons end in an area of the thalamus named for its location, the **ventral posterolateral (VPL) nucleus**.

Third-order neurons connect the thalamus to the sensory cortex. The axons form part of the thalamocortical radiations, fibers connecting the thalamus to the cerebral cortex. Thalamocortical axons travel through the internal capsule.

Discriminative Touch Information From the Face

Sensory innervation for the face is supplied by the three divisions of the **trigeminal nerve** (see Figure 6-9) (see Chapter 13 for more details on the trigeminal nerve). Some of the neurons in the trigeminal nerve are the first-order neurons for discriminative touch information from the face. Their cell bodies are in the trigeminal ganglion, and the proximal axons end in the **trigeminal main sensory nucleus**. Second-order neuron cell bodies are located in the trigeminal main sensory nucleus, and the axons cross the midline in the pons and end in the **ventral posteromedial (VPM) nucleus** of the thalamus. Third-order axons continue to the cerebral cortex. Details regarding sensation from the face are presented in Chapter 13. The effects of lesions in the discriminative touch/conscious proprioception pathways are illustrated in Figure 6-11.

Somatotopic Arrangement of Information

Although the axons in the dorsal column are arranged segmentally as they enter the dorsal columns, the axons are rearranged into a somatotopic organization as they ascend. The somatotopic arrangement is maintained throughout the second- and third-order neurons, so that the area of cerebral cortex devoted to discriminative somatosensation, the **primary sensory (primary somatosensory) cortex,** receives somatotopically organized information. The primary sensory cortex is located in the gyrus posterior to the central sulcus, that is, the postcentral gyrus.

The size of the area of primary sensory cortex devoted to a specific part of the body is represented by the **homunculus** surrounding the cortex in Figure 6-12. The homunculus is a map, developed by recording the responses of awake individuals during surgery. Small areas of the cerebral cortex are electrically stimulated, and the people report what they feel. When the sensory cortex is stimulated, people report feeling sensations that

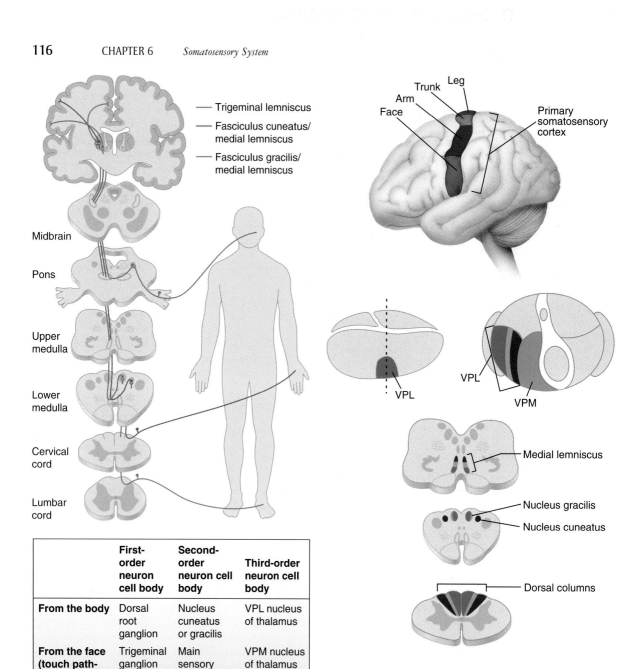

Trigeminal lemniscus

Fasciculus cuneatus/
medial lemniscus

Fasciculus gracilis/
medial lemniscus

Midbrain

Pons

Upper
medulla

Lower
medulla

Cervical
cord

Lumbar
cord

Leg

Trunk

Arm

Face

Primary
somatosensory
cortex

VPL

VPL

VPM

Medial lemniscus

Nucleus gracilis

Nucleus cuneatus

Dorsal columns

	First-order neuron cell body	Second-order neuron cell body	Third-order neuron cell body
From the body	Dorsal root ganglion	Nucleus cuneatus or gracilis	VPL nucleus of thalamus
From the face (touch pathway only)	Trigeminal ganglion	Main sensory nucleus of trigeminal nerve	VPM nucleus of thalamus

FIGURE 6-9

Discriminative touch and conscious proprioceptive information pathways. *Left,* A coronal section of the cerebrum, shown above horizontal sections of the brainstem and spinal cord. *Right,* The distribution of information from the face, arm, trunk, and leg. At top right, a lateral view of the cerebrum is shown. Below the cerebrum are lateral and coronal views of the thalamus. The lateral view of the thalamus shows the location of the VPL (ventroposterolateral nucleus). The dotted line indicates the plane of the coronal section of the thalamus. The coronal section of the thalamus reveals the VPM (ventroposteromedial nucleus). The medulla and the spinal cord are shown in horizontal section on the right. Color coding is indicated at top right.

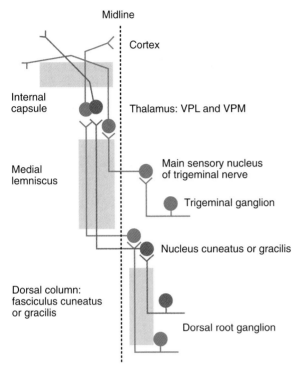

Midline

Cortex

Internal
capsule

Thalamus: VPL and VPM

Medial
lemniscus

Main sensory nucleus
of trigeminal nerve

Trigeminal ganglion

Nucleus cuneatus or gracilis

Dorsal column:
fasciculus cuneatus
or gracilis

Dorsal root ganglion

FIGURE 6-10
Schematic diagram of the discriminative touch and conscious
proprioceptive pathways. Blocks of color indicate groups of
axons, as labeled on the left side. Compare with Figure 6-9.

seem to originate from the surface of the body. For
example, stimulation of the medial postcentral gyrus
elicits sensations that seem to originate in the contralateral lower limb. Another method of testing is to stimulate
areas on the body and record from the cerebral cortex. For
example, touching a fingertip activates neurons in the
superolateral postcentral gyrus. The homunculus illustrates the proportions and arrangement of cortical areas
that contain representations of the surface of the body.
The fingers and lips of the homunculus are much larger
than their proportion of the body would indicate. The
large cortical representation corresponds to the relatively
high density of receptors in these regions and the associated degree of fine-motor control.

Somatosensory Areas of the Cerebral Cortex

The primary sensory cortex discriminates the size,
texture, or shape of objects. Another area of the cerebral
cortex, the **somatosensory association area,** analyzes
the information from the primary sensory area and the

thalamus and provides stereognosis and memory of the
tactile and spatial environment.

> Sensory information essential for identifying objects by pal-
> pation, distinguishing between closely spaced stimuli, and
> controlling fine movement and smoothness of movement
> travels in the dorsal columns, then in the medial lemniscus,
> to the primary sensory cortex. Tactile information from the
> face travels in the trigeminal nerve, then to the thalamus, then
> to the sensory cortex.

Discriminative Pain and Temperature, Coarse Touch

Anterolateral Columns

The anterolateral white matter in the spinal cord contains
axons that transmit discriminative information about
pain and temperature and also about coarse touch. Coarse
touch conveys less information than the dorsal column/
medial lemniscus system, and thus coarse touch cannot
be tested independently when discriminative touch is
intact. Coarse touch is involved with pleasant touch and
skin-to-skin contacts (Wessberg et al., 2003).

Several parallel tracts ascend in the anterolateral
spinal cord. One of the tracts, the **spinothalamic tract,**
is part of a three-neuron conscious relay pathway called
the spinothalamic pathway. Phylogenically older, slower
conducting divergent pathways include the spinolimbic,
spinoreticular, and spinomesencephalic.

Temperature Sensation

Warmth and cold are detected by specialized free nerve
endings of small myelinated and unmyelinated neurons.
$A\delta$ fibers carry impulses produced by cooling, and C
fibers carry information regarding heat. In the spinothalamic pathway, the proximal axon of the first-order
neuron branches to spread vertically to adjacent segments
of the spinal cord, then synapses with the second-order
neurons in the dorsal horn. The second-order axons cross
the midline and then ascend contralaterally to project to
the VPL nucleus of the thalamus. The axons of third-
order neurons project from the thalamus to the sensory
cortex.

Pain

Pain is an extremely complex phenomenon. Persistent pain affects emotional, autonomic, and social

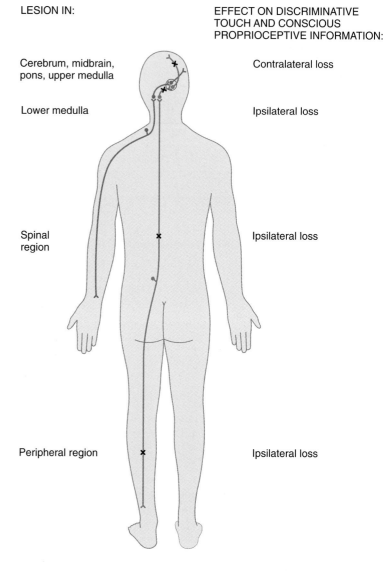

LESION IN:

Cerebrum, midbrain, pons, upper medulla

Lower medulla

Spinal region

Peripheral region

EFFECT ON DISCRIMINATIVE TOUCH AND CONSCIOUS PROPRIOCEPTIVE INFORMATION:

Contralateral loss

Ipsilateral loss

Ipsilateral loss

Ipsilateral loss

FIGURE 6-11

The effect of lesion location on transmission of discriminative touch and conscious proprioceptive information.

functioning. Pain is composed of both protective sensation and the emotional response to this sensation. The term *nociceptive* describes receptors or neurons that receive or transmit information about stimuli that damage or threaten to damage tissue. Nociceptive information travels in several different pathways.

A common patient report of back pain secondary to lifting a heavy object consists of an initial immediate sharp sensation that indicates the location of the injury; this is called fast or **spinothalamic pain.** Fast pain is often followed by a dull, throbbing ache that is not well localized. The latter pain is called slow or **spinolim-**

bic pain (also known as paleospinothalamic pain). Both types of pain occur in acute pain. Impulses conveying both fast and slow pain travel together in the antero-lateral section of the spinal cord, and then their paths become separate in the brain (Figure 6-13). Fast pain uses a conscious relay pathway and therefore is discussed in this section; slow pain is discussed in a subsequent section on divergent pathways.

Fast, Localized Pain: Lateral Pain System

Fast pain uses a three-neuron system (Abelson, 2005; see Figures 6-13, *A* and 6-14):

divisions of the spinal cord gray matter. The neurotransmitter released is glutamate.

The cell body of the second-order neuron is in lamina I, II, or V of the dorsal horn. The axon of the second-order neuron crosses the midline in the anterior white commissure, then ascends to the thalamus via the **spinothalamic tract.** Most spinothalamic tract neurons end in the VPL nucleus of the thalamus. The name *lateral pain system* derives from this termination of the tract in the lateral thalamus. The third-order neurons arise in the VPL nucleus and project to the primary and secondary sensory cortex. A lesion in the VPL nucleus interrupts the pathway to the cortex, causing inability to localize painful stimuli despite feeling the affective (emotional) aspects of pain.

> Information that enables people to localize noxious sensations and to consciously distinguish between warmth and cold travels to the cerebral cortex via spinothalamic pathways.

Comparison of the Dorsal Column/ Medial Lemniscus and Spinothalamic Systems

The spinothalamic and the dorsal column systems are anatomically similar, consisting of three neuron relay pathways. Unlike the dorsal columns, containing axons of primary neurons and ascending ipsilaterally, the ascending axons in the anterolateral columns are second-order neurons, and most ascend contralaterally. In both the dorsal column paths and the spinothalamic tract, the second-order axon crosses the midline. However, in the dorsal column path the crossing occurs in the medulla, while in the spinothalamic pathway the crossing occurs in the spinal cord before the axon ascends. The second neuron in both dorsal column and spinothalamic paths ends in the VPL nucleus of the thalamus. In both pathways, third-order neurons project from the thalamus to the primary sensory cortex, where the information can be localized.

In contrast to the discriminative touch and conscious proprioceptive information traveling in the dorsal columns, the anterolateral white matter contains axons transmitting information about pain, temperature, and coarse touch. However, functions of the dorsal and anterolateral columns are not rigidly segregated; information about nondiscriminative (coarse) touch travels in the anterolateral system, and some pain and temperature information ascends in the dorsal columns (Palecek et al., 2003).

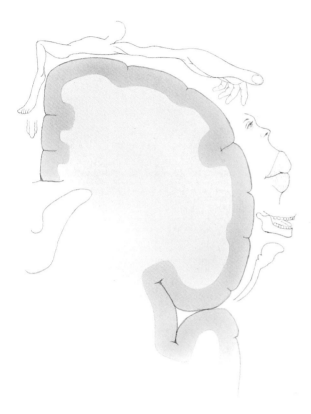

FIGURE 6-12
Primary sensory cortex. The areas of cortex responding to somatosensory stimulation are indicated by the homunculus.

- The first-order neuron brings information into the dorsal horn of the spinal cord.
- The axon of the second-order neuron crosses the midline and projects from the spinal cord to the thalamus.
- The third-order neuron projects from the thalamus to the cerebral cortex.

The primary neuron in the fast pain pathway is a small myelinated Aδ fiber. Aδ fibers transmit information from free nerve endings in the periphery to the spinal cord. The endings respond to noxious mechanical stimulation (high-threshold mechanoreceptor afferents) or to mechanical or thermal stimulation (mechanothermal afferents). The peripheral axon brings an impulse to the cell body in the dorsal root ganglion. The central axon enters the cord, then branches to several levels in the **dorsolateral tract** (Lissauer's marginal zone) before entering and terminating in lamina I, II, and/or V of the dorsal horn (Figure 6-15). *Lamina* are histologic

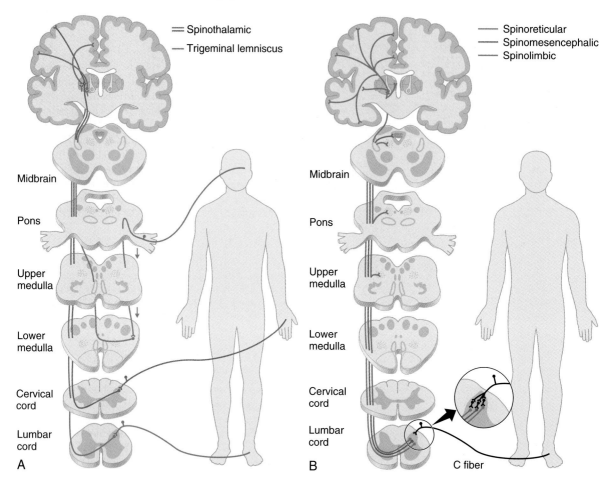

Spinothalamic
Trigeminal lemniscus

Spinoreticular
Spinomesencephalic
Spinolimbic

Midbrain

Pons

Upper
medulla

Lower
medulla

Cervical
cord

Lumbar
cord

A

Midbrain

Pons

Upper
medulla

Lower
medulla

Cervical
cord

Lumbar
cord

B

C fiber

	First-order neuron cell body	Second-order neuron cell body	Third-order neuron cell body
From the body	Dorsal root ganglion	Dorsal horn of spinal cord	VPL nucleus of thalamus
From the face	Trigeminal ganglion	Spinal nucleus of trigeminal nerve	VPM nucleus of thalamus

FIGURE 6-13

Pathways for nociceptive information. **A,** Sharp, localized pain travels in a three-neuron pathway. All sections are horizontal except the coronal section of the cerebrum at the top. The box below **A** lists the location of the cell bodies in this pathway. **B,** Slowly conducted nociceptive information from the body travels in the spinoreticular, spinomesencephalic, and spinolimbic tracts. Efferents from the thalamic nuclei project to widespread areas of the cerebral cortex and to the striatum.

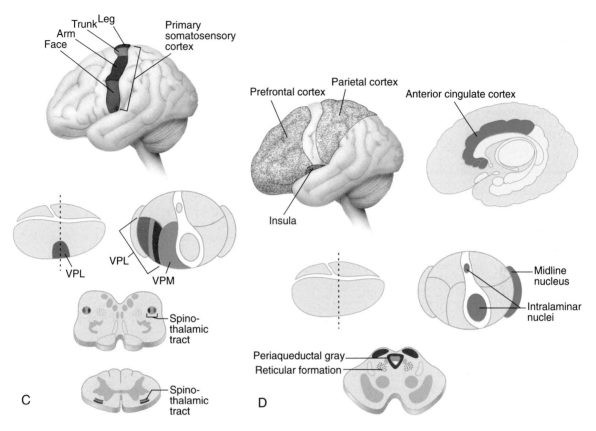

FIGURE 6-13, cont'd
C, The distribution of fast pain information from the face, arm, trunk, and leg. *Top,* A lateral view of
the cerebrum. Below the cerebrum is a lateral view of the thalamus, showing the location of the VPL
(ventroposterolateral nucleus). The dotted line indicates the plane of the coronal section of the thalamus.
The coronal section of the thalamus reveals the VPM (ventroposteromedial nucleus). The upper medulla
and cervical spinal cord are shown in horizontal sections. **D,** Sites of synapse and termination for slowly
conducted nociceptive information. Lateral and midsagittal views of the cerebrum, lateral and coronal views
of the thalamus, and a horizontal view of the midbrain are illustrated. Stippled blue in the cerebral cortex
and blue in the anterior cingulate cortex indicate the termination of the spinolimbic pathway. The blue
areas in the midline and intralaminar nuclei of the thalamus indicate sites of synapse of the spinolimbic
tract. Red indicates the termination of the spinomesencephalic tract in the superior colliculus and the
periaqueductal gray. Green indicates the termination of the spinoreticular tract in the midbrain reticular
formation.

Fast Pain Information From the Face

Afferent information interpreted as fast pain from the face
travels in the **trigeminal nerve.** Fibers in this pathway
enter the pons, then travel down into the medulla and
upper cervical cord in the descending tract of the trigeminal nerve before synapsing in the spinal nucleus
of the trigeminal nerve (see Figure 6-13, *A*). Second-
order fibers cross the midline and ascend to the VPM

nucleus of the thalamus. Third-order neurons project to
the cerebral cortex. Figure 6-16 summarizes the effect
of various lesions on transmission of fast pain and discriminative temperature information. Lesions that interrupt the pathways conveying nociceptive information
produce analgesia. **Analgesia** is the absence of pain in
response to stimuli that would normally be painful. The
term **crossed analgesia** indicates that a single lesion can
cause pain sensation to be lost on the side of the face

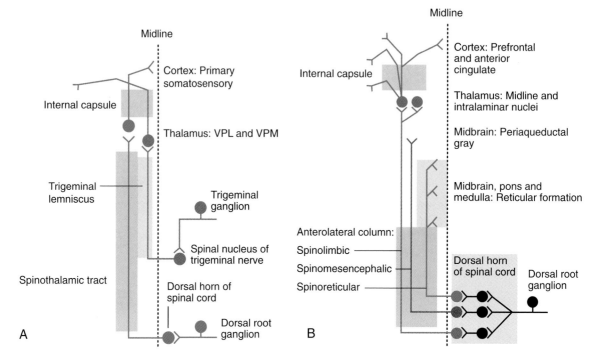

FIGURE 6-14

A, Schematic diagram of the fast nociceptive pathways: the spinothalamic and trigeminothalamic systems. (Compare with Figure 6-13, *A.*) **B,** Schematic diagram of the slow nociceptive pathways. (Compare with Figure 6-13, *B.*)

ipsilateral to the lesion and on the opposite side of the body (contralateral to the lesion).

Fast versus Slow Pain

When fast pain information reaches the somatosensory cortex, a person is consciously aware of sharp pain in a specific location. If tissue damage has occurred, the fast pain is followed by slow, aching pain. The onset of slow pain is later than fast pain because the impulses travel on smaller, unmyelinated axons. The difference in conduction velocities results in a C fiber's requiring about 0.5 second to transmit information to the spinal cord, while Aδ fibers require as little as 0.03 second.

DIVERGENT PATHWAYS

Medial Pain System

Many responses to nociception depend on a divergent ascending network of neurons called the *medial pain*

system. Activity of the medial pain system elicits affective, motivational, withdrawal, arousal, and autonomic responses. Most of the medial pain system projection neurons synapse in medial locations in the central nervous system (Brooks and Tracey, 2005; Almeida et al., 2004). The medial pain system uses several pathways with variable numbers of projection neurons, not a three-neuron pathway like fast pain. The information from the medial pain system is not somatotopically organized, so slow pain cannot be precisely localized.

First Neuron

The first neuron is a small, unmyelinated C fiber. The receptors are free nerve endings, sensitive to noxious heat, chemical, or mechanical stimulation (polymodal afferents). High-threshold C fiber endings become **sensitized** with repeated stimulation. Thus, after injury, these neurons can be fired with less stimulation than is usually required. Tissue damage also results in release of chemicals—histamine, prostaglandins, and others—that

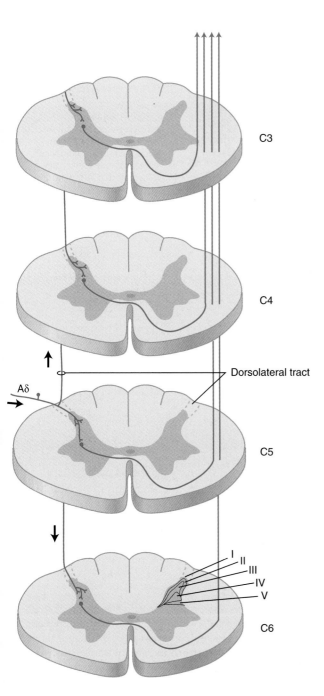

FIGURE 6-15
Four segments of the cervical spinal cord are illustrated. The numbered areas are the lamina in the dorsal horn. The dorsolateral tract conveys nociceptive information from one dermatome to adjacent levels of the spinal cord. Thus nociceptive information that enters the C5 cervical segment is conveyed to the C3, C4, and C6 segments via the dorsolateral tract. After synapse in the dorsal horn, the information crosses the midline in the tract neurons and ascends to the brain.

C3

C4

Dorsolateral tract

Aδ

C5

I
II
III
IV
V

C6

branches in the dorsolateral tract, and then synapses with interneurons in lamina I, II, and/or V of the dorsal horn. Lamina I is also called the *marginal layer,* and lamina II is also called the *substantia gelatinosa.* The neurotransmitter is **substance P.** Axons from the interneurons synapse with cell bodies of ascending projection neurons in laminae V to VIII.

Ascending Projection Neurons

The axons of ascending projection neurons reach the midbrain, reticular formation, and limbic areas via three tracts in the anterolateral spinal cord (see Figure 6-13, *B*):

- Spinomesencephalic
- Spinoreticular
- Spinolimbic

These three tracts are parallel ascending tracts. Of these tracts, only information in the spinolimbic tract is perceived as pain. Information in the other tracts serves arousal, motivational, and reflexive functions and/or activates descending projections that control the flow of sensory information (Brooks and Tracey, 2005).

Spinomesencephalic Tract This tract carries nociceptive information to two areas in the midbrain, the superior colliculus and to an area surrounding the cerebral aqueduct, the periaqueductal gray (Almeida et al., 2004). The spinomesencephalic tract is involved in turning the eyes and head toward the source of noxious input and in activating descending tracts that control pain. The periaqueductal gray is part of the descending pain control system (discussed in Chapter 7).

Spinoreticular Tract. These ascending neurons synapse in the brainstem reticular formation. The **reticular formation** is a neural network in the brainstem that includes the reticular nuclei and their connections. Arousal, attention, and sleep/waking cycles are modulated by the reticular formation. Thus severe pain commands attention and interferes with sleep. From the reticular formation, axons project to the midline and intralaminar nuclei of the thalamus.

sensitize pain receptors. For example, a gentle touch on sunburned skin can be painful.

Information from free nerve endings in the periphery travels in peripheral axons to the cell body in the dorsal root ganglion. The central axon enters the cord,

LESION IN:

Cerebrum, midbrain, upper pons

Lower pons, medulla

Spinal region

Peripheral region

EFFECT ON FAST PAIN AND TEMPERATURE SENSATION:

Entirely contralateral loss

Crossed analgesia, involving contralateral body and ipsilateral face, occurs when trigeminal and spinothalamic axons are interrupted. (Contralateral loss from the face if the trigeminal lemniscus axons are interrupted).

Loss of pain and temperature sensation from contralateral body one or two levels below lesion

Ipsilateral loss

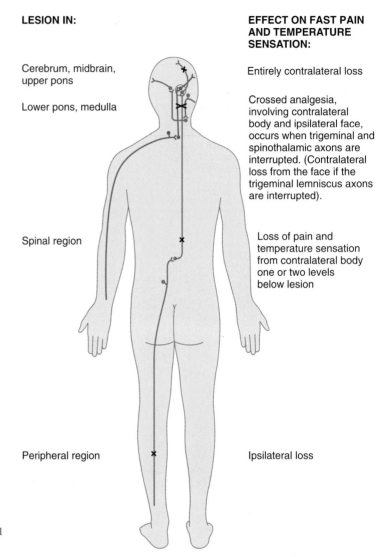

FIGURE 6-16
Effects of lesion location on the transmission of fast pain and discriminative temperature information. Crossed analgesia occurs with lesions in the lower pons and medulla because axons conveying fast pain information from the face (compare with Figure 6-11) descend ipsilaterally near the spinothalamic tract carrying pain information from the contralateral body.

Spinolimbic Tract. Axons of the spinolimbic tract transmit slow pain information to the medial and intralaminar nuclei in the thalamus. The neurons located in these thalamic nuclei have large receptive fields, sometimes from the entire body. Their axons project to the anterior cingulate cortex and the posterior insula (Price, 2002). Direct electrical stimulation of the posterior insula evokes pain in humans (Ostrowsky et al, 2002). When the anterior cingulate gyrus is removed as a treatment for chronic pain, the pain intensity is unchanged but patients report that the pain no longer bothers them (Lagraize et al., 2005). The ability to localize painful stimuli remains intact, but the affective dimension is eliminated. Eventually spinolimbic information projects to areas of the cerebral cortex involved with emotions, sensory integration, personality, and movement, as well as to the basal ganglia, the amygdala, and the hypothalamus. Activity in the spinoreticular and spinolimbic tracts results in arousal, withdrawal, autonomic, and affective responses to pain (Almeida et al., 2004; Price 2002).

If someone breaks a bone in the hand, the divergent pain pathways provide information that contributes to automatically directing the eyes and head toward the injury, automatically moving the hand away from the cause of injury, becoming pale, and feeling faint, nauseous, and emotionally distressed. The information provided by the divergent pathways is not well localized so that the entire hand seems to hurt.

> The slow pain pathways provide information that produces automatic movements and autonomic and emotional responses to noxious stimuli.

Trigeminoreticulolimbic Pathway

Slow pain information from the face proceeds in the **trigeminoreticulolimbic pathway** (van Bijsterveld, et al, 2003). The first neurons are C fibers in the trigeminal nerve, which synapse in the reticular formation with ascending projection neurons. These neurons project to the intralaminar nuclei. The projections from the intralaminar nuclei are similar to the spinolimbic pathway, with projections to many areas of the cerebral cortex.

Although an intact sensory cortex is required for the localization of pain, crude awareness of slow pain can be achieved in many cortical areas and possibly in the thalamus and basal ganglia.

Temperature Information

Temperature information is also transmitted in phylogenetically older pathways to the reticular formation, to the nonspecific nuclei of the thalamus, to subcortical nuclei, and to the hypothalamus. This temperature information that does not reach conscious awareness contributes to arousal, provides gross localization, and contributes to autonomic regulation.

UNCONSCIOUS RELAY TRACTS TO THE CEREBELLUM

Information from proprioceptors and information about activity in spinal interneurons are transmitted to the cerebellum via the **spinocerebellar tracts.** Information relayed by these tracts is critical for adjusting movements. For example, one of the complications of diabetes is dysfunction of proprioceptive neurons. If, as often occurs in diabetes, proprioceptive information from the ankle is decreased, sway during stance increases. Inadequate proprioceptive input can also cause ataxia (uncoordinated movement) because the loss of sensory feedback disrupts movement control (see Chapter 10 regarding types of ataxia).

Two of the spinocerebellar pathways deliver information from receptors in muscles, tendons, and joints from peripheral neurons to the cerebellum. These two neuron pathways relay high-fidelity, somatotopically arranged information to the cerebellar cortex. In contrast, two other spinocerebellar tracts are specialized to provide feedback to the cerebellum about the activity in spinal interneurons and in the descending motor tracts. These one-neuron internal feedback tracts do not directly convey information from any peripheral receptors.

High-Fidelity Pathways

There are two pathways that relay high-fidelity, somatotopically arranged information to the cerebellar cortex (Figure 6-17):
- Posterior spinocerebellar pathway
- Cuneocerebellar pathway

Posterior Spinocerebellar Pathway

The **posterior** (dorsal) **spinocerebellar pathway** transmits information from the legs and the lower half of the body. The proximal axon of the first-order neuron travels in the dorsal column to the thoracic or upper lumbar spinal cord, then synapses in the area of the dorsal gray matter called the **nucleus dorsalis** (Clarke's nucleus). The nucleus dorsalis extends vertically from spinal segments T1 to L2. Second-order axons form the posterior spinocerebellar tract. The tract remains ipsilateral and projects to the cerebellar cortex via the inferior cerebellar peduncle.

Cuneocerebellar Pathway

The **cuneocerebellar pathway** begins with primary afferents from the arm and upper half of the body; the central axons travel via the posterior columns to the lower medulla. The synapse between the first- and second-order neurons occurs in the **lateral cuneate nucleus,** a nucleus in the medulla analogous to the nucleus dorsalis in the spinal cord. The second-order neurons form the cuneocerebellar tract, enter the ipsilateral inferior cerebellar peduncle, and end in the cerebellar cortex. The target neurons for both the posterior spinocerebellar and cuneocerebellar tracts are arranged somatotopically in the cerebellar cortex.

Internal Feedback Tracts

The two internal feedback tracts monitor the activity of spinal interneurons and of descending motor signals from the cerebral cortex and brainstem (see Figure 6-17):

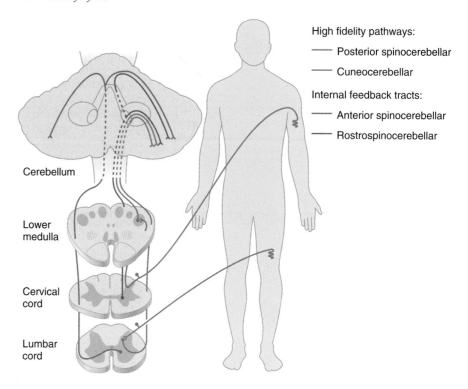

FIGURE 6-17

Tracts transmitting unconscious proprioceptive information. The high-fidelity pathways are the posterior spinocerebellar, from the lower body, and the cuneocerebellar, from the upper body. Internal feedback tracts are the anterior spinocerebellar, from the lower spinal cord, and the rostrospinocerebellar, from the cervical cord. *Inset:* Location of the three cerebellar peduncles.

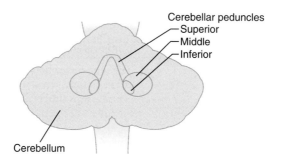

- Anterior spinocerebellar tract
- Rostrospinocerebellar tract

Anterior Spinocerebellar Tract

The **anterior spinocerebellar tract** transmits information from the thoracolumbar spinal cord. The tract begins with cell bodies in the lateral and ventral horns, in the area of the spinal cord containing the most interneurons. The axons cross to the opposite side and ascend in the contralateral anterior spinocerebellar tract to the midbrain. Leaving the midbrain, the axons enter the cerebellum via the superior cerebellar peduncle. Most fibers recross the midline before entering the cerebellum, so each side of the cerebellum gets information from both sides of the lower body. The bilateral projection may reflect the normally automatic coordination of lower limb activities, as opposed to the typically more voluntary control of the upper limbs.

Rostrospinocerebellar Tract

The **rostrospinocerebellar tract** transmits information from the cervical spinal cord to the ipsilateral cerebellum and enters the cerebellum via both the inferior and superior cerebellar peduncles.

The anterior and rostrospinocerebellar tracts apprise the cerebellum of the descending commands delivered to the neurons that control muscle activity via interneurons located between descending motor tracts and motor neurons that innervate muscles. The internal feedback tracts also convey information about the activity of spinal reflex circuits.

Function of Spinocerebellar Tracts

Information that travels in the spinocerebellar tracts is not consciously perceived. Damage to the spinocerebellar tracts can be differentiated from lesions of the cerebellum by comparing the coordination of movement with vision to movements without vision. In spinocerebellar tract lesions, movements are more coordinated when vision is present and more clumsy when the eyes are closed. Imaging studies can also distinguish between spinocerebellar and cerebellar lesions. The information in the spinocerebellar tracts is used for unconscious adjustments to movements and posture. Because the internal feedback tracts convey descending motor information to the cerebellum prior to the information reaching the motor neurons, and the high-fidelity pathways convey information from muscle spindles, tendon organs, and cutaneous mechanoreceptors, the cerebellum obtains information about movement commands and about the movements or postural adjustments that followed the commands. Thus the cerebellum can compare the intended motor output with the actual movement output. The cerebellum uses this information to make corrections to the neural commands via its connections with other brain areas (see Chapter 9).

Information in the spinocerebellar tracts is from proprioceptors, spinal interneurons, and descending motor pathways. This information, which does not reach conscious awareness, contributes to automatic movements and postural adjustments.

SUMMARY

Somatosensory pathways provide information about the external world, information used in movement control and to prevent or minimize injury. Conscious information about external objects can be provided by all four types of discriminative sensation: touch, proprioception, pain, and temperature. Discriminative sensations require analysis of sensory signals by the somatosensory area of the cerebral cortex. The dorsal column/medial lemniscus and spinothalamic pathways deliver the high-fidelity, somatotopically arranged information to the cerebral cortex. This conscious information contributes to our understanding of the physical world and to the control of fine movements. Unconscious information that contributes to the control of posture and movement is delivered to the cerebellum by the spinocerebellar tracts. Unconscious nociceptive information provides information about stimuli that threaten to damage or have damaged tissue. Spinolimbic, spinoreticular, and spinomesencephalic tracts deliver information to the thalamus, reticular formation, and midbrain that elicits automatic responses to nociceptive stimuli.

REVIEW QUESTIONS

1. What are the three types of somatosensory receptors?
2. What are nociceptors?
3. To what do the primary and secondary sensory endings in muscle spindles respond?
4. How is the sensitivity of sensory endings in a muscle spindle maintained when the muscle is shortened?
5. What type of information is transmitted by large-diameter type Ia and Ib axons?
6. What classes of axons convey nociceptive and temperature information?
7. What are the three types of pathways that convey information to the brain?
8. High-fidelity, somatotopically arranged somatosensory information is conveyed to what area of the cerebral cortex?
9. Neural signals that are interpreted as dull, aching pain travel in what pathway?

10. All of the unconscious relay tracts end in what part of the brain?
11. Where do synapses occur between neurons conveying discriminative touch information from the left lower limb?
12. Where do synapses occur between neurons conveying discriminative pain information from the left lower limb?
13. Name the tracts that relay unconscious proprioceptive information to the cerebellum. Name the tracts that provide unconscious information about activity in spinal interneurons and descending motor commands.

References

Abelson K (2005). Acetylcholine in spinal pain modulation. School of Medicine. Uppsala, Uppsala University, 1-56.

Almeida TF, Roizenblatt S, et al. (2004). Afferent pain pathways: A neuroanatomical review. Brain Research, 1000(1-2), 40-56.

Brooks J, Tracey I (2005). From nociception to pain perception: Imaging the spinal and supraspinal pathways. Journal of Anatomy, 207(1), 19-33.

Chalmers G (2004). Re-examination of the possible role of Golgi tendon organ and muscle spindle reflexes in proprioceptive neuromuscular facilitation muscle stretching. Sports biomechanics/International Society of Biomechanics in Sports, 3(1), 159-183.

Lagraize et al. (2005). In press.

Nallegowda M, Singh U, et al. (2003). Balance and gait in total hip replacement: A pilot study. American Journal of Physical Medicine & Rehabilitation/Association of Academic Physiatrists, 82(9), 669-677.

Ostrowsky K, and Magnin M et al. (2002). Representation of pain and somatic sensation in the human insula: a study of responses to direct electrical cortical stimulation. Cerebral Cortex, 12(4):376-385.

Palecek J, Paleckova V, et al. (2003). Fos expression in spinothalamic and postsynaptic dorsal column neurons following noxious visceral and cutaneous stimuli. Pain, 104(1-2), 249-257.

Price DD (2002). Central neural mechanisms that interrelate sensory and affective dimensions of pain. Molecular Interventions, 2(6), 392-403, 339.

Sacks O (1984). A leg to stand on. New York: Harper & Row.

Taylor A, Durbaba R, et al. (2004). Direct and indirect assessment of gamma-motor firing patterns. Canadian Journal of Physiology and Pharmacology, 82(8-9), 793-802.

Vallbo AB (1995). Single-afferent neurons and somatic sensation in humans. In MS Gazzaniga (Ed.). The cognitive neurosciences (pp. 237-252). Cambridge, Mass.: M.I.T. Press.

van Bijsterveld OP, Kruize AA, et al. (2003). Central nervous system mechanisms in Sjogren's syndrome. British Journal of Ophthalmology, 87(2), 128-130.

Van der Werf YD, Witter MP, et al. (2002). The intralaminar and midline nuclei of the thalamus. Anatomical and functional evidence for participation in processes of arousal and awareness. Brain Research. Brain Research Reviews, 39(2-3), 107-140.

Wessberg J, Olausson H, et al. (2003). Receptive field properties of unmyelinated tactile efferents in the human skin. Journal of Neurophysiology, 89(3), 1567-1575.

Suggested Reading

Gardner E, Kandel ER (2000). Touch. In ER Kandell, JH Schwartz, TM Jessell (Eds.). Principles of neural science, ed 4. New York: Elsevier.

7 Somatosensation: Clinical Application

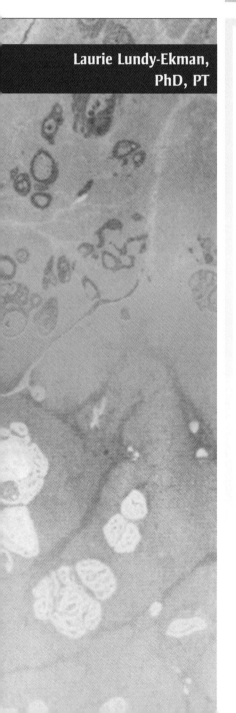

Laurie Lundy-Ekman,
PhD, PT

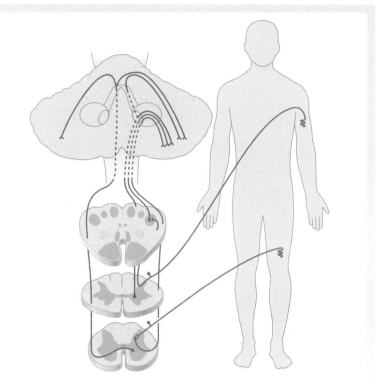

I am 69 years old, retired from working for the county, and the mother of three children. Nine years ago I awoke with sciatica, a severe pain extending from the left buttock, down the back of my leg, and into my big toe. I could not bend over to put on shoes or socks. A myelogram, an x-ray study of the spinal region in which dye is injected into the spinal region, showed a herniated intervertebral disk. I developed an excruciating headache secondary to the myelogram, and the scheduled surgery to remove part of the disk was cancelled. After two months of bed rest, I recovered.

One year later I again developed sciatic pain in my left leg that rapidly intensified. I couldn't walk at all because of the pain. I had to crawl. The pain was unbelievable. This time, magnetic resonance imaging revealed that two intervertebral disks had herniated. One month later, surgery was performed and when I awoke the sciatic pain was completely gone. Two years later, I was vacuuming and abruptly developed agonizing pain in my left leg. Surgery again repaired the disk. Since then I have had several deep cortisone shots that effectively relieved the pain.

Throughout this time, I didn't have any lack of sensation, weakness, or other problems. My ability to move was curtailed during the periods when I had sciatica. I could only move in ways that didn't hurt, so I couldn't drive or use stairs. The only time I wasn't in pain was when I was lying down, perfectly still. The pain completely dominated my life.

In physical therapy following the second surgery, I learned two exercises that I do daily. The first exercise is back extension. I lie on the floor on my stomach, my palms on the floor under my shoulders, then slowly push with my arms to raise my head and upper trunk off the floor. I hold this position for 20 seconds, then lie flat again. The other exercise is done lying on my side. If I am lying on my left side, I clasp my hands in front of me, then slowly raise both arms in an arc toward the ceiling and then to the floor on my right. When I began this exercise I could only move through half of the arc with my arms, but now I can reach across to the opposite side. This rotation of my spine works very well. I am much more limber now than when I began these exercises. I am free of pain now, except for a dull ache upon awakening that is relieved by the exercises. Also, I am careful not to lift more than ten pounds and I've learned to take breaks when I'm gardening.

—Pauline Schweizer

However, Taub et al. (1973) tested the effects of bilateral deafferentation. His group deafferented both forelimbs in newborn monkeys and sewed their eyelids closed to eliminate vision. These monkeys were able to ambulate, climb, and pick up some objects, although their performance was very clumsy and motor development was retarded. The monkeys were permanently unable to use their fingers individually, and thus could not pick up small objects.

The functional problems of a person with a severe peripheral sensory loss were reported by Rothwell et al. (1982). Motor power was nearly normal, and the subject could move individual fingers separately. Without vision, he could move his thumb accurately at different speeds and with different levels of force. Yet he could not write, hold a cup, or button his shirt. These difficulties were due to lack of somatosensation, depriving him of normal, automatic corrections to movement. When he tried to hold a pen to write, his grip did not automatically adjust because he lacked unconscious somatosensory information about the appropriate changes in pressure.

> Somatosensation is necessary for accurate control of movements.

INTRODUCTION

Somatosensation contributes to smooth, accurate movements, to the prevention or minimization of injury, and to our understanding of the external world. The first two of these topics are considered in this chapter. Perception, the ability to interpret somatosensation as meaningful information, is discussed in Chapters 16 and 17.

Contribution of Somatosensory Information to Movement

The role of sensation in movement is complex. In the early 1900s, Sherrington (1900) performed an experiment on a monkey to determine the effect of loss of information conveyed by the dorsal roots. He cut the dorsal roots entering the spinal cord from one arm, severing the sensory axons. Sherrington found that even after recovery from the surgery, the monkey avoided using that limb. This experimental outcome reinforced the assumption that sensation is essential for movement. Similarly, people who lack sensation in one upper limb tend to avoid using the limb, substituting with the unimpaired limb whenever possible.

Somatosensory Information Protects Against Injury

People with somatosensory deficits are prone to pressure-induced skin lesions, burns, and joint damage because they are unaware of excessive pressure, temperature, or stretch. Children with congenital insensitivity to pain have major musculoskeletal complications early in life from self-injury and repetitive trauma (Tsirikos, 2004).

TESTING SOMATOSENSATION

Clinically, the sensory examination covers conscious relay pathways:
- Discriminative touch
- Conscious proprioception
- Fast pain
- Discriminative temperature

These pathways are tested because the findings give information that can be used to localize a lesion.

The purpose of the sensory examination is to establish if there is sensory impairment and, if so, its location, type of sensation affected, and severity of the deficit. The following guidelines serve to improve the reliability of sensory testing.

1. Administer the tests in a quiet, distraction-free setting.
2. Position the subject seated or lying supported by a firm, stable surface to avoid challenging balance during the testing.
3. Explain the purpose of the testing.
4. Demonstrate each test prior to administering the test. During the demonstration, allow the subject to see the stimulus.
5. During testing, block the subject's vision by having the subject close the eyes or wear a blindfold or by placing a barrier between the part being tested and the subject's eyes.
6. Apply stimuli near the center of the dermatomes being tested. Record the results after each test. The time interval between stimuli should be irregular to prevent the subject from predicting the stimulation. Comparing the subject's responses on the left and right sides is often informative, especially if one side of the body or face is neurologically intact.

An important limitation of sensory testing is the reliance on conscious awareness of the sensory stimulation. Most somatosensory information is used at subconscious levels. For example, massive amounts of somatosensory information are processed by the cerebellum; however, there is no conscious awareness of this processing. Thus, testing proprioception by having the patient report whether he or she can sense the position of a limb tests conscious awareness of proprioception, but not the ability to use proprioceptive information to adjust movements.

Quick Screening

Quick screening for sensory impairment consists of testing proprioception and vibration in the fingers and toes and testing fast pain sensation in the limbs, trunk, and face with pinprick. This quick screening evaluates the function of some large-diameter and some small-diameter axons. Because of the possibility of spreading blood-borne diseases, care should be taken during pinprick testing to prevent puncturing the skin, and each pin should be discarded after use on a single person. A paper clip or plastic toothpick may serve as an alternative to the pin and is less likely to puncture the skin. If loss or impairment of sensation is found, additional testing is performed to determine the precise pattern of sensory loss.

Indications for more thorough testing include the following:

- Any complaints of sensory abnormality or loss
- Nonpainful skin lesions
- Localized weakness or atrophy

Complete Somatosensory Evaluation

A complete sensory evaluation includes measuring **sensitivity** and **thresholds** for stimulation of each conscious sensation (except proprioceptive thresholds are not measured). For example, a measure of conscious touch sensitivity is the ability to distinguish between two closely applied points on the skin; threshold is the lowest intensity of a stimulus that can be perceived, as when the person barely perceives being touched. Table 7-1 explains the testing procedures. Figure 7-1 shows normal values for touch sensitivity (two-point discrimination) on various parts of the body. A sensory assessment form is shown in Figure 7-2.

Interpreting Test Results

The results from these testing procedures can be used to map a person's pattern of sensory loss. The resulting map can be compared with standardized maps of **peripheral nerve distribution** and of dermatome distributions to determine if the person's pattern of sensory loss is consistent with a peripheral nerve or a spinal region pattern (see Figure 6-5). Because every individual is unique and adjacent dermatomes overlap one another, the maps presented represent common but not definitive nerve distributions. The overlap of adjacent dermatomes also ensures that if only one sensory root is severed, there is not complete loss of sensation in any area.

The primary somatosensory cortex is essential for two-point discrimination, graphesthesia, stereognosis, and simultaneous awareness of stimulation on both sides of the body. For predicting hand function from sensory tests, only two-point discrimination scores correlate well with hand function. People on ventilators or with communication disorders may present unusual challenges to sensory testing. The therapist may be able to establish a communication system using eye blinks (one for yes, two for no) or finger movements with cooperative people.

> Caveat: All somatosensory testing requires that the client has conscious awareness and cognition. These tests do not test the ability to use somatosensation to prepare for and during movements.

Table 7-1   TESTING THE SOMATOSENSORY SYSTEM

Discriminative Touch: Primary Sensation

Location of Touch

Test: Before testing touch, ask subject to "Say yes when you feel the touch and then to point to or tell me where you feel it." Lightly touch the pad of the subject's fingertips or toes with your fingertip or a wisp of cotton. If answers are accurate, assume that proximal location of touch is normal. If distal touch location is impaired, test dermatomes.* Once the extent of the impairment has been mapped, test peripheral nerve distributions (Figure 6-5) to determine whether the loss is in a dermatomal or peripheral nerve distribution.

Interpretation: If subject's responses are accurate, this indicates that the pathway for discriminative touch (dorsal column/medial lemniscus system) is intact from the periphery to the cerebral cortex. Failure to localize fine touch despite accurately reporting when touched indicates a lesion superior to the thalamus.

Tactile Thresholds

Test: Ask subject to "Say yes if you feel the touch." Touch a monofilament (nylon filaments available in sets of 5 to 10; bending pressure ranges from 0.02 to 40.0 g) to the subject's skin. The monofilament must be applied perpendicular to the skin. Press so that the filament bends. If answers are accurate, assume that proximal location of touch is normal. If distal touch location is impaired, test dermatomes.* Once the extent of the impairment has been mapped, test peripheral nerve distributions (Figure 6-5) to determine whether the loss is in a dermatomal or peripheral nerve distribution.

Interpretation: Normal response: able to feel the 2.83 filament anywhere on the face and upper limbs. The filaments that apply greater force are used to quantify decreased tactile sensitivity. Inability to sense filaments finer than 3.62 indicates diminished light touch; inability to sense the 4.31 filament indicates loss of stereognosis and protective sensation (Bell-Krotoski et al., 1993).

Discriminative Touch: Cortical Sensation

(Because these tests depend on touch sense, they cannot be performed when primary touch sensation is abnormal.)

Two-Point Discrimination

Test: Ask subject to "Tell me whether you feel one point or two points." Using calipers, apply light, equal pressure to two points. Begin with the points of the calipers farther apart than the mean value for the body part being tested. With each trial, move the points closer together until the subject cannot distinguish two points as separate. Measure the distance between the points with a ruler. To prevent anticipation, randomly stimulate with a single point. Typically, only test subject's hands.

Interpretation: Ability to accurately discriminate in normal ranges (see Figure 7-1) indicates that the pathway for discriminative touch (dorsal column/medial lemniscus system) is intact from the periphery to the cerebral cortex. However, problems producing a consistent amount of pressure make this test less sensitive and reliable than tactile threshold testing (Bell-Krotoski and Buford, 1997).

Bilateral Simultaneous Touch

Test: Ask subject to say "left" if the left side is touched, "right" if right side is touched, and "both" if both sides are touched. Lightly touch one limb, the opposite limb, or both sides of the body simultaneously. Typically test the forearms and the shins.

Interpretation: Tests for sensory extinction. Used to determine whether a person can attend to stimuli on both sides of the body simultaneously. If a person can accurately report stimuli presented on each side of the body separately but not when presented simultaneously, this indicates a lesion in the parietal lobe contralateral to the side of the body where sensory extinction occurs.

Table 7-1　TESTING THE SOMATOSENSORY SYSTEM—cont'd

Graphesthesia

Test: Ask subject to "Tell me what letter I draw in the palm of your hand." The subject's palm should be positioned facing the examiner, with the fingers pointing upward as if signaling "stop." Using a key or similar object, draw a letter in the palm of subject's hand.

Interpretation: Tests the dorsal column/medial lemniscus system and parietal lobe. Normal response: able to identify numbers or letters. If touch sensation is intact yet the person cannot perform this task, this indicates a lesion in the contralateral parietal cortex or adjacent white matter.

Conscious Proprioception

Joint Movement

Test: Ask subject to "Tell me whether I am bending or straightening your joint." Firmly hold the sides of the phalange (usually big toe or a finger), and passively flex or extend the joint approximately 10°. Randomize the order of flexions/extensions.

Interpretation: Normal response: no errors. Errors indicate dysfunction in the peripheral nerves, spinal cord, brainstem, or cerebrum.

Joint Position

Test: Tell subject you are going to move a joint. After the movement has stopped, either ask the subject to match the final joint position with the opposite limb or to report the position of the joint. Passively flex or extend the joint (usually elbow or ankle). Maintain a static position before asking subject to respond.

Interpretation: Normal response: no errors. Errors indicate dysfunction in the peripheral nerves, spinal cord, brainstem, or cerebrum.

Vibration

Test: Use a tuning fork with a frequency of 128 Hz. 1. Ask subject to "Tell me when the vibration stops," then touch a vibrating tuning fork to a bony prominence, *or* 2. Ask subject to "Tell me if the tuning fork is vibrating or not," then randomly apply a vibrating or non-vibrating tuning fork to a bony prominence. Test distal interphalangeal joint of the index fingers and big toes; if finger vibration sense is impaired, test wrists, elbows, clavicles. If toe vibration sense is impaired, test medial malleoli, patellas, and anterior superior iliac spines.

Interpretation: Primarily tests the large, A_β peripheral nerve fibers and the dorsal column/medial lemniscus neurons. Typically lesions superior to the thalamus do not impair vibration sensation.

Discriminative Touch and Conscious Proprioception

Stereognosis

Test: Ask subject to "Tell me what this is. You can move the object around in your hand." Place an object (key, paper clip) in subject's hand.

Interpretation: Normal response: able to identify object. If touch sensation is intact yet person cannot identify the object, this indicates a lesion in the contralateral parietal cortex or adjacent white matter.

Fast Pain (Lateral Pain System)

Sharp, Prickling Pain

Test: Ask subject to report "sharp" or "dull." If subject reports feeling the stimulus, ask where the stimulus was felt. Gently poke subject with a pin or touch with blunt end of a pin (or use a toothpick). To map an area of decreased or lost sensation, drag a pinwheel lightly along the skin to determine regions of normal and abnormal sensitivity. To use the pinwheel on a limb, circle the circumference of the limb.

Interpretation: Normal response: able to differentiate accurately between sharp and dull stimuli. Complete peripheral nerve lesions produce loss of all sensations in the region supplied by the nerve. Lesions of the anterolateral tracts or thalamocortical radiations produce inability to distinguish sharp from dull. Lesions of the primary sensory cortex interfere with ability to localize the stimulus, although the subject may be able to distinguish sharp versus dull.

Continued

Table 7-1 TESTING THE SOMATOSENSORY SYSTEM—cont'd

Discriminative Temperature	
Heat or Cold	
Test: Ask subject to report temperature as either hot or cold. Touch subject with test tubes filled with warm (40°C) and cool (10°C) water. Maintain contact with subject's skin for about 3 seconds before asking for a response.	**Interpretation:** Normal response: accurate identification of warm or cold. Usually used to map areas of deficiency to determine whether the sensory loss fits a peripheral or dermatomal pattern.

*To test upper limb dermatomes (see Figure 6-5), begin distally and test lateral, then posterior, then medial. For the hand, touch the thumb (C6), middle finger (C7), and little finger (C8). For the forearm, touch lateral (C6), posterior (C7), and medial (C8). For the upper arm, touch anterolateral (C5), lateral (C6), posterior (C7), posteromedial (C8), and anteromedial (T1).
For the lower limb, begin distally. On the sole of the foot, touch the big toe (L4), middle toe (L5), little toe (S1), and medial heel (S2). Midcalf: posteromedial (L3), anteromedial (L4), anterolateral (L5), posterolateral (S1), and posterior calf (S2). Anterior knee: L4. Thigh: medial proximal (L2), medial distal (L3), anterior distal (L4), lateral (L5), posterior (S1), and posteromedial (S2). Mnemonic for landmarks in lower limb: Stand on L4-S2; L3 medial knee.

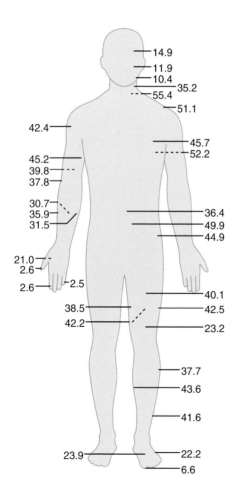

FIGURE 7-1

Normal two-point discrimination values, in millimeters, for various locations on the body. (Values from: Nolan MF (1982). Two-point discrimination assessment in the upper limb in young adult men and women. Physical Therapy, 62, 965; idem [1985]; Nolan, MF (1983). Limits of two-point discrimination ability in the lower limb of young adult men and women. Physical Therapy, 63(9), 1424; idem [1982]; and Nolan, MF (1985). Quantitative measure of cutaneous sensation: Two-point discrimination values for the face and trunk. Physical Therapy, 65(2), 181-185. With permission of APTA.)

ELECTRODIAGNOSTIC STUDIES

Recording the electrical activity from nerves reveals the location of pathology and is often diagnostic. Two methods of examining sensory nerve function are as follows:

- Nerve conduction studies (NCSs)
- Somatosensory evoked potentials (SEPs)

Nerve conduction studies only evaluate the function of peripheral nerves. Somatosensory evoked potentials test transmission of sensory information in both peripheral nerves and central nervous system pathways. In both NCS and SEP testing, the electrical stimulation is applied to the peripheral nerve so that all axons are depolarized simultaneously. In electrodiagnostic studies, measurements of the latencies, amplitudes, and conduction velocities obtained can be compared with unaffected nerves in the same patient or with published normal values. Some physical therapists specialize in performing NCSs, but therapists typically do not perform SEPs.

Diagnosis _____

Limb _____

Sketch the distribution of signs and symptoms.

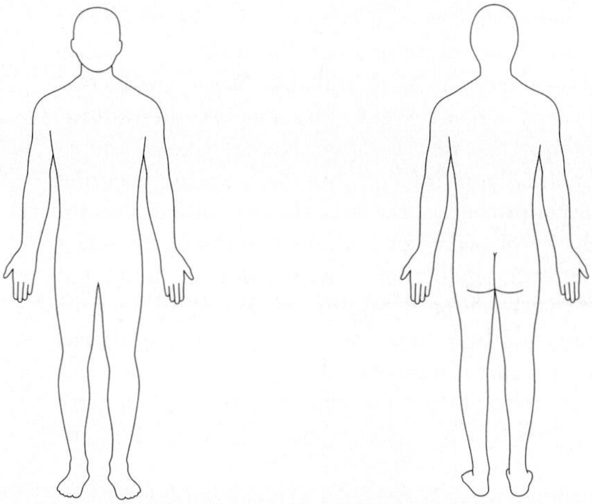

SYMPTOMS	Right	Left
Numbness		
Abnormal sensations (paresthesia or dysesthesia)		
SIGNS		
Light Touch		
Two-point discrimination		
Static proprioception		
Kinesthesia		
Vibration		
Pinprick		
Warmth		
Cold		

For symptoms, record the person's report. For signs, record as WNL (within normal limits), I (impaired), or A (absent).

FIGURE 7-2
Sensory examination form.

Sensory Nerve Conduction Studies

To test nerve conduction, surface recording electrodes are placed along the course of a peripheral nerve, and then the nerve is electrically stimulated. Nerve conduction studies only quantify the function of the fastest-conducting axons. Because large-diameter axons conduct fastest normally, in intact nerves NCS testing measures only the performance of the large-diameter fibers. Because the velocity of nerve conduction depends on an intact myelin sheath, conduction velocity is slowed throughout a nerve that has been demyelinated. If myelin has only been damaged by a focal injury, conduction is slowed only at the injured segment.

The function of the sensory fibers in the median nerve can be tested by electrically stimulating the skin of the middle finger and recording the electrical activity evoked in the median nerve at the wrist and elbow (Figure 7-3). The conduction velocity equals the distance between electrodes divided by the amount of time from the stimulus to the first depolarization at the recording electrode. The amplitude of the depolarization is also measured. Amplitude serves as an indicator of the number of axons conducting. Often the results from two recording sites are compared; for example, the amplitude and latency recorded at the wrist are compared with measurements at the elbow.

To determine if an NCS is normal, three numerical values are compared:
- Distal latency
- Amplitude of the evoked potential
- Conduction velocity

Distal latency is the time required for the depolarization evoked by the stimulus to reach the distal recording site. The results of an NCS in a normal nerve and in an abnormally functioning nerve are illustrated in Figure 7-3. Sensory nerve conduction may also be studied by stimulating proximal to the recording site. In this method, the recording electrode is picking up impulses that were propagated in the direction opposite to the normal physiological direction of sensory nerve impulse propagation.

Somatosensory Evoked Potentials

Somatosensory evoked potentials evaluate the function of the pathway from the periphery to the upper spinal cord or to the cerebral cortex. The skin over a peripheral nerve is electrically stimulated, and the resulting electrical activity is recorded from the skin over the upper cervical spinal cord or from the scalp over the primary somatosensory cortex. Again, the velocity is determined by dividing the distance between the stimulating and recording electrodes by the time required for the action potential to be transmitted. Somatosensory evoked potentials are used to verify subtle signs and locate lesions of the dorsal roots, posterior columns, and brainstem. For example, SEPs may be used in people with multiple sclerosis to determine the location of a lesion.

SENSORY ABNORMALITIES

Proprioceptive Pathway Lesions: Sensory Ataxia

Ataxia is incoordination that is not due to weakness. There are three types of ataxia: sensory, vestibular, and cerebellar. Lesions that produce sensory ataxia are located in peripheral sensory nerves, dorsal roots, dorsal columns of the spinal cord, or medial lemnisci. The Romberg test is used to distinguish between cerebellar ataxia (see Chapter 10) and sensory ataxia. The person is asked to stand with the feet together, first with eyes open, then with eyes closed. People with cerebellar ataxia have difficulty maintaining their balance regardless of whether their eyes are open or closed. People with sensory ataxia have better balance when their eyes are open but become unsteady when their eyes are closed (Romberg sign). Thus, people with sensory ataxia are able to use vision to compensate for decreased or lost somatosensory information. People with sensory ataxia often report that their balance is better when they watch their feet while walking, and that their balance is worse in the dark. Sensory ataxia can also be differentiated from cerebellar ataxia because conscious proprioception and vibratory sense are impaired in sensory ataxia yet intact in cerebellar ataxia. Differentiating vestibular ataxia from cerebellar or sensory ataxia is discussed in Chapter 15.

Peripheral Nerve Lesions

The general term for dysfunction or pathology of one or more peripheral nerves is **neuropathy.** Peripheral nerves are subject to trauma and disease. Complete severance of a peripheral nerve results in lack of sensation in the distribution of the nerve, pain may occur, and the sensory changes are accompanied by motor and reflex loss. Compression of a nerve affects large myelinated fibers preferentially, with initial relative sparing of the smaller pain, thermal, and autonomic fibers. For example, when one stands up after prolonged sitting with the legs crossed, occasionally one finds that part of a limb has "fallen

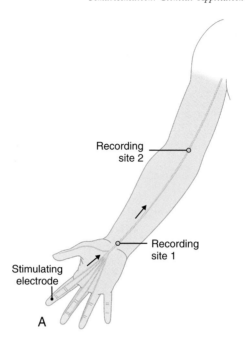

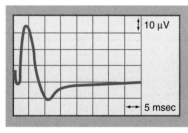

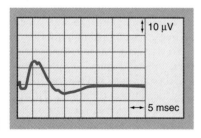

	Latency (ms)	Amplitude (µV)	Distance (cm)	Velocity (m/s)
Normal	2.44	34	12	49.1
Abnormal	6.5	18	13	20

FIGURE 7-3

Sensory nerve conduction study (NCS): median nerve. **A,** Sites of electrodes for stimulation of index finger and for recording from skin over the median nerve at the wrist and elbow. **B,** Graphic results from a normal median NCS recording at the wrist. **C,** Graph of recording at the wrist from a demyelinated nerve. **D,** Numerical results of the NCS.

asleep." The sensory loss proceeds in the following order:

1. Conscious proprioception and discriminative touch
2. Cold
3. Fast pain
4. Heat
5. Slow pain

When the compression is relieved, tingling or prickling sensations occur as the blood supply increases. After compression is removed, sensations return in the reverse order that they were lost. Thus, aching pain occurs first, then a sensation of warmth, then sharp, stinging sensations, then cold, and finally a return of discriminative touch and conscious proprioception.

Demyelination of axons in a peripheral nerve often affects proprioception and vibratory sense most severely because the large axons are the most heavily myelinated, resulting in diminished or lost proprioception. Neuropathy is discussed further in Chapter 11.

> Neuropathy is dysfunction or pathology of one or more peripheral nerves.

Spinal Region Lesions

Common causes of dysfunction of the spinal region include the following:

- Trauma to the spinal cord, completely or partially severing the cord
- Diseases that compromise the function of specific areas within the spinal cord (These diseases are discussed in Chapter 12.)
- A virus infecting the dorsal root ganglion

Complete Transection of the Spinal Cord

Complete transection of the cord prevents all sensation one or two levels below the level of the lesion from ascending to higher levels in the cord. Clinically, the observed complete loss of sensation begins in dermatomes one or two levels below the level of the lesion because of the overlap of nerve endings in adjacent dermatomes. Voluntary motor control below the lesion is also lost.

Hemisection of the Spinal Cord

A hemisection, that is, damage to the right or left half of the cord, interrupts pain and temperature sensation from the contralateral body because the axons transmit-

ting nociceptive and temperature information cross to the opposite side of the cord soon after entering the cord. As a result of collateral branching of nociceptive axons in the dorsolateral tract (Lissauer's marginal zone; see Figure 6-15), the complete loss of pain sensation occurs two to three dermatomes below the level of the lesion. Because discriminative touch and conscious proprioception information ascends on the same side of the cord as it entered, these sensations are lost ipsilateral to the lesion. Paralysis also occurs ipsilaterally. The pattern of loss is called Brown-Sequard's syndrome.

Posterior Column Lesions

In posterior column lesions, conscious proprioception, two-point discrimination, and vibration sense are lost below the level of the lesion. Immediately after the lesion, movements are uncoordinated, that is, ataxic. If the lesion is above C6, the person may be unable to recognize objects by palpation because ascending sensory information from the hand has been lost.

Infection

An infection of a dorsal root ganglion or cranial nerve ganglion with varicella-zoster virus causes **varicella zoster,** also called shingles or herpes zoster. The varicella-zoster virus causes chickenpox. After a chickenpox infection, the sensory ganglia hold latent components of the varicella-zoster virus. Occasionally, some of the virus reverts to infectiousness. If the level of circulating antibodies is inadequate, the virus begins to multiply and is transported antidromically down sensory peripheral axons. The virus irritates and inflames the nerve, causing pain. The virus is released into the skin around the sensory nerve endings, causing painful eruptions on the skin. The infection is usually limited to one dermatome or trigeminal nerve branch (Figure 7-4). If treated effectively very early, the duration and severity of varicella zoster can usually be limited (Box 7-1). However, in severe or inadequately treated cases, **postherpetic neuralgia** develops. Postherpetic neuralgia is severe pain that persists more than 1 month after the zoster infection.

Brainstem Region Lesions

Because the axons carrying sensory information from the body and face cross the midline at various levels, lesions in the brainstem usually cause a mix of ipsilateral and contralateral signs. Only in the upper midbrain, after all discriminative sensation tracts have crossed the midline, will sensory loss be entirely contralateral. Throughout the brainstem, a lesion of trigeminal nerve proximal

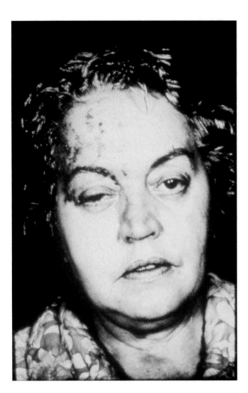

FIGURE 7-4
Varicella zoster (shingles) eruptions on the skin. One branch of the trigeminal nerve is affected.

axons or of the trigeminal nerve nuclei causes an ipsilateral loss of sensation from the face.

A lesion in the posterolateral medulla or lower pons can cause a mixed sensory loss consisting of ipsilateral loss of pain and temperature sensation from the face combined with contralateral loss of pain and temperature information from the body (Figure 7-5). This occurs because the trigeminal nerve pain information is uncrossed in the medulla and lower pons, while ascending pain information from the body crosses in the spinal cord. Discriminative touch and proprioceptive information from the body is not affected because the tracts conveying this information travel in the medial medulla and pons. Discriminative touch and proprioceptive information from the face is not affected because these tracts and nuclei are superior to the medulla.

A lesion in the medial medulla or lower pons may cause impairment of pain sensation from the contralateral face owing to interruption of some second-order axons conveying information from the trigeminal nerve, combined with the loss of discriminative touch and

---

BOX 7-1   VARICELLA ZOSTER

Pathology
Infection of sensory root cell bodies, causing inflammation of sensory neurons

Etiology
Varicella-zoster virus

Speed of Onset
Acute or subacute

Signs and Symptoms
Consciousness
Normal
Communication and Memory
Normal

Sensory
Itching, burning, or tingling may precede eruption of vesicles by up to five 5 days (Gnann and Whitley, 2002); pain is often severe
Autonomic
Normal
Motor
Normal
Region Affected
Usually limited to one dermatome (often thoracic) or one branch of trigeminal nerve

Demographics
Both genders equally affected; incidence increases with aging

Incidence and Prevalence
Varicella Zoster
140 per 100,000 people population per year; affects up to ½ of all people who live to the age of 85 years (Johnson and Dworkin, 2003)
Postherpetic Neuralgia
Incidence 11 per 100,000 people population per year; prevalence: 0.7 per 1000 people population (MacDonald et al., 2000)

Prognosis
Pain usually lasts 1-4 weeks but may persist longer and may progress to postherpetic neuralgia; ultimately, the pain resolves. Early treatment with medications shortens the course of varicella zoster and decreases the duration and pain of postherpetic neuralgia (Johnson and Dworkin, 2003).

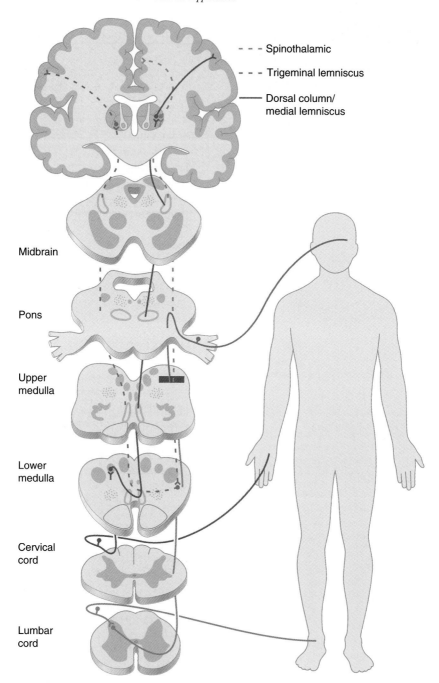

FIGURE 7-5

Mixed sensory loss due to a lesion in the posterolateral medulla. Black bar indicates the lesion site. Dotted lines indicate pathways that no longer transmit information. Pain and temperature information is lost from the ipsilateral face and contralateral body. The lesion does not affect discriminative touch and conscious proprioception because the medial lemniscus is medial to the site of the lesion.

conscious proprioceptive information from the contralateral body. The contralateral loss occurs because the medial lemniscus axons have crossed the midline in the lower medulla.

A lesion in the posterolateral upper pons or midbrain, after the trigeminothalamic tracts (except proprioceptive) and all of the tracts from the body have crossed the midline, causes contralateral sensory loss from the face (except proprioceptive) and entirely contralateral loss from the body because all tracts have crossed the midline below the lesion.

> Lesions in the brainstem often cause mixed sensory impairments, affecting the contralateral body and ipsilateral face.

Cerebral Region Lesions

Thalamic Lesions

Lesions in the ventral posterolateral (VPL) or ventral posteromedial (VPM) nucleus of the thalamus result in decreased or lost sensation from the contralateral body or face. Rarely, people who have strokes that affect the VPL or VPM nucleus have severe pain in the contralateral body or face.

Somatosensory Cortex Lesions

The sensory effects of a cortical lesion are contralateral and include decrease or loss of discriminative sensations:

- Conscious proprioception
- Two-point discrimination
- Stereognosis
- Localization of touch and pinprick (nociceptive) stimuli

Cortical processing is essential for discriminative sensation, although crude awareness of sensation is possible at the thalamic level.

In cases of **sensory extinction** (also called *sensory inattention*), the loss of sensation is only evident when symmetrical body parts are tested bilaterally. For example, if both hands are touched or pricked simultaneously, the person may only be aware of stimulation on the same side of the body as the cortical lesion. If stimuli are not simultaneous, people with sensory extinction are aware of stimulation on either side of the body. Sensory extinction is a form of unilateral neglect because the person neglects stimuli on one side of the body if the

other side of the body is stimulated simultaneously. Unilateral neglect is discussed in Chapter 17.

CLINICAL PERSPECTIVES ON PAIN

Pain is an unpleasant sensory and emotional experience (IASP Task Force on Taxonomy, 1994). Pain is frequently associated with tissue damage or potential tissue damage, although pain can be experienced independently of tissue damage. Nociceptors signal injury, yet nociceptor activity is insufficient to cause pain. Pain is a perception.

Nociception from Muscles and Joints

Both Aδ and C fibers are found in skeletal muscle and joints, so signals interpreted as both fast and slow pain can occur with musculoskeletal injuries. Under normal circumstances, many nociceptors are "sleeping" (Willis and Westlund, 1997). When tissue is injured or ischemic, biochemicals are released that awaken the sleeping nociceptors. The awakened nociceptors are excessively reactive to stimuli; this is called *peripheral sensitization.* The sensitized neurons fire in response to normally innocuous stimuli, even with slight movements, and may fire spontaneously. For example, after an ankle sprain, partial weight bearing may be painful and the ankle may ache while at rest.

Unlike superficial pain, which encourages withdrawal (movement to escape the source of pain), deep pain usually occurs after tissue has been damaged. The function of deep pain may be to encourage rest of the damaged tissue. After a lower limb injury, the pain on weight bearing often produces a modified gait. The modified gait is called *antalgic* and is characterized by a shortened stance phase on the affected side.

Referred Pain

Referred pain is perceived as coming from a site distinct from the actual site of origin. Usually pain is referred from visceral tissues to skin. For example, during a heart attack, the brain may misinterpret the nociceptive information as arising from the skin or the medial left arm. Similarly, gallbladder pain is often referred to the right subscapular region.

Referred pain is explained by convergence and facilitation of nociceptive information from different sources. Referred pain occurs when branches of nociceptive fibers from an internal organ and branches from nociceptive fibers from the skin converge on the same second-order neurons in the spinal cord or in the thalamus and the central neurons become sensitized (Giamberardino, 2003).

Common patterns of referred pain are illustrated in Figure 7-6.

> Identifying referred pain is important in preventing misdiagnoses and malpractice, so that people with disorders not amenable to occupational or physical therapy can be referred to the appropriate practitioner.

The Pain Matrix

The pain matrix consists of brain structures that process and regulate pain information and are capable of creating pain perception in the absence of nociceptive input. The pain matrix includes parts of the brainstem, amygdala, hypothalamus, thalamus, and areas of the cerebral cortex (Zambreanu et al., 2005). When peripheral nociceptors are stimulated, the signals travel up the pain matrix (Figure 7-7). The person perceives the location and intensity of the tissue damage or potential tissue damage

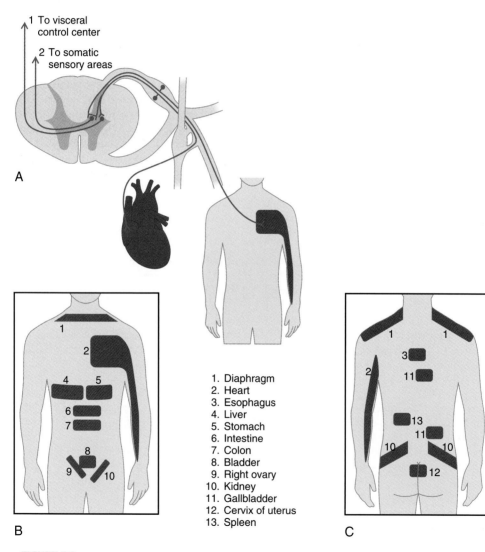

1. Diaphragm
2. Heart
3. Esophagus
4. Liver
5. Stomach
6. Intestine
7. Colon
8. Bladder
9. Right ovary
10. Kidney
11. Gallbladder
12. Cervix of uterus
13. Spleen

FIGURE 7-6

A, Theoretical mechanisms of referred pain. Some visceral afferents synapse with the same second-order neurons as somatosensory afferents. **B** and **C,** Common patterns of referred pain.

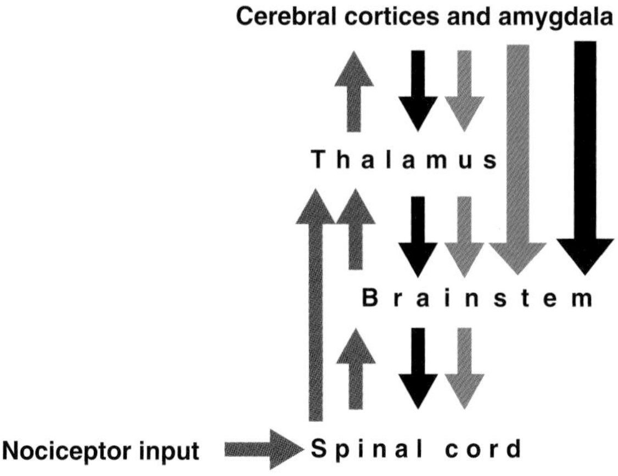

Cerebral cortices and amygdala

T h a l a m u s

B r a i n s t e m

Nociceptor input ➡ S p i n a l   c o r d

FIGURE 7-7

The pain matrix. Ascending arrows represent the medial and lateral nociceptive pathways. Descending arrows represent the top-down control of nociceptive signals by the pain matrix. Black arrows indicate antinociception. Green arrows indicate pronociception. The structures that process nociceptive information include in the brainstem: periaqueductal gray, locus ceruleus, dorsal raphe nucleus, and reticular formation; in the thalamus: ventroposterolateral, ventroposteromedial, midline and intralaminar nuclei; in the cerebrum: hypothalamus, amygdala, and somatosensory, insular, cingulate, and prefrontal cortex.

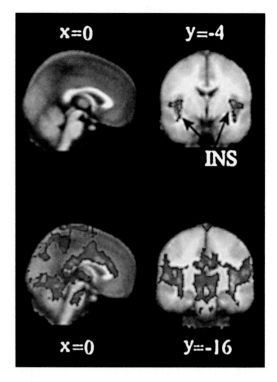

FIGURE 7-8

Brain activation in neurologically normal subjects during pressure on the skin with a stiff nylon filament (Frey hair). Left scans: midsagittal. Right scans: coronal. Top scans: stimulation of normal skin. Only the insula, part of the lateral pain system, was activated. Bottom scans: stimulation in the area of secondary hyperalgesia. The area of skin stimulated was adjacent to an area that had previous application of heat and a topical irritant, capsaicin. Both the lateral and medial pain systems responded. *(From Zambreanu L, Wise RG, et al. (2005). A role for the brainstem in central sensitisation in humans. Evidence from functional magnetic resonance imaging. Pain, 114(3), 397-407.*

(lateral pain system) and has affective and cognitive responses to the signals (medial pain system). Brain scans show differential activation of the medial and lateral systems of the pain matrix (Figure 7-8).

The experience of pain is strongly linked to emotional, behavioral, and cognitive phenomena (Nicholson and Martelli, 2004). Thus understanding pain requires consideration of multiple aspects of the pain experience: discriminative, motivational-affective, and cognitive-evaluative components (Nicholson and Martelli, 2004). The discriminative aspect refers to the ability to localize the site, timing, and intensity of tissue damage or potential tissue damage. This information travels in the spinothalamic tract and is processed in the somatosensory and insular cortex (lateral pain system). The motivational-affective aspect refers to the effects of the pain experience on emotions and behavior, including increased arousal and avoidance behavior. Nociceptive information that impacts emotions and motivation travels in the spinolimbic and spinoreticular tracts, to the medial and intralaminar nuclei of the thalamus, then to the limbic system. The cognitive-evaluative aspect refers to the meaning that the person ascribes to the pain. Is the pain

conceived as a punishment, an unfair burden, a signal of a life-threatening disorder? Cognitive factors, including focusing exclusively on the pain and worry regarding the pain, can increase distress (Craig, 1999). The separation of the discriminative system from the other systems is verified by the fact that cingulotomy (electrical destruction of the anterior cingulate gyrus and callosum) reduces the emotional and cognitive aspects of chronic pain but does not modify the sensory-discriminative aspects (Ingvar and Hsieh, 1999).

In reaction to nociceptive signals, the pain matrix generates a top-down response that regulates the ascending pain signals (see Figure 7-7). The top-down response depends upon psychological, physiological, social, and genetic factors and may suppress or amplify the nociceptive signals. Thus the pain matrix determines whether ascending nociceptive processing will be normal, suppressed, sensitized, or reorganized. **Antinociception** is the top-down inhibition of pain signals. **Pronociception** is the biological amplification of pain signals.

How is Pain Controlled?

What is a typical response to hitting one's thumb with a hammer? A common sequence is to withdraw the thumb, yell (via limbic connections), and then apply pressure to the injured thumb. The first scientific explanation of how pressure and other external stimuli inhibit pain transmission was the **gate theory of pain,** proposed by Melzack and Wall in 1965. They hypothesized that information from first-order low-threshold mechanical afferents and from first-order nociceptive afferents normally converges onto the same second-order neurons. They proposed that the preponderance of activity in the primary afferents determines the pattern of signals the second-order neuron transmits. Thus, if the low-threshold mechanical afferents are more active than the nociceptive afferents, the mechanoreceptive information is transmitted and the nociceptive information inhibited. According to the theory as initially presented, transmission of pain information is blocked in the dorsal horn, closing the gate to pain.

Although later investigations demonstrated that some details of the original gate theory proposal are incorrect, the original gate theory is important because it inspired inquiry into the mechanics and control of pain. One result of these investigations was the clinical application of transcutaneous electrical nerve stimulation (TENS). TENS uses electrical current applied to the skin to interfere with the transmission of pain information.

Counterirritant Theory

A theory that has incorporated findings from research stimulated by the gate theory is the **counterirritant theory.** According to the counterirritant theory, inhibition of nociceptive signals by stimulation of non-nociceptive receptors occurs in the dorsal horn of the spinal cord (Figure 7-9). For example, pressure stimulates mechanoreceptive afferents. Theoretically, proximal branches of the mechanoreceptive afferents activate interneurons that release the neurotransmitter **enkephalin.** Enkephalin binds with receptor sites on both the primary afferents and interneurons of the pain system. Enkephalin binding depresses the release of Substance P

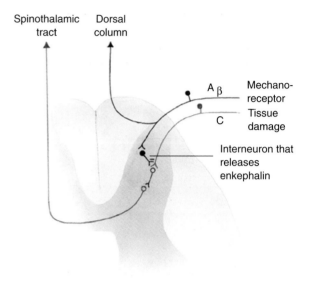

FIGURE 7-9

Counterirritant mechanism. Circuits in the dorsal horn that may produce inhibition of nociceptive signals. Collaterals of mechanoreceptive afferents stimulate interneurons that release enkephalins. Enkephalin binding inhibits the transmission of nociceptive messages by primary afferents and interneurons in the nociceptive pathway.

and hyperpolarizes the interneurons, thus inhibiting the transmission of nociceptive signals.

Dorsal Horn Processing of Nociceptive Information

Processing of somatosensory information in the dorsal horn can be altered by abnormal neural activity or by tissue injury. Four states of dorsal horn processing occur: normal, suppressed, sensitized, and reorganized (Doubell, 1999; Table 7-2). In the normal state, signals resulting from stimuli are accurate. For example, touch sensation is interpreted as touch, and nociceptive information is interpreted as painful. In the suppressed state, touch, pressure, and vibration information is transmitted normally but nociceptive impulses are inhibited. Medications, TENS, counterirritants, excitement, distraction, and placebo effects can produce the inhibition. In the sensitized state, changes in the quantity and type of neurotransmitters and receptors produces painful responses to both A_β and A_δ/C activity. In the reorganized state, the structure of the dorsal horn has changed due to cell death, degeneration of nociceptive axon terminals, and the sprouting of new A_β axon terminals that synapse with neurons in the nociceptive pathways. The

Table 7-2   STATES OF SENSORY PROCESSING IN THE DORSAL HORN OF THE SPINAL CORD

State of Dorsal Horn	Response to Activation of Primary Afferent Fibers	Mechanism
Normal	A_β: sensation of touch, pressure, vibration $A_\delta C$: nociceptive pain	Normal, physiologic activity
Suppressed nociception	A_β: normal A_δ/C: reduced response	Activity of segmental and descending inhibition on dorsal horn; includes counterirritation, medications, and psychological factors
Sensitized (temporary)	A_β: allodynia A_δ/C: excessive response	Additional types of neurotransmitters active, plus increased number and types of receptors
Reorganized (persistent increased pain sensibility)	A_β: allodynia A_δ/C: excessive response	Structural reorganization, including death of neurons, degeneration of C-fiber axon terminals, and sprouting of new A_β axon terminals to form abnormal synapses with neurons in the nociceptive pathways

sensitized and the reorganized states are both neuropathic states. That is, the pain experienced in these states is due to abnormal neural processing.

> Neuropathic pain results from changes in neuronal activity. Thus, neuropathic pain is produced by neuroplasticity, not by stimulation of nociceptors.

Antinociceptive Systems

Antinociception is suppression of pain in response to stimulation that would normally be painful. The endogenous, or naturally occurring, substances that activate antinociceptive mechanisms are called **endorphins**. Endorphins include enkephalins, dynorphin, and β-endorphin. Opiates, drugs that block nociceptive signals without affecting other sensations, bind to the same receptor sites as endorphins. Because opiates bind to the receptor sites, the receptors are sometimes called *opiate receptors*.

The transmission of nociceptive information can be inhibited by pain matrix activity (Figure 7-10). Brainstem areas that provide intrinsic antinociception form a neuronal descending system, arising in the following:
- **Raphe nuclei** in the medulla
- **Periaqueductal gray** (PAG) in the midbrain
- **Locus ceruleus** in the pons

When the raphe nuclei are electrically stimulated, axons projecting to the spinal cord release the neurotrans-

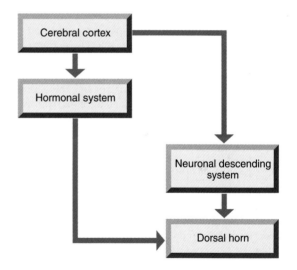

FIGURE 7-10
Flowchart of supraspinal antinociceptive systems. Cerebral cortical output activates the hormonal and neuronal descending systems that inhibit the transmission of nociceptive information in the dorsal horn.

mitter serotonin in the dorsal horn, inhibiting the tract neurons and thus interfering with transmission of nociceptive messages. Stimulation of PAG produces antinociception via activation of the raphe nuclei (Abelson, 2005). The third descending system, the ceruleospinal (from locus ceruleus), inhibits spinothalamic activity in the dorsal horn but is non–opiate-mediated; instead, binding of the transmitter norepinephrine on the primary afferent neuron directly suppresses the release of nociceptive transmitters (Lipp, 1991).

Narcotics, drugs derived from opium or opium-like compounds, bind to opiate receptor sites in the PAG, raphe nuclei, and dorsal horn of the spinal cord. By activating the receptor sites, narcotics induce antinociception and stupor (a state of reduced consciousness). If the descending tracts from the raphe nuclei are severed, administration of morphine or other opiates results only in slight antinociception because the lesion of the raphespinal tracts blocks descending inhibition. The slight antinociception that occurs is the result of morphine binding to opiate receptors in the dorsal horn.

The pain-inhibiting centers do not lie dormant waiting for an electrode or a drug to stimulate them. How are they normally activated? People injured in accidents, disasters, or athletic contests sometimes don't feel pain until after the emergency or game is over. Stress during an emergency or competition may trigger the antinociception systems. **Stress-induced antinociception** requires activation of the raphe nuclei descending tracts plus release of hormonal endorphins from the pituitary gland (β-endorphins) and adrenal medulla (similar to enkephalins). The hormonal endorphins bind to opiate receptors in the pain matrix and spinal cord. β-endorphins are the most potent endorphins, and their effects last for hours. Stress-induced antinociception may be triggered by cortical input to the descending antinociception systems.

Sites of Antinociception

The transmission of nociceptive information can be altered at several locations in the nervous system. The phenomenon of **antinociception** is summarized with a five-level model (Figure 7-11).

- **Level 1** occurs in the **periphery.** Non-narcotic analgesics (e.g., aspirin) decrease the synthesis of prostaglandins, preventing prostaglandins from sensitizing nociceptors.
- **Level II** occurs in the **dorsal horn,** via local inhibitory neurons releasing enkephalin or dynorphin. This is the level of counterirritant effects; examples are superficial heat and high-frequency, low-intensity TENS. Activity in collateral branches of non-nociceptive afferents decreases or prevents the transmission of nociceptive information to the second-order neuron in the spinal cord.
- **Level III** is the fast-acting **neuronal descending system,** involving the PAG, raphe nuclei, and locus ceruleus.

- **Level IV** is the **hormonal system,** involving the periventricular gray matter (PVG) in the hypothalamus, the pituitary gland, and the adrenal medulla. Direct electrical stimulation of the PVG results in antinociception with a 10-minute latency, and the effect lasts for hours after the stimulation has stopped. Low-frequency TENS may act on this level because its pattern of action has a similar latency and lasting effect.
- **Level V** is the **cortical level.** Here, expectations, excitement, distraction, and placebos all play a role in adjusting the transmission of nociceptive signals. Placebo antinociception activates the same higher order cognitive and brainstem areas that are activated by opiate drugs (Wager et al., 2004).

> Transmission of nociceptive information can be inhibited by binding of endorphins or of analgesic drugs to receptor sites in the dorsal horn, PAG, PVG, and raphe nuclei. Norepinephrine binding to primary afferents in the dorsal horn also inhibits transmission of nociceptive information. In the periphery, signals from nociceptors can be inhibited by non-narcotic analgesics.

Pronociception: Biological Amplification of Nociception

Pain transmission can also be intensified at several levels. Edema and endogenous chemicals can sensitize free nerve endings in the periphery. For example, following a minor burn injury, stimuli that would normally be innocuous can cause exquisite pain. Pronociception may occur when a person is anxious or depressed (Brooks and Tracey, 2005). Pronociceptive pain matrix activity can also produce pain perception in the absence of any nociceptive input (Brooks and Tracey, 2005). An example of pain perception without nociceptive input is the Eisenberger et al. (2003) study of social exclusion. Subjects played a virtual ball game and were eventually excluded. Scans during the experience indicated that the brain activity changes in the prefrontal and anterior cingulate cortex that occur during physical pain are the same during social distress.

CHRONIC PAIN

Therapists must distinguish between acute pain and chronic pain and between pain and activity limitations so appropriate treatment can be administered. Pain is an

Table 7-3 CHARACTERISTICS OF ACUTE AND CHRONIC PAIN

	Acute Pain	Chronic Pain
Causes	Threat of or actual tissue damage	Continuing tissue damage Environmental factors (operant conditioning) Sensitization of nociceptive pathway neurons Dysfunction of endogenous pain control systems
Client report	Clear description of location, pattern, quality, frequency, and duration	Vague description
Function	Warning of tissue damage, enforce rest of healing tissue	If tissue damage is not continuing, no biologic benefit; may have social or psychological benefit
Consequences	Excessive autonomic activity Excessive neuroendocrine activation If not adequately treated, can be as harmful as disease (Liebeskind, 1991) and may progress to chronic pain	Severe financial, emotional, physical, and/or social stresses on the person and family Physiologic consequences of inactivity

unpleasant subjective experience, while activity limitation is the lack of ability to perform normal tasks. Characteristics of acute and chronic pain are compared in Table 7-3.

Chronic pain can be classified according to etiology as follows:

• Nociceptive
• Neuropathic
• Chronic pain syndrome

Nociceptive Chronic Pain

Nociceptive chronic pain is due to continuing stimulation of nociceptive receptors. Examples are chronic pain resulting from tissue damage by cancer or by a vertebral tumor pressing on nociceptors in the meninges surrounding the spinal cord. The neurons are functioning normally, sending appropriate signals regarding tissue damage. The chemical changes in damaged tissue awaken sleeping peripheral nociceptors. Activity of the awakened nociceptors results in **primary hyperalgesia,** excessive sensitivity to stimuli in the injured tissue. An example is the pain caused by mild heat on burned skin. If a fingertip is burned, picking up a hot plate is more painful than if the skin were uninjured. Nociceptive chronic pain serves a useful biological function as a warning to protect the injured tissue.

Neuropathic Chronic Pain

Neuropathic pain is produced by pathologic neural activity. In neuropathic pain, the pain is a disease because the pain is independent of stimulation of nociceptive endings (Nicholson, 2003). Neuropathic pain is similar to a malfunctioning burglar alarm system: there is no

burglar, yet the alarm siren blasts a warning. Often, neuropathic pain has no beneficial biological function. For example, chronic low back pain may be caused by abnormal pain processing rather than current musculoskeletal injury. The neurons are pathologically active.

Symptoms of Neuropathic Pain

Symptoms of neuropathic pain include: paresthesia, dysesthesia, allodynia, and secondary hyperalgesia.

Paresthesia is a painless abnormal sensation in the absence of nociceptor stimulation. Paresthesias arise from dysfunction of neurons. Typically, paresthesias are experienced as tingling or prickling sensations. Lesions anywhere along the nociceptive pathways, from peripheral nerves to somatosensory cortex, can produce paresthesia.

Dysesthesia is an unpleasant abnormal sensation, whether evoked or spontaneous. Often spontaneous dysesthesia is described as a sensation of burning pain, or shooting or electrical sensations. A similar shooting pain is elicited by striking the ulnar nerve at the elbow. Allodynia and hyperalgesia are specific types of dysesthesia evoked by stimuli.

Allodynia is pain evoked by a stimulus that normally would not cause pain. For example, the normally nonpainful stimulus of touch produces pain if skin is sunburned.

Secondary hyperalgesia is excessive sensitivity to stimuli that are normally mildly painful in uninjured tissue.

See Box 7-2. Table 7-4 lists the tests for neuropathic pain.

Five Mechanisms Produce Neuropathic Pain

Neuropathic pain is produced by five mechanisms:
- Ectopic foci
- Ephaptic transmission
- Central sensitization
- Structural reorganization
- Altered top-down modulation

Ectopic Foci. When myelin is damaged, signals from the exposed axon alter the gene activity in the cell body, stimulating excessive production of mechanosensitive and chemosensitive ion channels. These channels are inserted into the demyelinated membrane, producing abnormal sensitivity to mechanical and chemical stimuli. The demyelinated region takes on a new, pathologic role:

the generation of action potentials in addition to the normal role of conducting action potentials. The sensitivity of ectopic foci to circulating catecholamines may contribute to the development of pain syndromes (Harden, 2005).

Ephaptic Transmission. Also called *cross-talk,* ephaptic transmission occurs in demyelinated regions as a result of lack of insulation between neurons. An action potential in one neuron may induce an action potential in another neuron.

Central Sensitization. Excessive responsiveness of central neurons, called central sensitization, develops in response to ongoing nociceptive input, yet the alterations in central neural activity outlast the tissue injury. Normally, when a brief, mild nociceptive message is

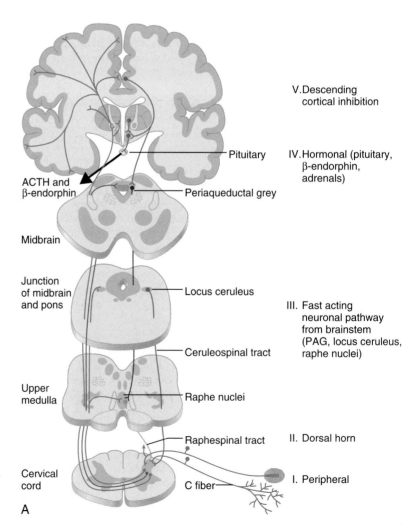

FIGURE 7-11

Antinociceptive systems. **A,** Tracts that convey ascending slow nociceptive information are shown on the left: the spinolimbic (blue), spinomesencephalic (red), and spinoreticular (green) tracts. The five levels of the nervous system involved in pain inhibition are shown on the right. All tracts are bilateral. Signals in the spinoreticular tract facilitate the locus ceruleus neurons.

Labels in figure:

V. Descending cortical inhibition

Pituitary

IV. Hormonal (pituitary, β-endorphin, adrenals)

ACTH and β-endorphin

Periaqueductal grey

Midbrain

Junction of midbrain and pons

Locus ceruleus

III. Fast acting neuronal pathway from brainstem (PAG, locus ceruleus, raphe nuclei)

Ceruleospinal tract

Upper medulla

Raphe nuclei

Raphespinal tract

II. Dorsal horn

Cervical cord

C fiber

I. Peripheral

A

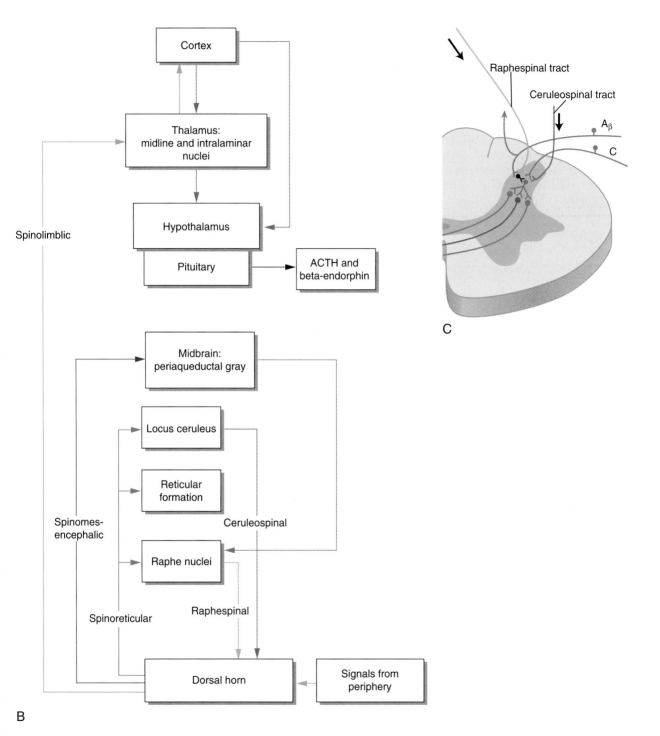

FIGURE 7-11, cont'd
B, Flowchart illustrating the same pathways as in **A.** The flow of slow pain information upward is shown on the left, and the descending antinociceptive pathways are shown on the right. **C,** A segment of the spinal cord. The raphespinal tract synapses with an interneuron (black) that inhibits the transmission of nociceptive information in the dorsal horn of the spinal cord. The ceruleospinal tract directly inhibits the primary nociceptive afferent.

BOX 7-2 NEUROPATHIC PAIN

Pathology
Ectopic foci, ephaptic transmission, abnormal connections of large afferents (Aβ) with nociceptive projection neurons in the dorsal horn, increased number of excitatory receptors and availability of transmitters in the nociceptive pathways, expansion of receptive fields, and/or malfunction of the pain matrix

Etiology
Trauma, inflammation, metabolic disorders, infection, tumor, toxin, autoimmune disorders (e.g., multiple sclerosis), pain matrix malfunction

Speed of Onset
Chronic

Signs and Symptoms
Consciousness, Communication, and Memory
Normal

Sensory
Paresthesia, dysesthesia, allodynia, and secondary hyperalgesia

Autonomic
May be impaired

Motor
May be impaired

Region Affected
Peripheral, spinal, brainstem, and/or cerebral

Demographics
One year prevalence: 19 per 1,000 people (Berger et al., 2004)

Prognosis
Variable, depending on genetic and environmental factors, type of neuropathic pain, and treatment

Table 7-4 DETECTING NEUROPATHIC PAIN

Cold Allodynia

Test: Ask patient "How does this feel?" Place a cold object, for example the metal handle of a reflex hammer, on the skin.	**Normal response:** perception of cold. **Neuropathic response:** perception of pain.

Brush Allodynia

Test: Ask patient "How does this feel?" Lightly stroke the skin with a 1-inch-wide foam brush. The stroke should be 3-5 cm (1.5-2 inches) long and require about 1 second (Lynch et al., 2005).	**Normal response:** perception of light touch. **Neuropathic response:** perception of pain.

Abnormal Temporal Summation

Test: Tell patient that you are going to tap on the skin with a nylon filament; ask "How does this feel?" For 5 to 10 seconds, repeatedly stimulate the same location on the skin with a stiff nylon filament, using the same amount of force each time.	**Normal response:** perception of the intensity of the stimulus remains constant. **Neuropathic response:** increasing perception of pain.

Secondary Hyperalgesia

Test: Ask patient "Does this feel the same on both sides?" Prick the skin with a sharp object on a normal area of the skin (contralateral to the affected area), and then prick the skin with the same object near the painful area on the affected side.	**Normal response:** perception is the same on both sides of the body. **Neuropathic response:** pain is more intense near the painful area.
Alternative test: Stimulate the normal side and ask "If this is worth one dollar," then stimulate the affected side and ask, "How much is this worth?"	**Normal response:** approximately one dollar **Neuropathic response:** significantly more than one dollar (e.g., $1.75)

conveyed into the central nervous system, a small amount of activity is generated in the central neurons, producing the usual level of output from the central neurons. However, peripheral injury can induce an abnormal increase in central nervous system responsiveness that persists after the peripheral injury has healed. The sensitization is created by increased availability of excitatory transmitters and an increased number of excitatory receptors. Central sensitization affects neurons throughout the nociceptive pathways, including cells in the dorsal horn, brainstem, thalamus, and cerebral cortex.

Intense signals from an injury in the periphery may cause central sensitization. In central sensitization, the central neurons produce neural output that is disproportionate to incoming nociceptive signals. Arnstein (1997) reported that if severe pain persists more than 24 hours, neuroplastic changes occur that are associated with intractable chronic pain. Figure 7-12 illustrates the process.

Cellular changes that reflect central sensitization include:

* Increased spontaneous activity
* Increased responsiveness to afferent inputs
* Prolonged afterdischarge (the part of the response to a stimulus that persists following the termination of the stimulus) in response to repeated stimuli
* Expansion of receptive fields (central neurons receive information from larger areas of tissue than normally)

The chemicals that produce these profound changes in physiology include glutamate and neuropeptides (Figure 7-13). Glutamate acts on both ligand-gated ion channels (AMPA and NMDA receptors) and G-protein–mediated receptors (metabotropic receptors) to increase cellular Ca^{++}. The peptides act via second-messenger systems to increase the activity of protein kinases. These changes lead to activation of genes, triggering increased cellular activity. For example, sensitized neurons in the spinothalamic tract are more easily excited, produce increased spontaneous activity, and undergo structural changes in neural connections (Willis, 2002). Thus, nociceptive information is not simply delivered to the brain. Instead, nociception can change the structure and function of the central nervous system.

The central sensitization process described is remarkably similar to long-term potentiation, the process vital for memory formation and learning. Therefore, although currently available NMDA antagonists have demonstrated efficacy in treating neuropathic pain, the side effects—primarily cognitive deficits—preclude the use of these agents to treat neuropathic pain. Because both peripheral inputs and central sensitization contribute to the maintenance of chronic pain, therapies must target both peripheral and central abnormalities. An anticonvulsant drug, gabapentin, has been reported to ease neuropathic pain with low toxicity and few side effects (Wetzel and Connelly, 1997).

> Central sensitization is a state of excessive excitability of central neurons in the nociceptive pathways. The critical events are NMDA receptor depolarization and an increase in intracellular Ca^{++}.

Structural Reorganization. Prolonged central sensitization leads to rewiring of connections in the central nervous system. In the dorsal horn, the structural changes include withdrawal of C-fiber axon terminals from the dorsal horn and growth of A_β-fiber axons into regions of the spinal cord that normally only receive C-fiber endings, with the formation of novel synapses between A_β fibers and central nociceptive neurons. Once the novel synapses have formed, stimulation of A_β fibers will produce impulses perceived as pain.

Altered Top-down Modulation. Antinociceptive signals are reduced, and pronociceptive signals are increased. People whose genetic code results in less production of an enzyme that regulates the levels of catecholamines and enkephalins are twice as likely to develop neuropathic pain as those who produce more of the enzyme (Diatchenko et al., 2005).

The mechanisms of nociceptive and neuropathic pain are summarized in Figure 7-14.

Sites That Generate Neuropathic Pain

Neuropathic pain can arise from abnormal neural activity in:

* The periphery (e.g., nerve compression in carpal tunnel syndrome)
* The central nervous system in response to loss of peripheral input (deafferentation or phantom limb pain)
* The dorsal horn and pain matrix

Peripheral Generation of Neuropathic Pain

Injury or disease of peripheral nerves often results in sensory abnormalities. A complete nerve section results in lack of sensation from that nerve's receptive field, but sometimes paresthesia and pain also occur in the denervated region. Partial damage to a nerve can result in allodynia and sensations like electric shock.

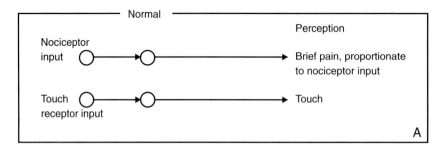

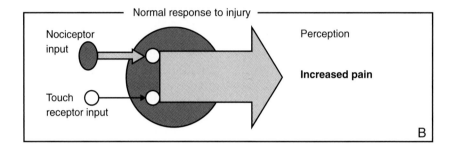

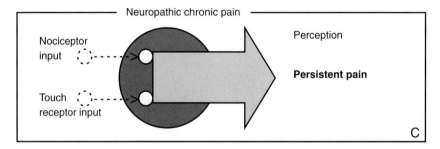

FIGURE 7-12

Contribution of both initial and ongoing central sensitization to excessive excitability of central nociceptive neurons. Open circles indicate the normal amount of activity in a neuron. Red circles indicate excessive neural activity due to sensitization. **A,** In the normal processing of brief, mild nociceptive inputs, there is a close correlation between the amount of input from peripheral nociceptors and the perception of pain. The neural output after central processing, indicated by the black arrow, is proportional to the input. Stimulation of touch receptors generates neural activity perceived as touch. **B,** Following injury, intensified, prolonged nociceptive input occurs due to peripheral sensitization. In turn, this abnormal input in response to injury produces sensitization of central neurons in the nociceptive pathway. The enlarged red oval for nociceptor input indicates sensitization of the nociceptive endings. The enlarged arrow from the peripheral nociceptor indicates increased input into the central nervous system. The large output arrow indicates the amplified output associated with central sensitization. Note that touch receptor information traveling on A_β fibers now activates increased pain. Prior to the injury, stimulation of the touch receptors produced only signals perceived as touch. **C,** In neuropathic chronic pain, the perception of pain may arise spontaneously, that is, without peripheral input. The central sensitization persists despite the lack of continuing signals from nociceptors. Alternatively, when a brief, small signal is sent from either nociceptors or touch receptors, the abnormal responses of the sensitized neurons produce an amplified perception of pain. In neuropathic chronic pain, no correlation exists between the amount of receptor stimulation and the perception of pain.

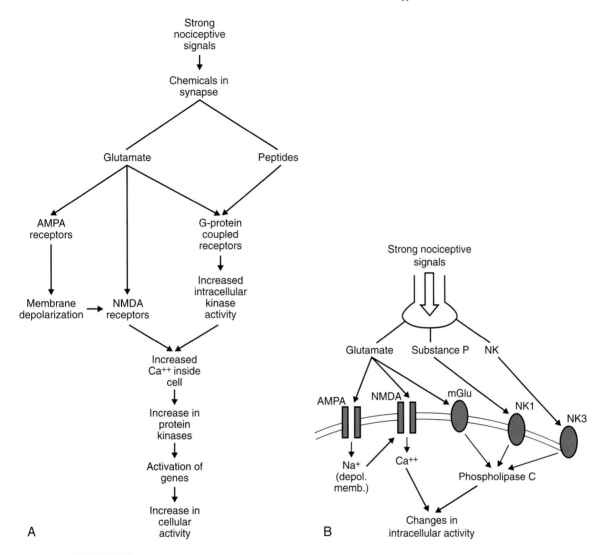

FIGURE 7-13

Central sensitization. **A,** Flowchart summarizing the sequence of events in central sensitization. **B,** Effects of intense activation of receptors involved in central sensitization. Strong nociceptive signals elicit the release of glutamate and the peptides substance P (SP) and neurokinin (NK). The binding of glutamate to the AMPA receptor depolarizes the postsynaptic neuron's membrane; then the combination of voltage change and binding of glutamate to the NMDA receptor opens the NMDA channel. Ca^{++} flows into the neuron through the NMDA channel. The remaining receptors involved in central sensitization act via second-messenger systems involving phospholipase C (an enzyme). Glutamate activates the metabotropic glutamate receptor (mGlu). Substance P and neurokinin activate neurokinin receptors (NKR). The effect of these second-messenger systems is to increase protein kinase activity, which in turn activates genes. The outcome is an increase in the activity of ion channels and intracellular enzymes, generating central sensitization.

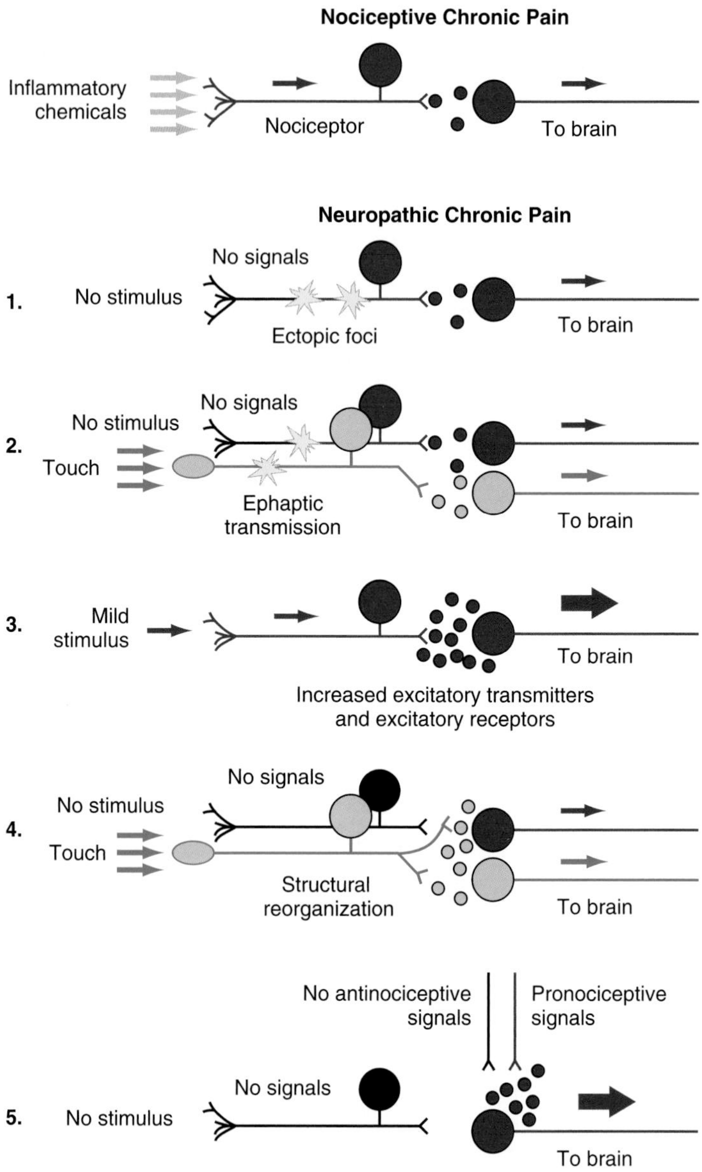

FIGURE 7-14

Mechanisms of nociceptive and neuropathic pain. The top panel illustrates normal physiologic function of the pain system: inflammatory chemicals at the site of injury have sensitized peripheral nociceptors, and signals indicating tissue damage travel to the brain. The numbered panels correspond to the sections in the text on neuropathic mechanisms: *1.* Ectopic foci, *2.* Ephaptic transmission from an A$_\beta$ tactile neuron to nociceptive fibers, *3.* Central sensitization, created by increased excitatory transmitter availability and an increased number of excitatory receptors, *4.* Structural reorganization, in this case the retraction of C-fiber proximal endings from nociceptive tract neurons and growth of A$_\beta$ tactile endings to synapse with nociceptive tract neurons, and *5.* Changes in pain matrix top-down regulation, with silence of the antinociceptive signals and excessive pronociceptive signals.

These unusual sensations are the result of aberrant activity in the peripheral nervous system, evoking abnormal responses in the central nervous system. Peripheral abnormalities causing neuropathic pain include the development of ephaptic transmission and ectopic foci in an injured nerve. Ephaptic transmission occurs in demyelinated regions. Ectopic foci can occur at the nerve stump, in areas of myelin damage, or in the dorsal root ganglion somas. These foci can become so sensitive to mechanical stimulation that tapping on an injured nerve can elicit pain or tingling (**Tinel's sign**). Examples of neuropathy that affect a single nerve (mononeuropathy) include median nerve entrapment in carpal tunnel syndrome and ulnar nerve compression at the elbow (see Chapter 11). Neuropathies that affect more than one nerve (polyneuropathies) include diabetic neuropathy and Guillain-Barré syndrome.

Centrally Generated Neuropathic Response to Loss of Peripheral Input

When peripheral sensory information is completely absent, as occurs in people with deafferentation or amputation, neurons in the central nervous system that formerly received information from the body part may become abnormally active. Avulsion of dorsal roots from the spinal cord produces **deafferentation** and causes people to feel burning pain in the area of sensory loss. Avulsion of dorsal roots of the brachial plexus sometimes occurs in motorcycle accidents. The extreme neck flexion when the head impacts the pavement pulls the dorsal roots out of the spinal cord.

Almost all people with amputations report sensations that seem to originate from the missing limb, called *phantom limb sensation.* Much less frequently, people with amputations report that their phantom sensation is painful. This condition is called phantom limb pain. Phantom limb pain must be differentiated from stump pain because some causes of stump pain can be successfully treated. Stump pain is caused peripherally by neuropathy, neuroma (a tumor of nerve tissue), a poorly fitting prosthesis, or nerve compression. In **phantom limb pain,** the absence of sensory information causes neurons in the central nociceptive pathways to become overactive. Maladaptive structural reorganization is found in the spinal cord, thalamus, and cerebral cortex. The cortex shows extensive overlap of cortical representations that are normally separate. For example, the thumb and finger representations overlap. Flor and Elbert (1998) demonstrated that massive cortical reorganization correlates with the severity of phantom limb pain. In some people with upper limb amputations, the abnormal representations can be reversed by anesthesia of the brachial plexus. Because this reversal occurs within minutes of the anesthesia administration, the mechanism of reorganization is probably unmasking of normally silent synapses (Flor and Elbert, 1998).

Pain Matrix Malfunction

When the pain matrix malfunctions, top-down regulation of pain is disturbed. Antinociception is reduced and/or pronociception is intensified. The result is increased pain. Fibromyalgia and complex regional pain syndrome involve disturbance of top-down regulation of pain.

Fibromyalgia. People with fibromyalgia have tenderness of muscles and adjacent soft tissues, stiffness of muscles, and aching pain. Mental or physical stress, trauma, and sleep disorders may contribute to the disorder. The painful area shows a regional rather than dermatomal or peripheral nerve distribution. Multiple reproducible tender points are found on palpation (Figure 7-15). The evidence that fibromyalgia is a neuropathic syndrome includes secondary hyperalgesia, allodynia, abnormal temporal summation to stimuli, and abnormal activation of the pain matrix.

Gracely et al. (2004) compared brain activation of people with and without fibromyalgia in response to 10 minutes of blunt, pulsing pressure to the base of the left thumbnail. When the same pressure intensity was used in both groups, (~2.5 kg/cm^2), people with fibromyalgia reported slightly intense pain and most of the pain matrix was activated. People without fibromyalgia reported that the stimulation was not painful and only part of the contralateral somatosensory cortex was activated. For control subjects to report slightly intense pain and to activate similar areas of the pain matrix required nearly twice as much pressure on the thumbnail. Thus the subjects with fibromyalgia demonstrated biological amplification of pain signals. The incidence of

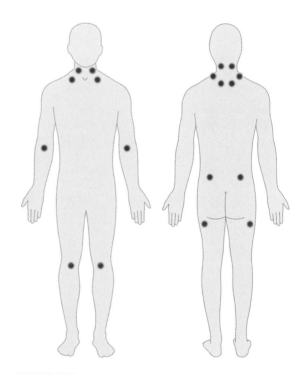

FIGURE 7-15
Tender points in fibromyalgia. The diagnosis of fibromyalgia requires that the person report pain with pressure at 11 or more of the 18 points indicated.

fibromyalgia is 35 per 100,000 people (Gallagher et al., 2004).

Complex Regional Pain Syndrome. **Complex regional pain syndrome** (CRPS) is a syndrome of pain, vascular changes, and atrophy (Figure 7-16). The term *regional* indicates that the signs and symptoms present in a regional distribution (upper limb or lower limb) rather than in a peripheral nerve or nerve root distribution. Typically the signs and symptoms are worst in the distal extremity, affecting the entire hand or foot. An aberrant response to trauma produces the syndrome. The trauma may be quite minor; for example, an ankle sprain that heals within a few days may precipitate the syndrome. The time between the trauma and the onset of CRPS is quite variable, from hours to weeks.

The primary complaint is severe, spontaneous pain, out of proportion to the original injury. The pain is aggravated by psychological as well as physical stimuli (sensitivity to cold, pressure, and touch). Early signs of CRPS include red or pale skin color, excessive sweating, edema, and skin atrophy. Later, the skin becomes dry and cold. If the condition progresses to its late stage, irreversible muscle atrophy, osteoporosis, and arthritic changes occur. Motor signs that may be associated include paresis, spasms, and tremor (Birklein, 2005). Formerly, reduction of signs and symptoms following injection of an anesthetic into sympathetic ganglia was considered diagnostic for CRPS. However, the response to sympathetic nerve block is not diagnostic, because later in the course of the disorder the pathology migrates into the central nervous system (Knobler, 2000).

Disuse of the limb is a primary precipitating factor in the development of CRPS. Classic theories postulate excessive activity of sympathetic efferents, but findings of low serum levels of norepinephrine in the affected limb indicate that sympathetic efferents are not

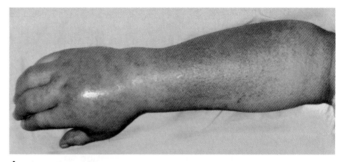

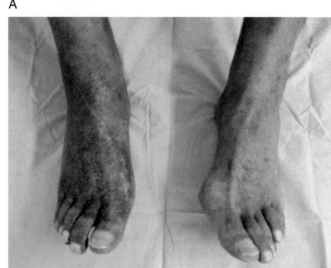

FIGURE 7-16

Complex regional pain syndrome (CRPS) causes intense pain in a limb, swelling, changes in skin color and temperature, and sweating. *(From Albrecht PJ et al {2006}. Pathological alterations of cutaneous innervation and vasculature in affected limbs from patients with complex regional pain syndrome. Pain, 120; p 246.)*

overactive. Pathologic processes in CRPS include increased levels of neurochemicals that produce neurogenic inflammation in the periphery, impairment of sympathetic regulation of blood flow and sweating, sensitization, and cortical reorganization (shrinkage of the hand or foot representation in the cortex; Birklein 2005, Pleger et al., 2005). The disorder affects children as well as adults: the youngest CRPS case documented in the literature is a 2½-year-old girl whose upper limb was affected (Güler-Uysal et al., 2003). The tendency to develop CRPS in response to trauma appears to be genetic (van de Beek et al., 2003) (Box 7-3).

Therapy is essential for complex regional pain syndrome (Birklein, 2005). Therapy consists of active and active-assisted exercise, including scrubbing and carrying activities, to tolerance (Li et al., 2005). Passive manipulation may aggravate CRPS. Despite the lack of efficacy of sympathetic nerve block for diagnosis, treatment during the early stage may be aided by sympathetic blockade. Thus, for lower limb CRPS, the lumbar sympathetic chain is blocked. For the upper limb, the stellate ganglion is blocked (see Figure 8-7). These sympathetic blocks are only effective in some people, and only during the early stage of the disorder. As CRPS progresses, the source of pain centralizes. That is, changes occur in the central nervous system that perpetuate the pain. Once the pain has centralized, sympathetic block has no effect on the signs and symptoms of CRPS. However, other drug treatments may be beneficial (Quisel et al., 2005).

The terms *causalgia, Sudeck's atrophy, sympathetically maintained pain,* and *reflex sympathetic dystrophy* are often used synonymously with complex regional pain syndrome, despite the attempts of some authors to distinguish among these terms. CRPS following stroke is often termed shoulder-hand syndrome. A prospective study demonstrated that a prevention program produced a reduction in post-stroke CRPS from 27% to 8%. The program consisted of daily physical therapy and instruction to all hospital staff and family members on methods to avoid trauma to the paretic upper limb (Braus et al., 1994).

Table 7-5 summarizes the difference between nociceptive and neuropathic pain.

Chronic Pain Syndromes

Migraine

Migraine is a neurogenic disorder. In migraine, a disorder of sensory processing produces pain matrix

---

BOX 7-3   COMPLEX REGIONAL PAIN SYNDROME

Pathology
Increased levels of inflammatory neurochemicals in the periphery, impairment of sympathetic regulation of blood flow and sweating, sensitization, and cortical reorganization

Etiology
Usually secondary to trauma; genetic predisposition

Speed of Onset
Chronic

Signs and Symptoms
  Consciousness
Normal
  Communication and Memory
Normal
  Sensory
Severe, spontaneous pain, often intensified by skin contact, heat, and cold
  Autonomic
Abnormal sweating, vasodilation in skin, atrophy (due to blood flow changes and disuse) of muscles, joints, and skin
  Motor
May have paresis, spasms, and tremor; muscle atrophy

Region Affected
Initially peripheral; as progresses, cortical reorganization occurs

Demographics
4 times more frequent in women
  Incidence
5.5 per 100,000 people (Sandroni et al., 2003)

Prognosis
Early intervention has best outcome; intensive physical therapy often required; some cases are intractable (Li et al., 2005)

---

malfunction that amplifies nociceptive signals in the trigemino-thalamo-cortical pathway (Goadsby, 2005).

Migraine headaches are characterized by at least two of the following: unilateral location, pulsating quality, severity that interferes with daily activities, and aggravation by routine physical activity. During the headache, nausea, vomiting, photophobia (fear and avoidance of light), and/or phonophobia (fear and avoidance of sound) are present (Martin et al., 2005). Untreated migraines last from 4 to 72 hours in adults and from 2 to 15 hours in children younger than 15 years old. Twenty-four

Table 7-5   CHRONIC SOMATIC PAIN: NOCICEPTIVE VERSUS NEUROPATHIC

Nociceptive Pain		
Neural activity is normal and appropriate. Normal transmission of information regarding tissue damage or threat of damage from nociceptors. Pain is a symptom.	Examples: Arthritis pain Cancer pain Mechanical low back pain	Patient description of pain: dull, aching, throbbing; rarely sharp. Clinical descriptors: primary hyperalgesia at location of injury

Neuropathic Pain		

Pathological neural activity. Pain is a disease, caused by neurochemical, gene expression, and anatomical changes in neurons.	Four types:
	1. Peripherally generated:
	   Painful mononeuropathies
	   Nerve entrapment
	   Trigeminal neuralgia
	   Painful polyneuropathies
	   Diabetic neuropathy
	   Guillain-Barré syndrome
	2. Centrally generated response to loss
	   of afferent information
	   Deafferentation pain
	   Phantom limb pain
	3. Pain matrix malfunction
	   Fibromyalgia
	   Complex regional pain syndrome
	   Postherpetic neuralgia
	   Migraine
	4. Other
	   Chronic low back pain syndrome
	   Episodic tension-type headache
		Patient description of pain: burning, shooting, tingling, electrical, lightning sensations. Clinical descriptors: paresthesia, dysesthesia, allodynia, and secondary hyperalgesia

percent of females and five percent of males have one or more migraines per year (Lyngberg et al., 2005a).

Some migraines are preceded, accompanied, or followed by an aura. An aura is a transient neurologic disorder that involves sensory, motor, or cognitive symptoms. Typically an aura develops over 5-20 minutes and lasts less than an hour. During visual aura, visual cortex neurons rapidly depolarize with a massive redistribution of ions across cell membranes. K+ and organic anions exit and Na^+, Ca^{++}, and Cl^- enter the neurons (Somjen, 2001). This depolarization produces visual illusions. Subsequently the neurons are temporarily unresponsive. The metabolic load during depolarization elicits dilation of the blood vessels in the meninges and activation of the nociceptive fibers that innervate the vessels.

Basilar migraine is a subtype of migraine with aura, affecting the territory of the basilar artery. The aura consists of at least two of the following: ataxia, visual symptoms in both hemifields of both eyes, double vision, vertigo (a spinning sensation), tinnitus (ringing in the ears), decreased hearing, dysarthria (disturbance of speech), bilateral paresthesia, bilateral paresis, and a decreased level of consciousness.

A once prevalent theory of migraine etiology, that initial vasoconstriction subsequently produced vasodilation and headache, has not been supported by blood flow studies. In people susceptible to migraine, cortical and brainstem neurons are hyperexcitable due to channelopathy (dysfunction of ion channels), mitochondrial abnormalities, or possibly excessive nitric oxide (Bigal et al., 2002). The tendency to have migraines is strongly influenced by genetic factors (Ulrich et al., 2004). The cascade of events in migraine (Aurora et al., 2005; Burstein and Jakubowski, 2005; Ramadan, 2005; Silberstein et al., 2005) is as follows:

1. Migraine trigger (bright light, loud noise, prostaglandins, emotional stress, hormonal changes, specific foods or drinks, or meteorologic changes)

2. Excitation of hyperexcitable brainstem neurons (Afridi et al., 2005)
3. Only in people who experience aura: Hyperexcitable cerebral cortex neurons cause increased metabolic load, eliciting vasodilation. The vasodilation stimulates trigeminal nociceptors in the blood vessels. Nociceptive signals in the trigeminal afferents trigger the trigeminal reflex: neurons antidromically release neurochemicals that inflame the meningeal blood vessels (neurogenic inflammation). This causes peripheral sensitization of the trigeminal nociceptors.

4. Activation of trigeminal afferents that synapse with trigeminal lemniscus neurons. Trigeminal lemniscus and thalamocortical neurons become sensitized during a migraine, due to pain matrix malfunction.

Figure 7-17 illustrates the sequence of events in migraine. The pain matrix malfunction disrupts antinociception and promotes pronociception affecting the trigemino-thalamo-cortical pathway (Goadsby, 2005). Estrogen cycles and changes in melatonin levels can interfere with function of the pain matrix. The neurogenic inflammation process can be inhibited by serotonin

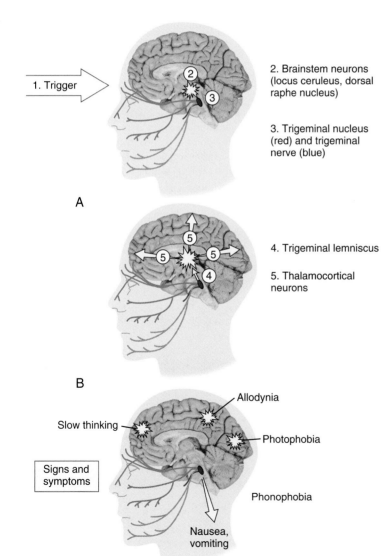

A

2. Brainstem neurons (locus ceruleus, dorsal raphe nucleus)

3. Trigeminal nucleus (red) and trigeminal nerve (blue)

B

4. Trigeminal lemniscus

5. Thalamocortical neurons

C

Allodynia

Slow thinking

Photophobia

Signs and symptoms

Phonophobia

Nausea, vomiting

FIGURE 7-17
Sequence of events in a migraine. **A,** Migraine begins when a trigger *(1)* activates hyperexcitable brainstem neurons *(2)* that activate the trigeminal nucleus and sensitize the trigeminal nerve *(3)*. **B,** Signals from the trigeminal nucleus sensitize the trigeminal lemniscus *(4)* and thalamocortical neurons *(5),* causing these neurons to fire excessively. **C,** The signs and symptoms of migraine imposed on a midsagittal section. Phonophobia is not indicated by a yellow flash because the auditory area is located in the lateral cerebral cortex.

agonists, including sumatriptan, rizatriptan, and other triptan drugs. The serotonin agonists also block synaptic transmission between the trigeminovascular afferents and the trigeminothalamic neurons (Burstein and Jakubowski, 2005).

Episodic Tension-Type Headache

The criteria for episodic tension-type headache (ETTH) include mild to moderate pain, usually bilateral, lasting 30 minutes to seven days, not aggravated by physical activity and not associated with nausea or vomiting. Photophobia or phonophobia but not both may accompany the headache. The mechanism of ETTH appears to be supersensitivity to nitric oxide, a molecule used in the transmission of nerve impulses. Nitric oxide sensitizes nociceptive pathways in the CNS (Ashina, 2004). The 1-year prevalence is 87% (Lyngberg, 2005b). Environmental factors appear to be much more important in ETTH than genetic factors (Ulrich et al., 2004). Environmental factors include volatile organic compounds (e.g., fumes from paint, lacquers, plastics), molds, lighting, noise, excessive heating, air conditioning, and psychosocial pressure (Woolhouse, 2005).

Chronic Low Back Pain Syndrome

Compared to people who either have subacute low back pain or are pain free, people with chronic low back pain syndrome have more emotional distress and less

endurance of the abdominal and back muscles (Brox et al., 2005). The transition from acute low back pain after injury to chronic low back pain has been characterized by Waddell et al. (1993) as a change in pain etiology from tissue damage to a physiologic impairment consisting of the following:

- Muscle guarding
- Abnormal movement
- Disuse syndrome

Subsequent research continues to support these physiologic impairments as significant factors in chronic low back pain syndrome (Barr et al., 2005). Figure 7-18 emphasizes the elements contributing to acute and chronic low back pain. In discussing chronic low back pain, Waddell (1987) cautions that "physical treatment directed to a supposed but unidentified and possibly nonexistent nociceptive source is not only understandably unsuccessful but failed treatment may both reinforce and aggravate pain, distress, disability, and illness behavior." For example, when a person complains of low back pain and magnetic resonance imaging (MRI) shows a bulging intervertebral disk, treatment may be directed toward the disk. However, Jensen and Brant-Zawadzki (1994) found that 64% of people *without* low back pain had abnormal findings on MRI of the lower spine, leading to the conclusion that disk bulges or protrusions may be coincidental rather than causative of low back pain. The emotional and cognitive aspects posited by

FIGURE 7-18
The differences between factors in acute and chronic low back pain. (*Redrawn from Waddell G, Newton M, et al. (1993). A fear-avoidance beliefs questionnaire (FABQ) and the role of fear-avoidance beliefs in chronic low back pain and disability. Pain, 52(2), 157-168.*)

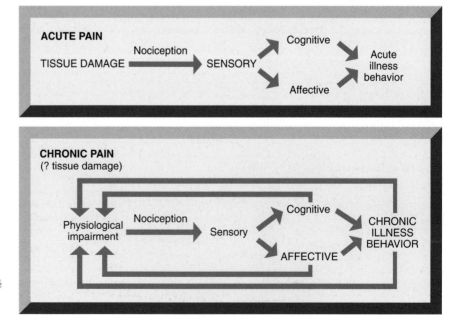

Waddell et al. are supported by the increasing acceptance of the biopsychosocial model (Pincus et al., 2002) and by the short-term effectiveness of behavioral treatment for chronic low back pain syndrome (Ostelo et al., 2003) (Box 7-4).

Brain scans show amplified pain signals in patients with idiopathic chronic low back pain. Giesecke et al. (2004) scanned the low back of patients for signs of musculoskeletal injury and eliminated patients from the study who had signs of disk, ligament, muscle, or joint damage. The pain threshold to blunt pressure on the thumbnail was compared between control and chronic low back pain subjects. At equal levels of pressure, those with chronic low back pain reported significantly greater pain and had more areas of the pain matrix activated than in the control subjects. Only part of the contralateral

somatosensory cortex was activated in the control subjects. This study also examined fibromyalgia patients, and reported similar outcomes to those reported by Gracely et al., 2002.

When pain persists, depression, sleep disturbance, preoccupation with pain, decreased activity, and fatigue are common.

> Chronic low back pain syndrome is a physiologic impairment consisting of muscle guarding, abnormal movement, and disuse syndrome.

Surgical Treatment of Chronic Pain

Theoretically, cutting selected dorsal roots (**dorsal rhizotomy**) or the spinothalamic tracts should eliminate pain sensation in people with pain that is resistant to other treatments. In practice, however, dorsal rhizotomy often fails to alleviate pain. The persistence of pain following spinothalamic tractotomy may be due to central nervous system changes in response to the original maintained pain or to pain-mediating fibers traveling in the dorsal columns (see Chapter 6).

RED FLAGS FOR HEADACHE

The following lists are compiled from Joubert (2005) and Dowson (2003).

Signs that headache may be caused by excessive pressure, including hydrocephalus or tumor:
- Headache present at wakening
- Pain triggered by coughing, sneezing, or straining
- Vomiting (may also indicate migraine)
- Worse when lying down

Sign that headache is caused by serious intracranial disease, including tumor, encephalitis, or meningitis:
- Progressive worsening over days or weeks
- Neck stiffness and vomiting (irritation of meninges)
- Rash and fever (bacterial meningitis or Lyme disease)
- History of cancer, HIV infection

Signs that headache may be caused by hemorrhage:
- Headache following head injury
- Abrupt onset

Headache associated with onset of paralysis or reduced level of consciousness (confusion, drowsiness, memory loss, loss of consciousness) is a strong indication for neuroimaging (Sobri et al., 2003).

BOX 7-4   CHRONIC LOW BACK PAIN SYNDROME

Pathology
Decreased endurance of abdominal and back muscles

Etiology
Deconditioning, pain matrix malfunction

Speed of Onset
Chronic

Signs and Symptoms
Consciousness
Normal
Communication and Memory
Normal
Sensory
Aching pain
Autonomic
Normal
Motor
Muscle guarding, disuse, abnormal movement patterns
Neural Region Affected
Central nervous system

Demographics
Incidence
10,000-15,000 per 100,000 people population per year
Prevalence
United States one 1-year prevalence of low back pain lasting at least one 1 month: 180 per 1000 people (Dillon et al., 2004)

Prognosis
Variable

RED FLAGS FOR LOW BACK PAIN

The following list is from Atlas and Deyo, 2001.
- No improvement with bed rest
- Age ≥50
- Previous or current history of cancer
- Unexplained weight loss
- Severe trauma
- History of osteoporosis
- Substance abuse
- Fever or chills
- Recent skin or urinary infection
- Immunosuppression
- Corticosteroid use
- Symptoms unrelated to activity
- Sciatica
- Leg pain that worsens with standing or walking and is relieved by sitting
- Urinary and/or bowel incontinence or retention
- Lower limb weakness

SUMMARY

Somatosensation is essential for smooth, accurate movements and to prevent injury. Testing of somatosensation includes testing discriminative touch, conscious proprioception, pinprick sensation (fast pain), and discriminative temperature sensations. Sensory nerve function can also be evaluated using nerve conduction studies and somatosensory evoked potentials.

Lesions of the proprioceptive pathway produce sensory ataxia. Peripheral nerve lesions may interrupt all somatosensation in the distribution of the nerve. Compression of a nerve primarily affects the function of large-diameter axons. Spinal region lesions affecting somatosensation include complete transection or hemisection of the cord, posterior column lesions, and infection. Varicella zoster selectively infects the cell bodies of somatosensory neurons, causing pain in a specific dermatome or trigeminal nerve branch.

Pain is a complex experience. The lateral pain system discriminates the location of actual or potential tissue damage. The medial pain system processes the motivational-affective and cognitive-evaluative aspects of pain.

Musculoskeletal injury or ischemia sensitizes peripheral nociceptors and thus causes pain in response to stimuli that are not normally painful. Sensitization can also occur in the dorsal horn and in the pain matrix. Pain matrix activity can cause pain perception in the absence of nociceptive input. Antinociception can occur in the periphery, dorsal horn, neuronal descending system, hormonal system, and the cerebral cortex.

Chronic pain can be caused by continuing stimulation of nociceptors, by neuropathic processes, or by chronic pain syndromes. The neuropathic processes include ectopic foci, ephaptic transmission, central sensitization, structural reorganization, and altered top-down pain modulation (Figure 7-19). Examples of neuropathic pain include mononeuropathies, polyneuropathies, deafferentation and phantom limb pain, fibromyalgia, and complex regional pain syndrome. Pain syndromes include migraine, episodic tension-type headache, and chronic low back pain.

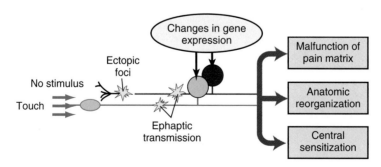

FIGURE 7-19

Mechanisms of neuropathic pain. Lesions of peripheral nerves cause changes in gene expression of the injured neurons, resulting in production of sodium channels that are inserted into the injured membrane and begin to generate ectopic action potentials. Lesions of peripheral nerves may also cause demyelination, resulting in ephaptic transmission. Pathologic changes in the central nervous system that cause neuropathic pain include changes in gene expression in the primary neuron cell bodies, central sensitization (gene activation in projection neurons), anatomic reorganization, and malfunction of the pain matrix.

CLINICAL NOTES

Case 1

A 25-year-old man sustained an incomplete spinal cord injury in an industrial accident. His left leg is paralyzed. With his eyes closed, the following sensory deficits are noted:

- Left lower extremity: Cannot report direction of passive joint movement of the hip, knee, ankle, and toes.
- Left side, below L2 level: Cannot distinguish between two closely spaced points applied to the skin or detect vibration.
- Right lower extremity below L4 level: Cannot distinguish between test tubes filled with warm or cold water, or between sharp and dull stimuli
- Reduced sensation in left L2 dermatome.
- Intact sensation: All sensations intact above L2 level.
- Left lower extremity: Can distinguish between test tubes filled with warm or cold water and can distinguish between sharp and dull stimuli.
- Right lower extremity: Can distinguish between two closely spaced points applied to the skin, can accurately report direction of passive movements of the joints, and can detect vibration.

Question

Explain the pattern of sensory loss seen in this person.

Case 2

A 42-year-old chef is unable to work because of weakness and altered sensation in her dominant right hand. She reports difficulty lifting heavy skillets that began 2 months ago. Tingling in the thumb, index, and middle fingers and half of the ring finger began 6 weeks ago. Currently, she is unable to stir anything for more than 5 minutes using her right hand. The thenar muscles are visibly atrophied. The results of motor and sensory testing of the right upper limb are as follows:

- Pinch grip on the right is 30 g (versus 120 g with left hand).
- Diminished sensation in the lateral three and a half digits.
- Strength, reflexes, and sensation are within normal limits throughout the remainder of the right upper extremity.

Question

What is the location and probable etiology of the lesion?

Case 3

A 73-year-old man was found unconscious on the floor at home 1 week ago. He is now lucid and cooperative. Sensation and movement are within normal limits on the right side of the body and face. He has sensory extinction on the left side. The lower half of the left side of his face appears to droop, and he cannot actively move the left limbs. When assisted to sitting, he collapses as soon as support is removed.

Question

What is the location and probable etiology of the lesion?

Case 4

A 24-year-old woman was stopped at a traffic signal when her car was struck from behind. She noted some stiffness of her neck the following day; within a week, her upper back was also stiff and becoming painful. X-rays were normal. During the next 2 weeks, she was free of pain. Now, 5 weeks after the accident, she is seeking treatment because the neck aching has returned, turning her head while driving is painful, and she has dull headaches. She denies having reinjured her neck but reports stressful deadlines at work. She has no motor or sensory loss. Active neck range of motion is as follows:

Continued

CLINICAL NOTES

- 20° forward flexion, 35° extension (30% and 70% of normal values)
- Lateral flexion: 15° to left, 24° to right (38% and 60% of normal)
- Rotation: 20° to left, 33° to right (36% and 60% of normal)

Question

What is the probable etiology of the problem?

Case 5

CM, a 42-year-old man, sustained mild soft tissue damage to his right wrist in a fall 4 months ago. Since the injury, he has completely stopped using his right upper limb. CM was initially evaluated in physical therapy 1 week ago. At that time he reported that he wears a sling, even while sleeping, and protects his entire right arm as much as possible. He also reported a constant burning sensation and that any stimulation, even putting on clothes or a breeze across the skin, evokes sharp pain. The therapist observed the following abnormalities in his fourth and fifth fingers: excessive sweating; shiny, red skin; and opaque, long fingernails. CM stated that he cannot tolerate cutting the nails because of pain. When asked to move his right arm, CM refused. He did allow passive flexion of the shoulder to 40°. CM refused to allow the therapist to touch his distal arm and refused to actively move his hand or wrist.

The following day, CM's doctor injected the right stellate ganglion with lidocaine, a drug that reversibly depresses neuronal function. After the injection, CM's upper eyelid drooped, his pupil was constricted, and sweating on the ipsilateral face and neck was absent. These side effects of the block indicate that the injection was successful in blocking sympathetic activity in the stellate ganglion. The intended result of the block, disrupting the pain in the right upper limb, ensued, and CM reluctantly moved his wrist and hand actively in therapy the same day. He requires vigorous daily physical therapy to move his hand and continues to protect his arm when not in therapy.

Questions

1. What is the most likely diagnosis? Why?
2. How was the diagnosis confirmed?

REVIEW QUESTIONS

1. How is a quick screening for somatosensory impairments performed?
2. What are the important limitations of sensory testing?
3. What signs and/or symptoms indicate that a thorough somatosensory evaluation should be performed?
4. What precautions are essential to ensure valid results of somatosensory testing?
5. How is a sensory nerve conduction study performed?
6. A patient describes spontaneous tingling and prickling in both feet. What clinical term corresponds to this description?
7. How can a clinician distinguish between sensory and cerebellar ataxia?
8. Which types of somatosensory information are usually most impaired by demyelination? Why?
9. What sensory and motor losses occur with a left hemisection of the spinal cord? Name the resulting syndrome.
10. What is varicella zoster?
11. Describe the sensory loss associated with a lesion in the left posterolateral lower pons.
12. What is sensory extinction?
13. How does the counterirritant theory explain the inhibition of pain messages by the application of pressure to an injured finger?
14. An inability to sleep due to nociception is an example of what aspect of the pain experience: discriminative, motivational-affective, or cognitive-evaluative?
15. List the origins of the three supraspinal analgesic systems.
16. How do narcotics induce their effects?
17. Name the levels of the antinociception model.

18. Define *referred pain.*
19. What is the difference between nociceptive chronic pain and neuropathic chronic pain?
20. What is central sensitization?
21. What happens when novel synapses form between Aβ afferents and central nociceptive neurons?
22. List four examples of neuropathic chronic pain.
23. Define paresthesia and dysesthesia.

24. What are ectopic foci?
25. What is phantom limb pain?
26. Often, people with chronic low back pain have no identifiable tissue damage. Waddell et al. (1993) propose that physiologic changes following acute low back injury may cause the chronic pain. What are the changes Waddell et al. cite as responsible for the continued pain?

References

Abelson K (2005). Acetylcholine in spinal pain modulation. Medicine. Uppsala, Uppsala University, 56.

Afridi S, Giffin NJ, et al. (2005). A positron emission tomographic study in spontaneous migraine. Archives of Neurology, 62(8), 1270-1275.

Arnstein PM (1997). The neuroplastic phenomenon: A physiologic link between chronic pain and learning. Journal of Neuroscience Nursing, 29(3), 179-186.

Ashina M (2004). Neurobiology of chronic tension-type headache. Cephalalgia, 24(3), 161-172.

Atlas SJ, Deyo RA (2001). Evaluating and managing acute low back pain in the primary care setting. Journal of General Internal Medicine, 16(2), 120-131.

Aurora SK, Barrodale P, et al. (2005). Cortical inhibition is reduced in chronic and episodic migraine and demonstrates a spectrum of illness. Headache, 45(5), 546-552.

Barr KP, Griggs M, et al. (2005). Lumbar stabilization: Core concepts and current literature, Part 1. American Journal of Physical Medicine & Rehabilitation/Association of Academic Physiatrists, 84(6), 473-480.

Bell-Krotoski JA, Buford WL Jr. (1997). The force/time relationship of clinically used sensory testing instruments. Journal of Hand Therapy, 10(4), 297-309.

Bell-Krotoski J, Weinstein S, et al. (1993). Testing sensibility, including touch-pressure, two-point discrimination, point localization, and vibration. Journal of Hand Therapy, 6(2), 114-123.

Berger A, Dukes EM, et al. (2004). Clinical characteristics and economic costs of patients with painful neuropathic disorders. Journal of Pain, 5(3), 143-149.

Bigal ME, Rapoport AM, et al. (2002). New migraine preventive options: An update with pathophysiological considerations. Revista do Hospital das Clínicas Sao Paulo, 57(6), 293-298.

Birklein F (2005). Complex regional pain syndrome. Journal of Neurology, 252(2), 131-138.

Braus DF, Krauss JK, et al. (1994). The shoulder-hand syndrome after stroke: A prospective clinical trial. Annals of Neurology, 36(5), 728-733.

Brooks J, Tracey I (2005). From nociception to pain perception: Imaging the spinal and supraspinal pathways. Journal of Anatomy, 207(1), 19-33.

Brox JI, Storheim K, et al. (2005). Disability, pain, psychological factors and physical performance in healthy controls, patients with sub-acute and chronic low back pain: A case-control study. Journal of Rehabilitation Medicine, 37(2), 95-99.

Burstein R, Jakubowski M (2005). Implications of multimechanism therapy: When to treat? Neurology, 64(10 Suppl 2), S16-S20.

Craig KD (1999). Emotions and psychobiology. In PD Wall and R Melzack (Eds.), Textbook of Pain (pp. 331-344). Edinburgh: Churchill Livingstone.

Diatchenko L, Slade GD, et al. (2005). Genetic basis for individual variations in pain perception and the development of a chronic pain condition. Human Molecular Genetics, 14(1), 135-143.

Dillon C, Paulose-Ram R, et al. (2004). Skeletal muscle relaxant use in the United States: Data from the Third National Health and Nutrition Examination Survey (NHANES III). Spine, 29(8): 892-896.

Doubell TP (1999). The dorsal horn: State-dependent sensory processing, plasticity, and the generation of pain. In PD Wall and R Melzack (Eds.), Textbook of Pain (pp. 165-182). Edinburgh: Churchill Livingstone.

Dowson AJ (2003). Casebook: Headache. Practitioner, 247(1642): 45-52.

Eisenberger NI, Lieberman MD, et al. (2003). Does rejection hurt? An FMRI study of social exclusion. Science, 302(5643): 290-292.

Flor H, Elbert T (1998). Maladaptive consequences of cortical reorganization in humans. NeuroScience News, 1(5), 4-11.

Gallagher AM, Thomas JM, et al. (2004). Incidence of fatigue symptoms and diagnoses presenting in UK primary care from 1990 to 2001. Journal of the Royal Society of Medicine, 97(12): 571-575.

Giamberardino MA (2003). Referred muscle pain/ hyperalgesia and central sensitization. Journal of Rehabilitation Medicine, May(41 Suppl), 85-88.

Giesecke T, Gracely RH, et al. (2004). Evidence of augmented central pain processing in idiopathic chronic low back pain. Arthritis and Rheumatism, 50(2), 613-623.

Gnann JW Jr., Whitley RJ (2002). Clinical practice. Herpes zoster. New England Journal of Medicine, 347(5), 340-346.

Goadsby PJ (2005). Migraine pathology. Headache, 45(Suppl 1), S14-S24.

Gracely RH, Geisser ME, et al. (2004). Pain catastrophizing and neural responses to pain among persons with fibromyalgia. Brain, 127(Pt 4), 835-843.

Gracely RH, Petzke F, et al. (2002). Functional magnetic resonance imaging evidence of augmented pain processing in fibromyalgia. Arthritis and Rheumatism, 46(5): 1333-1343.

Güler-Uysal F, Basaran S, et al. (2003). A 2½-year-old girl with reflex sympathetic dystrophy syndrome (CRPS type I): Case report. Clinical Rehabilitation, 17(2), 224-227.

Harden RN (2005). Chronic neuropathic pain. Mechanisms, diagnosis, and treatment. Neurologist, 11(2), 111-122.

IASP Task Force on Taxonomy (1994). Classification of Chronic Pain. In H Merskey and N Bogduk (Eds), Seattle, IASP Press, 209-214.

Ingvar M, Hsieh J-C (1999). The image of pain. In PD Wall and R Melzack (Eds.), Textbook of pain (pp. 215-234). Edinburgh: Churchill Livingstone.

Jensen MC, Brant-Zawadzki MN (1994). Magnetic resonance imaging of the lumbar spine in people without back pain. New England Journal of Medicine, 331(2), 69-73.

Johnson RW, Dworkin RH (2003). Treatment of herpes zoster and postherpetic neuralgia. BMJ, 326(7392), 748-750.

Joubert J (2005). Diagnosing headache. Australian Family Physician, 34(8). 621-625.

Knobler RL (2000). Reflex sympathetic dystrophy. In R W Evans, DS Baskin, et al. (Eds.), Prognosis of Neurological Disorders. New York: Oxford University Press.

Li Z, Smith BP, et al. (2005). Diagnosis and management of complex regional pain syndrome complicating upper extremity recovery. Journal of Hand Therapy, 18(2), 270-276.

Liebeskind JC (1991). Pain can kill. Pain, 44, 3-4.

Lipp J (1991). Possible mechanisms of morphine analgesia. Clinical Neuropharmacology, 14(2), 131-147.

Lynch ME, Clark AJ, et al. (2005). Topical 2% amitriptyline and 1% ketamine in neuropathic pain syndromes: A randomized, double-blind, placebo-controlled trial. Anesthesiology, 103(1), 140-146.

Lyngberg, AC, Rasmussen, BK, et al. (2005a). Incidence of Primary Headache: A Danish Epidemiologic Follow-up Study. American Journal of Epidemiology, 161(11), 1066-1073.

Lyngberg, AC, Rasmussen, BK, et al. (2005b). Has the prevalence of migraine and tension-type headache changed over a 12-year period? A Danish population survey. European Journal of Epidemiology, 20(3), 243-249.

MacDonald BK, Cockerell OC, et al. (2000). The incidence and lifetime prevalence of neurological disorders in a prospective community-based study in the UK (see comments). Brain, 123(Pt. 4), 665-676.

Martin VT, Penzien DB, et al. (2005). The predictive value of abbreviated migraine diagnostic criteria. Headache, 45(9), 1102-1112.

Melzack R, Wall PD (1965). Pain mechanisms: A new theory. Science, 150, 971-979.

Nicholson BD (2003). Diagnosis and management of neuropathic pain: A balanced approach to treatment. Journal of the American Academy of Nurse Practitioners, 15(12 Suppl), 3-9.

Nicholson K, Martelli MF (2004). The problem of pain. Journal of Head Trauma Rehabilitation, 19(1), 2-9.

Nolan MF (1982). Two-point discrimination assessment in the upper limb in young adult men and women. Physical Therapy, 62, 965-969.

Nolan, MF (1983). Limits of two-point discrimination ability in the lower limb in young adult men and women. Physical Therapy, 63, 1424-1428.

Nolan, MF (1985). Quantitative measure of cutaneous sensation. Two-point discrimination values for the face and trunk. Physical Therapy, 65(2), 181-185.

Ostelo RW, de Vet HC, et al. (2003). Behavioral graded activity following first-time lumbar disc surgery: 1-year results of a randomized clinical trial. Spine, 28(16), 1757-1765.

Pincus T, Burton AK, et al. (2002). A systematic review of psychological factors as predictors of chronicity/disability in prospective cohorts of low back pain. Spine, 27(5), E109-E120.

Pleger B, Tegenthoff M, et al. (2005). Sensorimotor retuning [corrected] in complex regional pain syndrome parallels pain reduction. Annals of Neurology, 57(3), 425-429.

Quisel A, Gill JM, et al. (2005). Complex regional pain syndrome underdiagnosed. Journal of Family Practice, 54(6), 524-532.

Ramadan NM (2005). Targeting therapy for migraine: What to treat? Neurology, 64(10 Suppl 2), S4-S8.

Rothwell JC, Traub MM, et al. (1982). Manual motor performance in a deafferented man. Brain, 105, 515-542.

Sandroni P, Benrud-Larson LM, et al. (2003). Complex regional pain syndrome type I: Incidence and prevalence in Olmsted county, a population-based study. Pain, 103(1-2), 199-207.

Sherrington, C S (1900). The muscular sense. In: E.A. Schafer (Ed.). Textbook of physiology. (pp 1002-1025). Edinburgh: Pentland. Vol 2.

Silberstein SD, Lipton RB, et al. (2005). From Migraine Mechanisms to Innovative Therapeutic Drugs. Neurology, 62(Suppl2), 81-83.

Sobri M, Lamont AC, et al. (2003). Red flags in patients presenting with headache: Clinical indications for neuroimaging. British Journal of Radiology, 76(908), 532-535.

Somjen GG (2001). Mechanisms of spreading depression and hypoxic spreading depression-like depolarization. Physiological Reviews, 81(3), 1065-1096.

Taub E, Perrella P, et al. (1973). Behavioral development after forelimb deafferentation on day of birth in monkeys with and without blinding. Science, 181(103), 959-960.

Tsirikos AI, Haddo O, et al. (2004). Spinal manifestations in a patient with congenital insensitivity to pain. Journal of Spinal Disorders & Techniques, 17(4), 326-330.

Ulrich V, Gervil M, et al. (2004). The relative influence of environment and genes in episodic tension-type headache. Neurology, 62(11), 2065-2069.

van de Beek WJ, Roep BO, et al. (2003). Susceptibility loci for complex regional pain syndrome. Pain, 103(1-2), 93-97.

Waddell G (1987). A new clinical model for the treatment of low-back pain. Spine, 12, 632-644.

Waddell G, Newton M, et al. (1993). A fear-avoidance beliefs questionnaire (FABQ) and the role of fear-avoidance beliefs in chronic low back pain and disability. Pain, 52(2), 157-168.

Wager TD, Rilling JK, et al. (2004). Placebo-induced changes in FMRI in the anticipation and experience of pain. Science, 303(5661), 1162-1167.

Wetzel CH, Connelly JF (1997). Use of gabapentin in pain management. Annals of Pharmacotherapy, 31(9), 1082-1083.

Willis WD (2002). Long-term potentiation in spinothalamic neurons. Brain Research. Brain Research Reviews, 40(1-3), 202-214.

Willis WD, Westlund KN (1997). Neuroanatomy of the pain system and of the pathways that modulate pain. Journal of Clinical Neurophysiology, 14(1), 2-31.

Woolhouse M (2005). Migraine and tension headache— A complementary and alternative medicine approach. Australian Family Physician, 34(8), 647-651.

Zambreanu L, Wise RG, et al. (2005). A role for the brainstem in central sensitisation in humans. Evidence from functional magnetic resonance imaging. Pain, 114(3), 397-407.

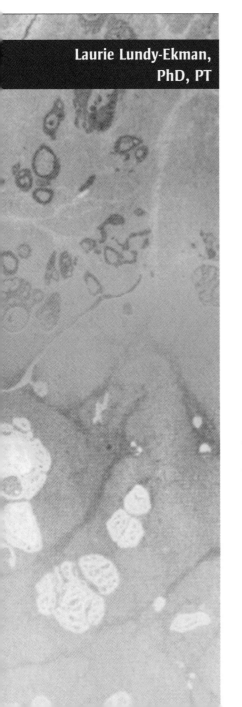

8 Autonomic Nervous System

Laurie Lundy-Ekman, PhD, PT

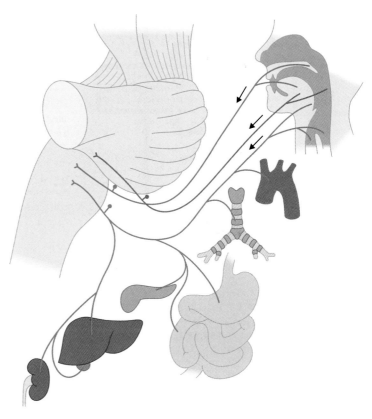

INTRODUCTION

The autonomic nervous system is critical for the survival of the individual and the species because it regulates homeostasis and reproduction. Homeostasis is the maintenance of an optimal internal environment, including body temperature and chemical composition of tissues and fluids. The autonomic nervous system maintains homeostasis by regulating the activity of internal organs and vasculature. Thus, the autonomic nervous system regulates circulation, respiration, digestion, metabolism, secretions, body temperature, and reproduction. The aspects of the autonomic nervous system considered in this chapter include receptors, afferent pathways, central regulation, and efferent pathways to the effectors (Figure 8-1). The autonomic efferent pathways are the sympathetic and parasympathetic divisions of the nervous system.

AFFERENT
PATHWAYS

CENTRAL
PROCESSING

EFFERENT
PATHWAYS

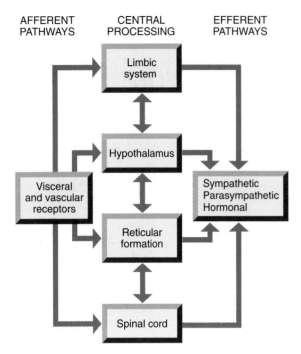

FIGURE 8-1
Flow of information in the autonomic nervous system.

> The autonomic system regulates the viscera, vasculature, and glands.

RECEPTORS

Receptors of the autonomic system include mechanoreceptors, chemoreceptors, nociceptors, and thermoreceptors. The **mechanoreceptors** respond to pressure and to stretch. Pressure receptors are found in the aortic baroreceptors, carotid sinuses, and lungs. Stretch receptors respond to distention of the veins, bladder, or intestines.

Chemoreceptors sensitive to chemical concentrations in the blood are located in the carotid and aortic bodies (respond to oxygen), medulla (respond to hydrogen ions and carbon dioxide), and hypothalamus (respond to blood glucose levels and to concentration of electrolytes). Chemoreceptors in the stomach, taste buds, and olfactory bulbs also respond to chemical concentrations.

Nociceptors, found throughout the viscera and in the walls of arteries, are typically most responsive to stretch and ischemia. Visceral nociceptors are also sensitive to irritating chemicals.

Thermoreceptors in the hypothalamus respond to very small changes in the temperature of circulating blood, and cutaneous thermoreceptors respond to external temperature changes.

AFFERENT PATHWAYS

The information from visceral receptors enters the central nervous system by two routes: into the spinal cord via the dorsal roots and into the brainstem via cranial nerves (Figure 8-2). Cranial nerves conveying autonomic afferent information include the facial (VII), glossopharyngeal (IX), and vagus nerves (X). All three of these cranial nerves transmit taste information, and the glossopharyngeal and vagus nerves transmit information from the viscera.

CENTRAL REGULATION OF VISCERAL FUNCTION

Most visceral information entering the brainstem via cranial nerves converges in the **solitary nucleus,** the main visceral sensory nucleus (Figure 8-3). In turn, information from the solitary nucleus is relayed to visceral control areas in the pons and medulla and to modulatory areas in the hypothalamus, thalamus, and limbic system. Modulatory areas regulate the activity of areas that directly control a particular function. For example, the limbic system does not directly control respiratory rate but instead influences the activity of respiratory control areas in the pons and medulla.

Visceral afferents entering the spinal cord synapse with visceral efferents (autonomic reflexes; see Chapter 12) and with neurons that ascend to regions of the brainstem, hypothalamus, and thalamus. Visceral nociceptive afferents have additional connections with the following:
- Somatosensory nociceptive afferents, contributing to referred pain (see Chapter 7)
- Somatic efferents, to produce muscle guarding (protective contraction of skeletal muscles)

Figure 8-4 illustrates the activity in these pathways during acute appendicitis.

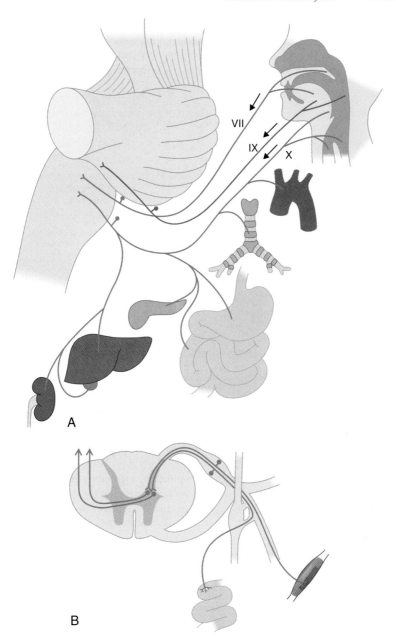

FIGURE 8-2
Afferent autonomic pathways into the brainstem and spinal cord. **A,** Visceral afferent information from the tongue and soft palate enters the brainstem through cranial nerves VII and IX. Information from the larynx and thoracic and abdominal viscera reaches the brainstem via cranial nerve X. **B,** Stretch of blood vessels in the periphery is registered by free nerve endings in the vessel walls. This information is conveyed via fibers in peripheral nerves into the spinal cord. Information from stretch receptors in the gastrointestinal tract passes through an autonomic ganglion, without synapsing, before entering the spinal cord.

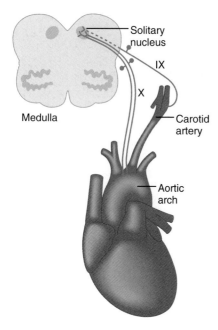

FIGURE 8-3

Visceral information converges in the solitary nucleus of the brainstem. An example is the convergence of blood pressure and blood chemical composition information, monitored by pressure and chemoreceptors in the carotid artery and the aortic arch. The information is transmitted to the solitary nucleus in the medulla.

> Afferent autonomic information is processed in the solitary nucleus, spinal cord, and areas of the brainstem, hypothalamus, and thalamus.

Control of Autonomic Functions by the Medulla and Pons

Areas within the medulla regulate heart rate, respiration, vasoconstriction, and vasodilation via signals to autonomic efferent neurons in the spinal cord and by signals conveyed in the vagus nerve. Areas in the pons are also involved in regulating respiration.

Role of the Hypothalamus, Thalamus, and Limbic System in Autonomic Regulation

The hypothalamus, thalamus, and limbic system modulate brainstem autonomic control. Visceral information reaching the hypothalamus, the master controller of homeostasis, is used to maintain equilibrium in the interior of the body. The hypothalamus influences cardiore-

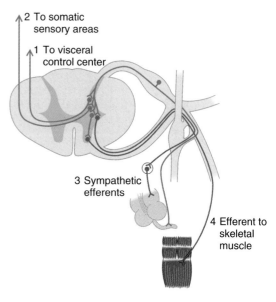

FIGURE 8-4

Pathways of afferent autonomic information in the spinal cord. The early stage of acute appendicitis is shown: the nociceptive signals enter the T10 spinal segment. Connections with

1. Autonomic tract fibers convey the information to areas in the brainstem, hypothalamus, and limbic system
2. Nociceptive second-order neurons results in pain sensation referred to the umbilical region
3. Sympathetic efferents inhibit peristalsis in the intestine
4. Somatic efferents elicit contraction of abdominal muscles

spiratory, metabolic, water reabsorption, and digestive activity by acting on the pituitary gland, control centers in the brainstem, and spinal cord (Jacobson, 2005; Matinyan, 2004, Toni et al., 2004). Visceral information reaching the thalamus is projected mainly to the limbic system, a collection of cerebral areas involved in emotions, moods, and motivation. Activation of limbic areas can produce autonomic responses; examples include increased heart rate due to anxiety, blushing with embarrassment, and crying (Morgane et al., 2005).

> Vital functions are controlled by areas in the medulla and pons. The hypothalamus, thalamus, and limbic system modulate the brainstem control.

Integration of Information

Autonomic regulation is often achieved by integrating information from peripheral afferents with information from receptors within the central nervous system. For example, if peripheral chemoreceptors in the carotid body signal a drop in oxygen content in the blood, the information is conveyed to the solitary nucleus (in the medulla) by the glossopharyngeal nerve. Then signals are sent to autonomic control areas to increase the depth and rate of respiration. If a specific group of neurons in the medulla, directly sensitive to the concentration of carbon dioxide and hydrogen ions (pH) in the blood, sense deviations from the optimum physiologic range, respiration is adjusted.

EFFERENT PATHWAYS

Autonomic efferent neurons are classified as sympathetic and parasympathetic. In general, the connections from the central nervous system to autonomic effectors use a two-neuron pathway, with the two neurons synapsing in a peripheral ganglion. The neuron extending from the central nervous system to the ganglion is called **preganglionic**; the neuron connecting the ganglion with the effector organ is called **post-ganglionic.**

Differences Between the Somatic Motor System and Autonomic Efferent System

All central nervous system output is delivered by somatic or autonomic efferent neurons. Somatic efferents innervate only skeletal muscle, and their activation is frequently voluntary. Autonomic efferents supply all other parts of the body that are innervated. The autonomic system is different from the somatic nervous system in three major ways:

1. Unlike the somatic nervous system, regulation of autonomic functions is typically nonconscious and can be exerted by hormones.
2. Unlike skeletal muscle, many internal organs can function independently of central nervous system input. Examples include independent activity of the heart and the gastrointestinal tract. The heart can continue to beat without neural connections. The gastrointestinal tract is unique in having an intrinsic nervous system, the enteric nervous system, so capable of operating independently of the central nervous system that the system has been called the abdominal brain (Holzer et al., 2001). This system of ganglia and sensory and motor neurons is located entirely within the walls of the digestive system. Because its function is purely digestive, further discussion of the enteric nervous system is beyond the scope of this text.

3. Somatic efferent pathways use one neuron; autonomic efferent pathways usually use two neurons, with a synapse outside the central nervous system.

Neurotransmitters Used by the Autonomic Efferent System

Autonomic neurons secrete the neurotransmitter acetylcholine, norepinephrine, or epinephrine. Neurons that secrete acetylcholine are called **cholinergic.** Neurons secreting norepinephrine or epinephrine are called **adrenergic.**

Cholinergic Neurons and Receptors

Autonomic neurons that secrete acetylcholine include the following (Figure 8-5):
- All preganglionic neurons in the autonomic nervous system
- Postganglionic neurons of the parasympathetic system
- Sympathetic postganglionic neurons that innervate sweat glands, and some sympathetic postganglionic neurons that innervate vessels in skeletal muscle

The effect of a neurotransmitter depends on the type of receptors activated by the transmitter. This is of particular importance in the autonomic nervous system, where differences in types of receptors are the key to the distinct physiologic effects of different drugs. Based on their ability to bind certain drugs, two groups of **cholinergic receptors** have been identified: muscarinic and nicotinic.

Muscarine, a poison derived from mushrooms, activates only the **muscarinic receptors** in the membranes of effectors. Acetylcholine binding to muscarinic receptors initiates a G-protein-mediated response, which can be either an excitatory postsynaptic potential (EPSP) or inhibitory postsynaptic potential (IPSP). Parasympathetic muscarinic acetylcholine receptors regulate glands, smooth muscles, and heart rate.

Nicotine, derived from tobacco, activates only the **nicotinic acetylcholine receptors.** Acetylcholine binding to nicotinic autonomic receptors, located on all postsynaptic autonomic neurons, the adrenal medulla, sweat glands, and vascular smooth muscle, causes a fast EPSP in the postsynaptic membrane. In addition to the effects on the autonomic system, nicotine activates acetylcholine receptors on skeletal muscle membrane and in limbic areas of the brain. Nicotine action in the limbic system induces feelings of alertness and arousal (Trimmel et al., 2004) and leads to addiction (Janhunen and Ahtee, 2006). In nonsmoking women, inhaling

SYMPATHETIC

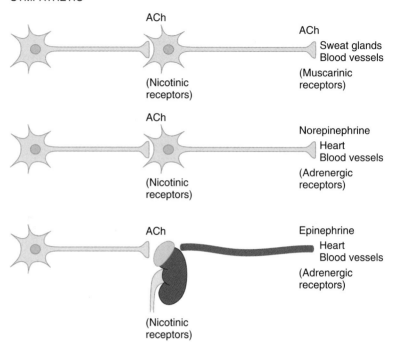

FIGURE 8-5
Neurochemicals secreted by autonomic neurons. The chemical is identified above the synapse, and the type of receptor is listed below the synapse. *ACh,* Acetylcholine.

nicotine improves mood and induces a feeling of calmness by increasing levels of dopamine in neural pathways that induce a feeling of pleasure and reduce anxiety. File and colleagues speculate that women may begin regular smoking as a form of stress self-medication. However, in nonsmoking males, nicotine enhances aggressive mood (File et al., 2001).

Adrenergic Neurons and Receptors

The transmitter released by most sympathetic postganglionic neurons is norepinephrine. The adrenal medulla, a part of the sympathetic system, is specialized to release epinephrine and norepinephrine directly into the blood. Receptors that bind norepinephrine or epinephrine are called adrenergic receptors. There are two groups of **adrenergic receptors,** designated α and β; each of

these has subtypes, indicated by subscripts: α_1, α_2, β_1, and β_2.

> Cholinergic neurons secrete acetylcholine. Nicotine and muscarine are exogenous chemicals that bind with subtypes of acetylcholine receptors. Adrenergic neurons secrete norepinephrine. Adrenergic receptors are classified as α or β.

SYMPATHETIC NERVOUS SYSTEM

Sympathetic Efferent Neurons

Cell bodies of the sympathetic preganglionic neurons are in the lateral horn of the spinal cord gray matter

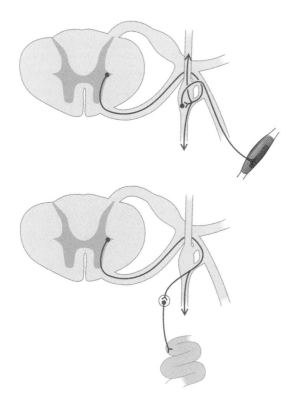

FIGURE 8-6
Sympathetic outflow innervating arterioles in skeletal muscle and in the walls of viscera.

(Figure 8-6). Because the cell bodies are located from the T1 to L2 levels, the sympathetic nervous system is often called the **thoracolumbar outflow.** Sympathetic efferent neurons innervate the adrenal medulla, vasculature, sweat glands, erectors of hair cells, and the viscera.

Sympathetic Efferents to the Adrenal Medulla

Direct connections are provided from the spinal cord to the adrenal medulla (Figure 8-7, *A*). The adrenal medulla can be considered a specialized sympathetic ganglion that secretes epinephrine and norepinephrine into the bloodstream.

Sympathetic Efferents to the Periphery and Thoracic Viscera

Sympathetic efferents to the limbs, face, body wall, heart, and lungs synapse in ganglia alongside the vertebral column, called *paravertebral ganglia* (Figure 8-7, *B*). The paravertebral ganglia are interconnected, forming sympathetic trunks. Preganglionic sympathetic axons leave the spinal cord through the ventral root, join the

spinal nerve, and then travel in a very short connecting branch to the paravertebral ganglia. The connecting branch, called the *white ramus communicans* (shown in Figure 8-6), is composed of sympathetic axons transferring from the spinal nerve to the paravertebral ganglion. The preganglionic axons either synapse in the paravertebral ganglion or travel up or down the sympathetic chain before synapsing in a ganglion.

The cell body of the postganglionic neuron is in the paravertebral ganglion. The postganglionic axon enters a peripheral nerve via a connecting branch, the *gray ramus communicans* (see Figure 8-6), then travels in either the ventral or dorsal ramus to the periphery.

Given that the head, except for the face, and most of the upper limbs are innervated by cervical spinal cord segments, and preganglionic sympathetic fibers arise only from thoracolumbar segments, how do sympathetic signals reach the head and upper limbs? Cervical paravertebral ganglia are supplied by preganglionic fibers that ascend from the upper thoracic cord. The cervical ganglia are named *superior, middle,* and *cervicothoracic* (Figure 8-7). The cervicothoracic ganglion, often called the **stellate ganglion** because of its star shape, is formed by the fusion of the inferior cervical and first thoracic ganglion. Postganglionic fibers from the superior and stellate ganglia innervate arteries of the face, dilate the pupil of the eye, and assist in elevating the upper eyelid. Other fibers from the cervicothoracic ganglion descend with fibers from the middle cervical ganglion to supply the heart and the blood vessels of the upper limb.

The lower lumbar and sacral paravertebral ganglia are supplied by preganglionic fibers that descend from the upper lumbar cord. Postganglionic neurons from the lower lumbar and parasacral paravertebral ganglia innervate blood vessels in the lower limbs.

Sympathetic Efferents to Abdominal and Pelvic Organs

The preganglionic sympathetic axons to abdominal and pelvic organs pass through the sympathetic ganglia without synapsing, then synapse in outlying ganglia near the organs (Figure 8-7, *C*). The preganglionic neurons travel in splanchnic nerves, which are peripheral nerves that innervate the viscera. Sympathetic signals to the gastrointestinal tract slow or stop peristalsis, reduce glandular secretions, and constrict sphincters within the digestive system.

Functions of the Sympathetic Nervous System

The primary role of the sympathetic nervous system is to maintain optimal blood supply in the organs.

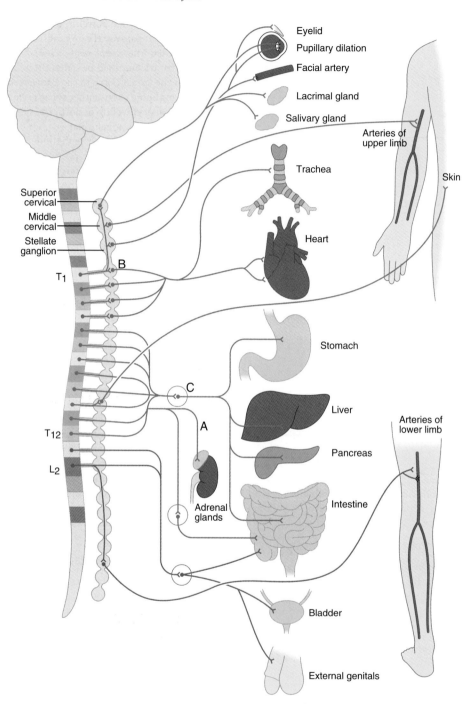

FIGURE 8-7

Efferents from the spinal cord to sympathetic effector organs: **A,** Direct, one-neuron connections to adrenal medulla. **B,** Two-neuron pathways to the periphery and thoracic viscera, with synapses in paravertebral ganglia. **C,** Two-neuron pathways to the abdominal and pelvic organs, with synapses in outlying ganglia.

Normally, moderate activity of the sympathetic system stimulates smooth muscle in the walls of blood vessels, maintaining some contraction of the vessel walls. Generally, increasing sympathetic activity further constricts the vessels, and decreasing sympathetic activity allows vasodilation. For example, when a person rises from supine to standing, blood pressure needs to be increased to prevent fainting. Firing of certain sympathetic efferents stimulates vasoconstriction in skeletal muscles, thus maintaining blood flow to the brain. However, when vigorous activity is demanded from skeletal muscles, firing of a different set of sympathetic efferents to blood vessels in skeletal muscles produces vasodilation. These opposing effects of sympathetic activation are possible because activation of the different subtypes of adrenergic receptors elicits different effects.

The role of the sympathetic nervous system is often illustrated by describing the physiologic responses to fear. When a person feels threatened, the sympathetic nervous system prepares for vigorous muscle activity, that is, for fight or flight. This is achieved by increasing blood flow to active muscles, increasing blood glucose levels, dilating bronchioles and coronary arteries, increasing blood pressure, and increasing heart rate. Simultaneously, sympathetic firing reduces activity in the digestive system.

Regulation of Body Temperature

Sympathetic activity regulates body temperature by effects on metabolism and on effectors in the skin. Epinephrine released by the adrenal medulla increases the metabolic rate throughout the body. In the skin, sympathetic signals control the diameter of the blood vessels, secretion of the sweat glands, and erection of hairs. Blood flow in the skin is controlled by α-adrenergic receptors in the smooth muscles of arterioles. Norepinephrine binding to α-adrenergic receptors in skin arterioles also stimulates precapillary sphincters to contract, forcing blood to bypass the capillaries and decreasing the radiation of heat from the skin. When the precapillary sphincters relax, blood enters the capillaries, and heat radiates from the skin. Sweating, activated when acetylcholine binds with muscarinic receptors on sweat glands, helps to dissipate heat. In humans, erection of hair cells probably contributes little to the retention of body heat.

Regulation of Blood Flow in Skeletal Muscle

Control of blood flow in skeletal muscle is more complex than in the skin. Skeletal muscle veins and venules are called **capacitance vessels** because blood pools in these vessels when their walls are relaxed. If pooling of blood in the lower limbs and abdomen is not prevented when a person assumes an upright position, the resulting drop in blood pressure can deprive the brain of adequate blood supply, causing **syncope** (fainting). Normally the pooling of blood is prevented by vasoconstriction of the capacitance vessels, prior to the change in position. This is accomplished by the release of norepinephrine to bind with α-adrenergic receptors in the walls of skeletal muscle venules and veins, causing vasoconstriction.

Arteriole walls in skeletal muscle contain α- and β_2- adrenergic and muscarinic cholinergic receptors. The action of norepinephrine on α-adrenergic receptors causes vasoconstriction of skeletal muscle arterioles. Binding of epinephrine to β_2-adrenergic receptors, or binding of acetylcholine to muscarinic receptors, vasodilates skeletal muscle arterioles during exercise or fight-or-flight situations. Local blood chemistry also affects the diameter of arterioles (Thomas and Segal, 2004).

> Sympathetic activity may either vasodilate or vasoconstrict arterioles supplying skeletal muscle. Sympathetic activity vasoconstricts arterioles in the skin.

Sympathetic Control in the Head

Sympathetic effects on blood flow, sweating, and erection of hair cells of the head are identical to sympathetic actions in the remainder of the body. In addition, sympathetic signals dilate the pupil of the eye and assist in elevating the upper eyelid. The levator palpebrae superioris muscle consists of both smooth and skeletal muscle fibers; only the smooth muscle fibers are innervated by the sympathetic nervous system. The skeletal muscle fibers are innervated by the facial cranial nerve. The sympathetic innervation of the head is shown in Figure 8-8. Sympathetic fibers also innervate salivary glands; their activation causes secretion of thick saliva, which causes a sensation of dryness in the mouth.

Regulation of the Viscera

Sympathetic effects on the thoracic viscera include increasing heart rate and contractility when β_1-adrenergic receptors are activated in cardiac muscle and dilation of the bronchial tree when β_2-adrenergic receptors are activated in the respiratory tract. The distribution of adrenergic receptor types is illustrated in Figure 8-9.

Drugs that bind with a receptor but do not activate the receptor are called *blockers*. Drugs that activate receptors are called *agonists*. α-blockers are used to decrease

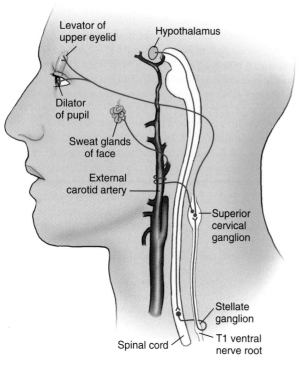

FIGURE 8-8

Sympathetic innervation of the head. The neural circuit begins in the hypothalamus, then synapses in the upper thoracic spinal cord and superior cervical ganglion. Axons from the superior cervical ganglion innervate facial sweat glands, vasculature of the face, the pupillary dilator muscle, the accessory levator muscle of the upper eyelid, and the lacrimal gland.

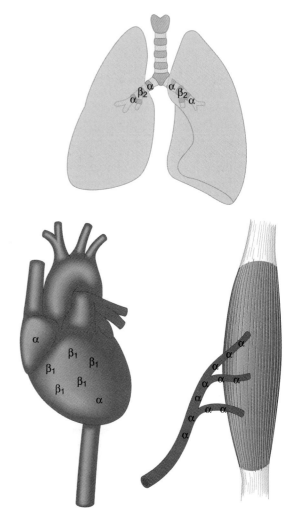

FIGURE 8-9

Distribution of adrenergic receptors. α-adrenergic receptors are most abundant in arterioles of peripheral smooth muscle but are also found in the heart and bronchial smooth muscle. β_1-adrenergic receptors are found primarily in the heart. β_2-adrenergic receptors are most numerous in bronchial smooth muscle but are also found in peripheral smooth muscle. The sympathetic nervous system optimizes blood flow to the organs, regulates body temperature and metabolic rate, and regulates the activity of viscera.

high blood pressure by blocking the action of norepinephrine on receptors in blood vessels, producing vasodilation. The differences between receptor subtypes (i.e., β_1 and β_2) allow the design of drugs that bind with one subtype of receptor and not another. β_1-blockers decrease heart rate and contractility without affecting the airways (Salpeter et al., 2003). β_2-agonists prevent constriction of the airways and thus are used to treat asthma and chronic obstructive pulmonary disease. However, β_2-agonists do not only affect airway function; heart ischemia, congestive heart failure, arrhythmias, and sudden death are associated with use of β_2-agonists (Salpeter et al., 2004).

In the gastrointestinal tract, sympathetic signals contract sphincters and decrease blood flow, peristalsis, and secretions. Sympathetic stimulation also inhibits con-

traction of the bladder and bowel walls and contracts internal sphincters.

Metabolism

When the adrenal medulla releases epinephrine into the bloodstream, the most significant effect is stimulation of metabolism in cells throughout the entire body. Epinephrine release usually coincides with a generalized release of norepinephrine from sympathetic postganglionic neurons because the sympathetic system is often activated as a whole. In addition to its effect on metabolism, epinephrine reinforces the effects of norepinephrine on most target organs.

> The sympathetic nervous system optimizes blood flow to the organs, regulates body temperature and metabolic rate, and regulates the activity of viscera.

PARASYMPATHETIC NERVOUS SYSTEM

The parasympathetic nervous system uses a two-neuron pathway from the spinal cord to the effectors. Because the preganglionic cell bodies are found in nuclei of the brainstem and the sacral spinal cord, this system is often called the **craniosacral outflow** (Figure 8-10). The ganglia of the parasympathetic nervous system are separate, unlike the interconnected ganglia of the sympathetic trunk. Parasympathetic ganglia are located near or in the target organs.

Parasympathetic information from the brainstem travels in cranial nerves to outlying ganglia. Postganglionic neurons are distributed to the eye, salivary glands, and viscera.

Parasympathetic fibers are distributed in cranial nerves III, VII, IX, and X. Seventy-five percent of the parasympathetic fibers in cranial nerves travel in cranial nerve X, the vagus nerve.

Parasympathetic fibers arising in the sacral spinal cord have cell bodies in the lateral horn of sacral levels S2-S4. Their axons travel in pelvic splanchnic nerves, distributed to the lower colon, bladder, and external genitalia. In contrast to the sympathetic nervous system, the parasympathetic system does not innervate the limbs or body wall.

The principal function of the parasympathetic nervous system is energy conservation and storage. Efferent fibers in the vagus nerve innervate the heart and the smooth muscle of the lungs and digestive system. Vagus nerve activity to the heart can produce either bradycardia (slowing of the heart rate) or decreased cardiac contraction force. Vagus stimulation in the respiratory system causes bronchoconstriction and increases mucus secretion. In the digestive system, vagus activity increases

peristalsis, glycogen synthesis in the liver, and glandular secretions.

Fibers in cranial nerves VII and IX, the facial and glossopharyngeal nerves, innervate salivary glands. Other fibers in cranial nerve VII innervate the lacrimal gland, providing tears to moisten the cornea and for crying. Fibers in cranial nerve III, the oculomotor nerve, constrict the pupil and increase the convexity of the lens of the eye for focusing on close objects.

The sacral parasympathetic efferents regulate emptying of the bowels and bladder and the erection of the penis or clitoris. Specific autonomic reflexes are discussed in the context of various regions of the nervous system. For example, reflexive control of the pupil is discussed in Chapter 13, and bladder and bowel reflexes are covered in Chapter 12.

> Parasympathetic activity decreases cardiac activity; facilitates digestion; increases secretions in the lungs, eyes, and mouth; controls convexity of the lens in the eye; constricts the pupil; controls voiding of the bowels and bladder; and controls the erection of sexual organs.

COMPARISON OF SYMPATHETIC AND PARASYMPATHETIC FUNCTIONS

In actions on the thoracic and abdominal viscera, the bladder and bowels, and the pupil of the eye, the effects of sympathetic and parasympathetic activity are synergistic: their opposing actions are balanced to provide optimal organ function. For example, immediately before a person begins to exercise, sympathetic signals increase heart rate and contractility, while parasympathetic signals that would slow heart rate decrease. Figure 8-11 illustrates the autonomic areas and pathways that regulate heart rate.

The autonomic efferent systems also have separate, unopposed effects: the sympathetic roles in regulating effectors in the limbs, face, and body wall and assisting elevation of the upper eyelid are not countered by parasympathetic innervation to these effectors. The role of the parasympathetic system in increasing the convexity of the lens of the eye is also unopposed. Tables 8-1 and 8-2 list the actions of the autonomic efferent systems. Table 8-3 summarizes the distribution of neurotransmitters and receptors in the autonomic efferent systems.

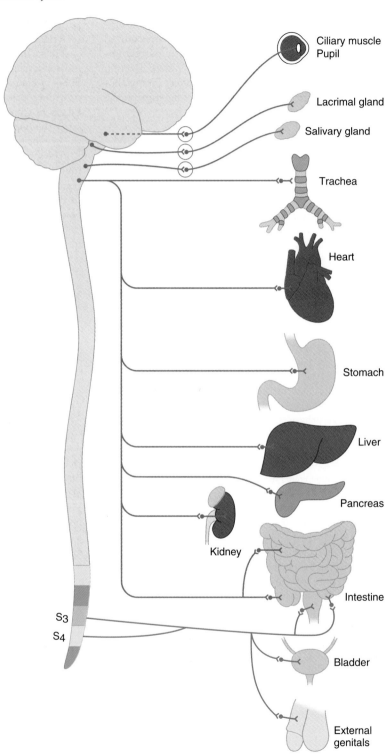

FIGURE 8-10
Parasympathetic outflow through cranial nerves III, VII, IX, and X and S2-S4. For simplicity, the neurons from cranial nerve VII to the salivary glands are omitted.

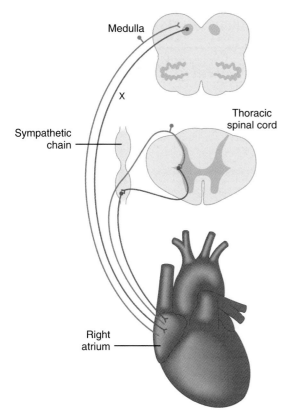

FIGURE 8-11
Autonomic regulation of heart rate. Sensory information enters both the medulla and spinal cord. Regulation is achieved by parasympathetic fibers in the vagus nerve and by sympathetic fibers from the thoracic spinal cord.

CLINICAL CORRELATIONS

Horner's Syndrome

If a lesion affects the sympathetic pathway to head, sympathetic activity on one side of the head is decreased. This leads to ipsilateral drooping of the upper eyelid, constriction of the pupil, and skin vasodilation, with absence of sweating on the ipsilateral face and neck. This constellation of signs is called **Horner's syndrome** (Figure 8-12) and occurs with lesions of the descending sympathetic tract, upper thoracic spinal cord, brachial plexus, or the cervical sympathetic chain (see Figure 8-8). Interruption of blood supply, trauma, tumor, or cluster headache may cause Horner's syndrome (Walton and Buono, 2003). Cluster headache is a severe headache on one side of the head, lasting a few minutes to three hours, and occurs as a series of headaches.

Peripheral Region

If a peripheral nerve is severed, interruption of sympathetic efferents causes loss of vascular control, temperature regulation, and sweating in the region supplied by the peripheral nerve. These losses may lead to trophic changes in the skin.

Spinal Region

A complete spinal cord lesion interrupts all communication between the cord below the lesion and the brain, disrupting ascending and descending autonomic signals at the level of the lesion. The severity of autonomic dysfunction depends on how much of the cord is isolated from the brain. Lower-level lesions allow the brain to influence more of the cord; higher-level lesions isolate more of the cord. Complete lesions above the lumbar level obstruct voluntary control of bladder, bowel, and genital function. Complete lesions above the midtho-

Table 8-1   EFFECT OF SYMPATHETIC ACTIVITY ON BLOOD VESSELS

Organ	Neurochemical	Receptor	Effect on Vessel Wall	Purpose
Skin	Adrenergic	α	Vasoconstriction of arterioles	↓ radiation of heat from skin
Skeletal muscle	Adrenergic	α	Vasoconstriction of venules and veins	↑ peripheral vascular resistance ↑ blood pressure
	Adrenergic	β_2	Vasodilation of arterioles	More blood available to muscle
	Acetylcholine	Muscarinic	Vasodilation of arterioles	More blood available to muscle
Heart	Adrenergic	β_1	Dilation	More blood available to heart

Table 8-2 COMPARISON OF SYMPATHETIC AND PARASYMPATHETIC EFFECTS ON ORGAN FUNCTION

Organ	Function	Sympathetic Effect	Parasympathetic Effect
Eye	Diameter of pupil	↑	↓
	Curvature of lens		↑
Heart	Contraction rate	↑	↓
	Force of contraction	↑	
Blood vessels	See Table 8-1		
Lungs	Diameter of bronchioles	↑	↓
	Diameter of blood vessels	↑	
	Secretions		↑
Sweat glands	Production of sweat	↑	
Salivary glands	Thick secretion	↑	
	Thin, profuse secretion		↑
Lacrimal glands	Production of tears		↑
	Vasomotor to blood vessels in lacrimal gland	↑	
Adrenal medulla	Secretion of epinephrine	↑	
Gastrointestinal tract	Peristalsis	↓	↑
	Secretions	↓	↑
Liver	Glucose release	↑	
	Glycogen synthesis		↑
Pancreas	Secretions	↓	↑
Bowel and bladder	Emptying	↓	↑
External genitalia	Erection of penis or clitoris		↑

Table 8-3 NEUROCHEMICALS AND RECEPTORS IN THE AUTONOMIC NERVOUS SYSTEM

Neurochemical	Site of Neurochemical Release	Receptor Type
Acetylcholine	Synapse between preganglionic and postganglionic neurons (both sympathetic and parasympathetic)	Nicotinic
	Parasympathetic postganglionic to smooth muscles and glands	Muscarinic
	Sympathetic postganglionic to sweat glands and some arterioles in skeletal muscle (dilates arterioles)	Muscarinic
Norepinephrine	Sympathetic postganglionic to constrict blood vessels in skeletal muscles, skin, and viscera, dilate pupil	α
	Sympathetic postganglionic to vasodilate arterioles in skeletal muscle, dilate bronchioles, decrease gastrointestinal activity, accelerate heart rate	β
Epinephrine	Adrenal medulla: release transmitter into bloodstream	α and β

Norepinephrine has a greater effect on α-adrenergic receptors than on β, epinephrine is equally effective in activating both α and β.

racic level isolate much of the cord from control by the brain, jeopardizing homeostasis by interfering with blood pressure regulation and the ability to adjust core body temperature. The autonomic consequences of spinal cord injury are discussed more fully in Chapter 12.

Brainstem Region

Lesions in the brainstem region may interfere with descending control of heart rate, blood pressure, and respiration. Brainstem lesions may also affect cranial

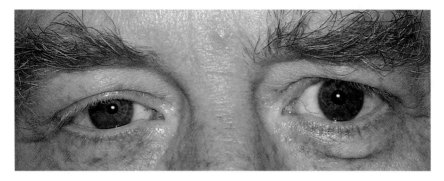

FIGURE 8-12

Horner's syndrome. A lesion of the sympathetic pathway (illustrated in Figure 8-8) to the face results in a drooping eyelid, pupil constriction, and dry, red skin of the face. Normally, activity in this sympathetic pathway facilitates the levator palpebrae muscle of the upper eyelid, the dilator muscle of the iris, constriction of blood vessels in the face, and the sweat glands of the face and neck. *(From Parsons M, Johnson M (2001). Diagnosis in Color: Neurology. Edinburgh: Mosby.)*

nerve nuclei, interfering with constriction of the pupil, production of tears, salivation, or regulation of thoracic and abdominal viscera.

Cerebral Region

Damage to certain nuclei in the hypothalamus disrupts homeostasis, with consequent metabolic and behavioral dysfunctions. Obesity, anorexia, hyperthermia, hypothermia, and emotional displays dissociated from feelings can occur. Activity in other limbic (emotional) areas can also interfere with homeostasis. For example, the response to perceived threat includes sympathetic activity that increases blood flow to skeletal muscles, accelerates cardiac rate, strengthens cardiac contraction, and decreases blood flow to skin, kidneys, and digestive tract.

Syncope

Syncope (fainting) is a brief loss of consciousness due to inadequate blood flow to the brain. If the cause of the syncope is powerful emotions, the attack is called vasodepressor syncope or neurogenic shock. Strong emotion can initiate sudden, active vasodilation of intramuscular arterioles, causing a precipitous fall in blood pressure. The blood flow to the head is temporarily reduced, leading to loss of consciousness and paleness of the face. Blood flow to the head is restored when the person is horizontal.

In some cases, particularly when syncope occurs in response to painful stimuli or on standing after prolonged bed rest, vagal stimulation to the heart follows the intramuscular vasodilation. The vagal activity slows the heart, further decreasing blood pressure, and elicits nausea, salivation, and increased perspiration. When vagal signs occur with vasodepressor syncope, called a vasovagal attack, excessive activity is occurring in both the sympathetic and parasympathetic systems (Mohan and Lavania, 2004).

Although vasodepressor syncope is the most common type of syncope, many different causes can produce syncope. As mentioned earlier in this chapter, assuming an upright posture can cause pooling of blood in the lower body, resulting in syncope. Other causes include insufficient cardiac output, hypoxia, and hypoglycemia.

Tests of Autonomic Function

The ability of the sympathetic nervous system to regulate blood pressure can be evaluated by measuring the person's blood pressure in the supine position, having the person stand, and measuring the blood pressure 2 minutes later. Abnormal responses include a drop of more than 30 mm Hg in systolic blood pressure or more than 15 mm Hg in diastolic blood pressure.

Sympathetic regulation of the skin can be tested by the sweat test or hand vasomotor test. For the sweat test, sweat is absorbed by small pieces of filter paper placed on the skin, and then the filter paper is weighed to determine the amount of sweat. For the vasomotor test, skin temperature is measured before and after the hands are immersed in cold water. This test is used to assess the amount of vasoconstriction.

SUMMARY

The autonomic nervous system regulates circulation, respiration, digestion, metabolism, secretions, body temperature, and reproduction. Receptors include mechanoreceptors, chemoreceptors, nociceptors, and thermoreceptors. Signals from the receptors travel via spinal nerves and cranial nerves VII, IX, and X into the central nervous system. Areas within the medulla and pons regulate vital functions (heart rate, respiration, and blood flow). The hypothalamus serves as the master controller of homeostasis via actions on the pituitary, brainstem centers, and the spinal cord.

The efferent pathways of the autonomic system are the sympathetic and parasympathetic systems. The sympathetic system regulates cardiac muscle, blood vessels, and sweat glands by activating adrenergic and muscarinic receptors on effectors. Sympathetic outflow arises in spinal segments T1-L2. Control of sympathetic functions in the head and neck is via cephalic extension of the sympathetic chain into the stellate, middle cervical, and superior cervical ganglia. Control of lower limb vasculature is via the caudal extension of the sympathetic ganglia. The parasympathetic nervous system regulates glands, smooth muscle, and cardiac muscle via muscarinic receptors on effectors. Parasympathetic outflow is through cranial nerves III, VII, IX and X, and S2-S4.

CLINICAL NOTES

Case 1

RD is a 23-year-old professional basketball player. While waiting to play in a championship game, he collapsed on the sidelines. His pulse could not be palpated, his blood pressure was 60/45 mm Hg, breathing was almost imperceptible, his pupils were dilated, and his face was pale. He was nonconscious for about 15 seconds; then color began to return to his face, and his breathing and pulse quickly returned to normal. RD regained his awareness of the environment on regaining consciousness. He reported feeling fine, although he felt weak; no headache or confusion followed the attack.

Question
What is the most likely diagnosis?

Case 2

BH, a 47-year-old man, had a myocardial infarction 3 weeks ago. He has been referred to physical therapy for cardiac rehabilitation. He is taking propranolol, a β-blocker.

Questions
1. What effect does blocking β-adrenergic receptors have on cardiovascular function?
2. Given that aerobic exercise prescriptions are based on a percentage of predicted age-related maximal heart rate, how will the β-blocker effects impact your exercise prescription?

REVIEW QUESTIONS

1. As a cardiac rehabilitation client begins treadmill exercise, which of his visceral and vascular sensory receptors would register changes? To what stimuli would the receptors be responding?
2. What is the function of visceral afferents?
3. What areas of the brain directly control autonomic function? What areas modulate activity in the autonomic control centers?
4. What are the differences between the autonomic and somatic efferent systems?

5. What are the sympathetic trunks? How do sympathetic fibers that leave the paravertebral ganglia reach effectors in the periphery, for example, blood vessels in skeletal muscle and in the skin?

6. What are splanchnic nerves?

7. What is the primary function of the sympathetic nervous system? How can sympathetic activation elicit vasodilation in skeletal muscles under certain conditions and vasoconstriction in the same vessels when conditions change?

8. What are capacitance vessels, and what is their significance? How is the blood flow in skeletal muscle arterioles controlled?

9. What would happen if the sympathetic fibers to the levator palpebrae superioris muscle and the pupil of the eye did not function?

10. What functions does the sympathetic nervous system regulate?

11. What functions are controlled by the parasympathetic nervous system?

12. A patient with CRPS (complex regional pain syndrome; see Chapter 7) arrives for an appointment with the following signs affecting the left side of the face: bright red dry skin, drooping of the eyelid, and a constricted pupil. What is your interpretation of these signs?

References

File SE, Fluck E, et al. (2001). Nicotine has calming effects on stress-induced mood changes in females, but enhances aggressive mood in males. International Journal of Neuropsychopharmacology, 4(4), 371-376.

Holzer P, Schicho R, et al. (2001). The gut as a neurological organ. Wiener Klinische Wochenschrift, 113(17-18), 647-660.

Jacobson L (2005). Hypothalamic-pituitary-adrenocortical axis regulation. Endocrinology and Metabolism Clinics of North America, 34(2), 271-292, vii.

Janhunen S, Ahtee L (2006). Differential nicotinic regulation of the nigrostriatal and mesolimbic dopaminergic pathways: Implications for drug development. Neuroscience and Biobehavioral Reviews. In press.

Matinyan LA (2004). Evolutionary aspects of the compensation for the functions of the damaged spinal cord. Neuroscience and Behavioral Physiology, 34(6), 525-533.

Mohan L, Lavania AK (2004). Vasovagal syncope: An enigma. Journal of the Association of Physicians of India, 52, 301-304.

Morgane PJ, Galler JR, et al. (2005). A review of systems and networks of the limbic forebrain/limbic midbrain. Progress in Neurobiology, 75(2), 143-160.

Salpeter SR, Ormiston TM, et al. (2003). Cardioselective beta-blockers for chronic obstructive pulmonary disease: a meta-analysis. Respiratory Medicine, 97(10), 1094-1101.

Salpeter SR, Ormiston TM, et al. (2004). Cardiovascular effects of beta-agonists in patients with asthma and COPD: A meta-analysis. Chest, 125(6), 2309-2321.

Thomas GD, Segal SS (2004). Neural control of muscle blood flow during exercise. Journal of Applied Physiology, 97(2), 731-738.

Toni R, Malaguti A, et al. (2004). The human hypothalamus: A morpho-functional perspective. Journal of Endocrinological Investigation, 27(6 Suppl), 73-94.

Trimmel M, Wittberger S (2004). Effects of transdermally administered nicotine on aspects of attention, task load, and mood in women and men. Pharmacology, Biochemistry, and Behavior, 78(3), 639-645.

Walton KA, Buono LM (2003). Horner syndrome. Current Opinion in Ophthalmology, 14(6), 357-363.

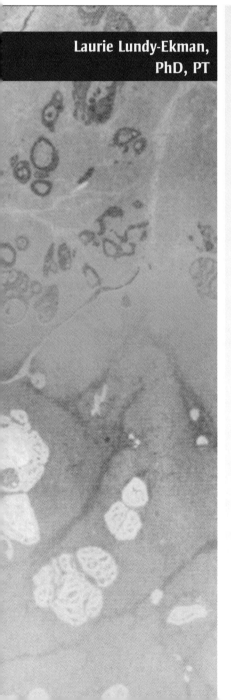

9 The Motor System: Motor Neurons

Laurie Lundy-Ekman, PhD, PT

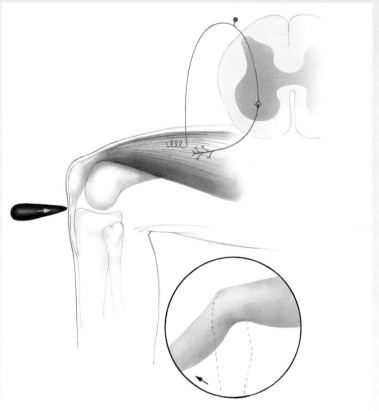

I am a 39-year-old woman. Before my stroke, I was very athletic. I ran every day. Two years ago I was at work, filling orders at a shoe warehouse, when I developed an excruciating headache. Prior to this, I never had headaches. My sister, who worked with me, asked if I needed an ambulance. I didn't think I needed an ambulance for a headache, so she drove me to a local emergency medical clinic. In the car on the way to the clinic, I had seizures. An aneurysm (a dilation of part of a wall of an artery, where the arterial wall is abnormally thin) had burst in my brain, causing bleeding into my brain. I underwent surgery to repair the damaged artery. People told me the doctor was amazed that I survived, and he repaired a second aneurysm during the surgery so that it would not rupture later. I had another surgery to insert a shunt about 2 weeks later because fluids were not draining normally from my brain.

I don't remember anything about the 2 months following the surgery. The stroke never affected my sensation or language abilities. The first thing I remember is that I couldn't recall how to chew or swallow. I couldn't plan the movements. I had to slowly figure out by trial and error how to eat by myself. Now I can do many things independently, except transfers and walking. Keeping my balance is difficult and fatiguing. When I am sitting, I use my arms for balance. My legs are very weak; I can move them a little when I'm lying down, but I cannot move them when I'm standing. I have had physical therapy since my hospitalization, focusing on balance, transfers, standing, and assisted walking. I take Dilantin to prevent seizures. I also take the antidepressants amitriptyline hydrochloride and nortriptyline hydrochloride. The amitriptyline hydrochloride also acts as an aid for sleeping, which I need because I am not active enough to get tired.

The stroke has profoundly altered my life. Before the stroke, I was vigorous, healthy, and independent. Now I live in a convalescent home, I use a wheelchair, and I need help to get into and out of the wheelchair. I think about when I could walk before the stroke, and I am planning on walking again.

—*Janet Abernathy*

INTRODUCTION

Every action we perform requires the motor system. Movement—which allows us to read, talk, walk, prepare dinner, and play musical instruments—is orchestrated by the coordinated action of the peripheral, spinal, brainstem/cerebellar, and cerebral regions, shaped by a specific context, and directed by our intentions. Consider how movement strategies change when we walk on an icy sidewalk: Our cadence, step length, and posture adjust to the differences. A young child may choose to sit and scoot rather than risk falling. We select these alternatives based on sensory information. As we saw in the example of Rothwell's patient (severe peripheral neuropathy, Chapter 7), normal motor performance and sensation are interdependent. Sensory information required varies with the task and is often used to prepare for movement in addition to providing information during and after movement.

SENSORY CONTRIBUTION TO MOVEMENT CONTROL

The anticipatory use of sensory information to prepare for movement is referred to as **feedforward.** An example of feedforward is the increase in hamstring activity prior to joint loading in people who have had an anterior cruciate ligament rupture (Riemann and Lephart, 2002).

The increased hamstring contraction prevents anterior tibial translation during acceptance of the load. **Feedback** is the use of sensory information during or after movement to make corrections either to the ongoing movement or to future movements. Feedback from proprioceptors, skin, vision, hearing, and vestibular receptors continually adapts walking to environmental constraints (Rossignol et al., 2006).

Proprioceptive information is analyzed to predict interaction torques and plan synchronization of multijoint movements. In people with normal nervous systems, joint movements are synchronized and the kinematics of most movements are the same regardless of whether the movements are performed slowly, at natural speed, or quickly. In people with complete loss of somatosensation below the neck, joint movements are not well synchronized and fast movements are decomposed. In movement decomposition, only one joint is moved at a time, to simplify control by eliminating interaction torques. For example, the person will keep the elbow joint in a fixed position and move only the shoulder (Messier et al., 2003).

Well-learned movements, including walking, eating, and driving, normally require little conscious attention. The smoothness of these practiced movements is remarkable, given the complexity of simultaneously coordinating the interacting torques produced by muscle actions with environmental conditions. The seeming effortlessness of automatic movement requires the continuous integration of visual, somatosensory, and vestibular information with motor processing.

Loss of any of the three senses integral to automatic movement interferes with ease and gracefulness. In the absence of vision, the act of reaching depends on somatosensation and proprioception to locate objects. Compared to visually guided reaching, movements without vision require more time and are less accurate. Loss of somatosensation in people with complete deafferentation disrupts positioning of limbs (Spencer et al., 2005). Complete, bilateral vestibular loss interferes with balance, yet visual or touch information from a stable surface can significantly improve balance despite complete absence of vestibular information (Horak et al., 2002). Smooth, accurate movement requires visual, tactile, and gravitational information.

PATIENT-CONTROLLED MOVEMENTS

My first experience as a therapist teaching wheelchair-to-car transfers to a person with quadriplegia (C7 level;

complete paralysis below shoulder level except for the biceps brachii) underscores the complexity of movement. Despite my attempt to instruct him, he didn't move from the wheelchair. He asked if he could try it his way, so I guarded as he placed his forehead on the dashboard, threw his forearm onto the roof using biceps brachii, momentum, and gravity, and then, contracting neck and elbow flexors, lifted himself into the car. Paralysis prevented a conventional car transfer, but he used biomechanics and environmental resources to solve the movement problem. As in most normal movements, he initiated and controlled the action; the movement was not in response to any external stimulus.

THE MOTOR SYSTEM

Even a simple motor act, such as picking up a pen, involves a complex sequence of events (Figure 9-1). Neural activity begins with a decision made in the anterior part of the frontal lobe. Next, motor planning areas are activated, followed by control circuits. Control circuits, consisting of the cerebellum and basal ganglia, regulate the activity in descending motor tracts. Descending motor tracts deliver signals to spinal interneurons and lower motor neurons (LMNs). LMNs transmit signals directly to skeletal muscles, eliciting contraction of the appropriate muscle fibers that move the upper limb and fingers.

Voluntary movement is controlled from the top down (brain to spinal cord to muscle). However, because understanding the function of higher levels depends on knowledge of lower levels, the following discussion begins with lower levels and progresses to higher levels of the nervous system.

Motor neurons are nerve cells that control skeletal muscles. LMNs directly innervate skeletal muscle fibers. In the spinal region, interactions among neurons determine the information conveyed by LMNs to muscles. Descending tracts deliver movement information from the brain to LMNs in the spinal cord or brainstem. The neurons whose axons travel in descending tracts are upper motor neurons (UMNs). Descending tracts are classified as postural/gross movement tracts, fine movement and limb flexion tracts, and nonspecific UMN tracts. The postural/gross movement tracts control automatic skeletal muscle activity, the fine movement and limb flexion tracts control movements of the limbs and face, and nonspecific UMNs facilitate all LMNs.

The control circuits are the basal ganglia and cerebellum. The control circuits adjust activity in the descend-

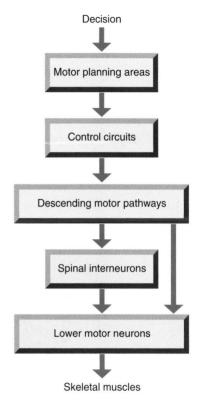

FIGURE 9-1
The neural structures required to produce normal movements. Although sensory information influences each of the neural structures involved in generating movements, the sensory connections have been omitted for simplicity.

ing tracts, resulting in excitation or inhibition of the LMNs. Thus, control circuits partially determine muscle contraction. In all regions of the central nervous system, sensory information adjusts motor activity. Therefore, the contribution of sensation to movement will be covered with each motor section.

LMNs have their cell bodies in the spinal cord or brainstem and synapse with skeletal muscle fibers. Connections in the spinal cord or brainstem determine the activity of LMNs. In contrast, UMNs arise in the cerebral cortex or brainstem, and their axons travel in descending tracts to synapse with LMNs and/or interneurons in the brainstem or spinal cord. Control circuits adjust the activity of the descending tracts.

SKELETAL MUSCLE STRUCTURE AND FUNCTION

Skeletal muscle is excitable, contractile, extensile, and elastic. To understand these properties, the structure and function of skeletal muscle must be considered. The plasma membrane of a muscle cell, called the *sarcolemma* (Figure 9-2), has projections that extend into the muscle, called *T (transverse) tubules.* Adjacent to the T tubules is the sarcoplasmic reticulum, a series of storage sacs for Ca^{++} ions. When acetylcholine (ACh) from an LMN binds with receptors on the sarcolemma, the sarcolemma depolarizes, inducing depolarization of the T tubules. This change in electrical potential elicits the release of Ca^{++} ions from their storage sacs in the sarcoplasmic reticulum. The Ca^{++} ions bind to receptors inside muscle fibers, initiating muscle contraction.

Individual muscle fibers consist of **myofibrils** arranged parallel to the long axis of the muscle fiber (Figure 9-3). Myofibrils consist of proteins arranged in **sarcomeres.** Sarcomeres are the functional units of muscle. Sarcomeres are composed of two types of proteins: structural and contractile. Proteins that provide

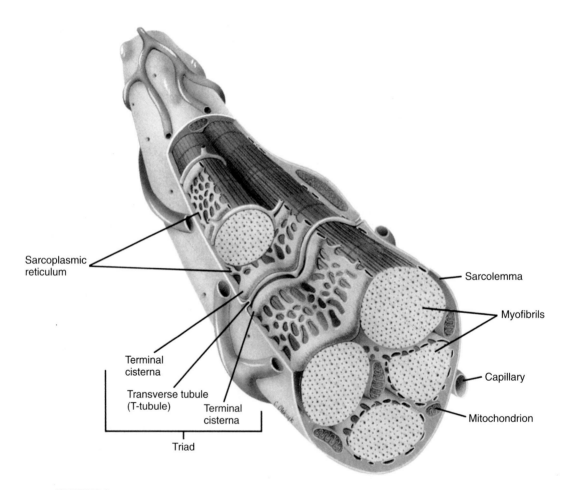

FIGURE 9-2

Sarcoplasmic reticulum and T tubules. The T tubules are continuations of the sarcolemma and are filled with extracellular fluid. On each side of a T tubule are terminal cisternae, part of the sarcoplasmic reticulum. The sarcoplasmic reticulum stores Ca^{++} and surrounds each myofibril. *(From Seeley RR, Stephens TD, et al. (Eds.) (1995). Anatomy and Physiology (ed. 3). New York: McGraw-Hill.)*

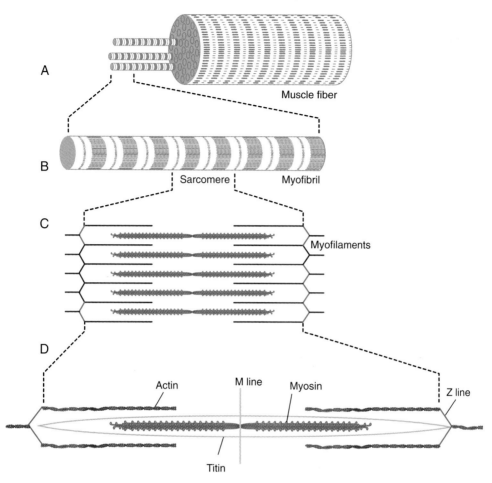

FIGURE 9-3
Structure of skeletal muscle. **A,** Muscle fiber, consisting of many myofibrils. **B,** Myofibril. The section of a myofibril between two Z lines is a sarcomere. **C,** Sarcomere. A sarcomere is composed of myofilaments, including actin and myosin. **D,** Proteins in a sarcomere. Actin is the thin filament, attached to the Z line. Myosin is the thick filament, attached to the M line. Titin is the elastic filament that anchors the M line to the Z line.

structure to the sarcomere include the Z line, M line, and titin. The Z line is a fibrous structure at each end of the sarcomere. The M line anchors the fibers in the center of the sarcomere. Titin, a large elastic protein in muscle, connects the Z line with the M line.

Myosin, actin, tropomyosin, and troponin are the proteins involved in muscle contraction. Myosin forms the thick filaments located in the central region of the sarcomere. The centers of the myosin filaments are connected by the M line. Myosin filaments have specialized projections called *crossbridges,* ending in myosin heads. These heads are capable of binding with active sites on actin. Actin is the primary component of the thin filaments. Actin filaments are anchored at each end of the sarcomere to Z lines. In resting muscle, most binding sites on actin are partially covered by tropomyosin, preventing myosin from binding at the sites. A small protein, troponin, maintains the blocking position of tropomyosin on actin. For muscle to contract, Ca^{++} binds to troponin, causing conformational change in troponin.

The alteration of troponin pulls tropomyosin away from the crossbridge binding sites on actin, allowing myosin to bind with actin.

Muscle is excited when ACh released by LMN at a neuromuscular junction binds with receptors on the sarcolemma. The neuromuscular junction is a synapse between a neuron and the sarcolemma. ACh binding to the receptors causes local depolarization of the muscle cell membrane. The resulting action potential is propagated along the T tubules, eliciting release of Ca^{++} from the sarcoplasmic reticulum. Ca^{++} binding to troponin initiates muscle contraction.

Contraction

Muscle contraction is produced when actin slides relative to myosin. This sliding is initiated when Ca^{++} binds to troponin, and a conformational change in troponin induces movement of the tropomyosin to uncover active sites on actin. This allows myosin heads to attach to these exposed active sites (Figure 9-4). Then the myosin heads swivel, pulling actin toward the center of the sarcomere. Repeated attachment, swiveling, and detachment of myosin heads produces contraction of the muscle (Figure 9-5).

The amount of tension generated by a contracting muscle depends on the length of the sarcomeres. When a sarcomere is at its optimal length, it generates maximal tension. At longer or shorter lengths, the overlap between actin and myosin declines, and less tension can be actively generated. This relationship between the maximal tension a sarcomere can generate and the sarcomere length is illustrated in Figure 9-6. At the shortest lengths, myosin filaments contact the Z line at the end of the sarcomere, hindering active force generation. At short lengths, actin filaments from one side of the sarcomere intrude into the territory of the actin filaments from the other side of the sarcomere, interfering with actin-myosin bonding. At longer than optimal sarcomere lengths, the decrease in overlap between actin and myosin results in fewer actin-myosin bonds, and thus less force can be generated actively.

Force Production

Force production is determined by muscle stiffness. Muscles behave somewhat like springs, in that the force they produce depends on their length. A stretched spring generates more force than the same spring when it is shortened. Resistance to stretch is called *stiffness*. Stiffness is technically defined as change in force per change in length. A stiff muscle generates more resistance to

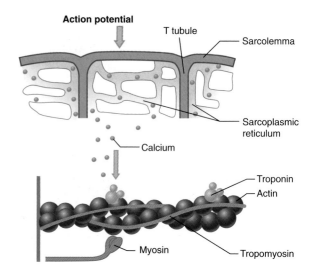

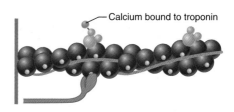

FIGURE 9-4

An action potential initiates muscle contraction. When an action potential depolarizes the sarcolemma, the depolarization spreads to the T tubules. This causes the sarcoplasmic reticulum to release Ca^{++} into the sarcoplasm. The Ca^{++} binds to troponin, and the tropomyosin moves to expose binding sites on actin. Myosin crossbridges bind to the sites on actin.

stretch than a less stiff muscle. Active, intrinsic, and passive factors determine the total stiffness of muscle (Figure 9-7). Active stiffness is initiated by neural signals to muscle: UMN firing and reflexes determine active stiffness. The UMN firing and reflexes both elicit LMN release of sufficient ACh to trigger the active process of muscle contraction. Intrinsic stiffness is produced by weak crossbridge attachments (weak actin-myosin bonds). Passive muscle stiffness arises primarily from the resistance provided by titin. Titin is an elastic, structural protein that maintains the position of myosin relative to actin and prevents the sarcomere from being pulled apart (Figure 9-8). The intrinsic and passive factors are discussed in the following sections.

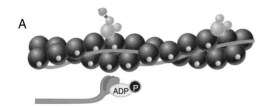

A

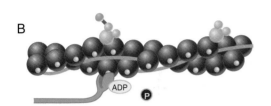

B

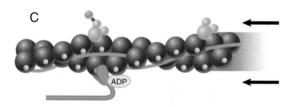

C

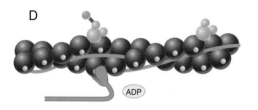

D

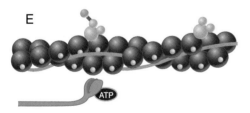

E

FIGURE 9-5
Muscle contraction. **A,** When active sites are exposed on actin, the myosin head is activated by the splitting of the attached ATP into ADP + P (adenosine triphosphate → adenosine diphosphate and phosphate). **B,** The myosin head binds to actin, and P is released from the myosin head. **C,** The crossbridge swivels, causing the actin to slide relative to the myosin. **D,** ADP detaches from the myosin head. **E,** A new ATP molecule binds to the myosin head, breaking the bond with actin.

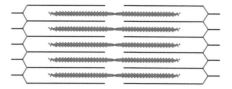

A Sarcomere at optimal length

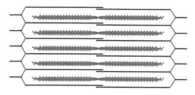

B Sarcomere at shortened length

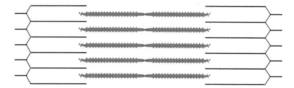

C Excessively lengthened sarcomere

FIGURE 9-6
Length-tension relationship in skeletal muscle. **A,** Muscle is at optimal length, allowing the maximum number of crossbridge connections between actin and myosin. Muscle actively generates maximum tension at this length. **B,** Muscle is in shortened position. The actin filaments intrude into each other's territory, interfering with actin-myosin bonding. The muscle generates little tension at this length. **C,** Muscle is in a lengthened position. Actin and myosin have little overlap, so only a few crossbridges can form. The muscle actively generates little tension at this length. However, lengthened muscle produces a large amount of tension owing to the stretching of titin.

Number of Sarcomeres Adapts to Muscle Length

When healthy, innervated muscle is continuously immobilized in a shortened position for a prolonged period of time, sarcomeres disappear from the ends of myofibrils. For example, if the elbow is maintained at 90° flexion by a cast for 2 months, the biceps will lose sarcomeres. Figure 9-9 illustrates contracture, the changes in muscle structure that occur secondary to prolonged muscle shortening. This loss of sarcomeres is a structural adaptation to the shortened position (Coutinho et al., 2004), so that the muscle can generate optimal force at the new resting length. When a structurally shortened muscle is

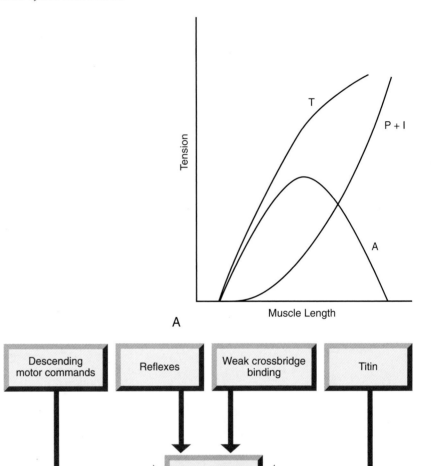

FIGURE 9-7

The relationship between length of a muscle and the tension generated by the muscle. **A,** Indicates the tension produced by active muscle contraction. P is the tension produced by passive stiffness, due to the elasticity of titin. I is intrinsic stiffness, created by weak crossbridge attachments. T is the total force generated by the muscle, produced by active, passive, and intrinsic muscle stiffness. **B,** Summary of the factors that contribute to muscle stiffness.

stretched, it will quickly reach the limits of its elasticity, and will therefore be very resistant to stretch. That is, the decreased amount of titin available to be stretched will limit the extensibility of the muscle. Conversely, if muscle is immobilized in a lengthened position, the muscle will add new sarcomeres (Caiozzo et al., 2002). Chronic loading of muscle, as in physical training, stimulates mechanoreceptors that switch on genes for producing collagen and extracellular matrix to improve the muscle's tensile strength (Kjaer, 2004).

Muscle Tone: Resistance to Passive Stretch

Muscle tone is the amount of stiffness in resting muscle. Clinically, passive range of motion is used to assess muscle tone. When muscle tone is normal, resistance to

passive stretch is minimal. Normal resting muscle tone is provided by intrinsic and passive stiffness. Even in relaxed standing, humans rely primarily on the loading of the skeleton, ligamentous structures, and intrinsic and passive stiffness of muscles; muscles are only slightly active or become active intermittently when sway exceeds tolerable limits.

Normal resistance to stretch is produced by:
- Weak binding of actin and myosin (intrinsic stiffness)
- Titin (passive stiffness)

In resting muscle some myosin heads are attached to actin (Nichols and Cope, 2004). However, these myosin heads do not swivel to produce a power stroke. Thus no muscle contraction occurs, yet mild resistance to stretch

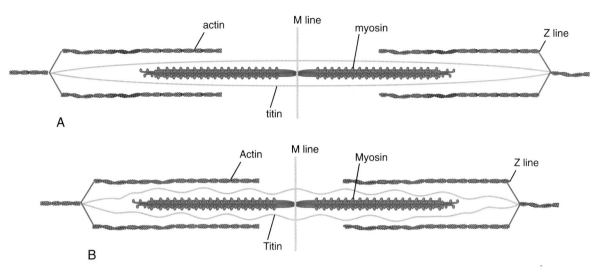

FIGURE 9-8
Actions of titin. **A,** Titin prevents the sarcomere from being pulled apart when the muscle is stretched. **B,** At normal sarcomere lengths, titin maintains the position of myosin in the center of the sarcomere.

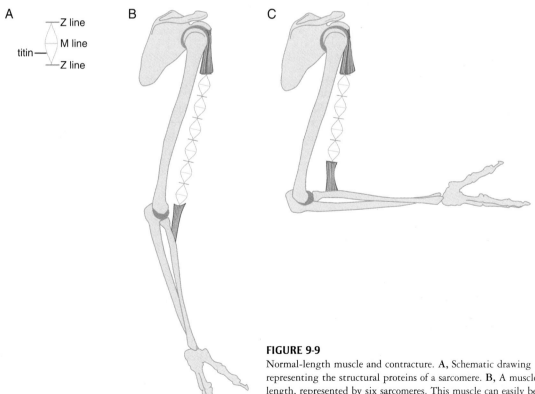

FIGURE 9-9
Normal-length muscle and contracture. **A,** Schematic drawing representing the structural proteins of a sarcomere. **B,** A muscle of normal length, represented by six sarcomeres. This muscle can easily be stretched to achieve full range of motion at the joint. **C,** Contracture, structurally shortened muscle, represented by four sarcomeres. This muscle cannot be stretched to a full range of motion without rupturing.

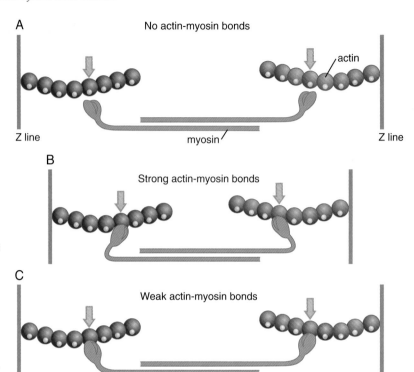

FIGURE 9-10
Actin and myosin bonds. **A,** Actin and myosin are dissociated (no actin-myosin bonds). **B,** Strong bonds between actin and myosin. When a strong bond is formed, the myosin heads swivel, pulling the actin (and the attached Z lines) closer together. This active contraction shortens the sarcomere. **C,** Weak actin-myosin bonds. The actin and myosin are attached, but because the myosin heads do not swivel, the sarcomere length is unchanged. However, a muscle with many weak actin-myosin bonds will produce more resistance to stretch than a muscle with fewer actin-myosin bonds.

is generated by these bonds (Figure 9-10). This weak binding between actin and myosin is somewhat similar to loosely attached Velcro strips, where relatively little force is required to separate the strips. In the relaxed state, when muscles are stretched slowly, individual crossbridges detach before generating large resistance to stretch. However, during fast stretches crossbridges do not have the opportunity to detach, making the muscle stiffer (Nichols and Cope, 2004). If a muscle remains immobile, weak actin-myosin bonds continue to form. Even in people with intact neuromuscular systems, stiffness of forearm muscles doubles during a few minutes of rest (Lakie and Robson, 1988), probably due to weak actin-myosin bonds. Thus, if a muscle is stretched following a prolonged period of immobility, the resistance of the muscle to stretch is increased. Also, in normally innervated muscle, stiffness increases briefly following a prolonged contraction. Sinkjaer (1997) demonstrated that nonreflex stiffness (stiffness intrinsic to the muscles) of the ankle dorsiflexors increases following a prolonged contraction. Intrinsic muscle stiffness is an important factor in standing ankle stability (Casadio et al., 2005).

Titin (see Figure 9-8) is the main contributor to passive resistance to stretch in relaxed muscles. Titin has two distinct elastic regions that respond differently to stretch. One elastic region produces very low levels of passive force at short sarcomere lengths. The other elastic region produces more resistance to force at moderate sarcomere lengths (Neagoe et al., 2003). Weak actin-myosin bonds and the elastic properties of titin together explain the stiffness of completely relaxed, healthy muscles.

> Muscle stiffness is regulated by intrinsic muscle properties (weak crossbridge attachments), passive muscle properties (titin), descending motor signals, and proprioceptive information (from muscle spindles, Golgi tendon organs, joint and cutaneous receptors).

Healthy muscle resistance to stretch has frequently been attributed to stretch reflexes and connective tissue. A stretch reflex is muscle contraction elicited by stretch of the spindle. However, the minimal change in muscle membrane electrical activity during slow stretch of relaxed muscle (Gajdosik et al., 2004) eliminates reflexes as a possible contributor to resting muscle tone because if the muscle membrane is not depolarizing the muscle does not contract. Extracellular connective tissue may play a minor role in the passive stiffness of some muscles (Neagoe et al., 2003).

> Normal relaxed muscle tone does not involve reflexes. Normal resistance to slow passive stretch in relaxed muscle is produced by weak actin-myosin bonds and by titin.

Joint Stiffness

The mechanical stiffness of a joint is the joint's resistance to movement, determined by the sum of muscle stiffness acting on the joint. Both the elastic and contractile forces of these muscles determine joint stiffness. Joint stiffness can be increased by **cocontraction,** the simultaneous contraction of antagonist muscles. Cocontraction stabilizes joints. In the upper limbs, this enables precise movements. An example is threading a needle. In the lower limbs, cocontraction allows a person to stand on an unstable surface, as on the deck of a ship or a moving bus. People frequently use cocontraction when learning a new movement skill (Osu et al., 2002).

Stretch Shortening Cycle

The stretch shortening cycle consists of an eccentric (lengthening) contraction, immediately followed by a concentric (shortening) contraction. The cycle is used to generate maximum muscle force. Athletes often use the stretch shortening cycle. For example, during a tennis serve, the triceps performs an eccentric contraction and then a concentric contraction. This optimizes the force output from the triceps. The energy of the stretch is stored by the elastic components of the muscle and tendon and used during the subsequent contraction. This technique is effective only if the concentric contraction immediately follows the eccentric contraction; otherwise the rebound effect is lost. The stretch shortening cycle is used to increase force in the plyometrics training procedure.

LOWER MOTOR NEURONS

LMNs are the only neurons that convey signals to extrafusal and intrafusal skeletal muscle fibers. There are two types of LMNs: alpha and gamma. Both types have cell bodies in the ventral horn of the spinal cord. Their axons leave the spinal cord via the ventral root, travel through the spinal nerve, then travel through the peripheral nerve to reach skeletal muscle.

Gamma Motor Neurons

Gamma motor neurons have medium-sized myelinated axons (Table 9-1). Axons of gamma motor neurons project to intrafusal fibers in the muscle spindle (see Chapter 6).

Alpha Motor Neurons

Alpha motor neurons have large cell bodies and large, myelinated axons. The axons of alpha motor neurons project to extrafusal skeletal muscle, branching into numerous terminals as they approach muscle.

Motor Units

An alpha motor neuron and the muscle fibers it innervates are called a **motor unit.** Whenever an alpha motor neuron is active, the neurotransmitter ACh is released at all of its neuromuscular junctions, and all muscle fibers innervated by that neuron contract (Figure 9-11). Motor units are classified as slow twitch or fast twitch, depending on the speed of muscle contraction in response to a

Table 9-1 CHARACTERISTICS OF LOWER MOTOR NEURONS

Axon Size and Myelination	Axon Type	Innervates
Large myelinated	Aγ	Extrafusal muscle fibers
Medium myelinated	Aγ	Intrafusal muscle fibers

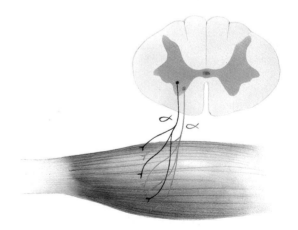

FIGURE 9-11
A motor unit consists of an alpha motor neuron and the muscle fibers it innervates. Two motor units are illustrated to show that muscle fibers innervated by a single neuron are distributed throughout the muscle.

single electrical shock. The neuron innervating the muscle determines the twitch characteristics of the muscle fibers. Smaller-diameter, slower-conducting alpha motor neurons innervate slow twitch muscle fibers; larger-diameter, faster-conducting alpha motor neurons innervate fast twitch muscle fibers.

Slow twitch fibers comprise the majority of muscle fibers in postural and slowly contracting muscles. For example, the soleus muscle has primarily slow twitch fibers and is tonically active in standing and phasically active in walking. The gastrocnemius muscle has more fast twitch muscle fibers than the soleus. Phasic contraction of the gastrocnemius produces fast, powerful movements, like sprinting. In most movements, slow twitch muscle fibers are activated first because the small cell bodies of the slow-conducting alpha motor neurons depolarize before the cell bodies of the larger alpha motor neurons do. Slow twitch muscle fibers typically continue to contribute during faster actions as fast twitch units are recruited. The order of recruitment from smaller to larger alpha motor neurons is called **Henneman's Size Principle.** However, the order of recruitment is modified depending upon the task and phase during human walking and running (Wakeling, 2004).

Motor units also vary in the number of muscle fibers innervated by a single neuron. The human gastrocnemius muscle has approximately 2,000 muscle fibers innervated by each motor neuron. In contrast, the lateral extraocular muscle averages 2.5 muscle fibers per motor neuron because precise control of eye movements is required (Shall et al., 2003).

> A motor unit is a single alpha motor neuron and the muscle fibers the alpha motor neuron innervates.

The activity of a motor unit depends on the convergence of information from peripheral sensors, spinal connections, and descending tracts onto the cell body and dendrites of the alpha motor neuron.

Peripheral Sensory Input to Motor Neurons

Golgi tendon organs (GTOs) and muscle spindles provide somatosensory input to motor neurons. This information is essential for accurate movement. The Golgi tendon organ converts muscle tendon tension into neural impulses. This information is conveyed into the spinal cord, and then, via collaterals and interneurons, to LMNs. Muscle spindles provide information regarding muscle length and velocity of changes in muscle length. Afferent

information from GTOs and muscle spindles is used to adjust movements via connections in the spinal cord and brainstem, and to provide proprioceptive information to the cerebral cortex and cerebellum. The sensitivity of the muscle spindle is adjusted by gamma motor neurons (see Chapter 6).

Alpha-Gamma Coactivation

During most movements, the alpha and gamma motor neuron systems function simultaneously. This pattern, called alpha-gamma coactivation, maintains the stretch on the central region of the muscle spindle intrafusal fibers when the muscle actively contracts. Excitatory signals sufficient to stimulate alpha motor neurons also stimulate gamma motor neurons to spindle fibers in the same muscle. Alpha-gamma coactivation occurs because most sources of input to alpha motor neurons have collaterals that project to gamma motor neurons and because gamma motor neurons, with their smaller cell bodies, require less excitation to reach threshold than do alpha motor neurons.

The activation of alpha and gamma motor neurons depends upon sensory information, spinal circuitry, and descending commands. Next we will consider how spinal region circuitry contributes to spinal region coordination and to spinal reflexes (simple movement responses to peripheral inputs).

SPINAL REGION

Movements are generated when somatosensory information is integrated with descending motor commands in the spinal cord. Networks of spinal interneurons act flexibly to elicit coordinated muscle contractions. As noted in Chapter 5, a group of muscles innervated by a single spinal nerve is called a myotome. Movements associated with specific myotomes are listed in Table 9-2. See Tables 12-1 and 12-2 for lists of specific muscles innervated by spinal nerves.

Motor Neuron Pools in the Spinal Cord

Motor neuron pools are groups of cell bodies in the spinal cord whose axons project to a single muscle. Motor neuron pools are located in the ventral horn. The actions of these pools correlate with their anatomical position: Medially located pools innervate axial and proximal muscles, and laterally located pools innervate distal muscles. Anteriorly located pools innervate extensors, whereas more posterior pools (still within the ventral horn) innervate flexors (Figure 9-12). Axons of descend-

Table 9-2   MOVEMENTS ASSOCIATED WITH SPECIFIC MYOTOMES

Myotome	Movements Produced
C5	Elbow flexion
C6	Wrist extension
C7	Elbow extension
C8	Flexion of tip of middle finger
T1	Finger abduction
L2	Hip flexion
L3	Knee flexion
L4	Ankle dorsiflexion
L5	Great toe extension
S1	Ankle plantar flexion

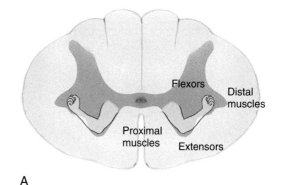

A

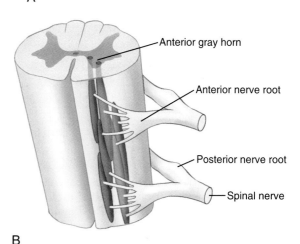

B

FIGURE 9-12
The cell bodies of LMNs are arranged in groups corresponding to each muscle innervated. **A,** The upper limb superimposed on the left anterior horn shows the arrangement of motor neuron pools. Medially located pools innervate axial and girdle muscles. Laterally located pools innervate distal limb muscles. Posterior pools (within the anterior horn) innervate flexor muscles. Anterior pools innervate extensor muscles. **B,** The pools may extend several spinal cord segments.

ing pathways from the brain are grouped according to their termination in the medial or lateral cord.

Spinal Region Coordination

Neuronal connections within the spinal cord contribute to coordination of movement. Reciprocal inhibition, muscle synergies, proprioceptive input, and stepping pattern generators are mechanisms that organize and synchronize muscle contractions to achieve smooth, flowing, effective movements.

Reciprocal Inhibition

Reciprocal inhibition, the inhibition of antagonist muscles during agonist contraction, is achieved by interneurons in the spinal cord that link motor neurons into functional groups. This process is used extensively during voluntary motion to prevent antagonist opposition to the movement. For example, reciprocal inhibition prevents hamstring muscle firing when the quadriceps femoris contracts (Figure 9-13). Reciprocal inhibition also prevents activation of antagonist muscles when an agonist is reflexively activated: A reflex hammer tap on the biceps tendon causes shortening of the biceps and abruptly stretches the triceps. Without a mechanism to prevent a triceps stretch reflex, the biceps contraction would be opposed by contraction of the antagonist muscle. To avert an antagonist stretch reflex, activity in collateral branches from type Ia afferents stimulate interneurons to inhibit the alpha efferent to the antagonist. A more complex example of spinal coordination is the activation of muscle synergies by type II afferents.

Muscle Synergies

Muscle synergy is a term describing coordinated muscular action. We use muscle synergies constantly. When we eat, finger and elbow flexion combine with supination of the forearm to bring food to the mouth. Type II afferents contribute to synergies by delivering information to spinal cord neurons from tonic receptors in muscle spindles, certain joint receptors, and cutaneous and subcutaneous touch and pressure receptors. Interneurons excited by type II afferents project to motor neurons of muscles acting at other joints, providing a spinal region basis for muscle synergies. Motor control researchers typically use the term *synergy* to describe the activity of

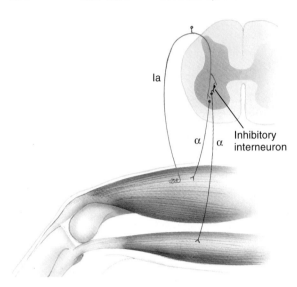

FIGURE 9-13

Reciprocal inhibition. Often, when a muscle is activated, opposition to the movement by antagonist muscles is prevented via inhibitory interneurons.

muscles that are often activated together by a normal nervous system. Clinicians often restrict the use of the term to pathologic synergies, for example when a person with a UMN lesion (due to head injury or stroke) cannot flex the shoulder without simultaneous, obligatory flexion of the elbow.

Proprioceptive Body Schema

The spinal cord creates a complete proprioceptive model, called a *schema,* of the body in time and space. This nonconscious schema is used to plan and adapt movements (Paillard, 1999; Shenton et al., 2004). For example, to hit a tennis ball, one must know the initial position of the arm in order to plan whether to move the racket hand up or down. Joint capsule and ligament receptors, muscle spindle receptors, and Golgi tendon organs provide the proprioceptive input required to generate the body schema.

> The spinal cord interprets proprioceptive information as a whole, and computes a complete proprioceptive image (schema) of the body in time and space. This schema is essential for adapting movements to the environment, based on proprioceptive feedback.

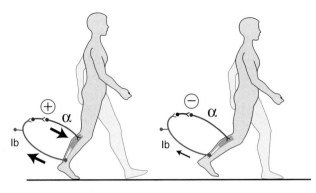

FIGURE 9-14

Golgi tendon organ. Stretch of a tendon activates type Ib afferents that synapse with interneurons. Depending upon the task, GTO input facilitates or inhibits LMN firing. For example, during stance phase of gait, GTO input facilitates LMNs to lower limb extensor muscles. During swing phase, GTO input inhibits LMNs to the same muscles.

Role of Golgi Tendon Organs in Movement

GTOs contribute to proprioception by registering tendon tension. This information is conveyed by type Ib afferents to the spinal cord, stimulating interneurons that excite or inhibit motor neurons to synergists and the muscle of origin (Figure 9-14). For example, stimulation of tendon organs in certain extensor muscles during weight bearing elicits autogenic excitation of the muscles of origin (Quevedo et al., 2000; Donelan and Pearson, 2004). Interneurons that receive signals from GTOs also receive signals from muscle spindles, cutaneous afferents, joint afferents, and descending pathways. In vivo, GTO signals are never isolated from the input of other proprioceptors, and GTO signals do not elicit responses independently from the responses to other proprioceptors. The role of GTOs in movement is to adjust muscle contraction, in concert with other proprioceptive signals and descending control.

Until recently, signals from GTOs were believed to protect muscles from excess loading injury by reflexively preventing excessive muscle contraction. However, the effect of GTO input is not powerful enough to inhibit voluntary muscle contraction. Maximal GTO activity occurs prior to 50% of maximal voluntary contraction (Pratt et al., 1995). Therefore, GTO activation cannot elicit sufficient inhibition to cause reflexive relaxation of overloaded muscle (Pratt et al., 1995). Decreased muscle contraction when muscles are severely overloaded may instead be a response to the integrated afferent information from musculoskeletal receptors, or may be a volitional response. Nor can GTO inhibition explain muscle relaxation following maximal muscle contraction, because when the muscle stops contracting the GTO firing rate decreases.

Effectiveness of Muscle Stretching Techniques Not Dependent on GTO Input. Two techniques commonly used to stretch tight muscles are *contract-relax* and *static stretching*. Contract-relax stretching (also known as *hold-relax*) involves three steps: The target muscle is (1) stretched and held at end range, (2) isometrically contracted against resistance, and (3) passively stretched. For example, a therapist might passively stretch a patient's hamstrings, then hold the limb while the patient contracts these muscles against the therapist's resistance, then stretch the relaxed muscles. Although this technique may briefly facilitate greater passive range of motion, recordings indicate that the hamstrings' electrical activity is the same before and after the procedure (reviewed by Chalmers, 2004). Therapists once believed the brief improvement in range of motion was due to inhibition of alpha motor neurons by Golgi tendon input, but this electrical evidence refutes that explanation. Instead, contract-relax may simply enhance a person's ability to tolerate muscle stretch (reviewed by Chalmers, 2004).

In static stretching, the target muscle is placed at end range and end range is held for a short period of time. Davis et al. (2005) found that a 4-week static stretching program for young adults with tight hamstrings increased hamstring length. The program consisted of a single stretch performed three times per week; participants placed the hamstrings at end range and held the position for 30 seconds. This effect is probably due to muscle viscoelastic properties (Chalmers, 2004).

Spinal Control of Walking: Stepping Pattern Generators

When a person is walking, each lower limb alternately flexes and extends. Circuits in the lumbar spinal cord provide neural processing that elicits stepping movements of the lower limbs. The neural circuits that control stepping movements at the hip and knee are called **stepping pattern generators (SPGs)**. SPGs are adaptable networks of spinal interneurons that activate LMNs to elicit alternating flexion and extension of the hips and knees. Each lower limb has a dedicated SPG (Yang et al., 2005). The cycles of the two SPGs are coordinated by signals conveyed in the anterior commissure of the spinal cord (Butt et al., 2002), so that when one leg flexes the other extends. In addition to generating repetitive

cycles, SPGs receive and interpret proprioception and predict the appropriate sequences of actions throughout the step cycle (Edgerton et al., 2004).

However, the alternating flexion/extension elicited by SPG activity is not the only mechanism responsible for walking. Postural control, cortical control of dorsiflexion (Capaday et al., 1999), and afferent information are also essential for human locomotion. Afferent input adjusts timing, facilitates the transition from stance to swing phase of gait, and reinforces muscle activation (Cattaert, 2004).

> Stepping pattern generators in the spinal cord contribute to walking in humans. However, descending input is normally required to activate SPGs, and the SPGs only provide bilaterally coordinated reciprocal hip and knee flexion/extension. Cortical control is essential for directing ankle dorsiflexion, and vestibulospinal and reticulospinal signals are required to maintain postural control during walking.

Reflexes

Most movement is automatic or voluntary and anticipatory, not reflexive. When a person decides to reach for a book, there is no external stimulus; this movement does not arise from reflex. However, clinical examination of reflexes provides important information about the peripheral and spinal circuits and the level of background excitation in the spinal cord. Spinal region reflexes require sensory receptors, primary afferents, connections between primary afferents and LMNs, and muscles. Spinal region reflexes can operate without brain input; however, normally signals from the brain influence spinal reflexes by adjusting the background level of neural activity in the spinal cord. In this section, stretch reflexes and cutaneous reflexes are discussed.

Stretch Reflexes: Muscle Spindles

There are two types of stretch reflexes: phasic and tonic. The term *phasic* indicates that the response to the stimulus is brief. *Tonic* refers to responses that last as long as the stimulus is maintained. Muscle contraction in response to quick stretch is called the **phasic stretch reflex**. A brisk tap with a reflex hammer on the quadriceps tendon elicits a reflexive contraction of the quadriceps muscle because quick stretch activates neural connections between muscle spindles and alpha motor neurons to the same muscle (Figure 9-15). Tapping the tendon delivers a quick stretch to the muscle and the spindles embedded parallel to the muscle fibers. The

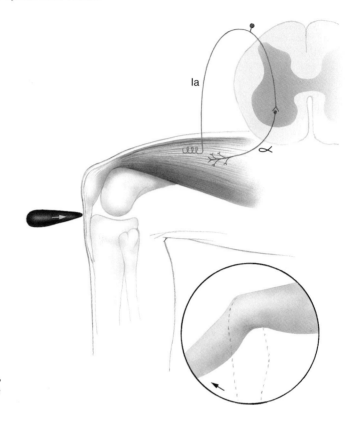

FIGURE 9-15

Phasic stretch reflex. Quick stretch of a muscle, elicited by striking the muscle's tendon, stimulates the type Ia afferents from the muscle spindle. Activity of type Ia afferents causes monosynaptic excitation of alpha motor neurons to the stretched muscle, resulting in abrupt contraction of the muscle fibers.

primary endings of the spindles are stimulated by the quick stretch. Type Ia afferents then transmit action potentials to the spinal cord and release neurotransmitters at synapses with alpha motor neurons. The alpha motor neurons depolarize, action potentials are propagated to the neuromuscular junctions, ACh is released and binds with muscle receptors, the muscle membrane depolarizes, and the muscle fibers contract. Only one synapse links the afferent and efferent neurons; thus the quick response to stretch is a monosynaptic reflex. The terms *myotatic reflex, muscle stretch reflex,* and *deep tendon reflex* are synonymous with phasic stretch reflex. The term *phasic* indicates that the frequency of action potentials in type Ia afferents is greatest during changes in spindle length and decreases when the spindle is maintained at a constant length.

At velocities of stretch used clinically to test muscle resistance to stretch, the **tonic stretch reflex** is only present following UMN lesions (Chou et al., 2005). In contrast to the phasic stretch reflex, the tonic stretch reflex continues as long as the stretch is maintained. The receptors for the tonic stretch reflex are primary and secondary endings in the muscle spindle. Maintained stretch of the central region fires the spindle endings, type Ia and II afferents conduct excitation into the spinal cord, and multiple interneurons link the afferent fiber terminals with LMNs (Figure 9-16). Following UMN lesions, loss of presynaptic inhibition allows slow or sustained stretch of the central spindle to elicit continual muscle contraction. In intact nervous systems, the information conveyed by type Ia and II afferents regarding sustained stretch is used to adjust muscle activity but does not elicit reflexive contraction because presynaptic inhibition and other inputs also influence the LMNs.

Cutaneous Reflexes

Cutaneous stimulation can also elicit reflexive movements. If a person steps on a tack, the withdrawal reflex automatically lifts the foot by flexing the lower limb, even before the person is consciously aware of pain (Figure 9-17). The circuitry responsible for the withdrawal reflex is located within the spinal cord. The withdrawal reflex and related reactions will be described in Chapter 12.

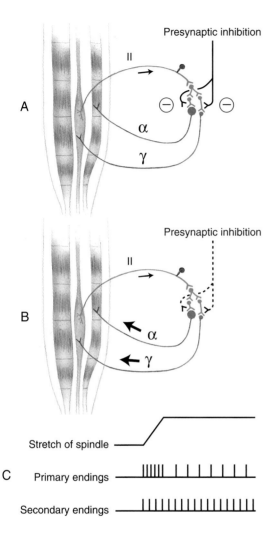

A

Presynaptic inhibition

II

α

γ

B

Presynaptic inhibition

II

α

γ

C Stretch of spindle

Primary endings

Secondary endings

> Activation of the Golgi tendon organ can inhibit or facilitate activity of the corresponding muscle. Reflexes can be elicited by stimulation of musculoskeletal or cutaneous receptors. Stimulation of muscle spindle receptors can result in phasic stretch reflexes, and in cases of UMN lesions, tonic stretch reflexes. Noxious cutaneous information can result in a withdrawal reflex.

Relationship Between Reflexive and Voluntary Movement

Classically, reflexes were considered to be responses to particular types of sensory information exciting only specific, isolated pathways within the spinal cord and resulting in stereotypic output. Voluntary movement

FIGURE 9-16

Tonic stretch reflex. At low or moderate velocities of joint rotation (less than 200° per second), this reflex is only present in people with UMN lesions (Thilmann et al., 1991). **A,** In an intact neuromuscular system, a muscle at rest is stretched passively and the stretch is maintained. Although the spindle afferents convey signals into the spinal cord, the LMNs do not fire because presynaptic inhibition prevents their activation. **B,** Following a complete spinal cord injury, maintained stretch of the muscle spindle elicits sustained firing of the spindle endings. Because presynaptic inhibition is absent, the spindle input is sufficient to activate LMNs, eliciting a tonic stretch reflex. For simplicity, the primary spindle endings are omitted from **A** and **B. C,** The firing frequency of primary endings is maximal while the spindle is being stretched, and the firing rate decreases when the spindle is maintained in a stretched position. The secondary endings fire at a high frequency during stretch of the spindle and while the spindle is maintained in a stretched position. In some UMN lesions, loss of presynaptic inhibition allows the input from secondary endings to elicit LMN firing and active muscle contraction (tonic stretch reflex). In an intact nervous system, input from secondary endings is used to adjust muscle contraction but does not elicit a tonic stretch reflex unless the velocity of stretch is extremely high.

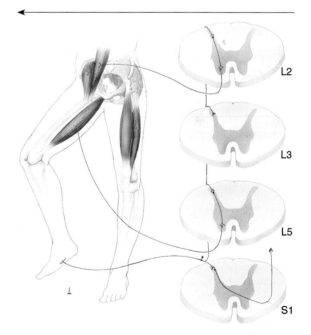

L2

L3

L5

S1

FIGURE 9-17

Withdrawal reflex. Usually in response to a painful cutaneous stimulus, muscles are activated to move the body part away from the stimulation. This action requires polysynaptic connections at multiple levels of the cord because various spinal segments innervate the active muscles.

was considered entirely separate from reflexes. Research has refuted this division. Most sensory stimuli act in an ensemble fashion, the involved interneurons can vary, and appropriate levels of the central nervous system interact to produce context-dependent movement. For example, changing a person's arousal, or alertness, level can modify the movement response to a tendon tap. If a person is relaxed, a quadriceps tendon tap tends to elicit a small movement. If the person is extremely anxious, a tendon tap using the same amount of force will probably elicit a much greater movement. Arousal changes the level of descending input to the spinal circuitry. Furthermore, muscle spindle output is modified by sensitivity adjustments and by the recent movements and contractions the muscle has undergone (Nichols and Cope, 2004). As a result, muscle spindle output is not linearly related to changes in muscle length or rate of change in length. Spindle information is integrated with other proprioceptive inputs to adjust muscle output.

H-reflexes

The H-reflex is a monosynaptic reflex elicited by electrically stimulating a nerve. The purpose is to quantify the level of alpha motor neuron facilitation or inhibition. H-reflex testing substitutes cutaneous electrical stimulation of a peripheral nerve for the tendon percussion of the myotatic reflex. For example, a stimulating electrode is placed over the tibial nerve in the popliteal fossa, and a recording electrode is placed on the inferomedial gastrocnemius (Figure 9-18). A weak current, adequate to stimulate only the largest axons (motor axons and type Ia and Ib afferents, which have the lowest electrical thresholds), is administered to the skin over the tibial nerve. Action potentials travel both toward the muscle (via motor axons) and toward the spinal cord (via type Ia and Ib afferents). The electrical stimulation produces two action potentials with different latencies that can be recorded from the skin over the muscle: the M wave and the H-reflex. The shorter-latency M wave is produced by impulses traveling along motor fibers, causing an almost immediate muscle contraction. The afferent fibers activity elicits the H-reflex. Action potentials in the large afferent fibers travel into the spinal cord, resulting in transmission across synapses to facilitate alpha motor neurons. If the central excitatory state of the alpha motor neurons is near threshold, activation of the alpha motor neurons will in turn cause depolarization of the calf muscle membranes. The H-reflex is slightly faster (by 10 milliseconds) than the tendon tap reflex because it does not require activation of spindle receptors.

UPPER MOTOR NEURONS

UMNs provide all of the motor signals from the brain to the spinal cord and from the cerebrum to the brainstem. UMNs project from cortical and brainstem centers to LMNs (alpha and gamma) and to interneurons in the brainstem and spinal cord. UMNs projecting to the spinal cord are classified according to whether they synapse medially, laterally, or throughout the ventral horn. Medial UMNs signal LMNs that innervate postural and girdle muscles. Lateral UMNs signal LMNs that innervate distally located muscles used for fine movement (Figure 9-19). The group ending throughout the ventral horn, the nonspecific UMNs, contributes to background levels of excitation in the cord and facilitates local reflex arcs.

Postural and Gross Movements: Medial Upper Motor Neurons

UMN activity controlling posture and gross movements usually occurs automatically, without conscious effort. Medial UMN activity can occur before a person is consciously aware of a stimulus. For example, if a loud noise occurs behind a person, the eyes and face turn toward the sound, before the person is consciously aware of the auditory stimulus. These coordinated, involuntary reactions are initiated in the brainstem. From there, medial UMNs convey the signals to the appropriate LMNs.

Four tracts from the brainstem and one from the cerebral cortex deliver signals controlling posture and gross movements to the medial motor neuron pools in the spinal cord. The axons of these tracts are located in the medial white matter of the spinal cord. The tracts include (Figure 9-20):
- tectospinal
- medial reticulospinal
- medial and lateral vestibulospinal
- medial corticospinal

Figure 9-21 shows connections between the medial UMNs and LMNs.

Medial Upper Motor Neuron Tracts

Tectospinal Tract. This tract arises in the superior colliculus section of the tectum (posterior midbrain). The superior colliculus processes visual, auditory, and somatic information. Neural activity in the superior colliculus stimulates neurons that project to the spinal cord in the tectospinal tract, activating LMNs in the cervical spinal cord to signal muscles that reflexively turn the head toward a sound or a visual stimulus.

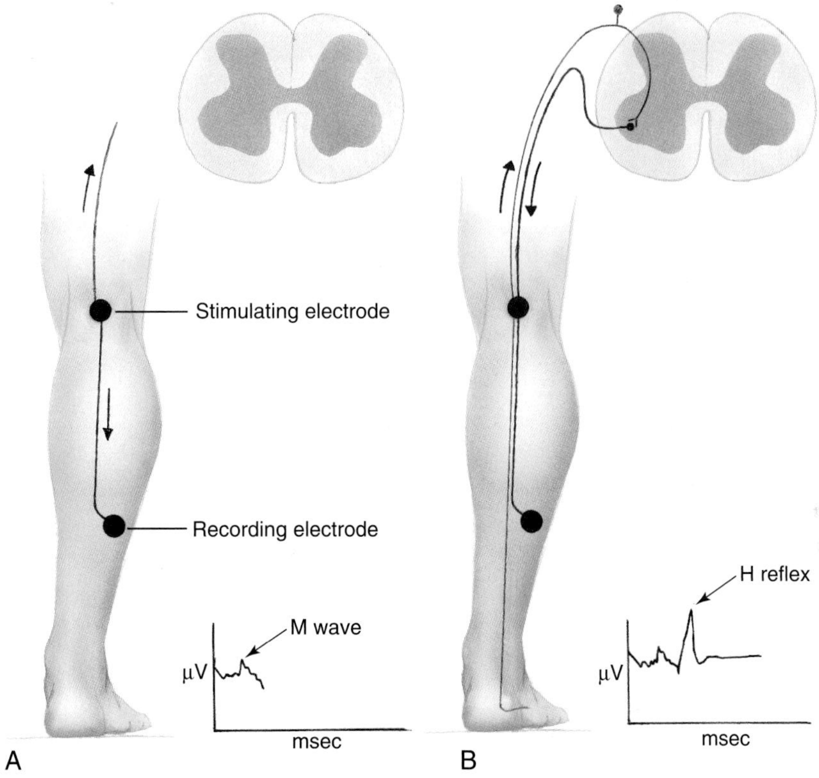

FIGURE 9-18

H-reflex electrode placement for quantifying the level of excitation in tibial nerve alpha motor neurons. **A,** Electrical stimulation applied to the skin in the popliteal fossa over the tibial nerve evokes action potentials in both sensory and motor axons. The action potentials are propagated proximally and distally from the site of stimulation. When the action potentials in alpha motor neurons reach the terminals, ACh is released and binds with receptors on the muscle membrane, and the muscle membrane depolarizes. The depolarization is recorded as the M wave. **B,** Action potentials evoked in the type Ia and Ib fibers are propagated into the spinal cord. Via synaptic connections, alpha motor neurons are stimulated. Then action potentials are propagated toward the muscle, and ACh is released at the neuromuscular junction and binds with receptors on the muscle membrane. When the muscle membrane depolarizes, the H-reflex is recorded.

Quickly turning the head destabilizes a person unless other automatic responses compensate for the change in weight distribution. Signals from the pontine reticular formation and vestibular nuclei activate LMNs to muscles that prevent loss of balance.

Medial Reticulospinal Tract. This tract begins in the pontine reticular formation. Stimulation of this tract facilitates ipsilateral LMNs innervating postural muscles and limb extensors. In addition to their activation by sensory input, the reticulospinal and tectospinal neurons are influenced by the cerebral cortex, forming corticoreticulospinal and corticotectospinal pathways.

Medial Vestibulospinal Tracts. Medial vestibular nuclei receive information about head movement and position from the vestibular apparatus, located in the inner ear. Axons projecting from these nuclei to the spinal cord, the medial vestibulospinal tracts, project bilaterally to cervical and thoracic levels and affect activity in LMNs controlling neck and upper back muscles.

Lateral Vestibulospinal Tracts. The lateral vestibular nucleus responds to gravity information from the vestibular apparatus. The pathways from the lateral vestibular nucleus, the lateral vestibulospinal tracts, project

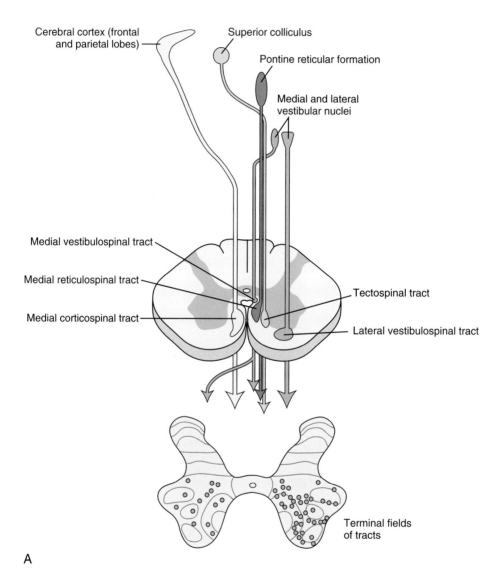

Cerebral cortex (frontal and parietal lobes)

Superior colliculus

Pontine reticular formation

Medial and lateral vestibular nuclei

Medial vestibulospinal tract

Medial reticulospinal tract

Medial corticospinal tract

Tectospinal tract

Lateral vestibulospinal tract

Terminal fields of tracts

A

FIGURE 9-19
Medial and lateral UMNs influence different groups of LMNs. **A,** Medial UMN tracts descend in the anterior column of the spinal cord and synapse with LMNs located in the anteromedial gray matter. These LMNs synapse with axial and girdle muscles.

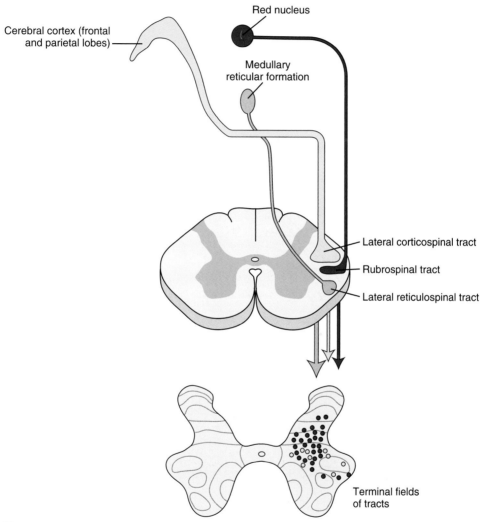

B

FIGURE 9-19, cont'd
B, Lateral UMN tracts descend in the lateral column of the spinal cord and synapse with LMNs located in the anterolateral gray matter. These LMNs synapse with limb muscles.

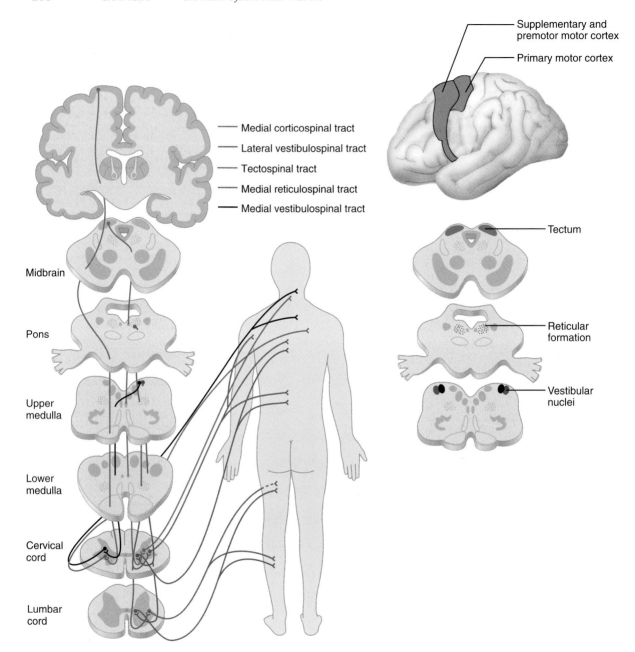

FIGURE 9-20
Medial UMNs adjust the activity in the axial and girdle muscles. The ipsilateral projection of the medial vestibulospinal tract has been omitted for simplicity. The illustrations on the right show the origins of each of the medial UMNs. All sections are horizontal except the coronal section of the cerebrum *(top left)* and the intact cerebrum *(top right)*. For the primary motor cortex, only the areas that control trunk and leg muscles are colored in the drawing at top right, because the areas that control face and distal arm movements do not contribute to control of axial and girdle muscles.

ipsilaterally and facilitate LMNs to extensors while inhibiting LMNs to flexors. When a person is upright, the lateral vestibulospinal tracts are continuously active to maintain the center of gravity over the base of support, responding to the slightest destabilization (Kennedy et al., 2004).

Medial Corticospinal Tract*. The direct connection from the cerebral cortex to the spinal cord, the medial corticospinal tract, descends from the cortex through the internal capsule and the anterior brainstem. The medial corticospinal axons synapse only in the cervical and thoracic cord (the tract does not reach the lower spinal cord), and convey information to LMNs that control neck, shoulder, and trunk muscles.

> Medial UMNs are involved primarily in control of posture and proximal movements. Medial UMNs include the medial corticospinal, medial reticulospinal, medial and lateral vestibulospinal, and tectospinal tracts.

*Evolving terminology: Corticospinal neurons are also known as corticomotoneuronal. Historically, *corticospinal* was an appropriate term because the sensory regulation function of some corticospinal neurons was undiscovered; now, *corticospinal* is a somewhat ambiguous term but remains the most commonly used term to describe UMNs that arise in the cerebral cortex and terminate in the spinal cord.

Most supraspinal control of posture and proximal movement is from brainstem centers. Cortical projections probably prepare the postural system for intended movements. In contrast to the postural and gross movement control of the medial UMNs, a different group of descending pathways controls distal limb movements.

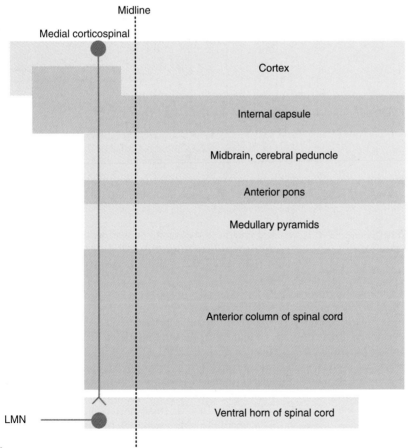

Midline

Medial corticospinal

Cortex

Internal capsule

Midbrain, cerebral peduncle

Anterior pons

Medullary pyramids

Anterior column of spinal cord

Ventral horn of spinal cord

LMN

A

FIGURE 9-21
Schematic diagram of the medial UMNs. The blocks of color indicate different parts of the nervous system, as identified on the right side. **A,** The medial corticospinal tract.

Continued

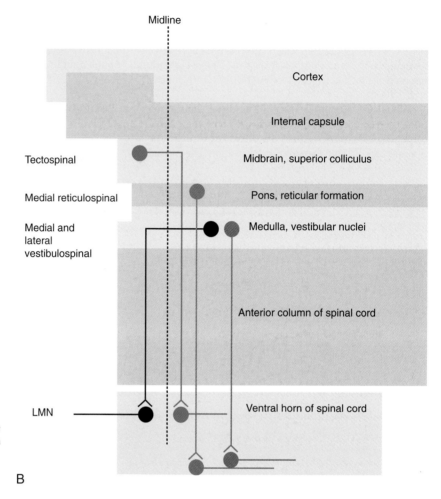

FIGURE 9-21, cont'd
B, Medial UMNs originating in the brainstem. The ipsilateral projection of the medial vestibulospinal tract has been omitted. Compare with Figure 9-20.

Limb Flexion and Fine Movements of Limbs and Face: Lateral Upper Motor Neurons

The UMNs that control limb flexion and fine movements synapse with LMNs in the lateral ventral horn of the spinal cord. Fine movements are precise muscle contractions, which produce movements ranging from the ability to button a button to the ability to simultaneously convey surprise and dismay via facial expression. The fine movement tracts for facial muscles, the corticobulbar tracts, synapse with LMNs in the brainstem. The corticobulbar tracts are discussed at the end of this section.

The three tracts controlling fine movements of the limbs and limb flexion descend in the lateral spinal cord and synapse with laterally located motor neuron pools in the ventral horn (Figure 9-22).

The lateral tracts that descend into the spinal cord are:
- Lateral corticospinal
- Rubrospinal
- Lateral reticulospinal

Figure 9-23 is a schematic of these pathways. The function of the lateral UMNs versus medial UMNs was discovered in a classic experiment: In monkeys, the only long-term deficit from severing the lateral corticospinal and rubrospinal tracts was the inability to use the fingers individually to pick small objects out of deep cavities in a board; balance, walking, running, and climbing abilities remained near normal (Lawrence and Kuypers, 1968).

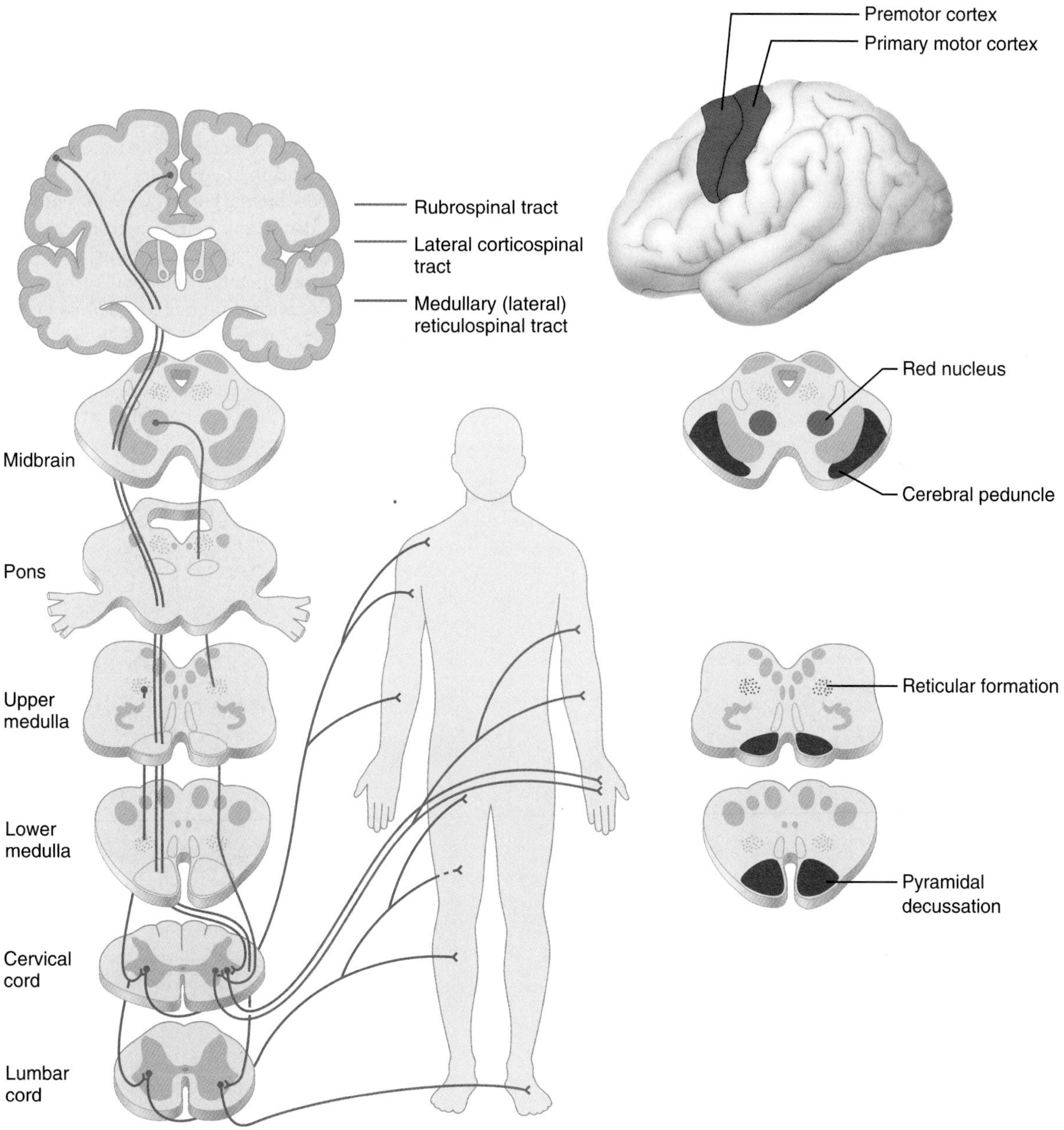

Premotor cortex

Primary motor cortex

Rubrospinal tract

Lateral corticospinal tract

Medullary (lateral) reticulospinal tract

Red nucleus

Cerebral peduncle

Midbrain

Pons

Reticular formation

Upper medulla

Lower medulla

Pyramidal decussation

Cervical cord

Lumbar cord

FIGURE 9-22
Lateral UMNs adjust the activity in limb muscles. The contralateral projection of the lateral reticulospinal tract has been omitted for simplicity. The illustrations on the right show the origins of each of the lateral UMN tracts and highlight areas of the brainstem *(in red)* that are composed of lateral corticospinal axons.

Lateral Upper Motor Neuron Tracts

Lateral Corticospinal Tract. The unique contribution of the lateral corticospinal tract* is fractionation of movement, the ability to activate individual muscles

---

*Clinical terminology: Historically, the corticospinal tract was considered to be the most important pathway, with other descending pathways playing minor supporting roles. Because the lateral corticospinal tract forms the medullary pyramids, this tract was called the *pyramidal system*. The remaining motor tracts were called *extrapyramidal*. The basal ganglia were mistakenly believed to exclusively control the extrapyramidal tracts, and thus, in clinical terminology, *extrapyramidal* became synonymous with *basal ganglia*. This terminology remains common in clinical use. The division of motor control into pyramidal/extrapyramidal is a false dichotomy because the basal ganglia are a major influence on cortical motor areas and so contribute to the control of the pyramidal tract, and because the cerebral cortex and cerebellum have great influence on the descending tracts that were formerly called *extrapyramidal*.

independently of other muscles. Fractionation is essential for normal movement of the hands, enabling us to tie knots, press individual piano or computer keyboard keys, and pick up small objects. Without fractionation, the fingers and thumb would act as a single unit, as they do when picking up a water bottle. This tract arises in motor planning areas and in the primary motor cortex. From their origin in the cerebral cortex, the axons project downward, passing first through the internal capsule, then the cerebral peduncles, the anterior pons, the pyramids of the medulla, and finally the lateral spinal cord to synapse with LMNs controlling fine distal movements (see Figure 9-22). The corticospinal tracts in the lower medulla form the pyramids, where, at the junction of the medulla and spinal cord, the lateral corticospinal axons cross to the contralateral side (the medial corticospinal axons remain ipsilateral; see Figure 9-20).

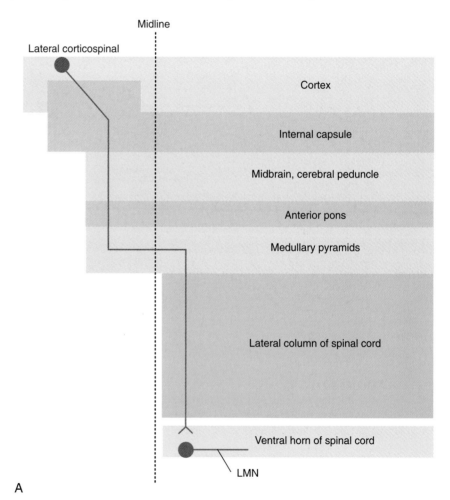

FIGURE 9-23
Schematic diagram of the lateral UMNs. The blocks of color indicate different parts of the nervous system, as identified on the right side. **A,** Schematic diagram of the lateral corticospinal tract.

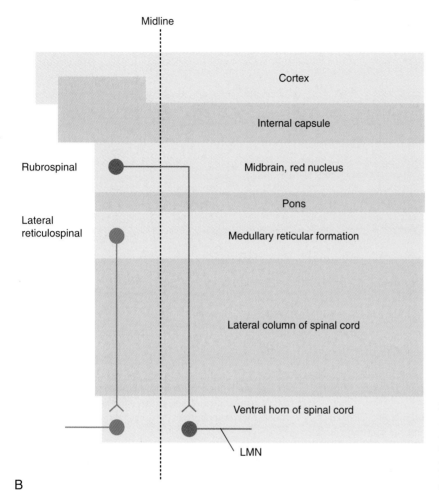

Midline

Cortex

Internal capsule

Rubrospinal

Midbrain, red nucleus

Pons

Lateral reticulospinal

Medullary reticular formation

Lateral column of spinal cord

Ventral horn of spinal cord

LMN

B

FIGURE 9-23, cont'd
B, Schematic diagram of the rubrospinal and medullary (lateral) reticulospinal tracts. The contralateral projection of the medullary reticulospinal tract has been omitted for simplicity. Compare with Figure 9-22.

Origin of Corticospinal Tracts. Lateral corticospinal fibers arise in the primary motor, premotor, and supplementary motor cortex. The primary motor cortex is located anterior to the central sulcus, in the precentral gyrus. This area of cortex provides precise, entirely contralateral control of movements of the hand, lower face, and foot. In contrast, muscles that are frequently activated bilaterally, including muscles of the back, receive signals from both primary motor cortices via the medial corticospinal tract. The corticospinal cell bodies in the primary motor cortex are arranged somatotopically, in an inverted homunculus similar to the cortical sensory representation (Figure 9-24).

Two regions anterior to the primary motor cortex are involved in preparing for movement: The lateral premotor area is on the lateral surface of the hemisphere,

and the supplementary motor area is on the superior and medial surface (Figure 9-25). The lateral premotor area is named for its position anterior to the primary motor cortex. Stimulation of the lateral premotor area produces muscle activity that spans several joints. Unlike in the lateral premotor cortex, many supplementary motor cortex cells are active prior to movements that require coordination of both hands (e.g., buttoning a button; Carson, 2005) and sequential movements that require actions to be accomplished in a specific order (e.g., putting on socks before shoes; Mushiake et al., 1990).

Rubrospinal Tract. The rubrospinal tract originates in the red nucleus of the midbrain, crosses to the opposite side, then descends through the pons, medulla, and lateral spinal cord to synapse with LMNs primarily

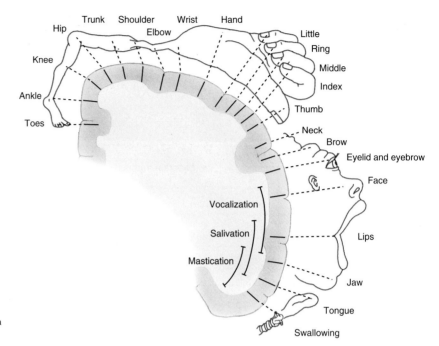

FIGURE 9-24
Motor homunculus. Map of the functional arrangement of neurons in the primary motor cortex.

innervating upper limb flexor muscles (see Figure 9-22).

Lateral (Medullary) Reticulospinal Tract. This tract usually facilitates flexor muscle motor neurons and inhibits extensor motor neurons. During some movements, particularly walking, the effect of lateral reticulospinal tract activity is reversed: the lateral reticulospinal tract inhibits flexor muscle motor neurons and facilitates extensor muscle motor neurons (Noga et al., 2003). The tract originates in the lateral reticular formation and descends bilaterally. The rubrospinal and lateral reticulospinal tracts both receive input from the cerebral cortex.

Attention affects the output of voluntary motor control. In a study of people with normal nervous systems, researchers assessing muscle activity using EMG found that attending to the active limb increases muscle activity, and attending to external factors (metronome beat or movement of apparatus, for example) decreases muscle activity (Vance et al., 2004).

Corticobulbar Tract. Corticobulbar fibers arise in the motor areas of the cerebral cortex, then project to cranial nerve nuclei in the brainstem. This tract facilitates LMNs innervating the muscles of the face, tongue, pharynx, and larynx, and the trapezius and sternocleidomastoid (Figures 9-26 and 9-27). LMNs to muscles of the lower face are controlled by contralateral corticobulbar fibers. LMNs to muscles of the upper face are bilaterally controlled by corticobulbar neurons.

> The lateral UMN tracts that direct limb movements via spinal LMNs are the lateral corticospinal, rubrospinal, and lateral reticulospinal tracts. The lateral corticospinal tract is unique in providing fractionation of distal movements. The corticobulbar tracts direct movements of facial muscles via LMNs in cranial nerves.

Nonspecific Upper Motor Neurons

Tracts descending from two bilateral nuclei in the brainstem enhance the activity of interneurons and motor neurons in the spinal cord. The locus ceruleus and raphe nuclei are the sources of the *ceruleospinal* and *raphespinal* tracts (Figure 9-28). The raphespinal tract releases serotonin, modulating the activity of spinal LMNs. The ceruleospinal tract releases norepinephrine, producing tonic facilitation of spinal LMNs (Palmeri et al., 1999). Both of these tracts are activated during excessive limbic activity. Holstege (1996) calls these tracts part of the

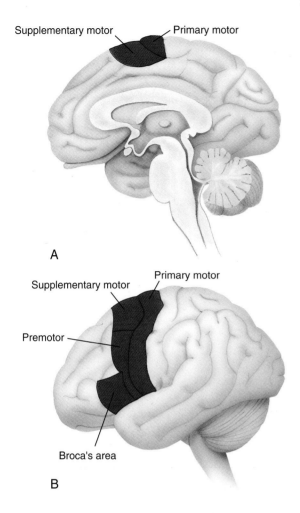

A

B

FIGURE 9-25
Location of the primary motor, premotor, and supplementary motor cortices. Broca's area plans the movements of speech.

emotional motor system. The motor effects of both tracts are general, not related to specific movements, and may contribute to poorer motor performance when anxiety is high. For example, climbers on a high wall move more slowly, make more exploratory movements, and use each hold longer than on a lower climbing wall, even when the traverse itself is identical (Pijpers et al., 2005). Similarly, in normal young adults, fear of falling (induced by standing at the edge of an elevated platform) reduces the magnitude and rate of postural adjustments (Adkin et al., 2002). Table 9-3 lists the UMN tracts.

SIGNS OF MOTOR NEURON LESIONS

Disorders of the motor system may cause the following:
- Paresis and paralysis
- Muscle atrophy
- Involuntary muscle contractions
- Abnormal muscle tone
- Abnormal reflexes
- Muscle hyperstiffness
- Disturbances of movement efficiency and speed (discussed in Chapter 10)
- Impaired postural control (discussed in Chapter 10)

The first four impairments listed are described in the following section. Muscle hyperstiffness and reflexes are discussed within the context of specific neurologic disorders.

Paresis and Paralysis

Decreased ability to generate muscle force and decreased muscle bulk are common consequences of motor neuron lesions. Although the terms *paresis* and *paralysis* are often used synonymously, technically *paralysis* refers to complete loss of voluntary contraction, while *paresis* refers to partial loss. Decreased muscle strength is commonly described by its distribution: *hemiplegia* is weakness affecting one side of the body, *paraplegia* affects the body below the arms, and *tetraplegia* affects all four limbs. A complete lesion of a peripheral nerve, interrupting all the axons in the nerve, produces paralysis because LMNs are the only pathway from the central nervous system to skeletal muscle. UMN lesions may cause paresis, because some of the descending motor tracts may be intact. For example, a stroke may interrupt the corticospinal tract neurons that synapse with LMNs to the right hand. The person may retain some voluntary control of hand movements via the lateral reticulospinal and tectospinal tracts.

Atrophy

Atrophy is the loss of muscle bulk. **Disuse atrophy** results from lack of muscle use, while **neurogenic atrophy** is caused by damage to the nervous system. Denervation of skeletal muscle produces the most severe atrophy, because frequent neural stimulation, even at a level inadequate to produce muscle contraction, is essential for the health of skeletal muscle. When LMNs no longer provide stimulation that influences genetic expression in muscles, muscle atrophy occurs rapidly because the pattern of protein production in the muscle

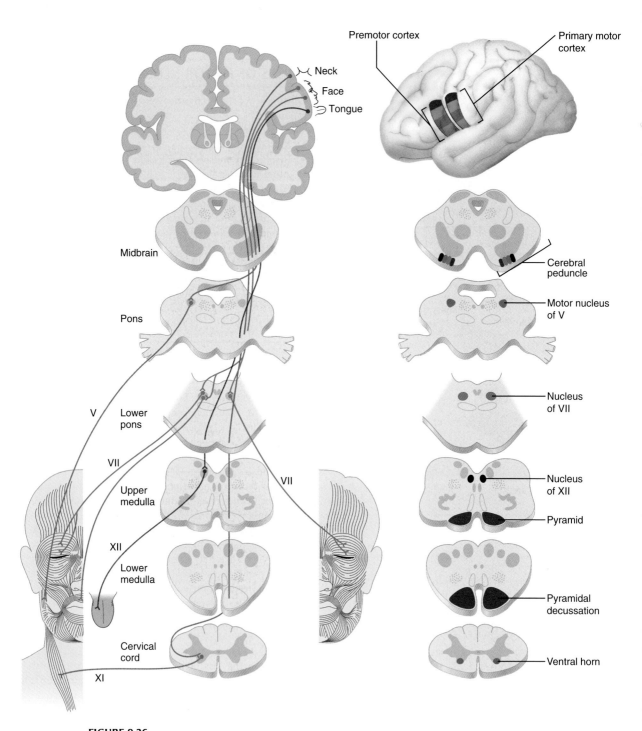

FIGURE 9-26

Corticobulbar tracts. Axons from the cerebral cortex transmit information to cranial nerve cell bodies; the cranial nerves project to muscles controlling movements of the head and neck. Descending input from the cortex influences all eight cranial nerves that innervate skeletal muscle. For simplicity, only four of the eight cranial nerves that innervate skeletal muscle are illustrated. The illustrations on the right show the origin of the corticobulbar tracts, areas composed of corticobulbar axons, and sites of synapse between corticobulbar neurons and LMNs. The sites of synapse illustrated are the nuclei of cranial nerves V, VII, XI, and XII.

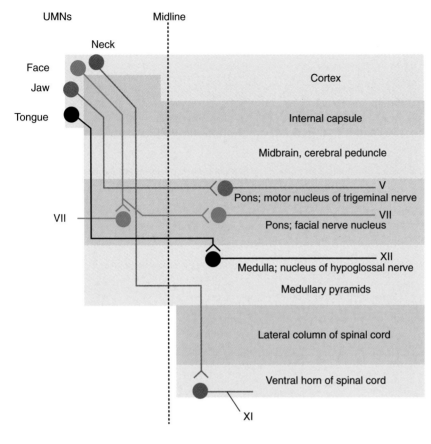

FIGURE 9-27
Schematic diagram illustrating the connections of UMNs with LMNs in cranial nerves V, VII, XI, and XII. In this case, the UMNs are corticobulbar neurons. The blocks of color indicate different parts of the nervous system, as identified on the right side. Compare with Figure 9-24.

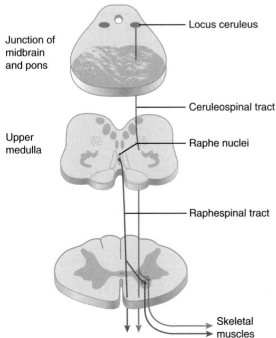

FIGURE 9-28
Nonspecific UMNs. When active, the ceruleospinal and raphespinal tracts facilitate LMNs to skeletal muscles.

Table 9-3   SUMMARY OF UPPER MOTOR NEURONS

Medial Upper Motor Neuron Tracts		
Tract	Origin	Function
Medial corticospinal	Supplementary motor, premotor, and primary motor cerebral cortex	Control of neck, shoulder, and trunk muscles
Tectospinal	Superior colliculus of midbrain	Reflexive movement of head toward sounds or visual moving objects
Medial reticulospinal	Pontine reticular formation	Facilitates postural muscles and limb extensors
Medial vestibulospinal	Vestibular nuclei in medulla and pons	Adjusts activity in neck and upper back muscles
Lateral vestibulospinal	Vestibular nuclei in medulla and pons	Ipsilaterally facilitates LMNs to extensors; inhibits LMNs to flexors
Lateral Upper Motor Neuron Tracts		
Lateral corticospinal	Supplementary motor, premotor, and primary motor cerebral cortex	Contralateral fractionation of movement, particularly of hand movements
Rubrospinal	Red nucleus of midbrain	Facilitates contralateral upper limb flexors
Lateral reticulospinal	Medullary reticular formation	Facilitates flexor muscle motor neurons, and inhibits extensor motor neurons
Nonspecific Upper Motor Neuron Tracts		
Ceruleospinal	Locus ceruleus in the brainstem	Enhances the activity of interneurons and motor neurons in the spinal cord
Raphespinal	Raphe nucleus in the brainstem	Same as ceruleospinal

changes. Normally innervated skeletal muscle produces 400 proteins. Following denervation, muscle production of 26 proteins decreases, and the production of 6 proteins increases (Jia et al., 2005). However, in UMN lesions, skeletal muscle continues to receive stimulation from the intact LMNs, and the rate of atrophy is slower than in LMN lesions.

Involuntary Muscle Contractions

Spontaneous involuntary muscle contractions include the following:
- Muscle spasms
- Cramps
- Fasciculations
- Myoclonus
- Fibrillations
- Abnormal movements generated by dysfunctional basal ganglia

Of these involuntary contractions, the first four occasionally occur in a healthy neuromuscular system, or they may be signs of pathology. **Muscle spasms** (sudden, involuntary contractions of muscle) and **cramps** (particularly severe and painful muscle spasms) are common following prolonged exercise, particularly if sweating has led to sodium depletion. **Fasciculations** (quick twitches of muscle fibers of a single motor unit that are visible on

the surface of the skin) are responsible for the eyelid twitches that sometimes accompany anxiety. **Myoclonus** (brief, involuntary contractions of a muscle or group of muscles) explains hiccups and the muscle jerks that some people experience when falling asleep.

Pathologic cramps, spasms, and fasciculations will be discussed within the context of specific lesions. Pathologic myoclonus occurs in epilepsy, brain or spinal cord injury, stroke, and chemical or drug poisoning. **Fibrillations** (brief contractions of single muscle fibers not visible on the surface of the skin) and abnormal movements are always pathologic. Fibrillations can result from UMN or LMN disorders. Abnormal movements due to basal ganglia disorders are considered within that context in Chapter 10.

Abnormal Muscle Tone

Muscle tone is defined as the stiffness (resistance to stretch) in resting muscle. Abnormally low resistance to passive stretch, called **hypotonia** or **flaccidity,** can be caused by:
- LMN lesions
- Acute UMN lesions (hypotonia is usually temporary in this case)
- Developmental disorders, usually caused by brain hypoxia/ischemia, intracranial hemorrhage, or genetic

or metabolic disorders (Paro-Panjan and Neubauer, 2004).

Hypertonia, abnormally strong resistance to passive stretch, can be caused by:
- Chronic UMN lesions
- Some basal ganglia disorders

There are two types of hypertonia: spastic and rigid. In velocity-dependent, or spastic, hypertonia (usually called *spasticity*), the amount of resistance to passive movement depends on the velocity of movement. Therefore spasticity is velocity-dependent hypertonia. In velocity-independent hypertonia, or *rigidity,* resistance to passive movement remains constant, regardless of the speed of force application. Thus rigidity is velocity-independent hypertonia. Decerebrate rigidity, caused by severe midbrain lesions, comprises rigid extension of the limbs and trunk, internal rotation of the upper limbs, and plantar flexion (Figure 9-29, *A*). Decorticate rigidity, caused by severe lesions superior to the midbrain, comprises flexed upper limbs, extended neck and lower limbs, and plantar flexion (Figure 9-29, *B*).

When an acute UMN lesion interrupts descending motor commands, the LMNs affected become temporarily inactive. This condition is called *spinal shock* or *cerebral shock,* depending on the location of the lesion. During nervous system shock, stretch reflexes cannot be elicited, and the muscles are hypotonic; that is, the muscles have abnormally low tone because facilitation of LMNs by descending UMNs has been lost. Following recovery from central nervous system shock, interneurons and LMNs usually resume activity, although their activity is no longer modulated (or is abnormally modulated) by UMNs. In many cases, during the months following a UMN lesion, muscle tone increases as a result of changes within the muscles, producing excessive resistance to muscle stretch (see later section on muscle hyperstiffness). See Chapter 12 for a discussion of spinal shock and recovery of reflexes.

DISORDERS OF LOWER MOTOR NEURONS

Trauma, infection (poliomyelitis), degenerative or vascular disorders, and tumors can damage LMNs. Interrupting LMN signals to muscle decreases or prevents muscle contraction. If LMN cell bodies and/or axons are destroyed, the affected muscles can undergo:
- Loss of reflexes
- Atrophy
- Flaccid paralysis
- Fibrillations

Traumatic injuries to LMNs are discussed in Chapter 11. An infection that only affects LMNs is poliovirus, which selectively invades LMNs and destroys some of them (Figure 9-30), denervating some muscle fibers. Polio survivors recover some muscle strength as surviving neurons sprout new terminal axons and innervate the

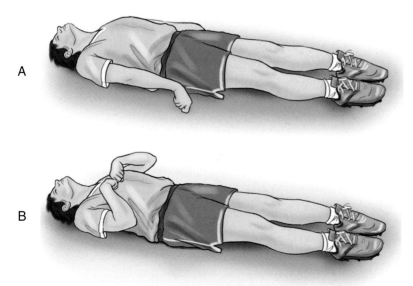

FIGURE 9-29
Rigidity. **A,** In decerebrate rigidity, the limbs and trunk are extended, the upper limbs are internally rotated, and the feet are plantarflexed. **B,** In decorticate rigidity, the upper limbs are flexed and the lower limbs are extended with the feet plantarflexed.

muscle fibers (Figure 9-31). In some polio survivors, post polio syndrome occurs years after the acute illness. The syndrome is not due to death of entire motor neurons; instead, the overextended surviving neurons cannot support the abnormal number of axonal branches, causing some distal branches to die.

Symptoms of post polio syndrome include increasing muscle weakness, joint and muscle pain, fatigue, and breathing problems. Grimby et al. (1998) reported that people who had polio more than 24 years previously had only 60% of the strength of age-matched control subjects, and showed signs of ongoing denervation/reinnervation of muscle fibers. This muscle weakness may be a normal age-related strength decline, more obvious in people who previously had polio because their muscles were previously weakened. Moderate intensity exercise has been demonstrated to be safe and beneficial in postpolio syndrome (Chan et al., 2003).

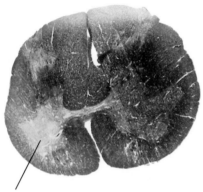

Loss of lower motor neuron cell bodies

FIGURE 9-30
Horizontal section of a spinal cord post polio. The section has been stained for myelin, so that the white matter appears dark. Loss of cell bodies is visible in the anterior horn. *(Courtesy Dr. Melvin J. Ball.)*

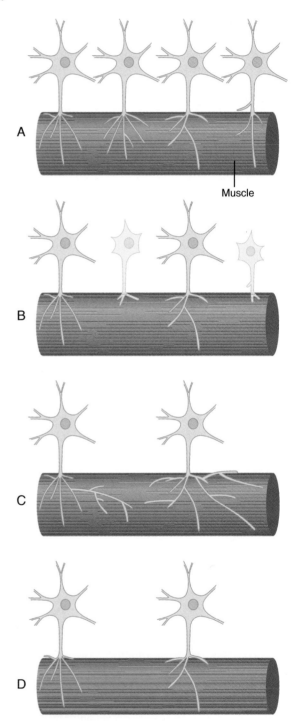

Muscle

FIGURE 9-31
Effects of polio on alpha motor neurons. **A,** Healthy motor units with normal innervation. **B,** Acute polio; death of some neurons leading to muscle fiber atrophy. **C,** Recovery; surviving neurons grow new distal branches to reinnervate surviving muscle fibers. **D,** Late postpolio; overextended neurons can no longer support the excessive number of distal branches. The newer distal branches atrophy, leaving some muscle fibers denervated.

UPPER MOTOR NEURON SYNDROME

UMNs can be damaged by spinal cord injury, cerebral palsy, multiple sclerosis, trauma, or loss of blood supply to part of the brain (stroke). UMN lesions can produce several changes in movement control, including:
1. Paresis
2. Loss of fractionation of movement
3. Abnormal reflexes
4. Muscle hyperstiffness

   Two other signs that typically occur only in specific types of UMN lesions, cocontraction (usually in spastic cerebral palsy) and abnormal muscle synergies (usually post stroke), will be discussed later in this chapter.

Paresis

Paresis occurs in UMN lesions as a consequence of inadequate recruitment of LMNs. Paresis is common following **stroke,** the sudden onset of neurologic deficits due to disruption of the blood supply in the brain (also called *cerebrovascular accident,* or *CVA*). Bobath (1977), the founder of neurodevelopmental therapy, contended that people post stroke do not lack muscle power on the affected side; she asserted that apparent weakness post stroke was due to antagonist muscle contraction opposing agonist muscle activity. However, research provides no evidence that antagonist opposition is a limiting factor in movement post stroke (Burne et al., 2005). Instead, paresis and loss of ability to fractionate movement are the major determinants of activity limitations (Sommerfeld et al., 2004). Gowland et al. (1992) recorded EMG activity during six different tasks in people post stroke, and found that decreased agonist activity was associated with inability to perform the tasks; no evidence for excessive antagonist activation was found.

   Paresis following UMN lesions leads to muscle disuse, causing secondary changes in muscles and the nervous system. Chronic muscle disuse often causes adaptive muscle contracture. Disuse also decreases the motor cortex representation of the disused body parts, leading to further paresis (Gracies, 2005).

Loss of Fractionation of Movement

As discussed earlier, fractionation is the ability to activate individual muscles independently of other muscles. Interruption of lateral corticospinal signals prevents fractionation, profoundly affecting the ability to use the hand. Loss of fractionation interferes with fine movements, including fastening buttons or picking up coins, because the fingers of the involved hand act as a single unit.

Abnormal Reflexes

Abnormal reflexes that may occur following UMN lesions include abnormal cutaneous reflexes, muscle stretch hyperreflexia, clonus, and the clasp-knife response.

Abnormal Cutaneous Reflexes

Changes in cutaneous reflexes include Babinski's sign (Figure 9-32) and muscle spasms in response to normally innocuous stimuli. **Babinski's sign** is extension of the great toe, often accompanied by fanning of the other toes. Firm stroking of the lateral sole of the foot, from the heel to the ball of the foot, then across the ball of the foot, elicits the sign. A key or the end of the handle of a reflex hammer is usually used as the stimulus. In infants until about 7 months of age, Babinski's sign is normal because the corticospinal tracts are not adequately myelinated. Although Babinski's sign is pathognomonic for corticospinal tract damage in people older than 6 months of age, the mechanism is not understood.

   In people with spinal cord injury, muscle spasms may occur in response to cutaneous stimuli. These spasms begin after recovery from spinal shock (**spinal shock,** caused by edema, is a temporary suppression of spinal cord function at and below the lesion following spinal cord injury). Following spinal shock, mild cutaneous stimulation, such as a gentle touch on the foot or putting on clothing, may result in abrupt flexion of the lower limb. Occasionally, a touch on one lower limb may elicit bilateral lower limb flexion. In rare cases the muscle spasms are severe enough to disturb the person's sitting balance, which can cause the person to fall out of a chair.

   The following three abnormal reflexes occur most often in people with chronic spinal cord injuries, although these signs may also occur in other types of UMN lesions.

Muscle Stretch Hyperreflexia

In tonic stretch hyperreflexia, absence of the moderating influence of UMNs onto the LMNs causes an excessive response to muscle spindle input. The result is excessive muscle contraction when spindles are stretched, due to the excessive firing of LMNs (see Figure 9-16).

Clonus

Involuntary, repeating, rhythmic muscle contractions are called **clonus.** Muscle stretch, cutaneous and noxious

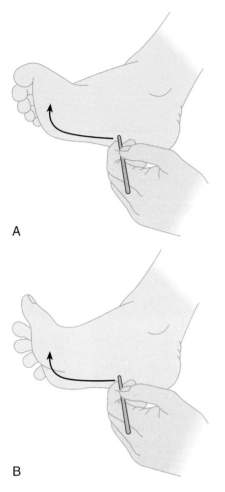

FIGURE 9-32

Babinski's sign. **A,** Normal. Stroking from the heel to the ball of the foot along the lateral sole, then across the ball of the foot, normally causes the toes to flex. **B,** Developmental or pathologic. Babinski's sign in response to the same stimulus. In people with corticospinal tract lesions or in infants less than 7 months old, the great toe extends, Although the other toes may fan out, as shown, movement of the toes other than the great toe is not required for Babinski's sign.

stimuli, and attempts at voluntary movement can induce clonus (Beres-Jones et al., 2003). Not all clonus is pathologic; rapid passive ankle dorsiflexion may elicit unsustained clonus in neurologically intact people. Unsustained clonus fades after a few beats, even with maintained muscle stretch (Campbell, 2005). Sustained clonus is always pathologic. Sustained clonus is produced when a lack of UMN control allows activation of oscillating neural networks in the spinal cord (Beres-Jones et al., 2003). In people with chronic spinal cord injury or other UMN lesion, sustained clonus of the soleus muscle may be triggered by placement of a foot on a wheelchair footrest.

Clasp-Knife Response

Occasionally when a paretic muscle is slowly and passively stretched, resistance drops at a specific point in the range of motion. This is called the **clasp-knife response** because the change in resistance is similar to opening a pocketknife: The initial strong resistance to opening the knife blade gives way to easier movement. When a therapist passively stretches a paretic biceps brachii muscle, resistance to passive movement is initially strong. However, if stretch is steadily applied, often the therapist will encounter an abrupt decrease in resistance. Type II afferents, including some joint capsule receptors and cutaneous and subcutaneous touch and pressure receptors, elicit the clasp-knife response (Ivanhoe and Reistetter, 2004).

Muscle Hyperstiffness

Excessive resistance to muscle stretch is called **hyperstiffness.** In contrast to hypertonia (which only refers to resistance to passive stretch), hyperstiffness refers to excessive resistance to both passive and active muscle stretch. Excessive muscle stiffness is caused by:

- Myoplasticity
- Overactive neural input to the muscles

Myoplasticity comprises adaptive changes within a muscle, in response to changes in activity level and to prolonged positioning. In a person with an intact nervous system, chronic muscle disuse and immobility (for example, wearing a cast for 6 weeks) results in increased numbers of weak actin-myosin bonds, atrophy, and contracture. The same changes also occur in muscles following UMN lesions, as a consequence of muscle paresis, paralysis, or hyperreflexia.

Two mechanisms produce neural overactivity: hyperreflexia and UMN overactivity. In hyperreflexia, muscle spindle stretch leads to overactivity in LMNs. Thus, in some cases, hyperreflexia contributes to hyperstiffness by the generation of active muscle contraction. In other cases, neural overactivity occurs without hyperreflexia. Overactive UMNs signal LMNs to cause excessive active muscle contraction. Figure 9-33 illustrates the factors that contribute to muscle hyperstiffness.

In UMN lesions, excessive muscle stiffness is frequently caused by myoplastic hyperstiffness, not by neural signals initiating muscle contraction.

	Post stroke	Chronic spinal cord injury	Spastic cerebral palsy
Neural factors			
UMN overactivity	✓	✓	✓
Tonic stretch hyperreflexia		✓	✓
Myoplastic factors			
Contracture	✓	✓	✓
Increased number of weak actin-myosin bonds	✓	✓	✓
Atrophy fast-twitch muscle fibers	✓		
Abnormal muscle development			✓

FIGURE 9-33

Factors contributing to muscle hyperstiffness during active movements. In people post stroke or with chronic spinal cord injury or spastic cerebral palsy, UMN overactivity, contracture, and increased number of weak actin-myosin bonds contribute to excessive muscle stiffness. The unique factor post stroke is the predominance of slow twitch muscle fibers contributing to muscle hyperstiffness. Note that post stroke, hyperreflexia typically does not contribute to muscle hyperstiffness during active movements. After spinal cord injury, tonic stretch hyperreflexia contributes to the increased resistance to stretch. In spastic cerebral palsy, the unique contributors to hyperstiffness are cocontraction and abnormal muscle development.

Myoplastic Hyperstiffness Post Stroke

After a stroke, paretic muscles exert excessive resistance to muscle stretch. Excessive resistance during active movement is due primarily to changes within the muscles (myoplasticity). These changes include:
- Contracture
- Increased weak binding of actin and myosin
- Selective atrophy of fast twitch muscle fibers

Contracture is normal in muscles maintained in shortened positions. When muscles are paretic, immobility often leads to structural shortening of specific muscles. For example, people who have had strokes may tend to rest their paretic arm for long periods in their lap when sitting (Ada and Canning, 1990). This sustained positioning, with the arm comfortable and somewhat protected, may predispose the elbow flexor muscles to contracture (O'Dwyer et al., 1996). This adaptive muscle shortening prevents normal range of motion at involved joints.

Contrary to a common misconception, most people post stroke do not have hyperactive stretch reflexes. Ada et al. (2006) found that only 42% of the post stroke patients they studied had hyperreflexia during the first year. In people who have hyperreflexia, the hyperreflexia contributes to the development of contracture for the first 4 months post stroke, and thereafter weakness is the only independent contributor to contracture (Ada et al., 2006). In the upper limb, neither contracture nor hyperreflexia of elbow flexors contribute significantly to activity limitations. For the elbow flexor group, the only independent contributor to upper limb activity limitations post stroke is weakness (Ada et al., 2006). Contracture of lower limb muscles contributes to the muscle shortening of the soleus and gastrocnemius muscles in adults with hemiplegia secondary to stroke, trauma, and cerebral palsy (Becher et al., 1998).

In any resting muscle (normal or paretic), weak bonds between actin and myosin produce resistance to stretch. These bonds produce the initial resistance that arises when muscle is stretched (Proske and Morgan, 1999). Weak actin-myosin bonds continue to form as long as the muscle remains immobile. Because paretic muscles seldom contract, prolonged immobility occurs frequently. Immobility allows excessive numbers of actin-myosin bonds to form, producing increased resistance to stretch.

Following the subacute phase post stroke, muscle fibers on the paretic side decrease in diameter and type

II muscle fibers selectively atrophy. The selective atrophy leads to predominance of type I fibers within the paretic muscles (Dietz et al., 1986, Hachisuka et al., 1997). Slow twitch muscle fibers (type I) are more resistant to stretch than fast twitch muscle fibers (type II) because of their contractile properties.

Post stroke muscle shortening and alteration of contractile properties in lower limb muscles may be functionally beneficial, allowing people to support their weight during gait despite lack of neural control (Dietz, 2002). Thus, according to Dietz, some muscle changes may compensate for decreased neural control, rather than cause disordered movement. Dietz cites the time lag between stroke onset and the alterations in paretic muscles as evidence that the changes are compensatory. However, even if the changes do give the person the ability to bear weight on the paretic limb, these post stroke muscle changes prevent fast, active movements.

In summary, when post stroke paretic muscle is stretched, the initial, strong resistance to stretch is produced by weak actin-myosin bonds (Proske and Morgan, 1999). The resistance encountered as the stretch continues is produced by titin (Linke et al., 1996). In muscles affected by contracture, this resistance is encountered earlier than in muscles that can be stretched to the full range of motion because contracture reduces the amount of titin. During active movements on the paretic side, hyperreflexia typically does not contribute to resistance to movement.

After stroke, myoplastic hyperstiffness produces excessive resistance to muscle stretch. This excessive stiffness is produced by contracture, increased weak binding of actin and myosin, and atrophy of type II muscle fibers. During active movements post stroke, hyperreflexia does not usually contribute to the hyperstiffness.

Spasticity

Spasticity has two definitions, one used in research and the other used by clinicians. The research definition of *spasticity* is: increase in muscle tone due to hyperexcitability of the tonic stretch reflex, characterized by a velocity-dependent increase in phasic stretch reflexes (Lance, 1980). Note that by this definition, the hyperstiffness during active movement following a stroke is not caused by spasticity, because muscle tone is only assessed passively. In contrast, the definition of spasticity used by clinicians is much broader, and often includes the entire

UMN syndrome (Sanger et al., 2003): paresis, myoplastic hyperstiffness, cocontraction, and hyperreflexia. The clinical definition is also used to describe specific clinical syndromes, including spastic cerebral palsy. In the clinical definition, paresis, myoplastic hyperstiffness, cocontraction, and hyperreflexia are not distinguished. Therefore, the term *spasticity* is enigmatic. With the misconceptions and multiple meanings, use of the term *spasticity* produces more confusion than clarity in both evaluation and intervention.

A prevalent misconception has been that hyperactive stretch reflexes are the only cause of excess muscle stiffness and the associated movement disorder following UMN lesions (Dietz, 1992). However, muscle hyperstiffness is independent of hyperactive stretch reflexes (Berger et al., 1984, Hiersemenzel et al., 2000). Although hyperactive phasic stretch reflexes* are sometimes associated with muscle hyperstiffness, hyperstiffness is often the result of nonreflexive factors: myoplasticity and/or muscle overactivity.

Causes of Excessive Muscle Stiffness

For optimal therapeutic intervention, precise terminology must be used to accurately describe pathology. *Myoplastic hyperstiffness* denotes contracture, excess weak actin-myosin binding, and selective muscle fiber atrophy. *Hyperreflexia* refers to muscle spindle stretch leading to overactivity in the LMNs and resulting in active muscle contraction. *Muscle overactivity* is excessive muscle contraction caused by excessive UMN activity. These terms differentiate among factors causing muscle stiffness, providing more accurate description of impairments than the term *spasticity*. Table 9-4 summarizes the terms used to describe common impairments in UMN lesions.

Independence of Phasic Stretch Hyperreflexia and Myoplastic Hyperstiffness

Dietz and Berger (1983) and Berger et al. (1984) have demonstrated that in adults with chronic hemiplegia, force generation in the nonparetic leg correlates with the level of EMG activity (as it does in people with intact neuromuscular systems). However, in the paretic leg, high levels of force generation are simultaneous with low

---

*Historical note: Hyperactive stretch reflexes were previously attributed to a hypersensitive spindle (excessive γ output); however, the fusimotor system is normal in hyperreflexia.

    Hyperactivity of monosynaptic stretch reflexes is probably due to decreased presynaptic inhibition of monosynaptic (type Ia) afferents and a decrease in inhibitory interneuron activity secondary to the reduced descending inputs to LMNs.

Table 9-4   TERMS DESCRIBING IMPAIRMENTS COMMON IN UPPER MOTOR NEURON LESIONS

Term	Definition and Comments
Abnormal synergy	Obligatory coupling of movements at adjacent joints due to stereotyped coactivation of muscles. An example is shoulder abduction and external rotation combined with elbow flexion when the person is attempting to reach forward.
Cocontraction	Temporal overlap of agonist and antagonist muscle contraction. Cocontraction is normal when learning a new motor skill and when stability is required. Cocontraction is abnormal only when it interferes with achieving the movement goal. Abnormal cocontraction is prevalent in spastic cerebral palsy.
Hyperreflexia	Excessive phasic and/or tonic stretch reflex response. Hyperreflexia often contributes to movement disorders post spinal cord injury and in spastic cerebral palsy. Hyperreflexia usually does not interfere with active movement post stroke.
Muscle contracture	Adaptive shortening of muscle, caused by the muscle remaining in a shortened position for prolonged periods of time. The decrease in length is caused by loss of sarcomeres.
Muscle hyperstiffness	Excessive resistance to muscle stretch, regardless of whether the stretch is active or passive. Produced by neural input to muscles (active muscle contraction) and/or by changes within the muscle (myoplastic hyperstiffness: contracture, selective atrophy of specific muscle fiber types, and weak actin-myosin bonding).
Muscle overactivity	Muscle contraction that is excessive for the task. Caused by excess neural input to the muscle(s). May be due to pain, anxiety, or lack of skill in performing the task.
Muscle tone	Amount of tension in resting muscle. Muscle tone is examined passively and is not an indicator of ability to move actively.
Myoplastic hyperstiffness	Excessive resistance to muscle stretch due to changes within the muscle secondary to UMN lesion. Produced by contracture and increased weak actin-myosin bonding. Post stroke, selective atrophy of type II muscle fibers also contributes to this excessive resistance.
Paresis	Decreased ability to generate the level of force required for a task. Prevalent in spina bifida, spinal cord injury, and post stroke.
Spasticity	1. Velocity-dependent increase in tonic stretch reflexes (muscle tone) with exaggerated tendon jerks, resulting from hyperexcitability of the stretch reflex (Lance, 1980). Note, by this definition, the hyperstiffness during active movement post stroke is not caused by spasticity, because muscle tone can only be assessed passively and because post stroke muscle hyperstiffness is usually not caused by hyperreflexia. 2. Entire UMN syndrome: paresis, myoplastic hyperstiffness, cocontraction, hyperreflexia. This meaning is frequently used by clinicians and is also used as a descriptor of specific clinical syndromes, including spastic cerebral palsy.

NOTE: Some of these terms are also used to describe impairments resulting from pathologies other than UMN lesions.

levels of EMG activity. This indicates that LMNs are less active than normal in the paretic limb. If hyperreflexia contributed to the hyperstiffness, EMG activity would be expected to increase with increased muscle force output. EMG, force, and goniometric readings comparing data from the paretic and nonparetic leg of a person with hemiplegia are shown in Figure 9-34.

In adult chronic hemiplegia, the clinically important impairments during movement are caused by decreased UMN input to LMNs (producing paresis), decreased fractionation of movement, and changes within muscle (myoplastic hyperstiffness). Becher et al. (1998) demon-

strated the dissociation of myoplastic hyperstiffness from neural influence. They found that people with chronic hemiplegia of cerebral origin had excessive stiffness in the triceps surae muscles. Following local anesthesia of the tibial nerve, there was no change in muscle stiffness, demonstrating that hyperstiffness was independent from hyperreflexia. Consistent with this concept, in the upper limb of people post stroke, after a passive elbow extension the stretch reflex amplitude was less than that in people with normal nervous systems, despite the increase in muscle stiffness post stroke (Salazar-Torres et al., 2004). Similarly, in some people with incomplete spinal

FIGURE 9-34

Gait recordings of a step cycle during slow gait of an adult with hemiparesis. The stiff leg is shown above and the normal one below. From top to bottom in each recording, changes in tension recorded from the Achilles tendon, tibialis anterior and gastrocnemius EMG, and goniometer signal from the ankle joint. Vertical lines indicate touchdown (↓) and liftoff (↑) of the foot. During pushoff (pushoff begins at 0.5 second), paresis of the gastrocnemius muscle is indicated by the decreased EMG amplitude: in the stiff limb, the gastrocnemius EMG amplitude is less than 50% that of the normal side. The increase in passive and intrinsic stiffness in the paretic limb during stance phase is indicated by the large, early increase in Achilles tendon force despite very little EMG activity of the gastrocnemius. *(From Dietz V, and Berger W (1983). Normal and impaired regulation of muscle stiffness in gait: A new hypothesis about muscle hypertonia. Experimental Neurology, 79(3), 680-687.)*

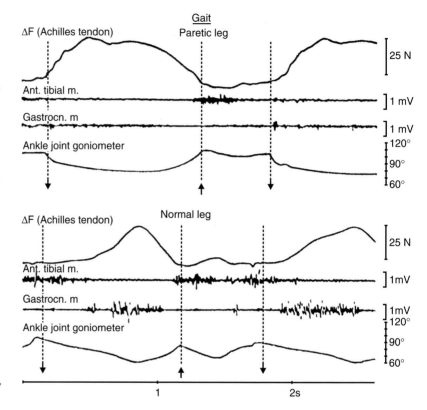

cord injury (iSCI), gastrocnemius muscle EMG activity during gait is minimal, yet the force exerted on the Achilles tendon is excessive (Figure 9-35).

For clarity in evaluation and diagnosis, and to assess the impact of interventions, hyperreflexia must be distinguished from myoplastic hyperstiffness (contracture, excess crossbridge binding, selective atrophy of type II muscle fibers). Rarely, following a stroke, phasic stretch hyperreflexia does occur when sufficient force can be generated quickly enough to produce a sufficient type Ia afferent volley. However, phasic stretch hyperreflexia during active movement is rare because most paretic muscles cannot generate sufficient force quickly enough to rapidly stretch antagonist muscles. Phasic stretch hyperreflexia is a far less important factor in movement impairment post stroke than paresis, decreased fractionation of movement, abnormal timing of muscle contraction, and muscular changes are, because people can avoid phasic stretch hyperreflexia by simply moving slowly.

In contrast to the relative unimportance of hyperreflexia post stroke, hyperreflexia often contributes to the

movement dysfunction in people with chronic iSCI. Excessive phasic stretch reflex activity may occur during both passive muscle stretch and during active movements in people with iSCI (Faist et al., 1999).

EVALUATION OF MOVEMENT IMPAIRMENTS IN CHRONIC UPPER MOTOR NEURON LESIONS

Passive testing provides little information about how a person performs actively, regardless of whether the person is neurologically intact or has a neurologic deficit. Clinically pertinent information can be obtained by using surface EMG to determine which of the following factors is contributing to movement impairment:

- Contracture
- Cocontraction
- Hyperreflexia
- Excessive UMN activity

Contracture produces decreased passive range of motion without increased EMG output. Cocontraction

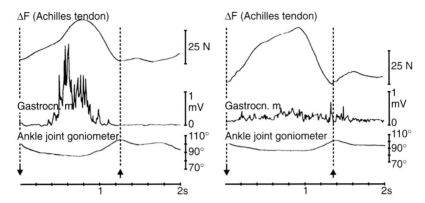

FIGURE 9-35

Averaged recordings (30 steps) of a step cycle during slow gait of a normal subject *(left)* and a subject with paraparesis *(right)* due to a spinal cord lesion. From top to bottom in each recording, changes in tension recorded from the Achilles tendon, gastrocnemius EMG, and goniometer signal from the ankle joint. Rectified EMG recordings are shown. In the normal subject, an increase in Achilles tendon tension correlates with an increase in gastrocnemius EMG activity. In the paraparetic subject, the increase in Achilles tendon tension does not correlate with an increase in EMG. Instead, the increase in Achilles tendon tension coincides with the stretch of the triceps surae during passive dorsiflexion of the foot in the stance phase. *(From Dietz V, and Berger W (1983). Normal and impaired regulation of muscle stiffness in gait: A new hypothesis about muscle hypertonia. Experimental Neurology, 79(3), 680-687.)*

produces temporal overlap of EMG activity in antagonist muscles (Figure 9-36).

Hyperreflexia is indicated by EMG activity occurring at a specific latency after the initiation of muscle stretch (Figure 9-37). Excessive UMN activity produces excessive EMG activity, causing increased muscle contraction that interferes with the desired movement.

EMG recordings and muscle stiffness should be considered within the context of functional tasks. Cocontraction and increased muscle stiffness are abnormal only if they interfere with achieving the goal of the task; people with intact neuromuscular systems often use cocontraction and increased muscle stiffness when learning a new movement or for stability (Hautier et al., 2000).

Paresis, decreased ability to generate appropriate force for a functional movement, is often an important contributor to movement impairment. However, paresis cannot be accurately assessed using EMG because functional tasks involve multiple muscles, and the force generated at a specific joint depends on the contributions of agonists, antagonists, and synergists. Assessing only the contribution of the agonist may be misleading, because antagonists and synergists may be deficient in providing stability or in reinforcing or opposing the agonist's activity at the appropriate time. There are also two technical

problems with using EMG to assess paresis. First, EMG amplitude must be normalized by comparing the EMG elicited by a maximal electrical stimulus to the motor nerve with the EMG elicited by a maximum voluntary contraction of the muscle. People with central paresis cannot completely activate their LMN pools; therefore, normalization cannot be accomplished. Second, because muscles slide under the skin, and electrical signals spread from adjacent muscles, there is no way to ascertain that the amplitude of EMG activity recorded from the skin above a particular muscle is produced only by that muscle.

The modified Ashworth scale (Table 9-5), a scale for measuring spasticity, does not actually measure spasticity because information from this test cannot be used to distinguish between contracture and hyperreflexia (Bakheit et al., 2003). The Ashworth score is the evaluator's subjective assessment of the resistance to passive stretch. For example, the evaluator passively stretches the biceps and assesses whether the resistance to stretch is normal or greater than normal. High scores on the modified Ashworth scale (MAS) are associated with contracture (Cooper et al., 2005). Mirbagheri et al. (2001) reported no correlation between objective measures (intrinsic stiffness and reflex stiffness) of muscle stiffness and the modified Ashworth scale in people with spinal

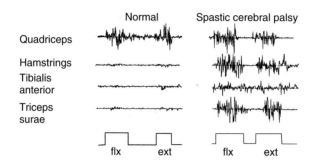

FIGURE 9-36

Electromyograms of gaitlike lower limb movements in supine children. **A,** Normal motor control; quadriceps muscle is contracting, and the other muscles are relatively inactive. **B,** Spastic cerebral palsy; abnormal cocontraction. Quadriceps, hamstrings, tibialis anterior, and triceps surae are cocontracting during the lower limb movements. The EMG data were selected specifically to show abnormal cocontraction, the simultaneous contraction of agonist and antagonists that interferes with performing tasks. Not all children with spastic cerebral palsy have abnormal cocontraction; in many cases paresis or hyperreflexia causes the gait abnormalities. *(Modified from Wong AM, Chen CL, et al. 2000. Motor control assessment for rhizotomy in cerebral palsy. American Journal of Physical Medicine and Rehabilitation, 79(5), 441-450, Figure 2, p. 443.)*

Table 9-5   MODIFIED ASHWORTH SCALE: MUSCLE RESISTANCE TO PASSIVE STRETCH

Grade	Description	Grade	Description
0	No increase in muscle tone	2	More marked increase in muscle tone through most of ROM, but affected part(s) easily moved
1	Slight increase in muscle tone, manifested by a catch or by minimal resistance at the end of the range of motion (ROM) when the affected part(s) is moved in flexion or extension	3	Considerable increase in muscle tone; passive movement difficult
		4	Affected part(s) rigid in flexion or extension
1+	Slight increase in muscle tone, manifested by a catch, followed by minimal resistance throughout the remainder (less than half) of ROM		

From Bohannon and Smith, 1987.

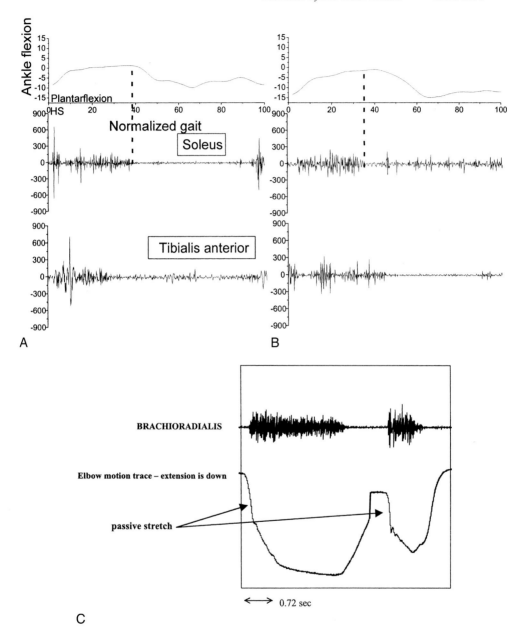

FIGURE 9-37

Hyperreflexia. **A,** Phasic stretch hyperreflexia. Electomyogram (EMG) of soleus muscle activity during gait in a 31-year-old subject with spastic cerebral palsy. When the foot begins to bear weight, soleus muscle stretch elicits a spike in EMG activity. **B,** After drug treatment to reduce spasticity, the phasic stretch hyperreflexia is absent. **C,** Tonic stretch hyperreflexia. Abnormal EMG activity continues for the duration of the muscle stretch. *(A and B modified from Remy-Neris O, Tiffreau V, et al. (2003). Intrathecal baclofen in subjects with spastic hemiplegia: Assessment of the antispastic effect during gait. Archives of Physical Medicine and Rehabilitation, 84(5), 643-650, Figure 4, p. 647. C from Mayer NH, Esquenazi A. (2003). Muscle overactivity and movement dysfunction in the upper motoneuron syndrome. Physical Medicine and Rehabilitation Clinics of North America, 14, 855-883.)*

cord injuries. Kim et al. (2005) reported no correlation between reflexive plantarflexor EMG activity post stroke and the modified Ashworth scale. Kim et al. noted that the modified Ashworth scale is highly subjective, its reliability is unacceptably low, and it is not valid at lower grades. Interrater reliability is reported to be unacceptably low in people post stroke (Blackburn et al., 2002) and in muscles other than the hamstrings and elbow flexors in children with hypertonia (Clopton et al., 2005). Functional improvement in people post stroke does not correlate with improvement on the MAS (Elovic et al., 2004), which is not surprising given that the MAS is purely passive.

Given that hyperreflexia and myoplastic hyperstiffness are independent of each other, it is not surprising that little correlation has been found among clinical measures of spasticity. Although measurement techniques vary, their validity is questionable. Scores on the measurements do not correlate well, and most measures do not differentiate between hyperreflexia and myoplastic hyperstiffness.

Levin and Hui-Chan (1993) have confirmed this lack of consistent results by using several different measures of spasticity on the same individuals. They tested resistance to passive ankle dorsiflexion, H-reflexes, H-reflexes obtained during tendon vibration, and EMG recording of stretch reflexes. Even though only passive evaluation techniques were used, the degree of spasticity was not consistently assessed. None of Levin and Hui-Chan's evaluations used active, functional movements (e.g., gait), which alter reflex responses even in people who are neurologically intact. Similarly, Priebe et al. (1996) found poor correlation among clinical scales used to measure spasticity in people with spinal cord injury.

TYPES OF UPPER MOTOR NEURON LESIONS

This section discusses spinal cord injury, stroke, and congenital lesions. Although head trauma, tumors, and multiple sclerosis can also damage UMNs, the affected structures and their clinical outcomes are so variable that a discussion of their motor effects is beyond the scope of this text. Because the etiology of each type of UMN lesion is different, research on movement disorders in one population cannot be generalized to the others; given the variety in size and location of lesions, research on one type of lesion cannot be indiscriminately applied to individuals. For this reason, analysis of surface EMG recordings is important to accurately evaluate the relative

contributions of each component of the movement disorder.

Spinal Cord Injury

A person with a complete spinal cord injury (SCI) loses all descending neuronal control below the level of the lesion. In complete SCI, stretch reflexes are hyperactive during passive movements yet during active movements stretch reflexes are the same as in people with intact nervous systems (Nielsen et al., 2005).

In iSCI, the function of some ascending and/or descending fibers is preserved within the spinal cord. The following conditions occur following iSCI:

1. Significant correlation between contracture and resistance to muscle stretch (Skold et al., 1999)
2. Predominance of type IIb muscle fibers and a reduction in type I muscle fibers (Lotta et al., 1991; Scelsi et al., 1986)
3. Excessive stretch reflexes in the quadriceps muscle during the swing phase of gait (Faist et al., 1999). In spinal cord injury, hyperreflexia is a major contributor to excess muscle stiffness and intrinsic stiffness increases significantly at end range, probably due to contracture (Mirbagheri et al., 2001).

> Following incomplete spinal cord injury, excessive stretch reflexes, muscle contracture, and increased crossbridge binding produce excessive resistance to muscle stretch.

Stroke

Stroke most frequently affects the middle cerebral artery (see Chapters 1 and 18), damaging corticospinal neurons and thus disrupting cortical connections with the spinal cord, brainstem, and cerebellum (Box 9-1). Because corticospinal neurons are affected, the impairments that limit activities are paresis and decreased fractionation of movement contralateral to the lesion. Stroke may alter output from all supraspinal motor areas, depending on the extent of the lesion. However, with the exception of direct cortical influences, other supraspinal motor areas continue to exert some control over LMN activity. Abnormal muscle activation occurs because corticospinal input is lost, and the lateral reticulospinal tract is deprived of its normal cortical facilitation, leaving the medial reticulospinal and vestibulospinal tracts to facilitate lower limb extension relatively unopposed. The medial reticulospinal and vestibulospinal tracts remain active because their activity is less dependent on cortical

BOX 9-1 STROKE, MIDDLE CEREBRAL ARTERY

Pathology
Interruption of blood supply

Etiology
Occlusion or hemorrhage

Speed of Onset
Usually acute

Signs and Symptoms
Consciousness
May be temporarily impaired
Affect
Emotional lability (pathological laughter or crying)
Communication and Memory
May be impaired
Sensory
Usually impaired contralateral to the lesion
Autonomic
May be impaired
Motor
Contralateral to the lesion: paresis, muscle atrophy, loss of fractionation of movement, decreased movement speed and efficiency, impaired postural control, Babinski's sign

Region Affected
Cerebrum

Demographics
Males and females affected equally; average age at onset approximately 72 years (Alter et al., 1993)
Incidence
First CVA (any artery): 205 per 100,000 population people per year (MacDonald et al., 2000)
Prevalence
9 cases per 1000 people population (MacDonald, et al., 2000)

Prognosis
About 20% percent die from stroke within the first 30 days; after first 30 days, risk of death approximately double the rate in the general population; after the first year, cardiovascular disease the most common cause of death (Dennis and Burn, 1993)

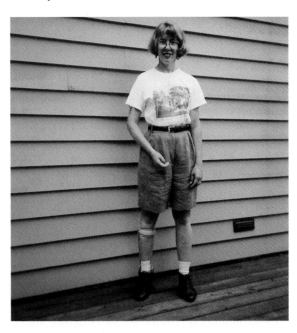

FIGURE 9-38
Typical posture of an adult who has sustained a left middle cerebral artery stroke. Note the flexed resting position of the right upper limb and the muscle atrophy in the right lower limb. Movement disorders post middle cerebral artery stroke are the consequences of paresis, decreased fractionation of movement, and myoplastic hyperstiffness.

stroke. As discussed in the section on myoplastic hyperstiffness, the resting posture of the hemiparetic arm is due to contracture, weak actin-myosin bonds, and atrophy of type II muscle fibers in the elbow flexors.

Gandevia (1993) summarized his research on adults with unilateral CVAs as follows: on the paretic side, weakness in one muscle group was usually associated with weakness in the antagonist muscle group; distal muscles were weaker than proximal muscles in both limbs; and muscle strength on the nonparetic side (particularly the shoulder) was weak in comparison to muscle strength in healthy subjects matched for age and sex.

facilitation. These neural activation changes, combined with paresis and myoplastic hyperstiffness in specific muscles of the lower extremity, contribute to excessive lower-extremity extension in standing and walking. Figure 9-38 shows a typical standing posture after a

Movement disorders post middle cerebral artery stroke are the consequences of paresis, decreased fractionation of movement, and myoplastic hyperstiffness. Rarely does hyperreflexia contribute significantly to the movement limitations.

In addition to movement consequences, approximately 34%-48% of people post stroke experience **emotional lability** (Kim and Choi-Kwon, 2000; Piamarta et al., 2004). Emotional lability is also called *pseudobulbar affect* (because emotional expression is less controlled by the corticobulbar neurons than normally) or *pathologic laughter* or *crying*. The emotional expression may or may not be congruent with the person's mood. For example, the person may laugh uncontrollably while he or she is feeling sad, or may cry excessively when only feeling slightly sad.

Spastic Cerebral Palsy

In spastic cerebral palsy, abnormal supraspinal influences, failure of normal neuronal selection, and consequent aberrant muscle development lead to movement dysfunction (see Chapter 5). Motor disorders in spastic cerebral palsy include paresis, abnormal tonic stretch reflexes both at rest and during movement, reflex irradiation (spread of reflex activity; e.g., tapping the biceps tendon causes finger flexor contraction in addition to biceps contraction), lack of postural preparation prior to movement, and abnormal cocontraction of muscles. Paresis of agonist postural muscles is the only impairment that interferes with balance recovery in children with spastic cerebral palsy (Roncesvalles et al., 2002).

Common Characteristics of Upper Motor Neuron Lesions

The force exerted by a muscle is produced by intrinsic factors (weak actin-myosin bonds), passive factors (amount of titin, predominant muscle fiber types), and active factors (contractile). In people with chronic UMN lesions, intrinsic and passive changes in muscle cause abnormal stiffness. When additional stiffness is actively generated by motor neuron input, causing active contraction of muscles, the muscles produce additional excessive force. Emotional agitation and pain lead to excessive muscle force in people with CVA, cerebral palsy, and iSCI via limbic action on motor cortical areas and via the nonspecific UMNs to LMNs.

In summary, common signs of UMN lesions include paresis, abnormal cutaneous reflexes, abnormal timing of muscle activity, and myoplastic hyperstiffness. Hyperreflexia of the phasic stretch reflex, clonus, and the clasp-knife phenomenon occur most commonly in chronic spinal cord injury. Reflex irradiation and abnormal cocontraction of antagonist muscles typically do not occur with damage to the mature nervous system (which includes most CVAs and spinal cord injuries); these signs typically accompanying UMN syndromes that arise during nervous system development (such as cerebral palsy). Reciprocal inhibition is preserved in adult CVA and in most spinal cord injuries because the damage occurs to a mature nervous system.

INTERVENTIONS FOR IMPAIRMENTS SECONDARY TO UPPER MOTOR NEURON LESIONS

Until recently, many therapists regarded spasticity (meaning hyperreflexia) as the primary problem in people post stroke or with spastic cerebral palsy. These therapists attempted to normalize muscle tone with therapy, assuming muscle hyperstiffness was produced by hyperreflexia and motor control would be normal if hyperreflexia were successfully reduced. These assumptions have been thoroughly disproved. Cahan et al. (1990) demonstrated that reduction of hyperreflexia (by selective dorsal rhizotomy), decreasing stretch reflexes without other intervention, does not improve function. Also, subjects with cerebral palsy who learn to decrease the sensitivity of the tonic stretch reflex during rest and active movement have no improvement in functional control (Neilson, 1993). These findings reflect the negligible impact of abnormal stretch reflexes on the performance of activities and tasks when compared with the effects of paresis, loss of fractionation, and abnormal cocontraction on the ability to perform desired actions.

Wolf and Catlin (1994) reported that in people with chronic hemiplegia, practicing elbow extension was as effective in improving range of motion as training that incorporated learning to inhibit biceps activity prior to elbow extension. As noted earlier, Dietz (1992) reported that in people with CVAs, neural activation of the calf muscles on the paretic side is less than normal. He attributed the muscle hyperstiffness to changes in muscle, not to reflexive muscle contraction. Dietz et al. (1991) reported similar findings in upper limb muscles. Paretic elbow flexor and extensor muscles in people with CVAs produce high torque during stretch with less EMG activity than normal. This demonstrates that factors other than excessive neural output are involved in the movement problems of people post stroke or with spastic cerebral palsy. Testing for and remediation of these deficits provide guidance for rehabilitation.

Improvement in Function Post Stroke

Laidler (1994) advocates avoiding effortful movements using paretic muscles, claiming these movements reinforce abnormal patterns of movement and increase spasticity. Contrary to Laidler's contentions, research has consistently demonstrated that forceful movement is beneficial in adults post stroke (Van Peppen et al., 2004) and does not increase spasticity. Improved movement in people post stroke has been demonstrated with:

- Movements against resistance
- Bicycling with high workloads
- Partial body weight support gait training

In a study comparing the effects of treatments for hand function in adults with hemiparesis, Butefisch et al. (1995) report that techniques focusing on spasticity reduction (techniques developed by Bobath [1977]) instead of on active movement produce no significant improvement in motor capabilities of the hand. In contrast, training of finger and hand flexion and extension against resistance results in significant improvement of grip strength, hand extension force, and other indicators of hand function.

Brown and Kautz (1998) demonstrated that people with post-stroke hemiplegia were able to ride a stationary bike with high workloads without generating increased inappropriate muscle activity; no change in abnormal movements nor increase in spasticity occurred. Also in people post stroke, walking using partial body weight support and a treadmill has been shown to produce a more symmetrical gait with more normal muscle activation patterns than training using overground walking (Hesse et al., 1999) (Figure 9-39). In partial body weight support training, an overhead harness is used to support up to 40% of the person's body weight (Figure 9-40). Barbeau and Visintin (2003) demonstrated that treadmill training with partial body weight support results in better walking abilities in people post-stroke than gait training while bearing full weight. Follow-up evaluations performed 3 months after training showed that the body weight support group continued to have significantly higher scores for overground walking speed and motor recovery than the group that practiced only overground walking.

However, forced movements too soon after a moderate or severe cerebral lesion may increase brain damage. Animal studies suggest that forced use induced by casting the nonparetic forelimb immediately following a lesion causes extension of that lesion (Humm et al., 1998). In rats forced to use a paretic forelimb during the 7 days immediately following a brain lesion, the lesion became significantly larger (Figure 9-41). This effect may be due to use-dependent release of glutamate by damaged neurons. When small lesions were induced in the hand area of the motor cortex in monkeys, early

restriction of the nonparetic hand (using a glove) had short-term deleterious effects on movement (Nudo et al., 1996). Despite this short-term effect, in the long term, use of this mild constraint enhanced use of the paretic forelimb and prevented loss of cortical representation of the hand area in the cortex. The extent of the lesion and the timing and extent of forced use are important considerations in using this technique.

In some cases, botulinum toxin (Botox) is a useful adjunct to occupational and physical therapy. Botox is injected directly into the muscles that produce excessive force. This allows the clinician to specifically target particular muscles without interfering with the contraction of other muscles. Botox inhibits the release of ACh at the neuromuscular junction, preventing active muscular contraction. Botox does not affect passive stiffness. Botox injection into calf muscles produces significant improvements in gait velocity, self-ratings of pain and gait function, manual muscle tests, and ankle clonus post stroke (Mancini et al., 2005). However, the long-term effects of this treatment have not been evaluated. If excessive intrinsic and passive stiffness arise secondary to paresis, then increasing the paresis by using Botox may have harmful long-term effects.

Treatment of Hyperreflexia Post Spinal Cord Injury

Baclofen is commonly used to decrease excessive muscle stiffness produced by hyperreflexia following spinal cord injury. Baclofen is administered systemically, either orally or via an implanted pump that delivers the drug into the subarachnoid or subdural space. Baclofen causes inhibition in spinal cord stretch reflex pathways, both presynaptically (by decreasing calcium influx into the presynaptic terminals of primary afferent fibers; Sakaba and Neher, 2003) and by stabilizing the postsynaptic membrane (Fairfax et al., 2004). Baclofen therefore inhibits hyperreflexia but does not have an effect on myoplastic hyperstiffness. Campbell et al. (1995) summarized the benefits and costs of baclofen in treating excessive muscle stiffness following spinal cord injury; their review of the literature reports decreased spasms, pain, and sleep disturbance, along with improved bladder function and increased mobility. However, baclofen may cause a decrease in function if reflexive muscle contraction is used functionally. For example, hyperreflexia may enable a person who is otherwise unable to sit upright to be stable in sitting, and baclofen would prevent this functionally beneficial use.

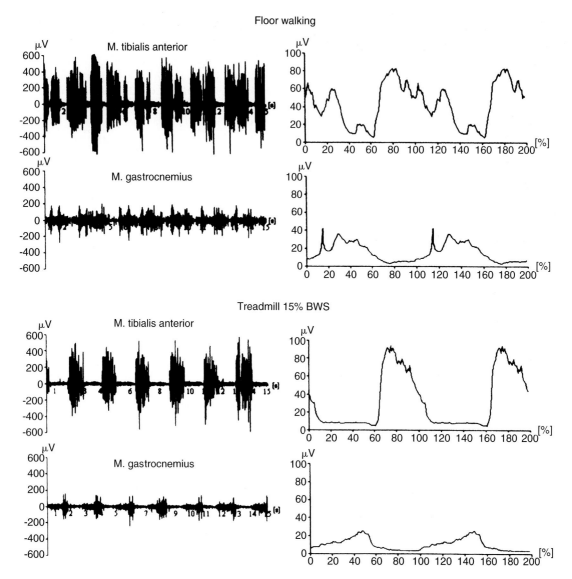

FIGURE 9-39

Recordings of EMG activity in the paretic limb of a person post stroke. The recordings on the left are raw EMGs, and those on the right are averaged EMGs. The upper recordings, made while the subject was walking on the floor, show more abnormal neural activity than the lower recordings, made while the subject was walking on a treadmill with 15% body weight support (BWS). The BWS recordings show a more phasic and smoother pattern of activation than the walking-on-the-floor recordings. *(From Hesse S, Konrad M, et al. (1999). Treadmill walking with partial body weight support versus floor walking in hemiparetic subjects. Archives of Physical Medicine and Rehabilitation, 80(4), 421-427.)*

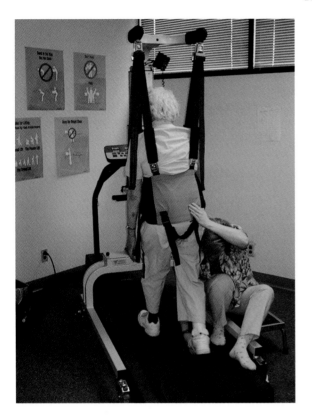

AMYOTROPHIC LATERAL SCLEROSIS

Amyotrophic lateral sclerosis (ALS) is a disease that destroys only somatic motor neurons. ALS destroys UMNs and brainstem and spinal cord LMNs bilaterally (Figure 9-42), resulting in both UMN and LMN signs. The disease leads to paresis, myoplastic hyperstiffness, hyperreflexia, Babinski's sign, atrophy, fasciculations, and fibrillations. The loss of LMNs in cranial nerves causes difficulty with breathing, swallowing, and speaking. Nearly 50% of people with ALS experience pathologic laughter or crying. Approximately 90% of cases are idiopathic, although the gene responsible for the familial type of ALS has been identified. Recent research indicates that brief, low to moderate intensity exercise is beneficial in muscles that are not profoundly weak (Simmons, 2005). People with ALS usually die of respiratory complications (Box 9-2).

FIGURE 9-40
Body weight support gait training. A harness, mounted overhead, supports part of the person's weight while the individual walks on a treadmill.

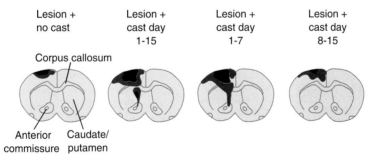

FIGURE 9-41
The effects of forced movement on brain lesion size in rats. Unilateral brain damage was induced in some of the rats, then some of the rats had the ipsilateral forelimb casted during recovery and others were not casted. The experimental groups were: no lesion, with or without cast; lesion without cast; lesion with cast on days 1 to 15; lesion with cast on days 1 to 7; and lesion with cast on days 8 to 15. In the group with no lesion, no effect of casting was found in the brain. The drawings of coronal sections indicate average lesions in each lesioned group. The black areas indicate minimum damage, and the red regions are the maximum extent of brain damage. Brain lesion size increased with constraint-induced movement that occurred on days 1 to 7 or days 1 to 15; constraint-induced movement on days 8 to 15 did not increase lesion size. However, in all cases constraint-induced movement produced behavioral deficits in use of the forelimb compared to the use of the forelimb by rats with brain lesions that did not undergo constraint-induced movement.
(Modified from Humm JL, Kozlowski DA, et al. (1998). Use-dependent exacerbation of brain damage occurs during an early post-lesion vulnerable period. Brain Research, 783(2), 286-292.)

BOX 9-2 AMYOTROPHIC LATERAL SCLEROSIS

Pathology

Bilateral degeneration of motor neurons (both upper and lower)

Etiology

Unknown; speculative: excessive levels of glutamate (Lipton and Rosenberg, 1994)

Speed of Onset

Chronic

Signs and Symptoms

Consciousness

Normal

Communication and Memory

Normal

Affect

Emotional lability (pathologic laughter or crying)

Sensory

Normal

Autonomic

Normal

Motor

Paresis, spasticity, clonus, Babinski's sign, hyper- or hyporeflexia, fasciculations, fibrillations, muscle

atrophy, difficulty with breathing, swallowing, speaking

Region Affected

Upper motor neurons in cerebrum, brainstem, and spinal cord; lower motor neurons in brainstem, spinal, and peripheral regions

Demographics

Onset is usually >50 years old; males outnumber females by 2:1

Incidence

1.7 cases per 100,000 population people per year (Sorenson et al., 2002)

Prevalence

0.05 cases per 1000 people

Prognosis

Progressive; average life span after diagnosis = 3 years; rarely live >20 years; death usually from respiratory complications

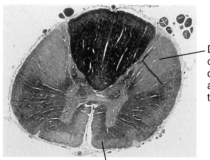

Degeneration of lateral corticospinal and rubrospinal tracts

Degeneration of medial activating pathways

FIGURE 9-42

Spinal cord section, stained for myelin, showing loss of descending UMNs in ALS. The loss is visible dorsolaterally, where the lateral corticospinal and rubrospinal axons should be, and ventromedially, where the medial UMNs should be. *(Courtesy Dr. Melvin J. Ball.)*

SUMMARY

For normal movement, motor planning areas, control circuits, and descending tracts must act together with sensory information to provide instructions to LMNs. Only LMNs deliver signals from the central nervous system to the skeletal muscles that generate movement. UMNs convey signals from the brain to LMNs and interneurons. To treat patients, a therapist must understand normal and impaired skeletal muscles and motor neurons. Because research regularly reveals new information about motor neurons and the effectiveness of different treatments, therapists should keep up-to-date with developments in this field.

CLINICAL NOTES

Case 1

MV is a 62-year-old man. While eating breakfast, he suddenly lost control of the left side of his body and face. He fell to the floor but did not lose consciousness. Now, 2 weeks later, he is examined in the hospital. The results are as follows:

- He has complete loss of sensation and voluntary movement of his left side.
- He requires assistance to move from supine to sitting and from sitting to standing.
- He cannot sit or stand independently.
- He has difficulty speaking because of lack of sensation and reduced control of the oral and pharyngeal muscles on the left side. The nursing staff reports he also has difficulty eating.
- Babinski's sign is present on the left side.

Question

What is the location of the lesion and probable etiology?

Case 2

AF is a 15-year-old girl who was thrown from a horse. She sustained fractures of the humerus and the C5 vertebra. Her coma lasted 2 days.

- Mentation and consciousness are normal.
- Except for the distal right upper limb, sensation, autonomic function, and movement are normal.
- Sensation and sweating are absent in the little finger, medial half of the ring finger, and the adjacent palm of the right hand. The skin is warm and red in the same distribution.
- Wrist flexion on the ulnar side and ulnar deviation are impaired. She cannot flex the distal interphalangeal joints in the fourth and fifth digits.

Question

What is the location of the lesion and probable etiology?

Case 3

PA is a 39-year-old woman, 1 month post injury from a 30-foot fall sustained while mountain climbing. She suffered multiple injuries, most prominently fractures of the right femur, right fibula, and the T10 vertebra.

- The right lower limb is in a cast, restricting evaluation, but sensation is absent in the L1 dermatome above the cast and in the toes. No voluntary movement of the right quadriceps or toes can be elicited.
- Sensation is absent throughout the left lower limb and bilaterally in the sacral region.
- No voluntary movement can be elicited in the left lower limb.
- The Achilles tendon reflex and Babinski's sign are present bilaterally.

Question

What is the location of the lesion and probable etiology?

Case 4

RJ is a 71-year-old man concerned about regaining his strength. Four months ago, he considered himself healthy and strong. He competed regularly in masters swimming events and walked several miles daily. Gradually he has become weaker; although he continues swimming, his times are not competitive, and he can walk only half a mile.

- Mentation, consciousness, sensation, and autonomic functions are normal. When asked, he mentions he has noticed muscle twitching.
- Throughout the body, skeletal muscles are visibly atrophied.
- Babinski's sign is present in both lower limbs.
- On passive movement, the therapist notes that faster movements meet with more resistance than slower movements. If RJ's limbs are moved slowly, the initially strong resistance gives way to easier movement.
- Diagnostic EMG studies reveal fasciculations and fibrillations in the muscles tested.

Question

What is the location of the lesion and probable etiology?

REVIEW QUESTIONS

1. After Ca^{++} binds to troponin, what is the sequence of events that leads to shortening of a sarcomere?
2. Why does a sarcomere at a shortened length produce less tension than the same sarcomere at its optimum length?
3. List the factors that contribute to muscle stiffness in an intact neuromuscular system.
4. Why do your hamstrings feel stiff when you stand after sitting for several hours?
5. When a person with an intact neuromuscular system is anxious, muscle resistance to passive movement increases. What produces this increase in resistance to passive movement?
6. What is the difference between an LMN and a UMN?
7. What is the general function of control circuits?
8. Why are slow twitch muscle fibers usually activated before fast twitch muscle fibers?
9. What factors determine the activity of a motor unit?
10. What is alpha-gamma coactivation?
11. What are the differences between the phasic and tonic stretch reflexes?
12. What roles does the Golgi tendon organ play?
13. How does changing a person's arousal level alter the response to a quadriceps tendon tap?
14. How is an H-reflex produced? What information does an H-reflex give?
15. What is the function of reciprocal inhibition?
16. How does the use of the term *synergy* differ between clinicians and motor control researchers?
17. What is a stepping pattern generator?
18. In an intact nervous system, how is the stepping pattern generator activated?
19. List each medial UMN tract and its function.
20. List each lateral UMN tract and its function.
21. List each nonspecific UMN tract and its function.
22. What is hemiplegia?
23. Which of the following signs always indicate pathology? Muscle spasms, cramps, fasciculations, fibrillations, abnormal movements.
24. What is hypertonia? What is the difference between the two types of hypertonia? How is hypertonia produced?
25. What is spinal shock?
26. If a person has loss of reflexes, muscle atrophy, flaccid paralysis, and fibrillations, what is the location of the lesion?
27. What does Babinski's sign in an adult indicate?
28. What is the location of a lesion that produces abnormal cutaneous reflexes, abnormal timing of muscle activation, paresis, and muscle hyperstiffness?
29. What factors contribute to muscle hyperstiffness post stroke?
30. Following a UMN lesion, if there is excessive resistance to active dorsiflexion yet very little EMG activity in the ankle plantar flexors, what is the source of the hyperstiffness?
31. What is clonus?
32. Post stroke, is muscle hyperstiffness primarily caused by hyperreflexia?
33. How can cocontraction, myoplastic hyperstiffness, and hyperreflexia be quantified using surface EMG?
34. What is the difference in effects on LMNs between a complete spinal cord lesion and a typical middle cerebral artery stroke?
35. What motor signs occur in spastic cerebral palsy that are not also seen in adult-onset UMN lesions?
36. What types of therapy have been shown to improve function in people post stroke? What do all of these types of therapy have in common?
37. In rats, what is the effect of 1 week of forced use of the paretic forelimb immediately following a cortical lesion?
38. What parts of the nervous system does ALS destroy?

References

Ada L, Canning C (1990). Anticipating and avoiding muscle shortening. In L Ada, and C Canning (Eds.), Key Issues in Neurological Physiotherapy (pp. 219-236). Oxford: Butterworth Heinemann.

Ada L, O'Dwyer N, O'Neill E (2006). Relation between spasticity, weakness and contracture of the elbow flexors and upper limb activity after stroke: An observational study. Disability and Rehabilitation, 28(13), 891-897.

Adkin AL, Frank JS, et al. (2002). Fear of falling modifies anticipatory postural control. Experimental Brain Research, 143(2), 160-170.

Alter M, Friday G, et al. (1993). The LeHigh Valley Recurrent Stroke Study: Description of design and methods. Neuroepidemiology, 12(4), 241-248.

Bakheit AM, Maynard VA, et al. (2003). The relation between Ashworth scale scores and the excitability of the alpha motor neurons in patients with post-stroke muscle spasticity. Journal of Neurology, Neurosurgery, and Psychiatry, 74(5), 646-648.

Barbeau H, Visintin M (2003). Optimal outcomes obtained with body-weight support combined with treadmill training in stroke subjects. Archives of Physical Medicine and Rehabilitation, 84(10), 1458-1465.

Becher JG, Harlaar J, et al. (1998). Measurement of impaired muscle function of the gastrocnemius, soleus, and tibialis anterior muscles in spastic hemiplegia: A preliminary study. Journal of Rehabilitation Research and Development, 35(3), 314-326.

Beres-Jones JA, Johnson TD, et al. (2003). Clonus after human spinal cord injury cannot be attributed solely to recurrent muscle-tendon stretch. Experimental Brain Research, 149(2), 222-236.

Berger W, Horstmann G, et al. (1984). Tension development and muscle activation in the leg during gait in spastic hemiparesis: Independence of muscle hypertonia and exaggerated stretch reflexes. Journal of Neurology, Neurosurgery and Psychiatry, 27, 1029-1033.

Blackburn M, van Vliet P, et al. (2002). Reliability of measurements obtained with the Modified Ashworth Scale in the lower extremities of people with stroke. Physical Therapy, 82, 25-34.

Bobath B (1977). Treatment of adult hemiplegia. Physiotherapy in Canada, 63, 310-313.

Bohannon RW, Smith MB (1987). Interrater reliability of a modified Ashworth scale of muscle spasticity. Physical Therapy, 67(2), 206-207.

Brown DA, Kautz SA (1998). Increased workload enhances force output during pedaling exercise in persons with poststroke hemiplegia. Stroke, 29(3), 598-606.

Burne JA, Carleton VL, et al. (2005). The spasticity paradox: Movement disorder or disorder of resting limbs? Journal of Neurology, Neurosurgery, and Psychiatry, 76(1), 47-54.

Butefisch C, Hummelsheim H, et al. (1995). Repetitive training of isolated movements improves the outcome of motor rehabilitation of the centrally paretic hand. Journal of the Neurological Sciences, 130(1), 59-68.

Butt SJ, Lebret JM, et al. (2002). Organization of left-right coordination in the mammalian locomotor network. Brain Research. Brain Research Reviews, 40(1-3), 107-117.

Cahan L, Adams J, et al. (1990). Instrumented gait analysis after selective dorsal rhizotomy. Developmental Medicine and Child Neurology, 32, 1037-1043.

Caiozzo VJ, Utkan A, et al. (2002). Effects of distraction on muscle length: Mechanisms involved in sarcomerogenesis. Clinical Orthopaedics, (403 Suppl), S133-S145.

Campbell WW (2005). DeJong's The Neurologic Examination. Philadelphia: Lippincott Williams & Wilkins.

Campbell S, Almeida G, et al. (1995). The effects of intrathecally administered baclofen on function in patients with spasticity. Physical Therapy, 75, 352-362.

Capaday C, Lavoie BA, et al. (1999). Studies on the corticospinal control of human walking. I. Responses to focal transcranial magnetic stimulation of the motor cortex. Journal of Neurophysiology, 81(1), 129-139.

Carson RG (2005). Neural pathways mediating bilateral interactions between the upper limbs. Brain Research. Brain Research Reviews, 49(3), 641-662.

Casadio M, Morasso PG, et al. (2005). Direct measurement of ankle stiffness during quiet standing: Implications for control modelling and clinical application. Gait Posture, 21(4), 410-424.

Cattaert D (2004). Studying the Nervous System Under Physiological Conditions. Focus on Contribution of Force Feedback to Ankle Extensor Activity in Decerebrate Walking Cats. Journal of Neurophysiology, 92(4), 1967-1968.

Chalmers G (2004). Re-examination of the possible role of Golgi tendon organ and muscle spindle reflexes in proprioceptive neuromuscular facilitation muscle stretching. Sports Biomechanics, 3(1), 159-183.

Chan KM, Amirjani N, et al. (2003). Randomized controlled trial of strength training in post-polio patients. Muscle Nerve, 27(3), 332-338.

Chou SW, Abraham LD, et al. (2005). Starting position and stretching velocity effects on the reflex threshold angle of stretch reflex in the soleus muscle of normal and spastic subjects. Journal of the Formosan Medical Association, 104(7), 493-501.

Clopton N, Dutton J, et al. (2005). Interrater and intrarater reliability of the Modified Ashworth Scale in children with hypertonia. Pediatric Physical Therapy, 17(4), 268-274.

Cooper A, Musa IM, et al. (2005). Electromyography characterization of stretch responses in hemiparetic stroke patients and their relationship with the Modified Ashworth scale. Clinical Rehabilitation, 19(7), 760-766.

Coutinho EL, Gomes AR, et al. (2004). Effect of passive stretching on the immobilized soleus muscle fiber morphology. Brazilian Journal of Medical and Biological Research, 37(12), 1853-1861.

Davis DS, Ashby PE, et al. (2005). The effectiveness of 3 stretching techniques on hamstring flexibility using consistent stretching parameters. Journal of Strength and Conditioning Research, 19(1), 27-32.

Dennis M, Burn JP (1993). Long-term survival after first-ever stroke: The Oxfordshire Community Stroke Project. Stroke, 24(6), 796-800.

Dietz V (1992). Spasticity: Exaggerated reflexes or movements disorder? In H Forssberg and H Hirshfeld (Eds.), Movement Disorders in Children (pp. 225-233). Basel: S. Karger.

Dietz V. (2002). Proprioception and Locomotor Disorders. Nature Reviews. Neuroscience, 3(10), 781-790.

Dietz V, Berger W (1983). Normal and impaired regulation of muscle stiffness in gait: A new hypothesis about muscle hypertonia. Experimental Neurology, 79(3), 680-687.

Dietz V, Ketelsen UP, et al. (1986). Motor unit involvement in spastic paresis: Relationship between leg muscle activation and histochemistry. Journal of the Neurological Sciences, 75(1), 89-103.

Dietz V, Trippel M, et al. (1991). Reflex activity and muscle tone during elbow movements in patients with spastic paresis. Annals of Neurology, 30, 767-779.

Donelan JM, Pearson KG (2004). Contribution of sensory feedback to ongoing ankle extensor activity during the stance phase of walking. Canadian Journal of Physiology and Pharmacology, 82(8-9), 589-598.

Edgerton VR, Tillakaratne NJ, et al. (2004). Plasticity of the spinal neural circuitry after injury. Annual Review of Neuroscience, 27, 145-167.

Elovic EP, Simone LK, et al. (2004). Outcome assessment for spasticity management in the patient with traumatic brain injury: The state of the art. Journal of Head Trauma Rehabilitation 19(2), 155-177.

Fairfax, BP, Pitcher JA, et al. (2004). Phosphorylation and chronic agonist treatment atypically modulate GABAB receptor cell surface stability. Journal of Biological Chemistry, 279(13), 12565-12573.

Faist M, Ertel M, et al. (1999). Impaired modulation of quadriceps tendon jerk reflex during spastic gait: Differences between spinal and cerebral lesions. Brain, 122(Pt. 3), 567-579.

Gajdosik RL, Vander Linden DW, et al. (2004). Slow passive stretch and release characteristics of the calf muscles of older women with limited dorsiflexion range of motion. Clinical Biomechanics (Bristol, Avon), 19(4), 398-406.

Gandevia SC (1993). Assessment of corticofugal output: Strength testing and transcranial stimulation of the motor cortex. In SC Gandevia, D Burke, and M Anthony (Eds.), Science and Practice in Clinical Neurology (pp. 76-88). Cambridge, England: Cambridge University Press.

Gowland C, deBruin J, et al. (1992). Agonist and antagonist activity during voluntary upper-limb movement in patients with stroke. Physical Therapy, 72, 624-633.

Gracies JM (2005). Pathophysiology of spastic paresis. I: Paresis and soft tissue changes. Muscle Nerve, 31(5), 535-551.

Grimby G, Stalberg E, et al. (1998). An 8-year longitudinal study of muscle strength, muscle fiber size, and dynamic electromyogram in individuals with late polio. Muscle and Nerve, 21(11), 1428-1437.

Hachisuka K, Umezu Y, et al. (1997). Disuse muscle atrophy of lower limbs in hemiplegic patients. Archives of Physical Medicine and Rehabilitation, 78(1), 13-18.

Hautier CA, Arsac LM, et al. (2000). Influence of fatigue on EMG/force ratio and cocontraction in cycling. Medicine and Science in Sports and Exercise, 32(4), 839-843.

Hesse S, Konrad M, et al. (1999). Treadmill walking with partial body weight support versus floor walking in hemiparetic subjects. Archives of Physical Medicine and Rehabilitation, 80(4), 421-427.

Hiersemenzel LP, Curt A, et al. (2000). From spinal shock to spasticity: Neuronaladaptations to a spinal cord injury. Neurology, 54(8), 1574-1582.

Holstege G. 1996. The somatic motor system. Progress in Brain Research, 107, 9-26.

Horak FB, Buchanan J, et al. (2002). Vestibulospinal control of posture. Advances in Experimental Medicine and Biology, 508, 139-145.

Humm JL, Kozlowski DA, et al. (1998). Use-dependent exacerbation of brain damage occurs during an early post-lesion vulnerable period. Brain Research, 783(2), 286-292.

Ivanhoe CB, Reistetter TA (2004). Spasticity: The misunderstood part of the upper motor neuron syndrome. American Journal of Physical Medicine & Rehabilitation, 83(10 Suppl), S3-S9.

Jia L, Xu L, et al. (2005). Protein abnormality in denervated skeletal muscles from patients with brachial injury. Microsurgery, 25(4), 316-321.

Kennedy PM, Cresswell AG, et al. (2004). Vestibulospinal influences on lower limb motoneurons. Canadian Journal of Physiology and Pharmacology, 82(8-9), 675-681.

Kim, DY, Park CI, et al. (2005). Biomechanical assessment with electromyography of post-stroke ankle plantar flexor spasticity. Yonsei Medical Journal, 46(4), 546-554.

Kim JS, Choi-Kwon S (2000). Poststroke depression and emotional incontinence: Correlation with lesion location. Neurology, 54(9), 1805-1810.

Kjaer M. (2004). Role of extracellular matrix in adaptation of tendon and skeletal muscle to mechanical loading. Physiological Reviews, 84(2), 649-698.

Laidler P (1994). Stroke rehabilitation: Structure and strategy. San Diego, Calif.: Singular.

Lakie M, Robson LG (1988). Thixotropic changes in human muscle stiffness and the effects of fatigue [published erratum appears in Quarterly Journal of Experimental Physiology, 73(5), following 808]. Quarterly Journal of Experimental Physiology, 73(4), 487-500.

Lance JW (1980). Symposium synopsis. Spasticity: Disorder of motor control, Miami, Symposia Specialists.

Lawrence D, Kuypers H (1968). The functional organization of the motor system in the monkey: I. The effects of bilateral pyramidal lesions. II. The effects of lesions of the descending brainstem pathways. Brain, 91(1), 1-36.

Levin MF, Hui-Chan, C. (1993). Are H and stretch reflexes in hemiparesis reproducible and correlated with spasticity? Journal of Neurology, 240, 63-71.

Linke WA, Ivemeyer M, et al. (1996). Towards a molecular understanding of the elasticity of titin. Journal of Molecular Biology, 261(1), 62-71.

Lipton SA, Rosenberg PA (1994). Excitatory amino acids as a final common pathway for neurologic disorders. New England Journal of Medicine, 330(9), 613-622.

Lotta S, Scelsi R, et al. (1991). Morphometric and neurophysiological analysis of skeletal muscle in paraplegic patients with traumatic cord lesion. Paraplegia, 29(4), 247-252.

MacDonald BK, Cockerell OC, et al. (2000). The incidence and lifetime prevalence of neurological disorders in a prospective community-based study in the UK [see comments]. Brain, 123(4), 665-676.

Mancini F, Sandrini G, et al. (2005). A randomised, double-blind, dose-ranging study to evaluate efficacy and safety of three doses of botulinum toxin type A (Botox) for the treatment of spastic foot. Neurological Sciences, 26(1), 26-31.

Messier J, Adamovich S, et al. (2003). Influence of movement speed on accuracy and coordination of reaching movements to memorized targets in three-dimensional space in a deafferented subject. Experimental Brain Research, 150(4), 399-416.

Mirbagheri MM, Barbeau H, et al. (2001). Intrinsic and reflex stiffness in normal and spastic, spinal cord injured subjects. Experimental Brain Research, 141(4), 446-459.

Mushiake J, Inase M, et al. (1990). Selective coding of motor sequence in the supplementary motor area of the monkey cerebral cortex. Experimental Brain Research, 82, 208-210.

Neagoe C, Opitz CA, et al. (2003). Gigantic variety: Expression patterns of titin isoforms in striated muscles and consequences for myofibrillar passive stiffness. Journal of Muscle Research and Cell Motility, 24(2-3), 175-189.

Neilson PD (1993). Tonic stretch reflex in normal subjects and in cerebral palsy. In

Ganderia SC, Burke D, Anthony M (Eds.), Science and Practice in Clinical Neurology (pp. 169-190). Cambridge, England: Cambridge University Press.

Nichols TR, Cope TC (2004). Cross-bridge mechanisms underlying the history-dependent properties of muscle spindles and stretch reflexes. Canadian Journal of Physiology and Pharmacology, 82(8-9), 569-576.

Nielsen J, Petersen NT, et al. (2005). Stretch reflex regulation in healthy subjects and patients with spasticity. International Neuromodulation Society, 8(1), 49-57.

Noga BR, Kriellaars DJ, et al. (2003). Mechanism for activation of locomotor centers in the spinal cord by stimulation of the mesencephalic locomotor region. Journal of Neurophysiology, 90(3), 1464-1478.

Nudo RJ, Wise BM, et al. (1996). Neural substrates for the effects of rehabilitative training on motor recovery after ischemic infarct [see comments]. Science, 272(5269), 1791-1794.

O'Dwyer NJ, Ada L, et al. (1996). Spasticity and muscle contracture following stroke. Brain, 119(Pt 5), 1737-1749.

Osu R, Franklin DW, et al. (2002). Short- and long-term changes in joint co-contraction associated with motor learning as revealed from surface EMG. Journal of Neurophysiology, 88(2), 991-1004.

Paillard J (1999). Body schema and body image—A double dissociation in deafferented patients. In GN Gantchev, S Mori, and J Massion (Eds.), Motor Control, Today and Tomorrow. Sofia, Bulgaria: Academic Publishing House.

Palmeri A, Sapienza S, et al. (1999). Modulatory action of noradrenergic system on spinal motoneurons in humans. Neuroreport, 10(6), 1225-1229.

Paro-Panjan D, Neubauer D (2004). Congenital hypotonia: Is there an algorithm? Journal of Child Neurology, 19(6), 439-442.

Piamarta F, Iurlaro S, et al. (2004). Unconventional affective symptoms and executive functions after stroke in the elderly. Archives of Gerontology and Geriatrics (9 Suppl), 315-323.

Pijpers JR, Oudejans RR, et al. (2005). Anxiety-induced changes in movement behaviour during the execution of a complex whole-body task. Quarterly Journal of Experimental Psychology. A, Human Experimental Psychology, 58(3), 421-445.

Pratt CA (1995). Evidence of positive force feedback among hindlimb extensors in the intact standing cat. Journal of Neurophysiology, 73(6), 2578-2583.

Priebe MM, Sherwood AM, et al. (1996). Clinical assessment of spasticity in spinal cord injury: A multidimensional problem. Archives of Physical Medicine and Rehabilitation, 77(7), 713-716.

Proske U, Morgan DL (1999). Do cross-bridges contribute to the tension during stretch of passive muscle? Journal of Muscle Research and Cell Motility, 20(5-6), 433-442.

Quevedo J, Fedirchuk B, et al. (2000). Group I disynaptic excitation of cat hindlimb flexor and bifunctional motoneurones during fictive locomotion. Journal of Physiology, 525(Pt 2), 549-564.

Riemann BL, Lephart SM (2002). The Sensorimotor System, Part II: The Role of Proprioception in Motor Control and Functional Joint Stability. Journal of Athletic Training 37(1), 80-84.

Roncesvalles MN, Woollacott MW, et al. (2002). Neural factors underlying reduced postural adaptability in children with cerebral palsy. Neuroreport, 13(18), 2407-2410.

Rossignol S, Dubuc R, et al. (2006). Dynamic sensorimotor interactions in locomotion. Physiological Reviews, 86(1), 89-154.

Sakaba T, Neher E (2003). Direct modulation of synaptic vesicle priming by GABA(B) receptor activation at a glutamatergic synapse. Nature, 424(6950), 775-778.

Salazar-Torres Jde J, Pandyan AD, et al. (2004). Does spasticity result from hyperactive stretch reflexes? Preliminary findings from a stretch reflex characterization study. Disability and Rehabilitation, 26(12), 756-760.

Sanger TD, Delgado MR, et al. (2003). Classification and definition of disorders causing hypertonia in childhood. Pediatrics, 111(1), e89-e97.

Scelsi R, Poggi P, et al. (1986). Skeletal muscle changes following myelotomy in paraplegic patients. Paraplegia, 24(4), 250-259.

Shall MS, Dimitrova DM, et al. (2003). Extraocular motor unit and whole-muscle contractile properties in the squirrel monkey. Summation of forces and fiber morphology. Experimental Brain Research, 151(3), 338-345.

Shenton JT, Schwoebel J, et al. (2004). Mental motor imagery and the body schema, evidence for proprioceptive dominance. Neuroscience Letters, 370(1), 19-24.

Simmons Z (2005). Management strategies for patients with amyotrophic lateral sclerosis from diagnosis through death. Neurologist, 11(5), 257-270.

Sinkjaer T (1997). Muscle, reflex and central components in the control of the ankle joint in healthy and spastic man. Acta Neurologica Scandinavica, (170 Suppl), 1-28.

Skold C, Levi R, et al. (1999). Spasticity after traumatic spinal cord injury, Nature, severity, and location. Archives of Physical Medicine and Rehabilitation, 80(12), 1548-1557.

Sommerfeld DK, Eek EU, et al. (2004). Spasticity after stroke, its occurrence and association with motor impairments and activity limitations. Stroke, 35(1), 134-139.

Sorenson EJ, Stalker AP, et al. (2002). Amyotrophic lateral sclerosis in Olmsted County, Minnesota, 1925 to 1998. Neurology, 59(2), 280-282.

Spencer RM, Ivry RB, et al. (2005). Bimanual coordination during rhythmic movements in the absence of somatosensory feedback. Journal of Neurophysiology, 94(4), 2901-2910.

Thilmann AF, Fellows SJ, et al. (1991). The mechanism of spastic muscle hypertonus. Variation in reflex gain over the time course of spasticity. Brain, 114(Pt 1A), 233-244.

Van Peppen RP, Kwakkel G, et al. (2004). The impact of physical therapy on functional outcomes after stroke: What's the evidence? Clinical Rehabilitation, 18(8), 833-862.

Vance J, Wulf G, et al. (2004). EMG activity as a function of the performer's focus of attention. Journal of Motor Behavior, 36(4), 450-459.

Wakeling JM (2004). Motor units are recruited in a task-dependent fashion during locomotion. Journal of Experimental Biology, 207(Pt 22), 3883-3890.

Wolf SL, Catlin PA (1994). Overcoming limitations in elbow movement in the presence of antagonist hyperactivity. Physical Therapy, 74, 826-835.

Yang JF, Lamont EV, et al. (2005). Split-belt treadmill stepping in infants suggests autonomous pattern generators for the left and right leg in humans. Journal of Neuroscience, 25(29), 6869-6876.

10 Basal Ganglia, Cerebellum, and Movement

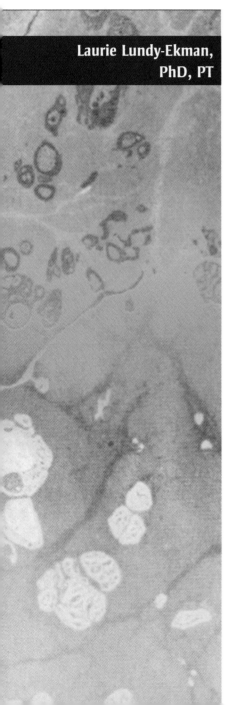

Laurie Lundy-Ekman, PhD, PT

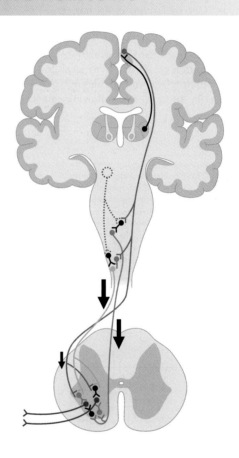

INTRODUCTION

The basal ganglia and cerebellum adjust activity in the descending tracts, despite a lack of direct connections with lower motor neurons. The basal ganglia and cerebellum influence movement via different pathways through the thalamus to motor areas of the cerebral cortex and by connections with upper motor neurons (UMNs). In this chapter, the basal ganglia and their clinical disorders will be discussed first, the cerebellum and clinical disorders affecting the cerebellum will be covered second, and the chapter will conclude with a summary of normal motor control and the three fundamental types of movement.

BASAL GANGLIA

The basal ganglia* regulate muscle contraction, muscle force, multijoint movements, and the sequencing of movements. The information for these functions is provided primarily by the cerebral cortex. The output of the basal ganglia is conveyed to UMNs via the motor areas of the cerebral cortex and the pedunculopontine nucleus (PPN; located in the brainstem). Stimulation of the **pedunculopontine nucleus** elicits rhythmical lower limb movements similar to walking or running.

The basal ganglia include the following nuclei (Figure 10-1):

---

*Historically, the term *basal ganglia* referred generically to deep gray matter in the cerebrum. Thus the amygdala and the thalamus were considered part of the basal ganglia, and the subthalamic nucleus and substantia nigra were excluded. Because subsequent research has established that the functions of the amygdala and most of the thalamus are not closely related to the functions of the striatum and globus pallidus, most authors now exclude the amygdala and thalamus. Similarly, because essential functional relationships have been confirmed among the substantia nigra, subthalamic nucleus, globus pallidus, and striatum, these structures are currently considered to constitute the basal ganglia.

- Caudate
- Putamen
- Globus pallidus
- Subthalamic nucleus
- Substantia nigra

The caudate, putamen, and globus pallidus are located within the cerebrum. Based on anatomic proximity, the cerebral basal ganglia have joint names: the globus pallidus and putamen together form the **lentiform nucleus;** the caudate and putamen together are the **striatum.** The lentiform nucleus is shaped like a broad, solid cone, with the putamen lateral (wide end of cone) and the globus pallidus medial (point of cone). The globus pallidus has an internus (medial) section and an externus (lateral) section. The caudate is joined with the putamen anteriorly. Their junction is called the **ventral striatum.** The **nucleus accumbens** (see Figure 10-1) is part of the ventral striatum.

During growth of the brain, the caudate assumes a *C* shape adjacent to the lateral ventricle (see Chapter 5). The large, anterior part of the caudate is the head, the adjacent section is the body, and the part on the edge of the inferior horn of the lateral ventricle is the tail of the caudate. Because the function of the caudate is primarily cognitive, not motor (Levy et al., 1997), and the function

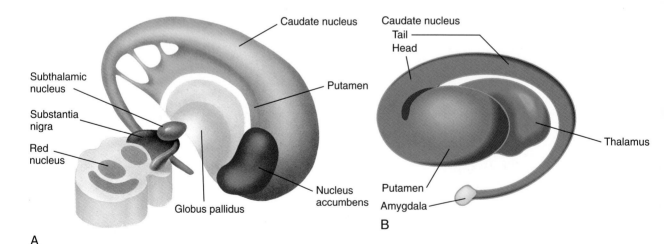

FIGURE 10-1
Basal ganglia. **A,** Three-dimensional view of the midbrain and the left caudate, putamen, and globus pallidus. *(Anterior shown on the right.)* The basal ganglia include the caudate, putamen, globus pallidus, substantia nigra, and subthalamic nucleus. The red nucleus, shown for anatomic reference, is not part of the basal ganglia. **B,** Lateral view of the left caudate and putamen, showing their anatomical relationship with the amygdala (part of the limbic system) and the thalamus. *(Anterior shown on the left.) (A Modified from Hendelman WJ (1994). Student's Atlas of Neuroanatomy (p. 39). Philadelphia: Saunders.)*

of the ventral striatum is primarily limbic, the caudate and ventral striatum will be covered in Chapter 16.

The **subthalamic nucleus** is located inferior to the thalamus and lateral to the hypothalamus (Figure 10-2). The substantia nigra is a nucleus in the midbrain named for the color of its cells. Some substantia nigra cells contain melanin, making the nucleus appear black. The substantia nigra has two parts: compacta and reticularis. The substantia nigra compacta provides essential dopamine to the striatum.

The **substantia nigra reticularis** and the **globus pallidus internus** are the output nuclei of the basal ganglia system. The output from these nuclei inhibits the motor thalamus and the PPN of the midbrain (Table 10-1, Figure 10-3). In addition to the motor circuit, the basal ganglia also have circuits that influence eye movements and emotions. These circuits are beyond the scope of this text.

Although functioning basal ganglia are vital for normal movement, they have no direct connections with lower motor neurons. Their influence is exerted through either of the following:

* Motor planning areas of the cerebral cortex
* PPN of the midbrain

The influence on motor planning areas of the cerebral cortex is indirect, via the thalamus. A major basal ganglia

Table 10-1   BASAL GANGLIA MOTOR CIRCUIT

Role	Structure
Receive input from premotor and sensorimotor cortex	Putamen
Process information within the basal ganglia circuit	Globus pallidus externus Subthalamic nucleus Substantia nigra compacta
Send output to motor areas of the cerebral cortex and PPN	Globus pallidus internus Substantia nigra reticularis (via the motor thalamus)

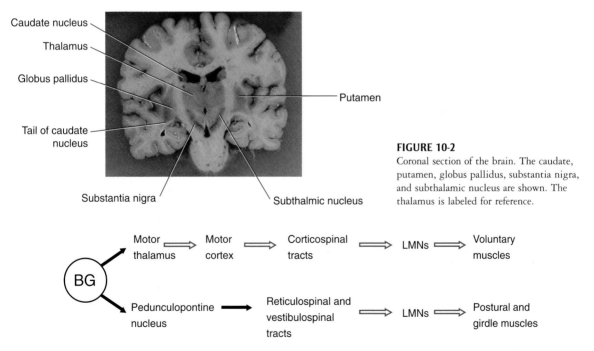

FIGURE 10-2
Coronal section of the brain. The caudate, putamen, globus pallidus, substantia nigra, and subthalamic nucleus are shown. The thalamus is labeled for reference.

FIGURE 10-3
Simplified summary of the role of the basal ganglia in movement. The output from the basal ganglia inhibits the motor thalamus, contributing to a normal level of activity in the motor cortex. Therefore the corticospinal tracts provide a normal level of facilitation to the lower motor neurons that innervate voluntary muscles. The output from the basal ganglia also inhibits the PPN. The PPN inhibits the reticulospinal and vestibulospinal tracts, providing the normal level of facilitation to the lower motor neurons that innervate postural and girdle muscles. Red arrows indicate facilitation; black arrows indicate inhibition.

circuit connects motor and somatosensory areas of the cerebral cortex → putamen → output nuclei → motor thalamus → motor areas of the cerebral cortex (Figure 10-4). The motor control exerted by the basal ganglia on the cortex is transmitted to lower motor neurons via the motor corticofugal tracts. **Motor corticofugal tracts** are the axons of upper motor neurons whose cell bodies are in the cerebral cortex: the corticospinal, corticopontine, and corticobulbar tracts. A second important basal ganglia motor circuit consists of connections from the basal ganglia output nuclei to the PPN, thence to the reticulospinal and to the vestibulospinal tracts.

Neurotransmitters in the Basal Ganglia Circuit

Of the many neurotransmitters and neuromodulators active in the basal ganglia circuitry, the actions of only

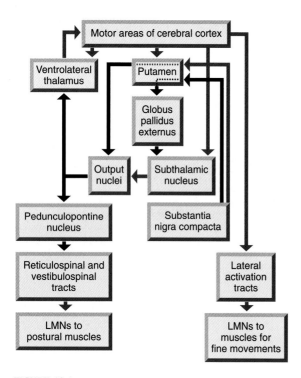

FIGURE 10-4
Basal ganglia functional connections during normal movement. Red arrows indicate that the connection is excitatory. Black arrows indicate that the connection is inhibitory. The direct route within the basal ganglia is from the putamen to the output nuclei. The indirect route is from the putamen to the globus pallidus externus, then to the subthalamic nucleus, and finally to the output nuclei. The output nuclei are the globus pallidus internus and the substantia nigra reticularis. LMNs, lower motor neurons.

a few are well understood. The effects are complex because often one structure will inhibit a second structure, whose output in turn inhibits a third structure. The result of this sequence is to disinhibit, or increase the activity in, the third structure, because inhibition of the second structure reduces its inhibitory output.

The cortical motor areas produce excitation of the putamen by delivering the transmitter glutamate. In the direct pathway (see Figure 10-4), the putamen inhibits the output nuclei by γ-aminobutyric acid (GABA) and Substance P. Because the output from the output nuclei is inhibitory to the motor thalamus and PPN (via GABA), the net effect of increasing input to the putamen is to increase the excitatory output from the motor thalamus to the cortical motor areas. Therefore the activity in the corticofugal pathways will increase.

The indirect route proceeds from the putamen inhibiting the globus pallidus externus (via GABA and enkephalins) to inhibition of the subthalamic nucleus (GABA), excitation of the substantia nigra reticularis (glutamate), inhibition of the motor thalamus (GABA), ending with less excitation of the motor areas of the cerebral cortex. Therefore, activity in the indirect route decreases the activity in corticofugal pathways.

Dopamine from the substantia nigra compacta enhances activity in the motor cortex by binding with two types of receptors in the basal ganglia circuit, D_1 and D_2. Binding of dopamine with the D_1 receptor facilitates activity in the direct pathway, while binding of dopamine with the D_2 receptor inhibits activity in the indirect pathway.

Function of the Basal Ganglia

The basal ganglia are involved with sequencing movements and regulating muscle tone and muscle force. The striatum initiates automatic, repetitive, overlearned skills. These skills include piano playing and the rules of syntax. The striatum is also part of the circuit involved in some cases of obsessive-compulsive disorder (Friedlander and Desrocher, 2006). The role of the basal ganglia in motor learning will be discussed in Chapter 16.

Basal Ganglia Pathology

Movement disorders in basal ganglia dysfunction range from hypokinetic disorders (too little movement, as in Parkinson's disease) to hyperkinetic (excessive movement, as in Huntington's disease, dystonia, or subtypes of cerebral palsy). The differences in abnormal movements are due to dysfunction in specific parts of the basal ganglia–thalamocortical motor circuit and in the basal ganglia–PPN output. The basal ganglia inhibit the motor thalamus and the PPN; excessive inhibition results in hypokinetic disorders, and inadequate inhibition results in hyperkinetic disorders.

Hypokinetic Disorders

Parkinson's Disease. The most common basal ganglia motor disorder is Parkinson's disease, characterized by muscular rigidity, shuffling gait, drooping posture, rhythmical muscular tremors, and a masklike facial expression. Parkinson's disease (paralysis agitans) interferes with both voluntary and automatic movements. People with Parkinson's disease have difficulty coming to standing from sitting, and their gait is characterized by a flexed posture, shuffling of the feet, and decreased or absent arm swing. The distinctive signs of Parkinson's disease are:

* Rigidity
* Hypokinesia (decreased movement)
* Resting tremor
* "Freezing" during movement
* Visuoperceptive impairments
* Postural instability and dementia

Rigidity is increased resistance to movement in all muscles. In contrast to myoplastic hyperstiffness, rigidity results from direct upper motor neuron facilitation of alpha motor neurons. Thus, in rigidity, output from the nervous system causes active muscle contraction, directly increasing resistance to movement.

Hypokinesia is manifested in decreased ranges of active motion and in the lack of automatic movements, including facial expression and normal arm swing during walking. Hypokinesia may be related to decreased ability to control the force output of muscles. Pope et al. (2006) demonstrated that people with Parkinson's disease are unable to control force production as well as people without neurologic disorders. People with Parkinson's disease are prone to falls because of their inability to generate adequate muscle force quickly. Their postural corrections may be too slow to be useful.

In contrast to the hypokinetic signs, a hyperkinetic sign of Parkinson's disease is resting tremor. **Tremor** is involuntary, rhythmic shaking movements of the limbs produced by contractions of antagonist muscles. Resting tremor of the hands is rhythmic movement as if using the thumb to roll a pill along the fingertips (pill-rolling tremor); the tremor is prominent when the hand is at rest and diminishes during voluntary movement. Resting tremor has a frequency of 3-6 per second and tends to affect the hands and feet. However, in some Parkinson's cases, tremor never presents.

People with Parkinson's disease often have episodes when their movements abruptly cease, called **freezing**. Freezing frequently interrupts gait. The phenomenon of freezing is not understood.

Visuoperceptive impairments are deficits in using visual information to guide movement. Visuoperceptive impairments produce impediments to action. For example, a walker, intended to assist a person with ambulation, may create a visual block, and movement ceases. A therapist standing near the person may also unwittingly interfere with the person's ability to move. People with Parkinson's disease frequently report difficulties moving past visual movement blocks, like doorways; if a marker is placed on the floor, the person can use the marker as a cue for getting through the doorway. Why the marker does not serve as an additional visual block is unknown.

Postural instability, secondary to the extreme stiffness of postural flexors and extensors, becomes a severe problem as Parkinson's progresses. The motor progression of Parkinson's disease occurs in predictable stages (Box 10-1). Clinical diagnosis of Parkinson's disease requires hypokinesia affecting the upper body combined with rigidity and/or resting tremor (Uitti et al., 2005).

Parkinson's disease also affects nonmotor systems. Often depression, psychosis (usually visual hallucinations), **Parkinson's dementia,** and autonomic dysfunction (constipation, orthostatic hypotension) further

---

BOX 10-1   STAGES OF PARKINSON'S DISEASE

1. *Stage One*
   Unilateral signs and symptoms, typically mild tremor of one limb
2. *Stage Two*
   Bilateral signs, posture and gait affected, minimal disability
3. *Stage Three*
   Moderately severe generalized dysfunction, significant slowing of body movements, early impairment of equilibrium on walking or standing
4. *Stage Four*
   Severe signs; able to walk to limited extent; rigidity, bradykinesia; unable to live alone
5. *Stage Five*
   Extreme weight loss, cannot stand or walk, requires constant nursing care (From Hoehn and Yahr, 1967.)

decrease the person's independence (Mark, 2005). Dementia is deterioration of intellectual function. Parkinson's dementia is different from Alzheimer's dementia. Alzheimer's dementia primarily affects memory. Parkinson's dementia interferes with the ability to plan, to maintain goal orientation, and to make decisions (Klinger et al., 2006).

The pathology in Parkinson's disease is the death of dopamine-producing cells in the substantia nigra compacta (Figure 10-5) and acetylcholine-producing cells in the PPN. Oxidative stress, mitochondrial dysfunction, and programmed cell death kill the cells (Mark, 2005). Cell death occurs long before clinical signs of Parkinson's disease become evident; about 80% of the dopamine-producing cells die before signs of the disease appear (Vatalaro, 2000).

The loss of dopamine in the basal ganglia direct pathway reduces activity in the motor areas of the cerebral cortex, decreasing voluntary movements. The loss of pedunculopontine cells, combined with increased inhibition of the PPN, disinhibits the reticulospinal and vestibulospinal tracts, producing excessive contraction of postural muscles (Figure 10-6). Figure 10-7 compares

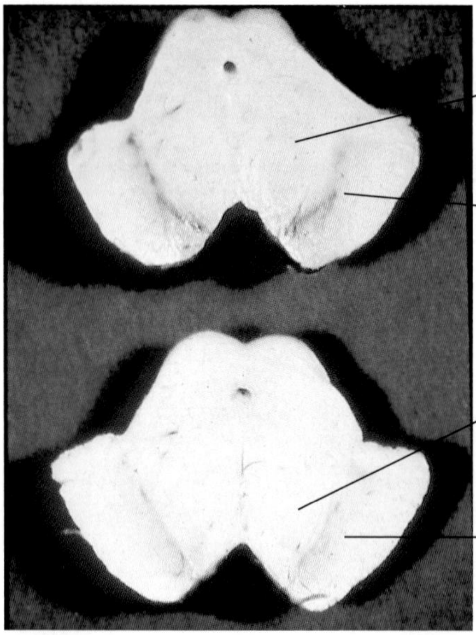

FIGURE 10-5
Horizontal sections of the midbrain. The upper section is normal, with darkly pigmented cells in the substantia nigra. The lower section is from a person with Parkinson's disease, with the characteristic loss of darkly pigmented, dopamine-producing cells. *Courtesy of Dr. Melvin J. Ball.*

the location and effects of upper motor neuron lesions with the location and effects of Parkinson's disease. (See Box 10-2.)

Treatments for Parkinson's Disease. Drugs, invasive procedures, and physical and occupational therapy are used to treat Parkinson's disease. Because Parkinson's disease involves loss of dopamine-producing cells in the substantia nigra, drug therapy that replaces dopamine (L-dopa) is initially effective in reducing signs of the disease. However, tolerance to L-dopa, side effects (including hallucinations, delusions, psychosis, and dyskinesia), and progression of the disease with involvement of other cells and neurotransmitters limit the effectiveness of L-dopa therapy. **Dyskinesia** is involuntary movement that resembles chorea (brisk, jerky movements) and/or dystonia (involuntary sustained postures or repetitive movements). Even with L-dopa therapy, people with Parkinson's disease may experience periods of near-normal mobility alternating with periods of immobility. This is called the *on-off phenomenon*. The duration of "on" times tends to decrease with continued use of L-dopa. Moreover, motor performance often varies at different times of day regardless of medication.

Invasive procedures, including deep-brain stimulation, neuronal transplantation, and destructive surgery, are sometimes used to treat the tremors and akinesia associated with Parkinson's disease. Akinesia, strictly defined, is the absence of movement. However, in clinical use, the term *akinesia* is used to describe paucity of movement.

For selected patients, deep brain stimulation (DBS) is an effective adjunct to drug therapy. DBS requires surgical implantation of a stimulator and electrodes. Typically the stimulator is implanted inferior to the clavicle. To treat tremors, electrodes are implanted into the thalamus (Volkmann, 2004). Continuous high-frequency electrical stimulation inhibits the firing of overactive thalamic neurons. Bilateral subthalamic nucleus DBS improves tremor, rigidity, and speed of movements and allows decreased L-dopa dosage. However, the surgery is only appropriate for relatively healthy, young, cognitively intact patients who are on optimal medications and have severe fluctuations of motor signs (Mark, 2005). Long term follow up demonstrates that thalamic deep brain stimulation is safe and effective for reducing tremors (Pahwa et al., 2006) and stimulation of the subthalamic nucleus provides a sustained improvement in motor function (Schupbach et al., 2005).

Researchers have also used neuronal transplantation to treat Parkinson's disease, placing fetal-donor dopamine-producing cells in the basal ganglia. This

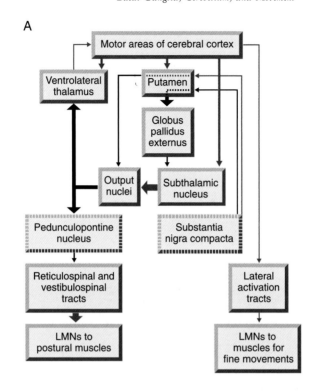

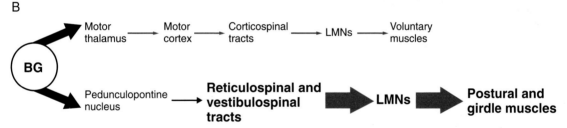

FIGURE 10-6

A, Changes in neural activity in Parkinson's disease. Compare to normal basal ganglia activity in Figure 10-4. Red arrows indicate that the connection is excitatory. Black arrows indicate that the connection is inhibitory. Thick arrows represent increased neural activity, and thin arrows represent decreased neural activity. A dotted outline surrounding a structure indicates the death of neurons within that structure. The output nuclei are the globus pallidus internus and the substantia nigra reticularis. Decreased dopamine from the substantia nigra compacta is the primary change leading to excessive activity of the output nuclei, in turn inhibiting the motor thalamus and thus reducing the output of motor areas of the cerebral cortex. Cells in the PPN die off. The death of cells in the PPN combined with excessive inhibition of the PPN by the output nuclei results in disinhibition of several of the medial upper motor neurons. **B,** Simplified summary of the changes that occur in Parkinson's disease. The sizes of the arrows and the letters symbolize the amount of activity in pathways and structures (for example, thick black arrows indicate excessive inhibition, and thin black arrows indicate insufficient inhibition). The basal ganglia provide too much inhibition to the motor thalamus, causing the motor cortex to be less active than normal. Therefore the corticospinal tracts provide less than the normal level of facilitation to the lower motor neurons that innervate voluntary muscles. The basal ganglia also provide excessive inhibition of the PPN. Therefore the PPN provides less inhibition of the reticulospinal and vestibulospinal tracts. In turn these tracts provide too much facilitation to lower motor neurons innervating postural muscles.

approach is based on the hypothesis that if the transplanted cells thrive in the brain environment, they will become internal sources of dopamine. However, to optimize transplantation, problems with culturing and delivering the cells and selecting locations need to be overcome (Fillmore et al., 2005).

Some specialized treatment centers perform destructive surgery for the treatment of severe tremor and akinesia associated with Parkinson's disease (Volkmann, 2004). In these surgeries, called *thalamotomy* and *pallidotomy,* surgery destroys a small, precise region of cells in the thalamus (for the treatment of tremor) and

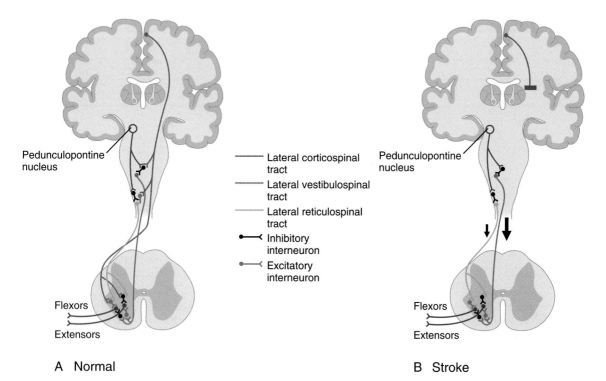

	Effect on Flexors	Effect on Extensors
Lateral corticospinal	++	––
Lateral reticulospinal	++	–
Lateral vestibulospinal	–	+

Lateral corticospinal also facilitates lateral reticulospinal and inhibits lateral vesibulospinal tracts.

	Effect on Flexors	Effect on Extensors
Lateral corticospinal		
Lateral reticulospinal	+	–
Lateral vestibulospinal	––	+++

Three changes occur as a result of interuption of the lateral corticospinal tract: loss of its direct input to lower motor neurons, loss of facilitation of lateral reticulospinal tract, and disinhibition of lateral vestibulospinal tract.

FIGURE 10-7

A-D, Comparison of the effects of stroke, complete spinal cord injury, and Parkinson's disease on activity in upper motor neurons and the resulting activity levels in skeletal muscles. Black interneurons are inhibitory; green interneurons are excitatory. The spinal cord section is a lumbar segment. In each table, a "+" sign indicates facilitation, and a "−" sign indicates inhibition. Thus, in an intact nervous system, the lateral corticospinal tract moderately facilitates lower motor neurons to flexor muscles and inhibits lower motor neurons to extensors. Also, in an intact nervous system, the lateral vestibulospinal tract weakly inhibits lower motor neurons to flexors and weakly facilitates lower motor neurons to extensors.

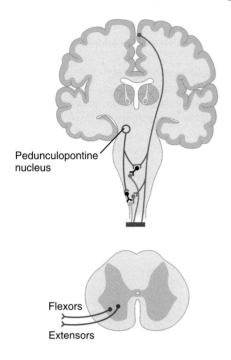

Pedunculopontine nucleus

Flexors

Extensors

C Complete spinal cord lesion

	Effect on Flexors	Effect on Extensors
Lateral corticospinal		
Lateral reticulospinal		
Lateral vestibulospinal		

All descending tracts are interrupted.

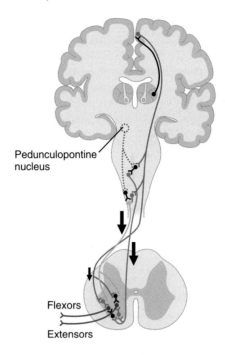

Pedunculopontine nucleus

Flexors

Extensors

D Parkinson's disease

	Effect on Flexors	Effect on Extensors
Lateral corticospinal	+	−
Lateral reticulospinal	+++	−
Lateral vestibulospinal	−	+++

Decreased activity of motor areas of cortex (due to inhibition of thalamus by globus pallidus) causes decreased output via the lateral corticospinal tract. Disinhibition of the lateral reticulospinal and lateral vestibulospinal tracts result from decreased activity of the pedunculopontine nucleus. These changes lead to muscle rigidity.

FIGURE 10-7, cont'd

in the globus pallidus of the basal ganglia (for the treatment of akinesia). Destruction of these cells, which are thought to be overactive in the disease process, may result in functional improvement. DBS, destructive surgery, and neural transplantation are also used to treat other movement disorders and for intractable chronic pain.

> Neural activity can be altered using a variety of neurosurgical approaches aimed at restoring more normal transmitter levels and neuron activity levels.

Physical and occupational therapy are reported to improve mobility and functional status in people with

---

BOX 10-2   PARKINSON'S DISEASE

Pathology
  *Death of dopaminergic neurons in substantia nigra
    compacta and in pedunculopontine nucleus (PPN)*
Etiology
  *Oxidative stress, mitochondrial dysfunction, and
    programmed cell death*
Speed of Onset
  Chronic
Signs and Symptoms
  Affect
  Depression is common
  Cognition
  Dementia and psychosis late in the disease
  Consciousness
  *Alterations in sleep/wake cycles cause excessive daytime
    sleepiness*
  Communication and Memory
  Normal; dementia may occur in late stages
  Sensory
  Normal
  Autonomic
  *Constipation, orthostatic hypotension, thermal
    dysregulation, bladder and sexual dysfunction*

Motor
  *Hypokinesia; rigidity; stooped posture; shuffling gait;
    difficulty initiating movements, turning, and stopping;
    resting tremor; visuoperceptive movement blocks;
    freezing during movements; decreased postural control*
Region Affected
  Basal ganglia nuclei in cerebrum and midbrain
Demographics
  *Onset typically between 50 and 65 years of age; men
    and women affected equally*
  Incidence
  *8-18 cases per 100,000 population people per year (de
    Lau and Breteler, 2006)*
  Lifetime Prevalence
  *3 cases per 1000 population people (de Lau and
    Breteler, 2006)*
Prognosis
  *Progressive; average life span after diagnosis is 13 years
    (Louis et al., 1995); death usually by heart disease
    or infection*

Parkinson's disease (Gage and Storey, 2004). Intense resistance training produces greater muscle hypertrophy and functional gains than standard exercise (Dibble et al., 2006).

Parkinsonism. Several other disorders cause signs similar to Parkinson's disease and must be distinguished from true idiopathic Parkinson's. Red flags indicating a different diagnosis other than Parkinson's disease include early postural instability, early dementia, lack of resting tremor, rapid progression, early autonomic dysfunction, and signs of cerebellar, corticospinal, or voluntary gaze dysfunction (Mark, 2005). *Parkinsonism* is the collective name for disorders that cause signs similar to Parkinson's disease.

Parkinsonism encompasses disorders of toxic, primary neurodegenerative, infectious, or traumatic etiology. Lesions of the lentiform nucleus are associated with parkinsonism. Parkinsonism is often a side effect of drugs that treat psychosis or digestive problems. Phenothiazine, thioxanthine, antiemetics, and other drugs that block central nervous system dopamine receptors may cause parkinsonism. Drug-induced parkinsonism frequently leads to misdiagnosis and unnecessary treatment

for Parkinson's disease in the elderly (Avorn et al., 1995). Signs that parkinsonism may be drug-induced include: subacute, bilateral onset with rapid progression, early postural tremor, and involuntary movements of the face and mouth (Adler, 1999).

The term *primary neurodegenerative disease* indicates that the cause is idiopathic or genetic. The primary neurodegenerative diseases that cause parkinsonism include progressive supranuclear palsy, dementia with Lewy bodies, and multiple system atrophy. The most common cause of death in people with primary parkinsonism is pneumonia.

Progressive supranuclear palsy (PSP) is characterized by early onset of gait instability with a tendency to fall backwards, axial rigidity, freezing of gait, depression, psychosis, rage attacks, plus supranuclear gaze palsy. Supranuclear refers to loss of descending neurons that synapse in the cranial nerve nuclei controlling eye movement. In supranuclear gaze palsy, the patient is unable to voluntarily control gaze. Vertical gaze is usually affected before horizontal gaze, so initially the patient may be unable to look downward or upward. Reflexive eye movements remain normal. The pathology is neurodegeneration with tauopathy (abnormal accumulation of the structural protein tau within neurons). The cause of PSP is unknown. PSP prevalence is 6.5 cases per 100,000 people (Nath et al., 2001).

Dementia with Lewy bodies causes cognitive decline, visual hallucinations, and parkinsonism. Lewy bodies are abnormal accumulations of proteins (tau and alpha-synuclein) within neurons. Unlike Alzheimer disease, memory is not disproportionately impaired compared with other cognitive functions. Prevalence estimates range from 0-5% and incidence is 0.1% per year (Zaccai et al., 2005).

Multiple system atrophy (MSA) is a progressive degenerative disease affecting the basal ganglia, cerebellar, and autonomic systems; the peripheral nervous system; and the cerebral cortex (Box 10-3).

MSA is characterized by:
- Parkinsonism
- Cerebellar signs
- Autonomic dysfunction

The parkinsonism features of MSA include slow movements and rigidity. Cerebellar aspects are **dysarthria** (uncoordinated speech) and truncal and gait ataxia. **Ataxia** is lack of coordination. The gait ataxia in MSA is not typical of cerebellar gait ataxia, because the ataxic gait in MSA is narrow-based. Autonomic features are postural hypotension, bladder and bowel incontinence, abnormal respiration, decreased sweating, tears, and saliva, and in men, impotence. A decrease in goal-oriented cognitive ability and difficulty with directing attention have been reported (Dujardin et al., 2003). In women, the first sign of MSA is usually difficulty urinating. In men, the first sign is usually impotence.

The diagnosis requires differentiating MSA from pure parkinsonism and from pure autonomic failure. The distinction between MSA and parkinsonism is made by exclusion; if no autonomic or cerebellar signs are present, the disorder is pure parkinsonism. In pure autonomic failure, orthostatic hypotension and other autonomic signs occur without signs of basal ganglia or cerebellar involvement. Another distinguishing feature is that pure autonomic failure primarily affects the postganglionic neurons of the sympathetic system, whereas MSA affects both the preganglionic and postganglionic neurons in the sympathetic and parasympathetic systems. In MSA, autonomic neurons are lost from brainstem nuclei, including the vagus, and from the spinal cord.

Because MSA initially manifests with signs of involvement of only one system, MSA is often misdiagnosed. Parkinson's disease is the most common misdiagnosis, and about one third of people with MSA die while still

---

BOX 10-3   MULTIPLE SYSTEM ATROPHY

Pathology
Progressive degenerative disease affecting the basal ganglia, cerebellar, and autonomic systems and the cerebral cortex

Etiology
Unknown

Speed of Onset
Chronic

Signs and Symptoms
Consciousness
Decreased goal-oriented cognition and difficulty with attention; may have dementia late in the disease process
Communication and Memory
May be impaired late in the disease process
Sensory
May have polyneuropathy that includes sensory fibers
Autonomic
Postural hypotension; hypotension after eating; bladder and bowel incontinence; abnormal respiration; decreased sweating, tears, and saliva; male impotence
Motor
Slow movements, rigidity, dysarthria, truncal ataxia, and narrow-based gait ataxia

Region Affected
Basal ganglia, cerebellar, and autonomic systems and the cerebral cortex

Demographics
Prevalence
0.6 cases per 100,000 people per year (Vanacore, 2005); males affected approximately twice as frequently as females
0.03 cases per 1000 population (Vanacore, 2005).

Prognosis
Progressive; average life span after diagnosis is 9.5 years (Wenning et al., 1994)

---

misdiagnosed (Quinn and Wenning, 1994). Signs indicating that MSA is a more likely diagnosis than Parkinson's disease include a poor response to L-dopa (Sinemet, a drug that is effective in Parkinson's disease), orthostatic hypotension, difficulty with urination, rapid progression of functional limitations, loud breathing, and impotence.

Because a variety of neural structures are involved in MSA, different varieties of MSA have been named for the structures predominantly affected. Thus, three names are synonymous with MSA: olivopontocerebellar atrophy, striatonigral degeneration, and Shy-Drager syndrome. When the initial signs of MSA are incoordination, dysarthria, and balance deficits, the disorder is often called **olivopontocerebellar atrophy.** When the most prominent signs initially are rigidity and bradykinesia, the disease may be called **striatonigral degeneration.** When the first signs are autonomic dysfunction, the disorder may be called **Shy-Drager syndrome.**

The cause of MSA is unknown. Treatment is symptomatic: fludrocortisone and midodrine to increase blood pressure, and pergolide, bromocriptine, and anticholinergic drugs to improve the movement disorder. Therapists advise people with MSA on methods to decrease orthostatic hypotension (slow position changes, avoiding prolonged standing, eating smaller meals, increasing the consumption of salt and caffeine, use of elastic garments, avoidance of warm temperatures) and on exercise programs to maintain strength and physiologic fitness as long as possible.

Hyperkinetic Disorders

Abnormal involuntary movements are characteristic of Huntington's disease, dystonia, and some types of cerebral palsy.

Huntington's Disease. **Chorea,** consisting of involuntary, jerky, rapid movements, and dementia are the signs of Huntington's disease. This autosomal dominant hereditary disorder causes degeneration in many areas of the brain, most prominently in the striatum and cerebral cortex (Figure 10-8). The degeneration decreases signals from the basal ganglia output nuclei, resulting in disinhibition of the motor thalamus and PPN. The result is excessive output from the motor areas of the cerebral cortex (Figure 10-9). Although the chorea decreases during sleep, people with Huntington's disease move more frequently and forcefully while sleeping than people without the disease (Hurelbrink et al., 2005). Onset is typically between 40 and 50 years of age, and the disease is progressive, resulting in death about 15 years after signs first appear. The prevalence of Huntington's disease is 5 to 10 cases per 100,000 people (Evans et al., 2000).

Dystonia. Dystonias are genetic, usually nonprogressive, movement disorders characterized by involuntary sustained muscle contractions causing abnormal postures or twisting, repetitive movements (Figure 10-10). Dystonia often increases during activity and emotional stress and vanishes completely during sleep (Adler, 2000). The most common are focal dystonias, limited to one part of the body (Table 10-2; Figure 10-11). An example of

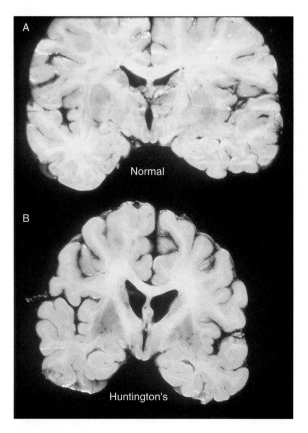

FIGURE 10-8
A, Coronal section of a normal cerebrum. Compare the size of the caudate nucleus and the overall size of the cerebrum to **B,** a cerebrum from a person with Huntington's disease. Atrophy of the caudate nucleus produces enlargement of the lateral ventricles. *(Courtesy Dr. Melvin J. Ball.)*

focal dystonia is spasmodic torticollis (also known as *cervical dystonia*). Torticollis is involuntary, asymmetrical contraction of neck muscles, causing abnormal position of the head. Not all torticollis is caused by dystonia: torticollis can also be caused by inflammatory, ocular, congenital, orthopedic, and other neurologic disorders. Focal hand dystonias usually occur only during a specific task. For example, writer's cramp is deterioration in handwriting due to involuntary muscle contractions in the upper limb. Similarly, musician's cramp most often involves the fourth and fifth fingers flexing involuntarily, interfering with the ability to play an instrument (Box 10-4). A sports-specific movement disorder, the yips in golf, can be caused by focal dystonia or by performance anxiety. Yips are abrupt, involuntary wrist movements that interfere with putting (Adler, 2005).

Byl (2000) has demonstrated that focal dystonia can be produced in some monkeys by requiring them to open and close one hand hundreds of times every day for several weeks. However, some monkeys spontaneously took breaks and performed the task more slowly than the other monkeys; these monkeys did not develop dystonia. In the monkeys that developed dystonia, neuronal activity in the primary somatosensory cortex was mapped. Receptive fields for the cortical neurons were 10 to 1000 times larger than normal, and many multiple receptive fields were documented.

In humans with focal dystonia, magnetic resonance imaging shows somatotopic degradation in the somatosensory cortex and in the somatosensory part of the thalamus (Byl, 2000; Lenz and Byl, 1999). Thus the loss of fractionation of movement results from maladaptive neural plasticity. Proprioception and stereognosis are impaired (McKenzie et al., 2003). A treatment protocol for musician's dystonia developed by Byl consists of cessation of abnormal movements, avoidance of heavy gripping of instruments (pens, musical instruments), sensory retraining, and mental rehearsal of the target movement

FIGURE 10-9

Changes in neural activity in Huntington's disease. Compare with normal basal ganglia activity in Figure 10-4. Red arrows indicate that the connection is excitatory. Black arrows indicate that the connection is inhibitory. Thick arrows represent increased neural activity, and thin arrows represent decreased neural activity. The output nuclei are the globus pallidus internus and the substantia nigra reticularis. Huntington's disease is characterized by excessive direct inhibition of the output nuclei by the putamen. The inhibitory output of the basal ganglia is inadequate, producing disinhibition of the motor thalamus and the PPN. This results in excessive activity of the motor areas of the cerebral cortex, producing hyperkinesias, combined with excessive output from the PPN, causing insufficient activity in several medial upper motor neuron tracts.

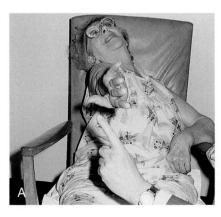
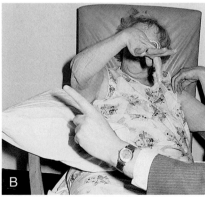

FIGURE 10-10

Generalized dystonia. Photograph of a 70-year-old woman exhibiting involuntary movements, including shoulder flexion, elbow extension, lateral flexion and extension of the neck, and trunk extension. *(From Parsons M, Johnson M (2001). Diagnosis in Color Neurology. St. Louis: Mosby.)*

Table 10-2   TYPES OF FOCAL DYSTONIA

	Body Region Affected	Differential Diagnosis
Cervical dystonia (spasmodic torticollis)	Neck	Congenital muscular torticollis; torticollis caused by inflammatory, ocular, other neurologic, and orthopedic disorders
Blepharospasm (involuntary closure of eyes)	Orbicularis oculi muscles	Irritation or inflammation of eyes or eyelids
Occupational dystonia: musician's cramp, writer's cramp	Upper limb	Carpel tunnel syndrome, apraxia
Oromandibular	Lower facial, masticatory, and tongue muscles	Dental problems, teeth grinding, drug side effect
Spasmodic dysphonia	Laryngeal muscles	Inflammatory conditions, vocal misuse, nodules, tumors, psychologic factors

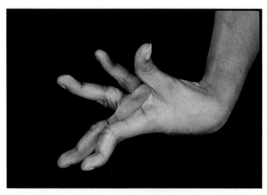

A

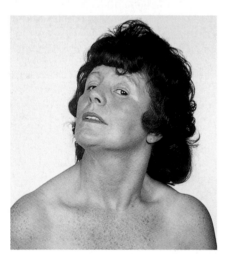

B

FIGURE 10-11
Focal dystonia. **A,** Sustained involuntary muscle contraction of the hand. **B,** Spasmodic torticollis. Involuntary contraction of neck muscles causes abnormal head posture. *(From Perkin GD (2002). Mosby's Colour Atlas and Text of Neurology. (2ⁿᵈ ed.). Edinburgh: Mosby.)*

BOX 10-4   FOCAL HAND DYSTONIA

Pathology
  Basal ganglia dysfunction
Etiology
  Genetic predisposition combined with highly repetitive movement patterns
Speed of Onset
  Chronic
Signs and Symptoms
  Consciousness
  Normal
  Communication and Memory
  Normal
  Sensory
  Impaired proprioception and stereognosis; degradation of the somatic representation in somatosensory cortex
  Autonomic
  Normal
  Motor
  Involuntary, sustained muscle contractions
Region Affected
  Cerebrum: basal ganglia
Demographics
  Average age at onset 45 years old; males and females affected equally
  Incidence
  Of hand dystonia: unknown. Focal dystonias including hand dystonia: 30 cases per 100,000 population people per year (Adler, 2000)
  Point prevalence: 10 cases per 100,000 population (Castelon-Konkiewitz et al, 2002)
Prognosis
  Normal life span

without overt body movement. After completing the protocol, all subjects in Byl's study showed improvement in strength, stereognosis, motor control, and other clinical measures. Improvement in motor control was accompanied by improvement in the organization of somatosensory cortex (Byl, 2000). Focal dystonia of the hand is frequently misdiagnosed as carpal tunnel syndrome, tennis elbow, strain, or a psychogenic disorder. Because the muscle contractions are caused by basal ganglia dysfunction, attempts at treating the disorder by stretching the muscles are ineffective. Heat, cold, and exercise may be helpful to relieve pain and/or spasms.

Generalized dystonia causes involuntary twisting postures of the limbs and trunk. In generalized dystonia, occasionally the prolonged muscle contractions are relieved by tactile stimulation applied to or near the affected body part. Medications that affect acetylcholine (ACh), GABA, and/or dopamine levels are effective in some cases. Severe dystonia can be alleviated by surgical lesion of the motor thalamus or by injection of botulinum toxin into the affected muscles. A very rare disorder, Segawa's dystonia, interferes with walking and may mimic the appearance of cerebral palsy; however, Segawa's dystonia progresses slowly and can be effectively treated with medications.

Choreoathetotic Cerebral Palsy. Abnormal involuntary movements are also observed in people with choreoathetosis, a type of cerebral palsy (the other major types of cerebral palsy are spastic and ataxic; see Chapter 5). The term *chorea* indicates abrupt, jerky movements, and the term *athetosis* identifies slow, writhing, purposeless movements. Choreoathetoid cerebral palsy is associated with lesions involving both the basal ganglia and ventrolateral thalamus (Krageloh-Mann et al., 2002).

> Basal ganglia disorders interfere with voluntary and automatic movements and produce involuntary movements. Hypokinesia is a decrease in the amount and speed of voluntary and automatic movements, characteristic of Parkinson's disease. However, Parkinson's signs are not purely hypokinetic because resting tremor is an increase in movement compared to normal. Hyperkinesia is abnormal excessive movement, seen in Huntington's disease, dystonia, and choreoathetotic cerebral palsy.

CEREBELLUM

The cerebellum coordinates movement and postural control by comparing actual motor output to the intended movement and then adjusting the movement as necessary. Information regarding intended movements is delivered to the cerebellum by corticopontine fibers that synapse in the pontine nuclei. Axons from the pontine nuclei project to the cerebellum. The cerebellum also receives information regarding activity in spinal interneurons via the internal feedback tracts (anterior spinocerebellar and rostrospinocerebellar tracts; see Chapter 6). Information about the actual movement is provided by information from muscle spindles, Golgi tendon organs, and cutaneous mechanoreceptors (posterior spinocerebellar and cuneocerebellar tracts; see Chapter 6). The cerebellum integrates information from these sources and adjusts the activity of upper motor neurons.

Massive amounts of sensory information enter the cerebellum, and cerebellar output is vital for normal movement. However, severe damage to the cerebellum does not interfere with sensory perception or with muscle strength. Instead, coordination of movement and postural control are degraded.

Anatomy of the Cerebellum

The outer layer of the cerebellum is gray matter, consisting of three cortical layers (Figure 10-12). The outer and inner layers contain interneurons (granule, Golgi, stellate, and basket cells), and the middle layer contains Purkinje cell bodies.

Deep to the cortex is white matter, and within the white matter are the cerebellar nuclei. Axons from the cerebellar nuclei project to vestibular, reticular, and red nuclei, and to the motor thalamus. Motor thalamus neurons project to motor areas of the cerebral cortex.

Purkinje cells are the output cells from the cerebellar cortex, and their projections inhibit the cerebellar nuclei and the vestibular nuclei. Two types of afferents enter the cerebellar cortex: mossy fibers, from the spinal cord, reticular formation, vestibular system, and pontine nuclei; and climbing fibers, from the inferior olivary nucleus in the medulla. The mossy fibers convey somatosensory, arousal, equilibrium, and cerebral cortex motor information to the cerebellum. The climbing fibers convey information regarding movement errors to the cerebellum. Climbing fibers synapse with Purkinje dendrites. Mossy fibers synapse with interneurons that convey information to Purkinje cells.

Three lobes form the cerebellum (Figure 10-13):

- Anterior
- Posterior
- Flocculonodular

The anterior lobe is superior and is separated from the larger posterior lobe by the primary fissure. The inferior

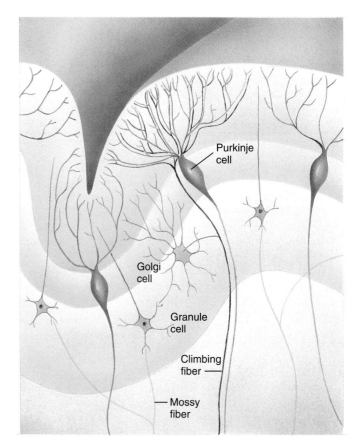

Purkinje
cell

Golgi
cell

Granule
cell

Climbing
fiber

Mossy
fiber

FIGURE 10-12
Three layers of the cerebellar cortex. In the middle layer are cell bodies of Purkinje cells, the output neurons of the cerebellar cortex. Climbing and mossy fibers are the input fibers to the cerebellar cortex. Most climbing fibers arise from the inferior olivary nucleus. Mossy fibers originate in the spinal cord (spinocerebellar tracts) and in the brainstem.

part of the posterior lobe is called the *cerebellar tonsil*. The cerebellar tonsils are clinically significant because increased intracranial pressure can force the tonsils into the foramen magnum, compressing vital brainstem structures that regulate breathing and cardiovascular activity. Tucked underneath the posterior lobe, touching the brainstem, is the small flocculonodular lobe.

Vertically, the cerebellum can be divided into sections (see Figure 10-13, *E*):

- Midline vermis
- Paravermal hemisphere
- Lateral hemisphere

Each of the vertical sections is associated with a specific class of movements, as we will see later. Each vertical section projects either to specific cerebellar nuclei or to vestibular nuclei. The cerebellar nuclei, from medial to lateral, are the fastigial, globose, emboliform, and dentate nuclei.

Fibers connecting the cerebellum with the brainstem form three cerebellar peduncles on each side of the brain-

stem. The superior cerebellar peduncle connects to the midbrain and contains most of the cerebellar efferent fibers. Fibers from the cerebral cortex synapse in the pons, and then the information travels via axons in the middle peduncle into the cerebellum. The inferior peduncle brings afferent information from the brainstem and spinal cord into the cerebellum and sends efferents from the cerebellum to the vestibular nuclei and reticular nuclei in the brainstem.

Input to the cerebellum is from the cerebral cortex (via pontine nuclei), the vestibular apparatus, vestibular and auditory nuclei, and from the spinal cord, via both high-fidelity pathways (proprioceptive information) and internal feedback tracts (information regarding activity in spinal interneurons and in descending motor tracts). The output of the cerebellum is via connections that influence vestibulospinal, reticulospinal, rubrospinal, corticobulbar, and corticospinal tracts.

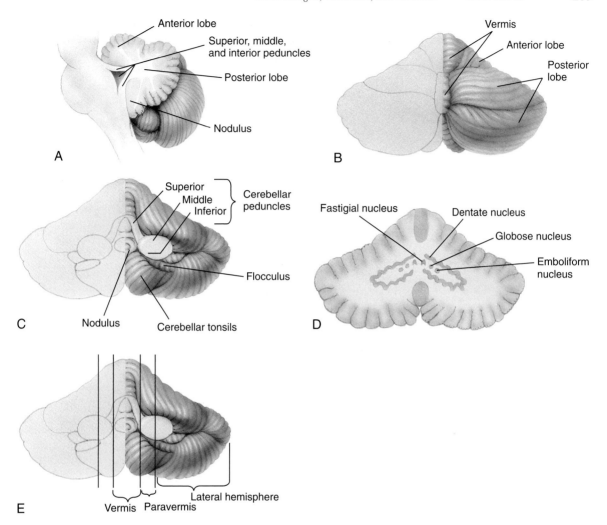

FIGURE 10-13
Anatomy of the cerebellum. **A,** Midsagittal section showing cerebellar peduncles and lobes of the cerebellum. **B,** Posterior view of cerebellum. **C,** Anterior view of the cerebellum with the brainstem removed. **D,** Coronal section of the cerebellum, revealing the cerebellar nuclei. **E,** Vertical divisions of the cerebellum.

Functional Regions of the Cerebellum

Human movements can be categorized into three broad classes:
- Equilibrium
- Gross movements of the limbs
- Fine, distal, voluntary movements

The cerebellum has specialized regions for controlling each of these classes of movement. Equilibrium is regulated by the vestibulocerebellum, named for its reciprocal links with the vestibular system. Gross limb movements are regulated by the spinocerebellum, named for its extensive connections with the spinal cord. Distal limb voluntary movements are regulated by the cerebrocerebellum, named for its connections with the cerebral cortex (Figure 10-14).

When a person reaches for a book from a high shelf, the vestibulocerebellum provides anticipatory contraction of lower limb and back muscles to prevent loss of balance. Otherwise, as the upper limb moves, altering

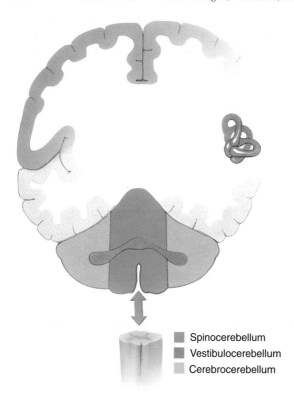

FIGURE 10-14

Conceptual diagram of the three functional divisions of the cerebellum and their connections. The purple part of the cerebellum is the flocculonodular lobe, the location of the vestibulocerebellum. The purple structure with three rings *(shown on the right)* is the vestibular apparatus, the sensory organ that detects head position relative to gravity and detects movement of the head. Much of the information processed by the vestibulocerebellum is from the vestibular apparatus. The blue part of the cerebellum is the spinocerebellum, and correspondingly the spinal cord is also blue. The green part of the cerebellum is the cerebrocerebellum, and correspondingly the cerebral cortex is also green.

- Spinocerebellum
- Vestibulocerebellum
- Cerebrocerebellum

the position of the body's center of mass, the person would fall forward. The upper limb reaching movement is coordinated by the spinocerebellum. Without the spinocerebellar contribution, the reach would be jerky and inaccurate. The cerebrocerebellum coordinates the finger and thumb movements to grasp the book.

Vestibulocerebellum is the functional name for the flocculonodular lobe because this area receives information

directly from vestibular receptors and connects reciprocally with the vestibular nuclei. The vestibulocerebellum also receives information from visual areas of the brain. Via connections with vestibular nuclei, the vestibulocerebellum influences eye movements and postural muscles.

Spinocerebellum is the functional name for the vermis and paravermal region because of extensive connections with the spinal cord. Somatosensory information, internal feedback from spinal interneurons, and sensorimotor cortex information converge in the spinocerebellum. This information is used to control ongoing movement via the brainstem descending tracts.

The vermal section of the spinocerebellum projects to the fastigial nucleus; the nucleus in turn adjusts activity in the medial upper motor neurons by direct action on brainstem nuclei and indirectly on the cerebral cortex via the motor thalamus. The paravermal area projects to the globose and emboliform nuclei; these nuclei influence the lateral upper motor neurons by action on brainstem nuclei and by projecting to the cerebral cortex via the motor thalamus.

The lateral cerebellar hemispheres connect indirectly with areas of the cerebral cortex controlling distal limb muscles; thus this section of the cerebellum is the *cerebrocerebellum*. Input to the cerebrocerebellum is from cerebral cortex (premotor, sensorimotor, and other cortical areas; see Chapter 16) fibers that synapse with neurons in the pons. Axons of the pontine neurons project to the cerebrocerebellum. Efferents from the lateral cerebellar hemispheres project to the dentate nucleus. The dentate is involved in motor planning. Prior to voluntary movements, alterations in dentate neural activity precede changes in activity in motor areas of the cerebral cortex. Efferents from the dentate nucleus project to the motor thalamus, then efferents from the motor thalamus project to the cerebral cortex. The functions of the cerebrocerebellum and dentate include the following:

- Coordination of voluntary movements via influence on corticofugal tracts
- Planning of movements
- Timing (Xu et al., 2006)

The connections of the functional divisions of the cerebellum are listed in Table 10-3 and illustrated in Figures 10-15 and 10-16.

Cerebellar Clinical Disorders

Unilateral lesions of the cerebellum affect the same side of the body. The cerebellar signs are ipsilateral because the output paths of the medial descending tracts remain ipsilateral and because cerebellar efferents project to the

Table 10-3   NEURAL CONNECTIONS OF THE CEREBELLAR FUNCTIONAL DIVISIONS

Functional Division (Anatomic Location)	Receives Input From	Sends Output To	Output Reaches Lower Motor Neurons Via
Vestibulocerebellum (flocculonodular lobe)	Vestibular apparatus Vestibular nuclei	Vestibular nuclei	Vestibulospinal tracts and tracts that coordinate eye and head movements (see Chapter 14)
Spinocerebellum			
Vermal section	Spinal cord (from trunk) Vestibular nuclei Auditory and vestibular information (via brainstem nuclei)	Vestibular nuclei Reticular nuclei (via fastigial nucleus) Motor cortex (via fastigial nucleus then thalamus)	Vestibulospinal tracts Reticulospinal tracts Medial corticospinal tract
Paravermal section	Spinal cord (from limbs)	Red nucleus (via globose and emboliform nuclei) Motor cortex (via fastigial nucleus then thalamus)	Rubrospinal tract Lateral corticospinal tract
Cerebrocerebellum (lateral cerebellar hemispheres)	Cerebral cortex (via pontine nuclei)	Motor and premotor cortices (via dentate nucleus and motor thalamus) Red nucleus	Lateral corticospinal and corticobulbar tracts Rubrospinal tract

contralateral cerebral cortex and red nucleus whose descending tracts cross the midline (see Figure 10-15).

Ataxia is the movement disorder common to all lesions of the cerebellum. Ataxia describes voluntary, normal-strength, jerky, and inaccurate movements that are not associated with hyperstiffness. Vermal and flocculonodular lobe cerebellar lesions result in truncal ataxia, paravermal lesions result in gait and limb ataxia, and lateral cerebellar lesions cause hand ataxia. The consequences of lesions in each of the functional regions of the cerebellum follow.

Lesions involving the vestibulocerebellum cause **nystagmus** (abnormal eye movements; see Chapter 15), dysequilibrium, and difficulty maintaining sitting and standing balance (truncal ataxia). Paravermal and cerebrocerebellar lesions result in **dysarthria**: slurred, poorly articulated speech (Schoch et al., 2006). Dysfunction of the spinocerebellum results in ataxic gait: a wide-based, staggering gait. In chronic alcoholism, the anterior lobe section of the spinocerebellum is often damaged because of malnutrition, resulting in the characteristic ataxic gait.

Spinocerebellar lesions result in limb ataxia, with the following manifestations:

- **Dysdiadochokinesia:** inability to rapidly alternate movements (e.g., inability to rapidly pronate and supinate the forearm, or inability to rapidly alternate toe tapping)

- **Dysmetria:** inability to accurately move an intended distance
- **Action tremor:** shaking of the limb during voluntary movement

Action tremor may arise because the onset and offset of muscle activity are delayed. Thus, in a rapid movement, the agonist burst is prolonged, and the onset of braking by the antagonist is delayed, causing overshoot of the target. As correction of the movement is attempted, the same dysfunctions cause repeated overshoot (Vilis and Hore, 1977). People with cerebellar lesions often compensate for limb ataxia using movement decomposition. This decomposition consists of maintaining a fixed position of one joint while another joint is moving. For example, when ascending a 30° incline, people with cerebellar lesions tend to maintain the ankle joint in a fixed position during early stance phase. In contrast, people with intact neuromuscular control extend the knee and flex the ankle simultaneously during early stance phase (Figure 10-17).

Cerebellar lesions interfere with the coordination of fine finger movements. This ataxia affects the ability to play musical instruments, fasten buttons, and type on a keyboard.

Not all ataxia is caused by cerebellar lesions. Interference with the transmission of somatosensory information to the cerebellum, either by lesions of the spinocerebellar

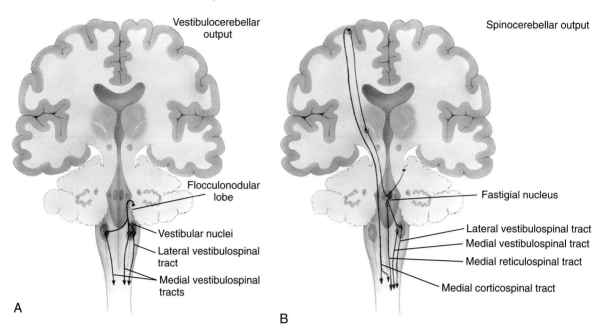

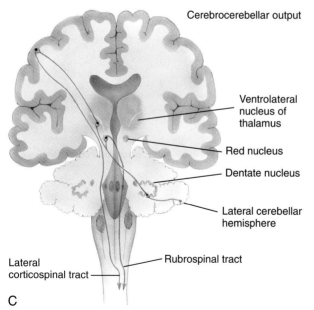

FIGURE 10-15

The efferents from each functional division of the cerebellum.
A, Vestibulocerebellar output. For simplicity, the tracts that
transmit signals for eye and head movements are omitted.
B, Spinocerebellar output. The connections with the red
nucleus and the rubrospinal tract are omitted for simplicity.
The red nucleus and rubrospinal tract are illustrated in part
C. C, Cerebrocerebellar output. The corticobulbar tracts are
omitted for simplicity.

tracts or by peripheral neuropathy, may also produce
ataxia. Ataxia in the lower limbs may be caused by
sensory deficits or by lateral cerebellar lesions. To differentiate between the two possibilities, test stance with
eyes open versus eyes closed, proprioception, vibration
sense, and ankle reflexes. People with **cerebellar limb
ataxia** will be unable to stand with their feet together,
with or without vision, and will have normal vibratory

sense, proprioception, and ankle reflexes. The opposite
results occur in **sensory ataxia:** the person is able to
stand steadily with the feet together with the eyes open,
but balance is impaired with the eyes closed. In sensory
ataxia, conscious proprioception and vibratory sense are
impaired, and ankle reflexes are decreased or absent.

The characteristics of the major types of motor control
disorders are compared in Table 10-4.

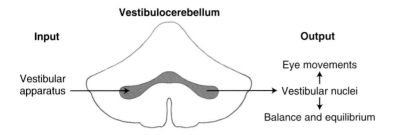

Vestibulocerebellum

Input

Vestibular apparatus →

Output

Eye movements ↑
→ Vestibular nuclei ↓
Balance and equilibrium

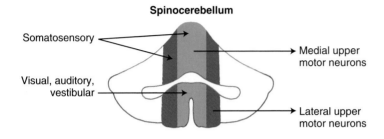

Spinocerebellum

Somatosensory →

Visual, auditory, vestibular →

→ Medial upper motor neurons

→ Lateral upper motor neurons

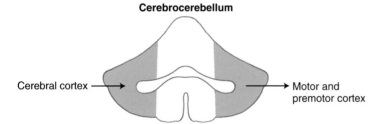

Cerebrocerebellum

Cerebral cortex →

→ Motor and premotor cortex

FIGURE 10-16

The inputs and outputs of the three functional divisions of the cerebellum.

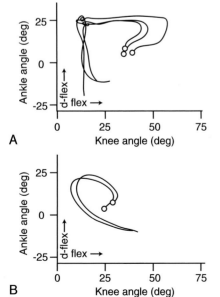

A

B

FIGURE 10-17

Movement decomposition. Plots of ankle angle versus knee angle during stance while walking up a 30° incline. Heel strike is indicated by a circle and is the starting point of the plot. **A,** Subject with a superior cerebellar artery infarct demonstrating movement decomposition. The horizontal line indicates that the ankle angle is maintained at approximately 25° dorsiflexion as the knee extends from 60° flexion to 15°. The vertical line indicates that the knee angle remains fixed at 15°, while the ankle plantarflexes from 25° to −25°. **B,** Normal movement composition. In a subject with normal neuromuscular control, the ankle and knee joints move simultaneously. During early stance the knee extends while the ankle dorsiflexes; then during late stance the knee flexes while the ankle plantarflexes. *(Modified from Earhart GM, and Bastian AJ (2001). Selection and coordination of human locomotor forms following cerebellar damage. Journal of Neurophysiology, 85(2), 759-769.)*

Table 10-4   CHARACTERISTICS OF MAJOR TYPES OF MOTOR CONTROL DISORDERS

Characteristic	Complete Severance of Peripheral Nerve (Lower Motor Neuron Lesions)	Upper Motor Neuron Lesions	Parkinson's Disease	Huntington's Disease	Cerebellar Lesions
Muscle strength	Absent (paralysis)	Decreased (paresis)	Normal	Normal	Normal
Muscle bulk	Severe atrophy	Variable atrophy	Normal	Normal	Normal
Involuntary muscle contraction	Fibrillations	Fibrillations	Resting tremor	Chorea	None
Muscle tone*	Decreased	Velocity-dependent increase (spasticity)	Velocity-independent increase (rigidity)	Variable, depending on stage of disease	Normal
Movement speed and efficiency	Absent	Decreased	Decreased	Abnormal	Ataxic
Postural control	Normal	Decreased or normal, depending on location of lesion	Excessive	Abnormal	Depends on location of lesion

*Muscle tone ratings are compared to muscle tone ratings in an alert person. Thus, muscle tone in a person with a complete peripheral nerve lesion would be similar to muscle tone in a completely relaxed person with an intact nervous system because titin would be the primary source of resistance to stretch in both cases.

MOVEMENT

Summary of Normal Motor Control

For normal movement, the motor planning areas, control circuits, and descending tracts must act in concert with sensory information to provide instructions to lower motor neurons. The basal ganglia receive most of their input from the cerebral cortex, and their influence on movement is via the cerebral cortex and PPN. In contrast, the cerebellum receives copious information from the spinal cord, vestibular system, and brainstem. The cerebellum influences movement via motor areas of the cerebral cortex and extensive connections with upper motor neurons that arise in the brainstem. Only lower motor neurons deliver the signals from the central nervous system to the skeletal muscles that generate movement. Figures 10-18 and 10-19 summarize the complex neural activity required to generate movement.

Three Fundamental Types of Movement

Movements can be classified into three types:
- Postural
- Ambulatory
- Reaching/grasping

Posture is primarily controlled by brainstem mechanisms, ambulation by brainstem and spinal regions, and reaching/grasping by the cerebral cortex; however, all regions of the nervous system contribute to each type of movement.

The contributions of each region of the central nervous system to an externally imposed movement can be assessed by electromyography (EMG) (Figure 10-20). For example, a subject is asked to support a light weight and to maintain a constant position of the elbow (flexion at 90°). Then a weight is unexpectedly added, resulting in displacement of the forearm and hand downward.

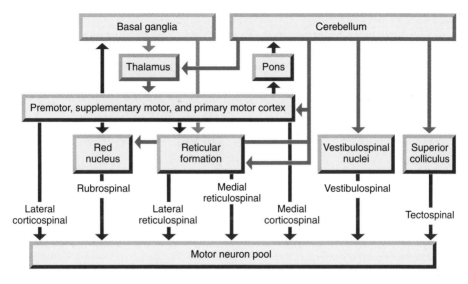

FIGURE 10-18

Flowchart summarizing the relationships among components of the motor system. Although sensory information is essential for normal movement, for simplicity sensory input is omitted from this chart.

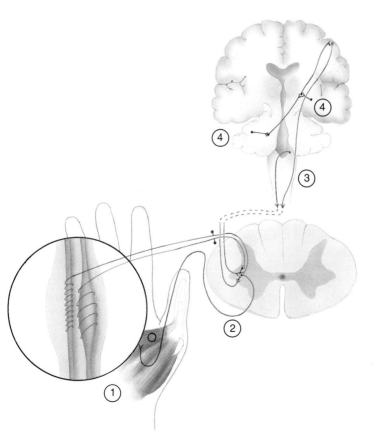

FIGURE 10-19

Simplified schematic diagram of the major influences on muscle activity. 1. Peripheral region. The alpha motor neurons innervate contractile fibers in skeletal muscle. Proprioception from muscle sensors *(muscle spindle shown)* affects motor output. 2. The spinal region integrates information from other spinal cord segments *(not shown)*, from local circuits within the cord, and from the brain. 3. The upper motor neurons provide information from the brain. The tracts illustrated are the lateral corticospinal and lateral reticulospinal. Although the lateral reticulospinal tract projects bilaterally, only the contralateral projection is shown. 4. The control circuits (cerebellum, basal ganglia) adjust the level of activity in the descending tracts.

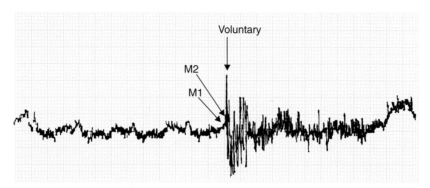

FIGURE 10-20

Surface EMG responses to displacement when a subject is instructed to maintain 90° of elbow flexion, then a weight is placed in the subject's hand. The first response, called M1, occurs 25-30 milliseconds after the weight is added. M1 is the EMG activity produced by the monosynaptic stretch reflex. The second response, called M2 or the long latency response, occurs 50-80 milliseconds after the weight is added. Production of M2 requires brainstem connections. The third response, the voluntary response, occurs 80-120 milliseconds after the weight is added.

After about 1/10 of a second, biceps contraction begins to restore the elbow angle to 90°. The EMG response to the displacement shows three distinct increases in activity occurring at 30 milliseconds, 50 to 80 milliseconds, and 80 to 120 milliseconds after the imposed biceps stretch.

The shortest latency response, M1, is the monosynaptic stretch reflex; this reflex does not generate enough force to restore the elbow position. The second response, M2, is the long loop response; this response generates enough force to begin to move the hand upward. The subject's intentions influence M2: if the instructions to the subject are to "let go" when the extra weight is added, the M2 response is attenuated or disappears. The final response, voluntary, completes the return of the elbow angle to 90°. The latencies provide clues to the central nervous system region involved in each response. The 30-millisecond latency of M1 is just enough time for the afferent conduction, transmission across one synapse in the spinal cord, and efferent conduction to activate the biceps. Fifty to eighty milliseconds allows enough time for transmission involving brainstem connections. The 120-millisecond response requires synapses in the cerebral cortex.

Postural Control

Postural control provides orientation and balance (equilibrium). Orientation is the adjustment of the body and head to vertical, and balance is the ability to maintain the center of mass relative to the base of support. Pos-

tural control is achieved by central commands to lower motor neurons; the central output is adjusted to the environmental context by sensory input.* The central commands are mediated by the tectospinal, medial reticulospinal, vestibulospinal, and medial corticospinal tracts. Sensory input is used in both feedback and feedforward mechanisms. Feedback is information about the state of the system. For example, if I slip on ice, I get feedback from proprioceptors, vestibular receptors, and vision that elicit equilibrium adjustments. Feed-forward is anticipatory motor impulses sent prior to movement that prepare for movement. Feed-forward control involves prediction and anticipation to prepare for upcoming hazards to stability. Before I lift my arms forward, I contract my gastrocnemii to prevent the change in center of gravity from causing me to lose my balance.

To orient in the world, we use three senses:

- Somatosensation
- Vision
- Vestibular

Somatosensation provides information about weight bearing and the relative positions of body parts. Vision

*Historical note: An earlier theory of postural control posited three separate control mechanisms: reflexive, reactive, and voluntary. The theory proposed that during development, reflexes and reactions were inhibited by the voluntary system: in the mature nervous system, the voluntary system controlled all normal movements. However, as noted in the text, reflexes and reactions help to restore stability before the voluntary system is aware of possible loss of balance and participate extensively in mature motor control.

provides information about movement and cues for judging upright. Vestibular input from receptors in the inner ear informs us about head position relative to gravity and about head movement. Visual and somatosensory information can predict destabilization; all three sensations can be used to shape the motor reaction to instability (Figure 10-21).

Head position in reference to gravity, to the neck, and to the visual world affects muscular activation. Head position in space is signaled by neck proprioception and vestibular and visual information (visual aspects will be covered in Chapter 15). In normal infants and in children and adults with extensive cerebral lesions, neck and vestibular reflexes can be elicited by neck movements or by changing head position. In children and adults with intact nervous systems, the same stimuli do not produce obvious responses.

Activity of cervical joint receptors and neck muscle stretch receptors elicits neck reflexes. The **symmetrical tonic neck** reflex results in flexion of the upper limbs and extension of the lower limbs when the neck is flexed and the opposite pattern in the limbs when the neck is extended (Figure 10-22, *A*). The **asymmetrical tonic neck reflex** is elicited by head rotation to the right or left; the limbs on the nose side extend, and limbs on the skull side flex (Figure 10-22, *B*).

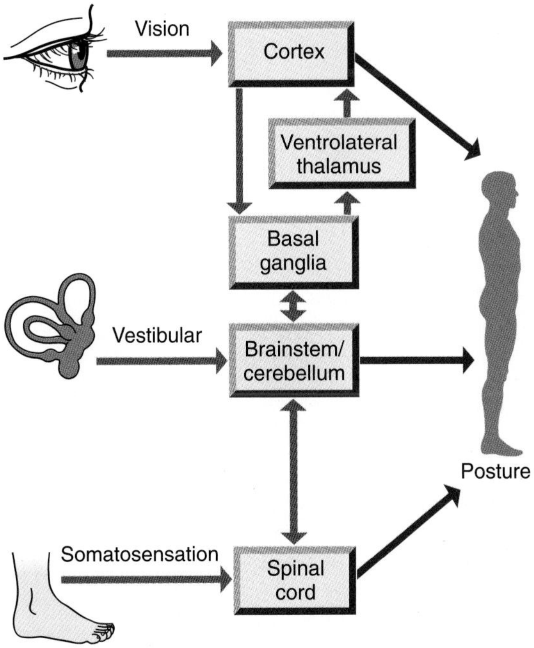

When the head is tilted, information from vestibular gravity receptors is used to right the head by contraction of neck muscles. Vestibular gravity receptors also influence limb muscle activity, in a manner opposite to the neck reflexes; for instance, tilting the head back causes flexion of the upper limbs and extension of the lower limbs if the position of the head relative to the neck is unchanged (eliminating the influence of neck reflexes). Because the vestibular receptors for gravity are in the labyrinthine part of the inner ear, the reflex is called the **tonic labyrinthine reflex** (Figure 10-22, *C*). Because vestibular and neck reflexes oppose each other, and normally head and neck movements occur together, the reflexes usually counteract each other. By canceling out these two reflexes, our limbs are not compelled to move when we turn or nod or shake our heads.

During stance, we sway continuously; to prevent falling, the postural control system makes adjustments to maintain upright posture. Sometimes inappropriate sensory information is selected, as when we rely on visual information regarding movement and a large object nearby moves. A person standing next to a bus that unexpectedly moves can misinterpret the moving visual information and make inappropriate postural adjustments to compensate for the illusory movement. The person's goal is to maintain upright posture, but reacting to deceptive sensory information leads to instability.

Posturography can be used to determine sensory organization (which sensory stimuli a person relies on preferentially) and muscle coordination (how postural adjustments are coordinated). The subject stands on a force platform, and surface EMGs are recorded from specific muscles. As indicated in Figure 10-23, six sensory conditions can be tested (Nashner et al., 1982). In the sensory conflict conditions, vision and/or proprioception is rendered inaccurate by having the visual field and/or the support surface move with the subject as the subject sways. Thus subjects have the visual and/or proprioceptive illusion that they are not swaying when in fact they are moving; under these conditions, a person without vestibular function will fall. The results of posturography can be compared to norms for different diagnostic groups. For example, the postural responses of an individual can be compared to those of people with Parkinson's disease and other disorders.

Posturography can also test motor coordination. If the platform moves forward, the subject sways backward; the

FIGURE 10-21
Sensory influences on postural control.

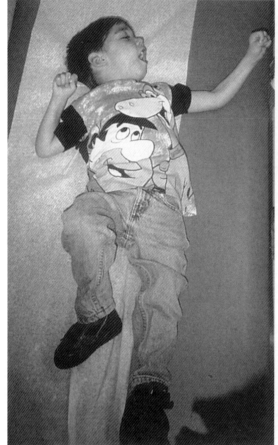

A

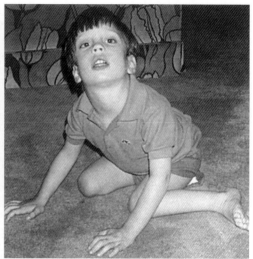

B

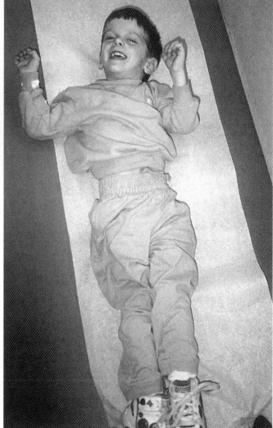

C

FIGURE 10-22

Neck and vestibular reflexes. **A,** Asymmetrical tonic neck reflex: when the head is rotated right or left, the limbs move into the fencer's position. **B,** Symmetrical tonic neck reflex: when the neck is extended, the upper limbs extend and the lower limbs flex. **C,** Tonic labyrinthine reflex: when the head is tilted back, the upper limbs flex and the lower limbs extend. These reflexes may be elicited with head and neck movements in infants with intact neuromuscular systems. The reflexes are obligatory only in people with cerebral damage. *(From Braddom RL (2001). Physical Medicine and Rehabilitation. (2ⁿᵈ ed.). Philadelphia: Saunders.)*

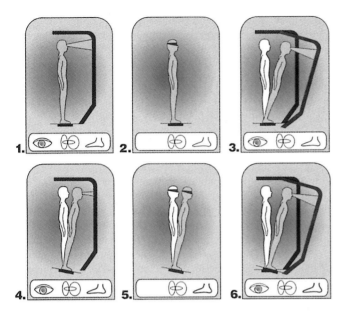

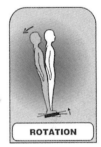

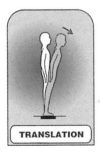

FIGURE 10-23

Posturography. Six sensory conditions are used to evaluate the relative contributions of vision, vestibular, and somatosensory input in balance function. The icons at the bottom of each figure indicate the eyes, vestibular system, and foot and ankle proprioceptors. If the eye icon is red, this indicates that the visual surround sways with the person's postural sway. In conditions 3 and 6, if the person sways forward, movement of the visual field matches the person's sway; this creates the visual illusion of lack of movement. If the foot icon is red, this indicates that the support surface moves with the person's postural sway, providing inaccurate information about orientation. In conditions 4-6, if the person sways forward, the support surface under the person's toes tilts downward, so proprioception from the distal lower limbs does not give accurate orientation information. *(Courtesy Neurocom International Inc., Clackamas, OR.)*

normal response is contraction of the tibialis anterior, then quadriceps, then abdominal muscles to return the subject to upright (Figure 10-24). If the platform moves backward, the gastrocnemius, then hamstrings, then back muscles contract to restore the person to upright. In both cases, distal to proximal muscle activation normally occurs.

When the platform moves backward, the subject's forward lean stretches the gastrocnemius muscle. An equivalent stretch of the gastrocnemius can be provided by dorsiflexing the subject's ankles by tilting the platform so that the anterior edge of the platform is higher than the posterior edge. However, in the platform tilt situation, contracting the gastrocnemius further destabilizes the subject. Because the subject's ankles are dorsiflexed, contracting the gastrocnemius pushes the person posteriorly. After a few trials, healthy subjects learn to reduce the response of the gastrocnemius, thus preserving their balance.

Although sophisticated, this type of testing is similar to the clinical practice of pushing a person off balance to test the equilibrium response. Both tests assess the ability to respond to externally imposed displacements; in daily life, these displacements are uncommon. The continual challenge in everyday posture is to anticipate and adjust for voluntary destabilization. For example, prior to a forward reach when a person is standing, the muscles of the opposite leg and back contract to provide stability before the deltoid contracts (Cordo and Nashner,

FIGURE 10-24

The gastrocnemius can be passively stretched by moving the support surface backward (translation) or by tilting the support surface to raise the toes (rotation). Illustration shows the body position at the end of platform movement in gray and the return to upright in white. If the support surface moves backward, the long latency stretch reflex helps return the body to upright. If platform rotation causes ankle dorsiflexion, the long latency stretch reflex will plantar flex the ankle and result in loss of balance backward. With repeated trials, the long latency reflex decreases as the nervous system learns to maintain posture efficiently when the platform tilts. *(Courtesy Neurocom International Inc., Clackamas, OR.)*

1982). If a standing person decides to walk, anticipatory adjustments must prepare for the movement of the center of mass. Posturography can also be used to assess these active conditions. A complete postural evaluation includes sensory and motor assessment under three conditions: imposed displacement, active reaching, and ambulation.

Certain nervous system dysfunctions produce recognizable postural abnormalities. People with Parkinson's disease have muscle rigidity and reduced central control. This combination of deficits results in flexed posture, lack of protective reactions, and weak anticipatory postural adjustments. The postural effects of cerebellar lesions depend on the cerebellar region involved. As noted earlier, cerebrocerebellar lesions have little effect on posture, spinocerebellar lesions result in gait and stance ataxia, and vestibulocerebellar lesions result in truncal ataxia. The sequence of muscle activation is normal in people with spinocerebellar lesions, but the duration and amplitude of postural adjustments are larger than normal, and anticipatory adjustments for predictable conditions are lacking.

People with intact nervous systems respond to movement of the supporting platform differently depending on instructions (Burleigh et al., 1994). If asked to maintain stance when the platform moves, the first response is to sway forward or backward. If asked to step when the platform moves, the first response is to weight shift laterally. This ability to switch motor response to identical stimuli demonstrates the importance of both instructions and the subject's intentions in sculpting motor output.

Ambulation

All regions of the nervous system are required for normal human ambulation. The cerebral cortex provides goal orientation and control of ankle movements, the basal ganglia govern generation of force, and the cerebellum provides timing, coordination, and error correction. Brainstem descending tracts (vestibulospinal and reticulospinal) adjust the strength of muscle contractions by two mechanisms: direct connections with lower motor neurons and adjusting transmission in spinal reflex pathways. Spinal locomotor pattern generators control the pattern of muscle activation. Sensory information is used to adapt motor output appropriately for environmental conditions.

During normal gait initiation, the swing limb first pushes downward and backward against the support surface. This pattern of force results in the center of mass being moved forward and onto the stance leg in preparation for foot-off and increases the magnitude of the subsequent movement. However, in adults with hemiplegia, the contribution of the paretic leg to weight transfer is much less than normal if the feet are parallel. When the foot of the swing limb is placed 10-15 cm behind the stance foot, normal weight transfer occurs, indicating that foot position is an important variable in weight transfer for gait initiation (Malouin et al., 1994). People with Parkinson's disease also fail to adequately move the center of mass prior to attempting stepping (Gantchev et al., 1996), causing inability to initiate gait.

Reaching and Grasping

Vision and somatosensation are essential for normal reaching and grasping. Vision provides information for locating the object in space, as well as assessing the shape and size of the object. Preparation for movement (feedforward) is the primary role of visual information; if the movement is inaccurate, vision also guides corrections (feedback). The stream of visual information used for movement ("action stream"; Goodale and Westwood, 2004) flows from the visual cortex to the posterior parietal cortex (Figure 10-25). The posterior parietal cortex contains neurons associated with both sensation and movement; these neurons project to premotor cortical areas controlling reaching, grasping, and eye movements. The premotor cortical areas for each action are somewhat distinct, with the result that reaching, grasping, and eye movements are controlled separately but coordinated by connections among the areas. Information from sensory and planning areas of the cerebral cortex projects to the basal ganglia and cerebellum, then via the thalamus to the sensorimotor cortex, the origin of the corticospinal tract. Proprioception is used similarly to vision, to prepare for movement and to provide information regarding movement errors. Proprioceptive and cutaneous

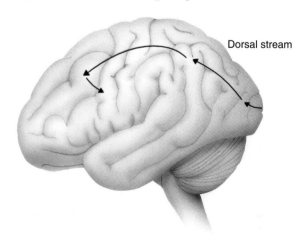

FIGURE 10-25

Visual action stream. Visual information traveling from occipital to parietal to premotor cortex helps control movement.

information also triggers changes in movement, as when contact with an object triggers the fingers to close around the object.

Before one can reach accurately, visual grasp (fixing the object in central vision) and proprioceptive information about upper limb position are required. This information allows successful prediction of task dynamics and control for the first phase of reaching: fast approach to the object, which is primarily a feed-forward process. The second phase of reaching is homing in, a slower, corrective adjustment to achieve contact with the target. Visual guidance (feedback) is necessary for homing in (Jeannerod, 1990). In contrast to classic concepts of proximal to distal muscle activation during reaching, proximal muscles move the hand toward the target; the muscles are controlled by the medial upper motor neurons. Simultaneously, distal muscles orient and pre-shape the hand for grasp; these actions are controlled primarily by feed-forward mechanisms via the lateral upper motor neurons. If fractionated movements are used, as in picking up a coin with the index finger and thumb, the neural activity that begins in the prefrontal cortex eventually activates the lateral corticospinal tract (Figure 10-26).

Grasping is coordinated with activity of the eyes, head, proximal upper limb, and trunk; orientation and postural preparation are integral to the movement. When the object is contacted, grip force adjusts quickly, indi-cating feed-forward control. After the object is grasped, somatosensory information corrects any error in grip force. Somatosensory information is also used to trigger shifts in movement, for example, to switch from touch to grasp or from grasp to lift (Castiello, 2005).

During development, normal infants grasp objects before they can control their posture, and the ability of infants to manipulate objects in their hands does not depend on proximal control (vonHofsten, 1992). In fact, early manual activity may be important in developing normal proximal control (Bradley, 1992).

Adults with parietal lobe damage have abnormal timing of reaching and grasp, lack anticipatory adjust-ments of the fingers, and use a palmar, rather than pincer, grasp (Freund, 2003). Pincer grasp requires corticospinal control, which explains the use of palmar grasp by infants prior to myelination of the corticospinal tracts as well as the palmar grasp of adults with parietal lobe damage.

In normal actions, feed-forward and feedback interact to create movement. Preparation for movement (feed-forward) is based on prediction, and the movement is adjusted according to the resulting sensory information (feedback) (Figure 10-27). The source of the signal to initiate movements is unknown.

Testing the Motor System

An evaluation of the motor system assesses strength, muscle bulk, muscle tone, reflexes, movement efficiency and speed, postural control, and abnormal movements (Table 10-5).

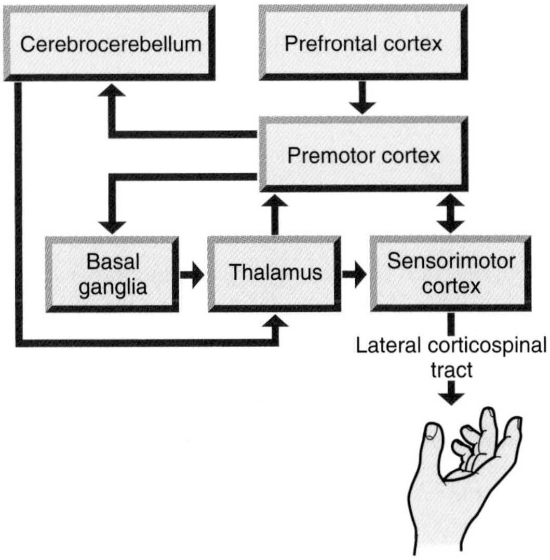

FIGURE 10-26
The motor circuit for fractionated finger movements.

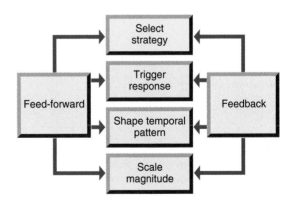

FIGURE 10-27
Interaction of feed-forward and feedback in determining movements. *(Modified from Horak FB: Somatosensory experience in adapting postural coordination. Presented at Sensory Mechanisms in Motor Coordination: Implications for Motor Control and Rehabilitation Symposium, Society for Neuroscience, Nov. 13, 1994.)*

Table 10-5   EVALUATION OF THE MOTOR SYSTEM

Test	Procedure and Interpretation
Strength	
Quick screening	Resist abduction, adduction, flexion, and extension at the shoulder, elbow, fingers, hip, and ankle. Resist flexion and extension at the elbow and knee. Paresis or paralysis usually indicates a lower or upper motor neuron lesion.
Manual muscle test	Position patient appropriately; see Kendall et al. (2005) or Hislop and Montgomery (2002); apply manual resistance to patient's movement.
Pronator drift	Patient flexes both shoulders 90°, extends elbows, fully supinates both forearms, and closes eyes. Gradual pronation and downward drift of one arm indicates an upper motor neuron lesion.
Muscle bulk	Visually inspect for disparity in muscle size. Measure the circumference of the limbs if a difference is suspected. More severe atrophy typically indicates a lower motor neuron lesion. Less severe atrophy indicates an upper motor neuron lesion or disuse.
Muscle stiffness	
Passive range of motion	Passively flex and extend patient's elbow, wrist, knee, ankle, and neck; note resistance to movement. Less resistance than normal may indicate a lower motor neuron lesion. Hyperstiffness may be a sign of upper motor neuron or basal ganglia lesion. Velocity-dependent hyperstiffness indicates an upper motor neuron lesion. Hyperstiffness that does not vary with the speed of the stretch, called *rigidity,* is characteristic of Parkinson's disease. Muscle guarding or contracture may also cause decreased passive range of motion.
Reflexes	
Phasic stretch reflex (also called *deep tendon reflex, muscle stretch reflex,* and *tendon jerk*)	Use a reflex hammer to tap the tendon of a relaxed muscle; muscle should contract. Indicates whether the reflex loop (spindle, afferents, spinal segment, efferent, and muscle) is functioning. Biceps, triceps, quadriceps, and triceps surae tendons are most commonly tested. The response of each muscle is compared to the response of the same muscle on the other side of the body. Asymmetrical hyperreflexia may indicate an upper motor neuron lesion. Asymmetrical hyporeflexia (or absence of reflex) indicates a peripheral or spinal region lesion. Sometimes no reflexes can be elicited even in people with intact nervous systems. The presence of more than four beats of clonus is always an abnormal sign.
Babinski's sign	Extend the patient's knee, then firmly stroke the outer edge of patient's foot with the handle of a reflex hammer. Babinski's sign is present if great toe extends; other toes may spread apart. Babinski's sign indicates an upper motor neuron lesion. The response is normal if no response occurs or all toes curl.
H-reflex*	Electrically stimulate skin over large fiber afferents; a reflexive contraction of muscle should occur. Indicates excitability of alpha motor neurons.
Movement efficiency and speed	
Rapid alternating movements	Patient taps both index fingers or both feet, then pronates and supinates forearms; note speed, smoothness, symmetry, and rhythm of movements. If patient has difficulty with these movements in the absence of weakness, cerebellar or proprioceptive dysfunction is indicated.
Accuracy and smoothness of movement	Patient performs the following movements several times: (1) finger-to-nose test—patient laterally abducts the arm with the elbow extended, then touches own nose; (2) finger-to-finger test—patient abducts the arm with the elbow extended, then touches examiner's fingertip; (3) heel-to-shin test—patient places heel on knee of opposite leg and slides the heel down the shin to the ankle while maintaining contact with the tibial crest; (4) walk heel-to-toe. Normal performance: all movements are smooth and precise. For example, the patient slows the finger movements as the finger approaches the target and stops the movement accurately. Observe for jerky movements (ataxia), tremor worsening with movement (action tremor), and inability to move the precise distance required (dysmetria). Difficulty indicates cerebellar or proprioceptive dysfunction.

Table 10-5   EVALUATION OF THE MOTOR SYSTEM—cont'd

Test	Procedure and Interpretation
Transcranial magnetic stimulation*	Currently experimental, not used clinically. Investigates possible upper motor neuron lesions by inducing magnetic activation of cortical neurons, then recording muscle activity.
Movements by surface EMG tests	
During active movement	
Hyperreflexia	Increase in EMG activity during active or passive muscle lengthening indicates hyperreflexia.
Cocontraction	Measure the amount of time antagonist muscles are contracting simultaneously. Cocontraction is only abnormal if it interferes with movement goals.
During muscle stretch	
Hyperstiffness	If EMG does not increase during stretch despite limitation in range of motion, restriction is due to nonneural factors, i.e., intrinsic changes in the muscle. If EMG increases, neural factors are contributing to decreased range of motion.
Postural control	
Romberg's test	Patient stands with arms folded across chest, feet together. Time how long patient can maintain balance with eyes open, then with eyes closed. Stop test if time exceeds 1 minute. If patient has difficulty maintaining balance with eyes open and eyes closed, a cerebellar problem is indicated. Better balance with eyes open than with eyes closed indicates a proprioceptive problem.
Sharpened Romberg	Same as Romberg's test, but with one foot in front of the other foot. Stop test if time exceeds 1 minute. Interpretation is the same as for Romberg's test.
Tinetti balance scale (Tinetti, 1986)	Balance in sitting, standing, moving from sit to stand and stand to sit, turning 360°, and in response to push on sternum is assessed. Score is used to predict likelihood of falls.
Clinical test for sensory interaction in balance	Three visual conditions—eyes opened, eyes closed, and vision altered by a dome covering the face—are combined with standing on firm surface or on foam. See Shumway-Cook and Horak (1986) for interpretation.
Functional reach	Patient stands with feet together, shoulder flexed 90°; then patient reaches as far forward as possible (Duncan et al., 1990). Distance reached is recorded. Score is used to predict likelihood of falls.
Computerized balance testing	Stationary posturography: Patient stands on force platform; variations in force exerted are recorded. May incorporate EMG recording. May vary foot position and eyes open, closed. Moving platform posturography: as previously noted, with movement of platform and different sensory conditions (see text).
Postural muscle EMG	During three conditions: external displacement (push on shoulder), prior to voluntary limb movement, and during walking.
Abnormal involuntary movements	Patient sits quietly; note any of the following: athetosis, chorea, dystonia. These involuntary movements indicate basal ganglia disorders. A more sensitive test is to have patient stand with eyes closed, arms stretched forward, forearms pronated, and fingers abducted; note any involuntary movements.

*Indicates a test used by researchers but not routinely used by therapists.

Electrodiagnostic Studies

Frequently the purpose of nerve conduction studies in motor disorders is to differentiate among three possible sites of dysfunction: nerve, neuromuscular junction, and muscle. In nerve conduction studies examining motor nerve, the skin over a nerve is electrically stimulated, and potentials are recorded from the skin over an innervated muscle. Diagnostic EMG, using a needle electrode inserted into muscle, is commonly used to distinguish between denervated muscle and myopathy. **Myopathy** is an abnormality or disease intrinsic to muscle tissue. The electrical activity of a muscle is recorded using an oscilloscope and loudspeaker.

Motor Nerve Conduction Studies. The function of motor fibers in the median nerve can be tested by electrically stimulating the median nerve at the wrist while recording from electrodes over the abductor pollicis brevis muscle and then stimulating at the elbow while recording from the same site. The depolarization of the muscle is recorded as a muscle action potential (MAP). The nerve conduction velocity equals the distance between the proximal and distal stimulation sites, divided by the difference between the latencies. MAP amplitude indicates the function of the neuromuscular junction and muscle fibers in addition to the conduction ability of the alpha motor neurons (Figure 10-28).

Electromyography. Diagnostic EMG requires inserting an electrode directly into muscle. Muscle electrical activity is recorded during four conditions: on insertion of the needle into the muscle (insertional activity), during rest, during minimal voluntary contraction, and during maximal voluntary contraction. Normal response

to needle insertion is a brief interval of depolarization, due to mechanical irritation of muscle fibers. At rest, normal muscle is electrically silent. Minimal voluntary contraction elicits single motor unit action potentials. Increasing voluntary contraction generates a full interference pattern, created by the asynchronous discharge of many muscle fibers.

If a muscle membrane is unstable, due to denervation, trauma, electrolyte imbalance, or upper motor neuron lesion, its fibers become hypersensitive to ACh, and fibrillation (random, spontaneous contraction of individual muscle fibers) ensues. Fibrillation occurs when the subject intends the muscle to be at rest. If muscle is reinnervated, larger than normal amplitude muscle potentials are recorded, owing to axons innervating a greater than normal number of muscle fibers. In primary disease of muscle (myopathy), axons innervate fewer than normal numbers of muscle fibers, resulting in a small-amplitude MAP. Myopathy is indicated by short-

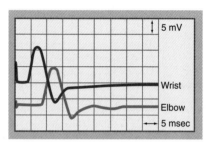

		Latency (ms)	Amplitude (mV)	Velocity (m/s)
Recorded values:				
	Stimulated at wrist	Distal 3.7	11.2	Between wrist and
	Stimulated at elbow	8.5	11.2	elbow 51.7
Norms for median nerve		Distal latency <4.2	>5.0	50

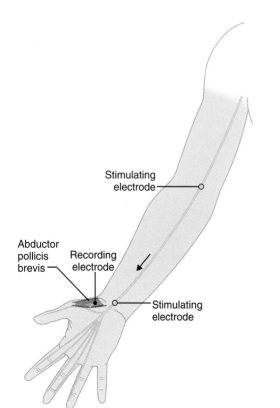

FIGURE 10-28

Normal medial nerve conduction study recording. Normal values for median nerve conduction are listed below the recorded values.

duration, low-amplitude potentials during voluntary contraction, lack of spontaneous muscle activity (fasciculations, fibrillations), and absence of sensory involvement.

> Nerve conduction studies differentiate among nerve, neuro-muscular junction, and muscle disorders. Diagnostic EMG distinguishes between denervated muscle and myopathy.

SUMMARY

The basal ganglia are a group of interconnected nuclei located in the cerebrum and midbrain. Together these nuclei regulate muscle force, muscle contraction, multi-joint movements, and movement sequencing. Basal ganglia pathology causes a spectrum of movement disorders, ranging from the hypokinesia of Parkinson's disease to the hyperkinesia of choreoathetoid cerebral palsy.

The cerebellum coordinates movement and postural control. Cerebellar dysfunctions can cause ataxia, nystagmus, and dysarthria.

Although all regions of the nervous system have some involvement in control of posture, ambulation, and reaching/grasping, specific neural areas provide the primary control for each of these fundamental types of movement. Posture is predominantly controlled by brainstem mechanisms, ambulation by brainstem and spinal circuits, and reaching/grasping by the cerebral cortex.

CLINICAL NOTES

Case 1

KL is a 73-year-old woman recently admitted to long-term care because she is unable to care for herself. Ten years ago she developed tremor in both hands; the tremor has gotten progressively worse. Her current status is as follows:
- Consciousness, mentation, sensation, and autonomic functions are intact.
- The tremor is worse when her hands are resting and improves when she is using her hands.
- She tends to remain in the position the staff leaves her in. She does not move spontaneously.
- She cannot independently change from sitting to standing, nor can she initiate walking. However, if someone assists her by leaning her forward, she can walk with a shuffling gait.
- During passive range of motion, all muscles show increased resistance compared to normal.

Question

What is the location of the lesion and probable diagnosis?

Case 2

LF is a 67-year-old retired man. During the past 5 years, he has complained of gradual onset of balance and gait problems, including dizziness when standing, difficulty with sit-to-stand, difficulty initiating gait, and frequent tripping and falling. Autonomic complaints include erectile dysfunction, urinary retention, chronic constipation, and occasional incontinence.
- Consciousness, mentation, and sensation are normal.
- Lacks facial expression.
- Posture: trunk and head are flexed forward.
- Strength is normal throughout the body.
- During passive range of motion, all muscles show increased resistance compared to normal
- Cranial nerve function is normal
- Babinski's sign: bilateral upgoing toe signs
- Coordination: lower limb ataxia; ataxia is equal in supine, standing, and sitting positions. Dysmetria bilaterally (finger-to-nose and heel-shin test). Bilateral dysdiadochokinesis.
- Narrow-based ataxic gait. Able to heel walk and toe walk with assistance. Unable to tandem walk.

Question

What is the location of the lesions and probable diagnosis?

Continued

CLINICAL NOTES

Case 3

BF is a 52-year-old accountant. His only complaint is right forearm muscle pain and cramping when writing.
- Normal right upper limb cutaneous sensation and autonomic function except: cannot distinguish between closely spaced tactile stimuli on fingertips and thumb pad, poor stereognosis, and impaired proprioception in the digits of the right hand.
- When the therapist palpates the muscles of the forearm, BF reports no pain in the wrist extensor muscles and deep, aching pain on palpation of the wrist and finger flexor muscles.
- Active range of motion is normal throughout the right upper limb.
- When BF is asked to write, after 2 minutes his forearm and finger flexor muscles cramp. To continue writing, he must use an abnormal upper limb position with the shoulder abducted 60°.

Question

What is the location of the lesion and probable diagnosis?

Case 4

RL, a 57-year-old man, complains of increasing right-sided clumsiness and shaking. Onset has been gradual, beginning 4 months ago.
- Somatosensation, autonomic function, and muscle strength are normal throughout the entire body.
- Coordination tests are normal in the left upper and lower limbs.
- On the right side: attempts at rapid alternating movements are slow and uncoordinated; action (intention) tremor occurs during finger-to-nose and heel-to-shin tests; dysmetria on finger-to-nose test.
- Abnormal involuntary eye movements.

Question

What is the location of the lesion and probable diagnosis?

REVIEW QUESTIONS

1. What are the two routes for information from the basal ganglia output nuclei to the lower motor neurons?
2. List the nuclei that form the basal ganglia.
3. What are the functions of the basal ganglia?
4. What disease is characterized by rigidity, hypokinesia, resting tremor, and isuoperceptive impairments? Cell death in which nuclei produce this disease?
5. What disease is characterized by Parkinsonism, cerebellar signs, and autonomic dysfunction?
6. List three disorders that cause hyperkinesia.
7. Involuntary abnormal postures or repetitive twisting movements are signs of what disorder?
8. What is the major function of the cerebellum?
9. What are the major sources of input to the cerebellum?
10. Which part of the cerebellum coordinates individual finger movements? Gross limb movements? Postural adjustments?
11. Ataxic gait indicates damage to what part of the cerebellum?
12. What is movement decomposition? Where is a lesion that produces movement decomposition?
13. List and define the signs of cerebrocerebellar lesions.
14. What is a long loop response?
15. What is an asymmetrical tonic neck reflex?
16. What information can posturography provide?
17. Give an example of a preparatory postural adjustment.
18. Give an example of identical stimuli eliciting different responses depending on instructions given to a person.

19. If a person with hemiplegia is having difficulty initiating gait, what simple adjustment might make gait initiation easier?
20. What are the two phases of reaching?
21. What is diagnostic EMG used for?
22. What is the difference in purpose between motor nerve conduction velocity studies and movement analysis by surface EMG tests?

References

Adler CH (1999). Differential diagnosis of Parkinson's disease. Medical Clinics of North America, 83(2), 349-367.

Adler CH (2000). Strategies for controlling dystonia. Overview of therapies that may alleviate symptoms. Postgraduate Medicine, 108(5), 151-152, 155-156, 159-160.

Adler CH, Crews D, et al. (2005). Abnormal co-contraction in yips-affected but not unaffected golfers: Evidence for focal dystonia. Neurology, 64(10), 1813-1814.

Avorn J, Bohn RL, et al. (1995). Neuroleptic drug exposure and treatment of parkinsonism in the elderly: A case-control study. American Journal of Medicine, 99(1), 48-54.

Braddom RL (2001). Physical medicine and rehabilitation. (2nd ed.). Philadelphia: Saunders.

Bradley NS (1992). What are the principles of motor development? In H Forssberg and H Hirschfeld (Eds.), Movement Disorders in Children (pp. 41-49). Basel, Switzerland: S. Karger.

Burleigh AL, Horak FB, et al. (1994). Modification of postural responses and step initiation: Evidence for goal directed postural interactions. Journal of Physiology, 76(6), 2892-2902.

Byl NN (2000). The neural consequences of repetition. Neurology Report, 24(2), 60-70.

Castellon Konkiewitz E, Trender-Gerhard I, et al. (2002). Service-based survey of dystonia in Munich. Neuroepidemiology. 21(4):202-206.

Castiello U (2005). The neuroscience of grasping. Nature Reviews. Neuroscience, 6(9), 726-736.

Cordo PJ, Nashner LM (1982). Properties of postural adjustments associated with rapid arm movements. Journal of Neurophysiology, 47, 287-302.

de Lau LM, Breteler MM (2006). Epidemiology of Parkinson's disease. Lancet Neurology, 5(6), 525-535.

Dibble LE, Hale TF, et al. (2006). High-intensity resistance training amplifies muscle hypertrophy and functional gains in persons with Parkinson's disease. Movement Disorders 21(9), 1444-1452.

Dujardin K, Defebvre L, et al. (2003). Executive function differences in multiple system atrophy and Parkinson's disease. Parkinsonism & Related Disorders, 9(4), 205-211.

Duncan P, Weiner DK, et al. (1990). Functional reach: A new clinical measure of balance. Journal of Gerontology, 45(6), 192-197.

Earhart GM, Bastian AJ (2001). Selection and coordination of human locomotor forms following cerebellar damage. Journal of Neurophysiology, 85(2), 759-769.

Evans RW, Baskin DS, et al. (2000). Prognosis of neurological disorders. New York: Oxford University Press.

Fillmore HL, Holloway KL, et al. (2005). Cell replacement efforts to repair neuronal injury: A potential paradigm for the treatment of Parkinson's disease. NeuroRehabilitation, 20(3), 233-242.

Freund HJ (2003). Somatosensory and motor disturbances in patients with parietal lobe lesions. Advances in Neurology, 93, 179-193.

Friedlander L, Desrocher M (2006). Neuroimaging studies of obsessive-compulsive disorder in adults and children. Clinical Psychology Review, 26(1), 32-49.

Gage H, Storey L (2004). Rehabilitation for Parkinson's disease: A systematic review of available evidence. Clinical Rehabilitation, 18(5), 463-482.

Gantchev N, Viallet F, et al. (1996). Impairment of posturo-kinetic coordination during initiation of forward oriented step in parkinsonian patients. Electroencephalography and Clinical Neurophysiology, 101(2), 110-120.

Goodale MA, Westwood DA, et al. (2004). Two distinct modes of control for object-directed action. Progress in Brain Research, 144, 131-144.

Hislop HJ, Montogomery J (2002). Daniels and Worthingham's Muscle testing: Techniques of manual examination. (7th ed.). Philadelphia: WB Saunders.

Hoehn MM, Yahr MD (1967). Parkinsonism: Onset, progression and mortality. Neurology. 17, 427-442.

Horak FB: Somatosensory experience in adapting postural coordination. Presented at Sensory Mechanisms in Motor Coordination: Implications for Motor Control and Rehabilitation Symposium, Society for Neuroscience, Nov 13, 1994.

Hurelbrink CB, Lewis SJ, et al. (2005). The use of the Actiwatch-Neurologica system to objectively assess the involuntary movements and sleep-wake activity in patients with mild-moderate Huntington's disease. Journal of Neurology, 252(6), 642-647.

Jeannerod M (1990). The neural and behavioral organization of goal-directed movements. Oxford: Clarendon Press.

Kendall FP, McCreary EK, et al. (2005). Muscles: Testing and Function with Posture and Pain. Baltimore: Lippincott Williams & Wilkins.

Klinger E, Chemin I, et al. (2006). Virtual action planning in Parkinson's disease: A control study. Cyberpsychology & Behavior, 9(3), 342-347.

Krageloh-Mann I, Helber A, et al. (2002). Bilateral lesions of thalamus and basal ganglia: Origin and outcome. Developmental Medicine and Child Neurology, 44(7), 477-484.

Lenz FA, Byl NN (1999). Reorganization in the cutaneous core of the human thalamic principal somatic sensory nucleus (ventral caudal) in patients with dystonia. Journal of Neurophysiology, 82(6), 3204-3212.

Levy R, Friedman HR, et al. (1997). Differential activation of the caudate nucleus in primates performing spatial and nonspatial working memory tasks. Journal of Neuroscience, 17, 3870-3882.

Louis ED, Goldman JE, et al. (1995). Parkinsonian features of eight pathologically diagnosed cases of diffuse Lewy body disease. Movement Disorders, 10(2), 188-194.

Malouin F, Menier C, et al. (1994). Dynamic weight transfer during gait initiation in hemiparetic adults and effect of foot position. Society of Neuroscience: Abstracts, 20, 571.

Mark M. (2005). Parkinson's disease: Pathogenesis, diagnosis, and treatment. Primary Psychiatry, 12(7), 36-41.

McKenzie AL, Nagarajan SS, et al. (2003). Somatosensory representation of the digits and clinical performance in patients with focal hand dystonia. American Journal of Physical Medicine & Rehabilitation, 82(10), 737-749.

Nashner LM, Black FO, et al. (1982). Adaptation to altered support and visual conditions during stance: Patients with vestibular deficits. Journal of Neuroscience, 2, 536-544.

Nath U, Ben-Shlomo Y, et al. (2001). The prevalence of progressive supranuclear palsy (Steele-Richardson-Olszewski syndrome) in the UK. Brain, 124(Pt 7), 1438-1449.

Pahwa R, Lyons KE, et al. (2006). Long-term evaluation of deep brain stimulation of the thalamus. Journal of Neurosurgery, 104(4), 506-512.

Pope PA, Praamstra P, et al. (2006). Force and time control in the production of rhythmic movement sequences in Parkinson's disease. European Journal of Neuroscience, 23(6), 1643-1650.

Quinn N, Wenning G (1994). Multiple system atrophy. British Journal of Hospital Medicine, 51(9), 492-494.

Schoch B, Dimitrova A, et al. (2006). Functional localization in the human cerebellum based on voxelwise statistical analysis: A study of 90 patients. Neuroimage, 30(1), 36-51.

Schupbach WM, Chastan N, et al. (2005). Stimulation of the subthalamic nucleus in Parkinson's disease: A 5 year follow up. Journal of Neurology, Neurosurgery, and Psychiatry, 76(12), 1640-1644.

Shumway-Cook A, Horak FB (1986). Assessing the influence of sensory interaction on balance. Physical Therapy, 66, 1548-1550.

Tinetti M (1986). Performance oriented assessment of mobility problems in elderly patients. Journal of the American Geriatrics Society, 40, 479.

Uitti RJ, Baba Y, et al. (2005). Defining the Parkinson's disease phenotype: Initial symptoms and baseline characteristics in a clinical cohort. Parkinsonism & Related Disorders, 11(3):139-145.

Vanacore N (2005). Epidemiological evidence on multiple system atrophy. Journal of Neural Transmission, 112(12), 1605-1612.

Vatalaro M (2000). Fly model of Parkinson's offers hope of simpler, faster research. NIH Record, L11(12), 3.

Vilis T, Hore J (1977). Effects of changes in mechanical state of limb on cerebellar intention tremor. Journal of Neurophysiology, 40, 1214-1224.

Volkmann J (2004). Deep brain stimulation for the treatment of Parkinson's disease. Journal of Clinical Neurophysiology, 21(1), 6-17.

vonHofsten C (1992). Development of manual actions from a perceptual perspective. In H Forssberg, H Hirschfeld (Eds.), Movement Disorders in Children (pp. 113-123). Basel, Switzerland: S. Karger.

Wenning GK, Ben-Shlomo Y, et al. (1994). Clinical features and natural history of multiple system atrophy: An analysis of 100 cases. Brain, 117(Pt 4), 835-845.

Xu D, Liu T, et al. (2006). Role of the olivo-cerebellar system in timing. Journal of Neuroscience, 26(22), 5990-5995.

Zaccai J, McCracken C, et al. (2005). A systematic review of prevalence and incidence studies of dementia with Lewy bodies. Age and Ageing, 34(6), 561-566.

11 Peripheral Nervous System

Laurie Lundy-Ekman, PhD, PT

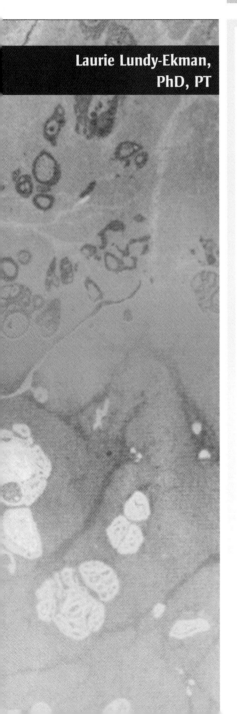

I was a 32-year-old woman working a 40-hour week as a chef's assistant. I first noticed pain in my wrist and hand while working. After work, my hand would be numb and have tingling sensations. As the problem progressed, it became difficult to grip a knife or cleaver.

When I first went to the doctor, the problem was diagnosed as tendonitis, and I was advised to use my other hand more. I kept working, and the condition worsened; on returning to the doctor, I received pain medication and a wrist brace. When these did not help, I was referred to an orthopedic specialist. Nerve conduction studies were performed by a physical therapist. The condition was diagnosed as carpal tunnel syndrome. I went to a physical therapist two times a week for heat treatments and exercises for about 3 months. I was told I could no longer continue my line of work. I ended up with a full cast for 6 weeks to prevent me from using my left arm and hand.

The pain in my wrist and hand continued to be intense, much worse at night. I could only sleep with my arm propped up on a pillow above my head. I ended therapy after having two cortisone shots into my wrist, which did not have any effect.

Today if I garden or use my left hand too long typing or playing tennis, I will have pain and know I need to lighten up.

—Genevieve Kelly

INTRODUCTION

The peripheral nervous system includes all neural structures distal to the spinal nerves. Thus, axons of sensory, motor, and autonomic neurons, along with specialized sensory endings and entire postganglionic autonomic neurons, form the peripheral nervous system. Examples of peripheral nerves include the median, ulnar, and tibial nerves. Although cranial nerves are also peripheral nerves, cranial nerves will be covered in Chapters 13 and 14 because their function can best be understood in the context of brainstem function. In this textbook, all nervous system structures enclosed by bone are considered parts of the central nervous system; nerve roots, dorsal root ganglia, and spinal nerves are therefore within the spinal region (Figure 11-1). Distal to the spinal nerve, the groups of axons split into posterior and anterior rami. Axons in the **posterior rami** innervate the paravertebral muscles, posterior parts of the vertebrae, and overlying cutaneous areas. Axons in the **anterior rami** innervate the skeletal, muscular, and cutaneous areas of the limbs and the anterior and lateral trunk. Axons in the rami communicantes connect the spinal nerve with the ganglia in the sympathetic chain.

Classifying nerve roots, dorsal root ganglia, and spinal nerves as spinal and the remaining axons as peripheral allows the clinical difference between spinal and peripheral lesions to be easily distinguished: sensory, autonomic, and motor deficits in spinal region lesions show a myotomal and/or dermatomal distribution; sensory,

autonomic, and motor deficits in peripheral lesions show a peripheral nerve distribution (see Figure 6-5). Signs of peripheral neuron lesions are paresis or paralysis, sensory loss, abnormal sensations, muscle atrophy, and reduced or absent deep tendon reflexes.

> Peripheral nerve lesions produce signs and symptoms in a peripheral nerve distribution. Spinal region lesions produce signs and symptoms in a myotomal and/or dermatomal distribution.

PERIPHERAL NERVES

Peripheral nerves consist of parallel bundles of axons surrounded by three connective tissue sheaths: endoneurium, perineurium, and epineurium. **Endoneurium** separates individual axons, **perineurium** surrounds bundles of axons called *fascicles,* and **epineurium** encloses the entire nerve trunk (Figure 11-2). An outer layer of connective tissue, the mesoneurium, surrounds the epineurium. The connective tissues protect the axons and glia and support the mechanical changes in length that nerves undergo during movements.

Peripheral nerves receive blood supply via arterial branches that enter the nerve trunk. Within the nerve, axons are electrically insulated from each other by endoneurium and by a myelin sheath. The myelin sheath is provided by Schwann cells, which either partially

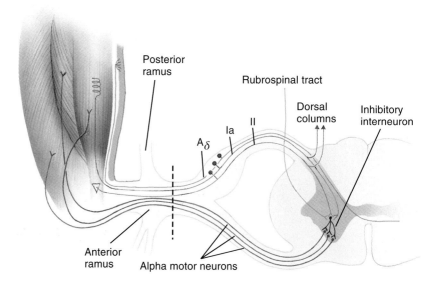

FIGURE 11-1
The vertical dotted line indicates the division between the peripheral and the central nervous system. Neural structures in the periphery include muscle spindle receptors (blue spiral in muscle), the Golgi tendon organ (blue triangle in the tendon), motor endings in muscle (red *V*s), and axons. The posterior rami innervate structures along the posterior midline of the body, the anterior rami supply structures in the lateral and anterior body, and the rami communicantes connect with the sympathetic ganglia.

Posterior ramus

Rubrospinal tract

Dorsal columns

Inhibitory interneuron

Ia   II

A$_\delta$

Anterior ramus

Alpha motor neurons

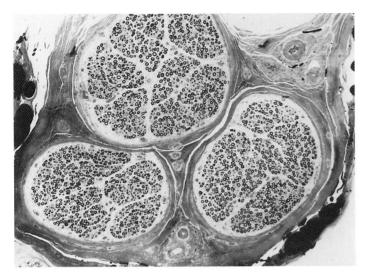

FIGURE 11-2

Cross section of a normal peripheral nerve, showing three fascicles. Within each fascicle are many darkly stained myelin sheaths, appearing as small oval structures enclosing the axons, which appear white. Endoneurium surrounds each axon. Perineurium surrounds each fascicle. External epineurium surrounds the three fascicles. Internal epineurium and blood vessels fill the areas between fascicles. *(From Richardson EP, Jr., DeGirolami U (1995). Pathology of the Peripheral Nerve. (p. 3). Philadelphia: Saunders.)*

surround a group of small-diameter axons or completely envelop a section of a single large axon. The small-diameter axons that share Schwann cells are called *unmyelinated* (although *partially myelinated* would be a more accurate term), while the large-diameter axons that are fully wrapped by individual Schwann cells are designated *myelinated*.

Peripheral nerves supply either viscera or somatic structures. The visceral supply, via splanchnic nerves, is discussed in Chapter 8.

Somatic peripheral nerves are usually mixed, consisting of sensory, autonomic, and motor axons. Cutaneous branches supply the skin and subcutaneous tissues; muscular branches supply muscle, tendons, and joints. Cutaneous branches are not purely sensory because they deliver the sympathetic efferent axons to sweat glands and arterioles. Muscular branches are not purely motor because they contain sensory axons from proprioceptive structures.

Peripheral axons are classified into groups according to their speed of conduction and their diameter (Table 11-1). Two classification systems for peripheral axons are in common use. The letter classification system (A, B, C) applies to both afferent and efferent axons; the Roman numeral system applies only to afferent axons.

Nerve Plexuses

The junctions of anterior rami form four nerve plexuses. The cervical plexus arises from anterior rami of C1-C4 and lies deep to the sternocleidomastoid muscle. The cervical plexus provides cutaneous sensory information from the posterior scalp to the clavicle and innervates the anterior neck muscles and the diaphragm. The phrenic nerve, whose cell bodies are in the cervical spinal cord (C3-C5), is the most important single branch from the cervical plexus because the phrenic nerve is the only motor supply and the main sensory nerve for the diaphragm.

The brachial plexus is formed by anterior rami of C5-T1. The plexus emerges between the anterior and middle scalene muscles, passes deep to the clavicle, and enters the axilla. In the distal axilla, axons from the plexus become the radial, axillary, ulnar, median, and musculocutaneous nerves. The entire upper limb is innervated by brachial plexus branches (Figure 11-3).

The lumbar plexus is formed by anterior rami of L1-L4; the plexus forms in the psoas major muscle. Branches of the lumbar plexus innervate skin and muscles of the anterior and medial thigh (Figure 11-4). A cutaneous branch from the plexus, the saphenous nerve, continues into the leg to innervate the medial leg and foot. Branches of the cervical, brachial, and lumbar plexuses provide sympathetic innervation via connections with the sympathetic chain.

The sacral plexus innervates the posterior thigh and most of the leg and foot. Unlike the other plexuses, which contain sympathetic axons, the sacral plexus contains parasympathetic axons.

Movement Is Essential for Nerve Health

Movement optimizes the health of nerves by promoting the flow of blood throughout the nerves and the flow of

Table 11-1 PERIPHERAL AXONS

Axon	Conduction Speed (m/sec)	Axon Diameter (μm)	Efferent Axons		Afferent Axons	
			Group	Innervates	Group	Innervates
Large myelinated	7-130	7-22	Aα	Extrafusal muscle fibers	Ia, Ib, II	Spindles, Golgi tendon organs, touch and pressure receptors
Medium myelinated	2-10	2-15	Aγ	Intrafusal muscle fibers		
Small myelinated	12-45	2-10			Aδ	Pain, temperature, visceral receptors
	4-25	1-5	B	Presynaptic autonomic		
Unmeylinated	0.2-2.0	0.2-0.5	C	Postsynaptic autonomic	C	Pain, temperature, visceral receptors

axoplasm through the axons. Normally, fascicles glide within the nerve and nerves glide relative to other structures. Adequate blood flow is necessary to supply nutrition and oxygen and remove waste from neural tissues. Axoplasm thickens and becomes more resistant to flow when stationary. Movement causes axoplasm to thin and flow more easily, facilitating retrograde and anterograde transport. Retrograde axoplasmic transport moves chemicals from the axons and surrounding structures to the cell body, providing information for the genetic machinery to adjust production of ion channels, transmitters, vesicles, and support structures. Anterograde axoplasmic transport delivers the new structural and signaling components to their proper locations in the neuron.

Connective tissues support the changes in length that nerves undergo during movements. For example, with the shoulder abducted to 90°, the median nerve is approximately 10 cm longer when the elbow and wrist are extended than when the elbow and wrist are flexed (Dilley et al 2003). This increase in nerve length without injury is made possible by axons wrinkling within the endoneurium when the nerve is not stretched (Figure 11-5), by connective tissue, and by fascicular plexuses. The fascicular plexuses are connections that spread tensile load among fascicles, preventing excessive loading on a single fascicle.

As a nerve is stretched, first the viscoelastic tubes formed by endoneurium, perineurium, and external epineurium stretch, axons unfold, and fascicles glide relative to each other. As stretching continues, the entire nerve slides relative to surrounding structures. As stretching continues and exceeds the capacity of these mechanisms, tensile stress develops in the neural tissues. As the nerve is shortened, the processes reverse: the tensile stress is relieved first, then the nerve slides relative to surrounding structures, the viscoelastic tubes recoil, and the axons fold. The nerve may also fold, as the median nerve does at the flexed elbow. See Millesi et al., 1995; Nee and Butler, 2003; Rempel and Diao, 2004; Sunderland, 1990; and Wright et al., 2001 for discussion of the mechanisms that permit nerves to lengthen and shorten without injuring either axons or their supporting structures.

NEUROMUSCULAR JUNCTION

Motor axons synapse with muscle fibers at neuromuscular junctions. This nerve-muscle synapse requires only depolarization of the motor axon, releasing acetylcholine (ACh), which diffuses across the synaptic cleft and binds with receptors to cause depolarization of the muscle membrane. Unlike neuron-neuron synapses, no summation of action potentials is required to depolarize the postsynaptic membrane. No inhibition is possible because only one branch of an axon synapses with a muscle fiber and the action of the neurotransmitter is always excitatory. In a normal motor unit, every

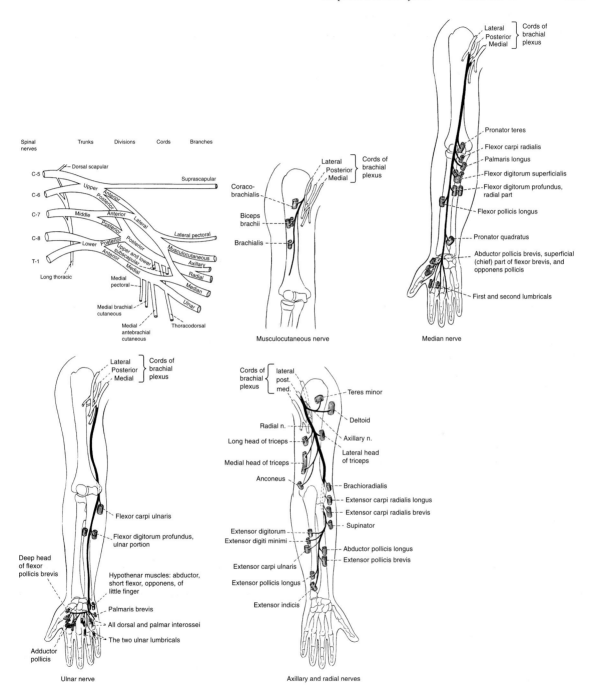

FIGURE 11-3

Brachial plexus and the distribution of the branches of the brachial plexus. *(From Jenkins DB (1991). Hollinshead's Functional Anatomy of the Limbs and Back. (6th ed., pp. 74, 116, 134, 135, 145). Philadelphia: Saunders.)*

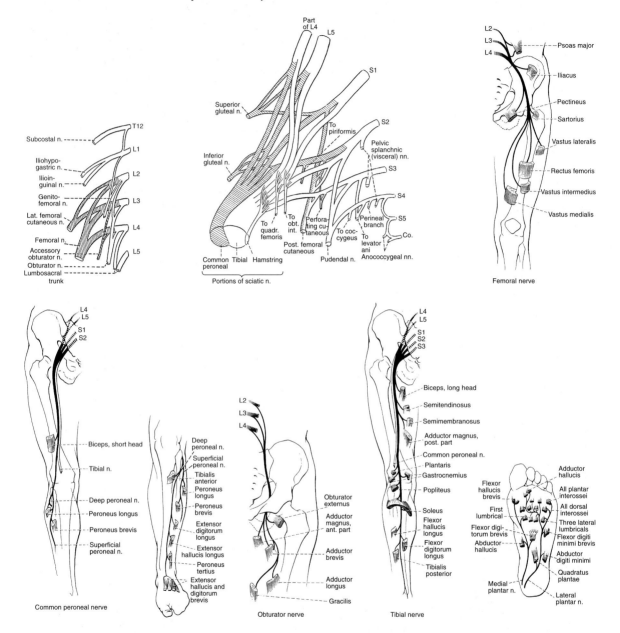

FIGURE 11-4

Lumbar and sacral plexuses and the distribution of their branches. *(From Jenkins, DB (1991). Hollinshead's Functional Anatomy of the Limbs and Back. (6th ed., pp. 239, 253, 256, 300, 304). Philadelphia: Saunders.)*

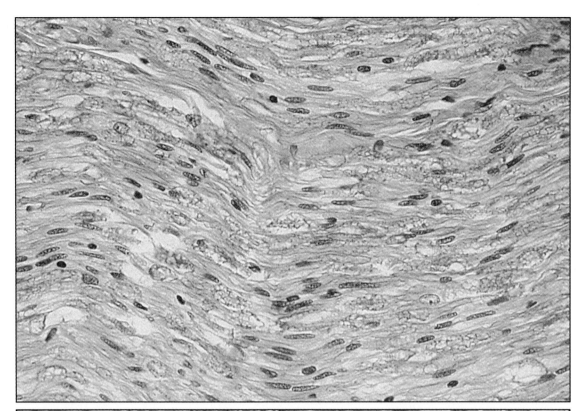

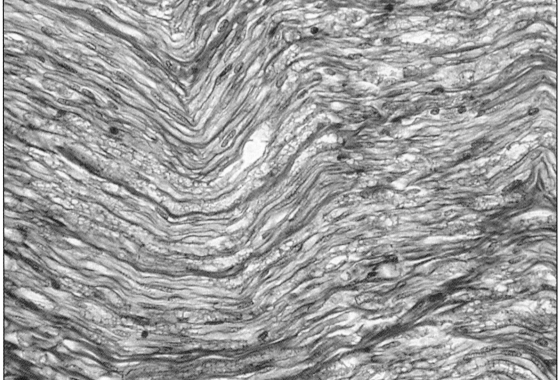

FIGURE 11-5
The normal folding of axons when a nerve is in the shortened position. Longitudinal section of femoral nerve, magnified 100X. Myelin is stained red and connective tissue is blue. *(From Warner JJ, 2001. Atlas of Neuroanatomy. (p. 343). Boston: Butterworth-Heinemann.)*

depolarization of the motor axon releases sufficient ACh to initiate action potentials in the innervated muscle fibers. Even when a lower motor neuron is inactive (no action potentials are occurring), it spontaneously releases minute amounts of ACh. Binding of the small quantity of ACh to the receptors on muscle membrane causes miniature end-plate potentials. These potentials, although not sufficient to initiate the process of muscle contraction, are believed to supply factors necessary to maintain muscle health. Without miniature end-plate potentials, muscles atrophy.

DYSFUNCTION OF PERIPHERAL NERVES

The signs of peripheral nerve damage include sensory, autonomic, and motor changes. All signs are in a peripheral nerve distribution.

Sensory Changes

Sensory changes include decreased or lost sensation and/or abnormal sensations: hyperalgesia, dysesthesia, paresthesia, and allodynia (see Chapter 7).

Autonomic Changes

Autonomic signs depend on the pattern of axonal dysfunction. If a single nerve is damaged, autonomic signs are usually only observed if the nerve is completely severed. These signs include lack of sweating and loss of sympathetic control of smooth muscle fibers in arterial walls. The latter may contribute to edema in an affected limb. If many nerves are involved, autonomic problems may include difficulty regulating blood pressure, heart rate, sweating, and bowel and bladder functions, and impotence.

Motor Changes

Motor signs of peripheral nerve damage include paresis (weakness) or paralysis. If muscle is denervated, electromyography (EMG) recordings show no activity for about 1 week following injury. Muscle atrophy progresses rapidly. Then muscle fibers begin to develop generalized sensitivity to ACh along the entire muscle membrane, and fibrillation ensues. Fibrillation is spontaneous contraction of individual muscle fibers. Fibrillation is only observable with needle EMG. Unlike fasciculation, fibrillation cannot be observed on the skin surface. Fibrillation is not diagnostic of any specific lesion; historically, fibrillation was considered diagnostic of muscle denervation (Johnson, 1980).

Denervation: Trophic Changes

When nerve supply is interrupted, trophic changes begin in the denervated tissues. Muscles atrophy, skin becomes shiny, nails become brittle, and subcutaneous tissues thicken. Ulceration of cutaneous and subcutaneous tissues, poor healing of wounds and infections, and neurogenic joint damage are common, secondary to blood supply changes, loss of sensation, and lack of movement.

CLASSIFICATION OF NEUROPATHIES

Peripheral neuropathy can involve a single nerve (mononeuropathy), several nerves (multiple mononeuropathy), or many nerves (polyneuropathy). Mononeuropathy is focal dysfunction, and multiple mononeuropathy is multifocal. Multiple mononeuropathy presents as asymmetrical involvement of individual nerves. Polyneuropathy is a generalized disorder that typically presents distally and symmetrically. Dysfunction can be due to damage to the axon, myelin sheath, or both. Table 11-2 summarizes the types, pathology, and prognosis of peripheral neuropathies.

Traumatic Injury to a Peripheral Nerve: Mononeuropathy

Various types of trauma, including repetitive stimuli, prolonged compression, or wounds, may injure peripheral nerves. Depending on the severity of damage, traumatic injuries to peripheral nerves are classified into three categories:
- Traumatic myelinopathy
- Traumatic axonopathy
- Severance

Traumatic Myelinopathy

Traumatic myelinopathy is a loss of myelin limited to the site of injury. Peripheral myelinopathies interfere with the function of large-diameter axons, producing motor, discriminative touch, proprioceptive, and phasic stretch reflex deficits and cause neuropathic pain. Unless the injury is unusually severe, autonomic function is intact and the axons are not damaged (if axons are damaged, the lesion is called an axonopathy; see below). Recovery from traumatic myelinopathy tends to be complete because remyelination can occur rapidly, before irreversible damage occurs in the target tissues.

Focal compression of a peripheral nerve causes traumatic myelinopathy. Repeated mechanical stimuli,

Table 11-2   PERIPHERAL NEUROPATHIES

Neuropathy	Usual Cause	Pathology	Typical Recovery
Mononeuropathy			
Traumatic myelinopathy	Trauma	Demyelination	Complete and rapid, by remyelination
Traumatic axonopathy	Trauma	Axonal damage	Slow, by regrowth of axons, but good recovery because Schwann cell and connective tissue sheaths intact
Traumatic severance	Trauma	Axon and myelin degeneration	Slow, with poor results, due to inappropriate reinnervation and traumatic neuroma
Multiple mononeuropathy	Complication of diabetes or blood vessel inflammation	Ischemia of neuron	Slow, by regrowth of axons, usually good recovery
Polyneuropathy	Complication of diabetes or autoimmune disorder (e.g., Guillain-Barré syndrome)	Metabolic or inflammatory	Diabetic may be stable, progressive, or improve with better blood sugar control; Guillain-Barré syndrome usually improves gradually

including excessive pressure, stretch, vibration, and/or friction may cause focal compression. The following sequence of events produces traumatic myelinopathy (Figure 11-6):

1. Nerve compression decreases axonal transport (Chang et al., 2004) and epineurial blood flow.
2. Decreased blood flow causes edema of the endoneurium and epineurium.
3. The edema further restricts blood and axoplasmic flow, interfering with axon function despite the axons being physically intact.
4. The external epineurium and perineurium thicken, causing myelin damage, leading to decreased nerve conduction velocity and the development of ectopic foci. Signals from the myelin deficient part of the nerve alter the gene activity in the cell body, stimulating the production of an excessive number of mechanosensitive and chemosensitive ion channels that are subsequently inserted into the myelin-deficient membrane, producing ectopic foci (Liu et al., 2000). Axons that previously only conveyed action potentials can now repeatedly generate action potentials (Devor and Seltzer, 1999).
5. The decreased nerve conduction velocity results in impaired discriminative touch, proprioception, and movements. Mechanical or chemical stimulation of ectopic foci generates neuropathic pain in the peripheral nerve distribution (Rempel et al., 1999).

Nerve entrapment, the mechanical constriction of a nerve within an anatomic canal, often causes traumatic myelinopathy. Entrapment is most common in the following nerves: median (carpal tunnel), ulnar (ulnar groove), radial (spiral groove), and peroneal (fibular head). Prolonged pressure from casts, crutches, or sustained positions (e.g., sitting with knees crossed) may compress nerves. Compression temporarily interferes with blood supply or, in the case of prolonged compression, may cause local demyelination. Local demyelination slows or prevents nerve conduction at the demyelinated site (Figure 11-7).

Carpal tunnel syndrome is a common compression injury of the median nerve in the space between the carpal bones and the flexor retinaculum (Box 11-1). Initially, pain and numbness are noted at night. Later, these symptoms persist throughout the day, and sensation is decreased or lost in the lateral three and one-half digits and adjacent palm of the hand. On the dorsum of the hand, the distal half of the same digits are involved. Paresis and atrophy of the thumb intrinsic muscles may follow (Figure 11-8). Pain from carpal tunnel syndrome may radiate into the forearm and occasionally to the shoulder (Kasdan et al., 1993a and 1993b). Provocative tests include Tinel's sign, tapping on the wrist to evoke paresthesia in the median nerve distribution. Direct pressure applied over the carpal tunnel to evoke symptoms has better specificity, that is, elicits fewer false-positive results, than Tinel's sign (Durkan, 1991).

Carpal tunnel syndrome is more prevalent in people whose occupations require repetitive hand movements or the gripping of vibrating tools than in the general

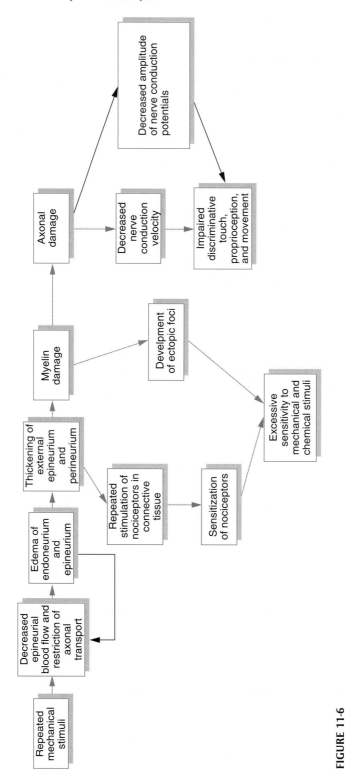

FIGURE 11-6

Sequence of events leading to the signs and symptoms of traumatic myelinopathy. Axonal damage occurs only in unusually severe cases.

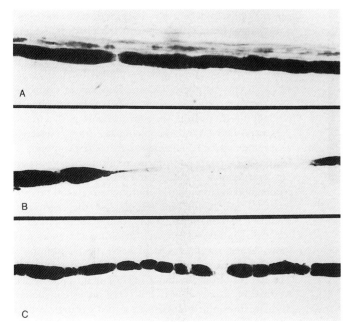

FIGURE 11-7
Nerve fiber with myelin stained to appear black.
A, Normal myelin. **B,** Segmental demyelination severe
enough to cause secondary axonal degeneration.
C, Remyelination, with abnormally short distance
between nodes of Ranvier. *(From Richardson EP, Jr.,
DeGirolami U (1995). Pathology of the Peripheral Nerve.
(p. 18). Philadelphia: Saunders.)*

BOX 11-1   CARPAL TUNNEL SYNDROME

Pathology
  Compression of median nerve in carpal tunnel

Etiology
  Repetitive finger movements, gripping vibrating tools

Speed of Onset
  Chronic

Signs and Symptoms
  Consciousness
  Normal
  Communication and Memory
  Normal
  Sensory
  *Numbness, tingling, burning sensation in median nerve
    distribution. Symptoms maybe evoked by compressing
    the median nerve or by stretching the nerve (neural
    tension test).*
  Autonomic
  *If unusually severe, lack of sweating in median nerve
    distribution*

  Motor
  Paresis and atrophy of thenar muscles

Region Affected
  Peripheral

Demographics
  *Most common in people over 30 years of age; women more
    often affected than men*
  Prevalence
  64 per 1000 population (Atroshi et al., 1999)
  Incidence
  *99 per 100,000 population per year (de Krom et al.,
    1992)*

Prognosis
  *Variable; according to the National Center for Health
    Statistics "carpal tunnel syndrome required the longest
    recuperation period of all conditions resulting in lost
    workdays, with a median 30 days away from work"
    (Rosenstock, 1996)*

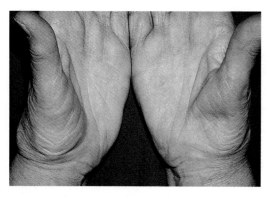

FIGURE 11-8
Carpal tunnel syndrome in the right hand. The thenar eminence
has atrophied as a result of compression of the medial nerve.
*(From Parsons M, Johnson M (2001). Diagnosis in Color Neurology.
St. Louis: Mosby.)*

population. Thus food service, factory, data entry, and
carpentry workers are at high risk. For mild cases,
often 1 month of rest, splinting, and antiinflammatory
medication (to reduce trauma and edema) followed by
exercises designed to promote gliding of the tendons in
the carpal tunnel (to improve blood flow and axonal
transport) are sufficient treatment. For more severe
cases, changing to a different occupation and surgical
release by severing the transverse carpal ligament may
be necessary.

Traumatic Axonopathy

Traumatic axonopathy disrupts axons, and wallerian
degeneration occurs distal to the lesion. Axonopathies
affect all sizes of axons, so reflexes, somatosensation, and
motor function are markedly reduced or absent. Subsequently, muscle atrophy ensues. Because the myelin and
the connective tissues remain intact, regenerating axons
are able to reinnervate appropriate targets. Axon regrowth
typically proceeds at a rate of 1 mm/day. Recovery from
axonopathies is generally good because the connective
tissue and myelin sheaths provide guidance and support
for axonal sprouts. Traumatic axonopathies usually arise
from crushing of the nerve secondary to dislocations or
closed fractures.

Severance

Severance occurs when nerves are physically divided, by
excessive stretch or laceration. The axons and connective
tissue are completely interrupted, causing immediate
loss of sensation and/or muscle paralysis in the area sup-

plied. Wallerian degeneration begins distal to the lesion
3 to 5 days later. Then axons in the proximal stumps
begin to sprout. If the proximal and distal nerve stumps
are apposed and scarring doesn't interfere, some sprouts
enter the distal stump and are guided to their target
tissue in the periphery. Other sprouts meet obstacles,
and their growth goes awry, with axons growing in
random directions from the proximal stump. In a mixed
peripheral nerve, the lack of guidance from connective
tissue and Schwann cells may allow the axon sprouts to
reach inappropriate end-organs, resulting in poor recovery. For example, a motor axon may innervate a Golgi
tendon organ; although the motor neuron could fire, the
tendon organ would not respond, so the connection
would be nonfunctional. If the stumps are displaced or
scar tissue intervenes between the stumps, sprouts may
grow into a tangled mass of nerve fibers, forming a
traumatic **neuroma** (tumor of axons and Schwann cells).
The recovery from severance injuries is initially similar
to that of axonopathies; however, nerve conduction
distal to the injury may never return because of poor
regeneration.

Multiple Mononeuropathy

Involvement of two or more nerves in different parts of
the body occurs most commonly from ischemia of the
nerves, either from diabetes or vasculitis. Vasculitis,
inflammation of blood vessels, may cause multiple mononeuropathy by restricting flood flow or by weakening
vessel walls, resulting in rupture. In multiple mononeuropathy, individual nerves are affected, producing a
random, asymmetrical presentation of signs. If vasculitis
is suspected, urgent referral should be made for an electrodiagnostic evaluation (England and Asbury, 2004).

Polyneuropathy

Symmetrical involvement of sensory, motor, and autonomic fibers, often progressing from distal to proximal,
is the hallmark of polyneuropathy. The symptoms typically begin in the feet and then appear in the hands, areas
of the body supplied by the longest axons. Degeneration
of the distal part of long axons may occur because of
inadequate axonal transport to keep the distal axons
viable. Demyelination is also likely to produce distal
symptoms first because the longer axons have more
myelin along their length and thus have a greater
chance of being affected by the random destruction of
myelin.

    In contrast to mononeuropathies, polyneuropathies
are not due to trauma or ischemia. The etiology can be
toxic, metabolic, or autoimmune. The most common

causes of polyneuropathies are diabetes, nutritional deficiencies secondary to alcoholism, and autoimmune diseases. A variety of therapeutic drugs, industrial and agricultural toxins, and nutritional disorders (including malnutrition secondary to alcoholism) can cause polyneuropathy. In severe polyneuropathy, trophic changes (poor healing, ulceration of skin, neurogenic joint damage) often occur; these changes probably occur because the person is unaware of injuries to the part, owing to lack of sensation (Olaleye et al., 2001). Thus, education regarding monitoring and care of insensitive areas is vital. Therapists are likely to treat people with diabetic (metabolic) and Guillain-Barré (autoimmune) polyneuropathies.

In **diabetic polyneuropathy** (Greene et al., 1990), axons and myelin are damaged. Usually sensation is affected most severely, often in a stocking/glove distribution (Figure 11-9). All sizes of sensory axons are damaged (Figure 11-10), resulting in decreased sensations and pain, paresthesias, and dysesthesias. Impaired vibration sense is often the first sign. Ankle reflexes are decreased. Unfortunately, physicians fail to diagnose peripheral neuropathy in approximately $\frac{2}{3}$ of cases (Herman and Kennedy, 2003). Loss of pain sensation often leads to damaged joints in the feet (Charcot's joints) and to foot ulcers. Proper diabetic foot care, including regular sensory testing with monofilaments (see Chapter 7), wearing of appropriate shoes, regular self-inspection of the feet, and proper care of the skin and toenails, may prevent or forestall limb amputations in people with diabetes. Exercise decreases the symptoms of diabetic neuropathy and improves balance (Richardson et al., 2001). Due to the risk of exercise-induced hypoglycemia or hyperglycemia, self-monitoring of blood glucose should be performed before, during, and after moderate to intense physical activity (Chipkin et al., 2001). Later in the disease process, muscle weakness and atrophy also tend to occur distally. Patients typically have difficulty walking on their heels but are able to walk on their toes (England and Asbury, 2004). All autonomic functions are susceptible to diabetic neuropathy: cardiovascular, gastrointestinal, genitourinary, and sweating dysfunction (lack of sweating distally, excessive compensatory sweating proximally) are common (Box 11-2). Glycemic control can limit the progression of diabetic neuropathy (Maji, 2004).

Although the incidence of peripheral polyneuropathy is particularly high in people with diabetes, older people without diabetes also develop peripheral neuropathy. Franklin et al. reported that among people 60-74 years of age, 7% of the normoglycemic, 11% of those with

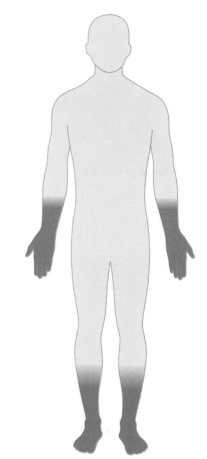

FIGURE 11-9
Stocking/glove distribution of sensory impairment in diabetic neuropathy.

impaired glucose tolerance, and 32%-50% of those with diabetes mellitus had peripheral neuropathy (Franklin et al., 1990).

The polyneuropathy in **Guillain-Barré syndrome** is characterized by more severe effects on the motor than sensory system (see Box 2-1). Contrary to the pattern in most polyneuropathies, paresis may be worse proximally. The onset is rapid, with progressive paralysis, requiring urgent diagnosis and treatment to prevent respiratory failure. One quarter to one third of Guillain-Barré patients require a ventilator (England and Asbury, 2004).

An inherited form of peripheral neuropathy is **hereditary motor and sensory neuropathy (HMSN),** also

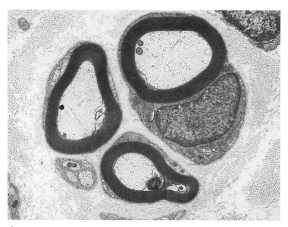

A

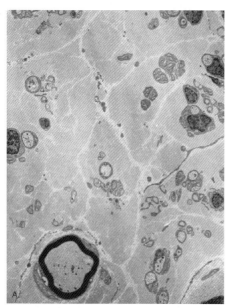

B

FIGURE 11-10

Sural nerve biopsies. The sural nerve is often used for biopsies because it is a purely sensory nerve, and thus the removal of a small section does not cause motor loss. **A,** Cross section of normal nerve, with three myelinated axons (surrounded by darkly stained rings of myelin) and a small group of unmyelinated axons to the left of the bottom myelinated axon. **B,** Cross section of a nerve with damage by diabetic neuropathy. All sizes of axons have been lost, only one myelinated fiber is present, and many axons have been replaced by collagen. *(From Richardson EP, Jr., DeGirolami U (1995). Pathology of the Peripheral Nerve. (pp. 5, 80). Philadelphia: Saunders.)*

BOX 11-2   DIABETIC POLYNEUROPATHY

Pathology
> *Demyelination and axon damage*

Etiology
> *Metabolic*

Speed of Onset
> *Chronic*

Signs and Symptoms
> *Distal more involved than proximal*
>
> Consciousness
> *Normal*
>
> Communication and Memory
> *Normal*
>
> Sensory
> *Numbness, pain, paresthesias (tingling, pins and needles), dysesthesias (burning, aching)*
>
> Autonomic
> *Orthostatic hypotension; impaired sweating; bowel, bladder, digestive, genital, pupil, and lacrimal dysfunction*
>
> Motor
> *Balance and coordination problems (secondary to sensory deficits); weakness*
>
> Cranial Nerves
> *Usually normal; occasionally cranial nerve III is involved, producing drooping of upper eyelid and paresis of four extraocular muscles*

Region Affected
> *Peripheral*

Demographics
> *Affects all ages; no gender predominance*
>
> Incidence
> *54 per 100,000 population per year*
>
> Lifetime Prevalence
> *2 per 1000 population (MacDonald et al., 2000)*

Prognosis
> *Stable or progressive; occasionally better control of blood sugar levels leads to improvement*

---

known as **Charcot-Marie-Tooth disease.** This disease generally causes paresis of muscles distal to the knee, with resulting foot drop, a steppage gait, frequently tripping, and muscle atrophy. As the disease progresses, muscle atrophy and paresis affect the hands. Despite the involvement of sensory neurons, significant numbness or pain is unusual. Instead, there is decreased ability to sense heat, cold, and pain. Onset typically occurs in adolescence or in young adults, but varies with the specific type of HMSN. The various types of HMSN are caused by different genetic mutations, affecting the production of different proteins essential to the structure and function of peripheral axons or myelin sheaths. The pattern of inheritance may be autosomal dominant, autosomal recessive, or X-linked (abnormal gene on the X chromosome). Rarely HMSN results from a spontaneous (nonhereditary) gene mutation. Therapy involves strengthening; stretching; conditioning; and joint, muscle, and skin protection.

DYSFUNCTIONS OF THE NEUROMUSCULAR JUNCTION

Two typical problems at the neuromuscular junction have similar effects. In myasthenia gravis, an autoimmune disease that damages ACh receptors at the neuromuscular junction, repeated use of a muscle leads to increasing weakness. In botulism, ingesting the botulinum toxin from improperly stored foods causes interference with the release of ACh from the motor axon. This produces acute, progressive weakness, with loss of stretch reflexes. Sensation remains intact. Botulinum toxin (botox) is used therapeutically in people with movement dysfunctions due to upper motor neuron syndromes or dystonia, to weaken overactive muscles by directly injecting the toxin into muscles. Although botox injections are commonly believed to treat "spasticity," botox actually interferes with release of ACh at the neuromuscular junction and thus does not treat the myoplastic component of muscle hyperstiffness. This treatment frequently improves function by improving the person's ability to control antagonistic and synergistic muscles.

MYOPATHY

Myopathies are disorders intrinsic to muscle. An example is muscular dystrophy; random muscle fibers degenerate, leaving motor units with fewer muscle fibers than normal. Activating such a motor unit produces less force than a healthy motor unit. Because the nervous system is not affected by myopathy, sensation and autonomic function remain intact. Coordination, muscle tone, and reflexes are unaffected until muscle atrophy becomes so severe that muscle activity cannot be elicited.

ELECTRODIAGNOSTIC STUDIES

Dysfunction of peripheral nerves and the muscles they innervate can be evaluated by electrodiagnostic studies. Recording the electrical activity from nerves and muscles by nerve conduction study (NCS) and EMG studies (see Chapters 7 and 10) reveals the location of pathology and is often diagnostic. Nerve conduction studies can be used to differentiate between the following:

- Processes that are primarily demyelinating (myelinopathy) and those that primarily damage axons (axonopathy). Myelinopathies produce marked slowing of velocity. Axonopathies produce decreases in the amplitude of nerve conduction potentials and may produce slowing of conduction velocity.
- Upper motor neuron and lower motor neuron paresis. Upper motor neuron lesions have no effect on peripheral nerve conduction, so NCS is normal. Lower motor neuron lesions produce abnormal NCS.
- Mononeuropathy and polyneuropathy (Williams et al., 2005).
- Local conduction block and wallerian degeneration. Local conduction block interferes with nerve conduction only at one site, whereas wallerian degeneration affects the entire axon distal to the lesion.

Electromyography differentiates between nerve and muscle disorders, thus distinguishing neuropathy from myopathy (see Chapter 10).

The effect of myelinopathy on nerve conduction is to slow or stop conduction across the site of damage, with normal conduction in the axon segments proximal to and distal to the injury (Figure 11-11). In axonopathy, axons lose their ability to conduct action potentials across the damaged site at the time of injury. Thus, the amplitude of the evoked potential is decreased (Figure 11-12). Nerve conduction velocity in the section of nerve distal to the injury gradually decreases over several days, eventually ceasing as a result of wallerian degeneration distal to the lesion. When a nerve is completely severed, nerve conduction may never return distal to the injury.

Generalized neuropathies (i.e., polyneuropathies) are characterized by slowed nerve conduction throughout the affected nerves and by decreased amplitude, particularly with increased distance between stimulation and recording sites. In myopathy, nerve conduction is normal, but the amplitude of the potential recorded from muscle is decreased.

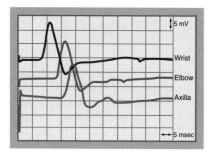

	Latency (ms)	Amplitude (mV)	Distance (mm)	Velocity (m/s)
Recorded values:				
Stimulated at wrist	8.0 (distal)	13.0		
Stimulated at elbow	12.8	13.2	240	49.6
Stimulated at axilla	15.2	11.5	145	62.1
Normal values for median nerve	Distal latency <4.2	>5.0		>50

A

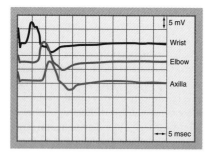

	Latency (ms)	Amplitude (mV)	Distance (mm)	Velocity (m/s)
Recorded values:				
Stimulated at wrist	3.0 (distal)	8.0		
Stimulated at elbow	6.7	7.5	205	55.9
Stimulated at axilla	8.8	7.8	150	69.2
Normal values for ulnar nerve	Distal latency <3.4	>5.0		>49.5

B

FIGURE 11-11

Motor nerve conduction study. **A,** Severe demyelination of the median nerve at the wrist. This is indicated by the 8.0 distal latency and the slow forearm conduction velocity, combined with normal amplitude of the recorded potential. **B,** Normal, ipsilateral ulnar NCS in the same person. *(Courtesy Robert A. Sellin, PT.)*

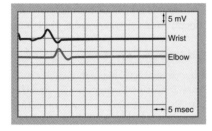

	Latency (ms)	Amplitude (mV)	Distance (mm)	Velocity (m/s)
Recorded values:				
Stimulated at wrist	9.2	3.3		
Stimulated at elbow	13.2	3.2	230	57.5
Normal values for median nerve	Distal latency <4.2	>5.0		>50

FIGURE 11-12

Median motor nerve conduction study, showing severely prolonged distal latency and a marked decrease in amplitude compared to normal. Conduction velocity between the wrist and elbow is normal. *(Courtesy Robert A. Sellin, PT.)*

CLINICAL TESTING

Richardson (2002) identified three clinical signs that detect peripheral neuropathy in outpatients 50 years of age and older. The presence of two or three of the signs correlates highly with electrodiagnostic evidence of peripheral neuropathy. The three signs are: absence of ankle jerk reflex despite facilitation, impaired vibration, and impaired position sense of the great toe. The ankle jerk was tested two ways: by striking the tendon and by striking the plantar surface of the foot as shown in Figure 11-13. The facilitory techniques for the ankle jerk reflex included having the patient gently plantarflex the foot, close the eyes tightly, or pull against the resistance of their own clasped hands just prior to the reflex hammer strike. For vibration testing, a 128-Hz tuning fork was struck, then placed until the patient reported that the vibration was gone. The sites tested, in order, were: the clavicle, just proximal to the nailbed of the index finger of the dominant upper limb, just proximal to the nailbed of each of the great toes, and at the medial malleolus. Position sense was tested on the dominant great toe. The examiner grasped the medial and lateral surfaces and flexed and extended the great toe. The patient's eyes were open for a few trials, then the patient closed the eyes and ten 1-second movements of approximately 1 cm were administered smoothly. Results that indicated a periph-

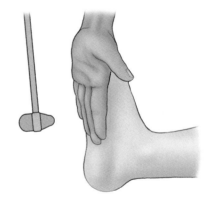

FIGURE 11-13

The plantar strike method of testing the ankle jerk reflex. The patient is supine with the knees extended. The examiner places the dorsum of the hand against the sole of the patient's foot, passively dorsiflexes the foot, then strikes their own fingers with the reflex hammer.

eral neuropathy included: absence of the ankle jerk reflex despite facilitation, decreased vibration sense at the great toe (vibration perceived for less than 8 seconds), and decreased position sense at the toe (correct perception less than 8 times in 10 trials).

CLINICAL APPLICATION

Evaluation

As the severity of peripheral neuropathy increases, so do reports of pins and needles sensation (Herman and Kennedy, 2003). Sensory, autonomic, and motor functions are evaluated as indicated in their respective chapters (see Chapters 7, 8, and 10). Signs of peripheral nervous system damage result from hypoactivity or hyperactivity of neurons. For example, neuronal hypoactivity, a decrease or loss of neuronal activity, may produce loss of proprioception. An example of neuronal hyperactivity is light touch eliciting a painful sensation.

Table 11-3 lists the signs and symptoms of mononeuropathy. In polyneuropathy, the same characteristics are found but in a symmetrical distribution, sometimes with additional autonomic signs: postural hypotension, bowel or bladder incontinence, and inability to have a sexual erection.

Clinically, making the distinction between peripheral neuropathy and central nervous system dysfunction is vital. Table 11-4 indicates factors that differentiate peripheral from central nervous system lesions.

Treatment

Results of sensory, manual muscle, and, if indicated, electrodiagnostic testing guide treatment decisions. Education is necessary to prevent complications from damage due to lack of sensation, disuse, or overuse. The person with peripheral neuropathy that affects sensation should be taught to visually inspect the involved areas daily, using mirrors if necessary, to monitor for wounds and for reddening of the skin that persists more than a few minutes. If the feet are involved, proper foot care should be taught. Interventions for edema include elevation of the limb, compression bandaging with an elastic wrap, and electrical stimulation. Contractures may be prevented by prolonged stretching or by daily activities.

Exercise beginning the day following a peripheral nerve crush injury has been demonstrated to enhance both sensory and motor recovery (vanMeeteren et al., 1997). Exercises should emphasize gradual strengthening and the functional use of individual muscles and

Table 11-3   SIGNS AND SYMPTOMS OF MONONEUROPATHY

	Neuronal Hypoactivity	Neuronal Hyperactivity
Sensory	Decrease or lack of sensation (touch, pressure, proprioception, or pain)	Pain, dysesthesia, allodynia, hyperesthesia
Autonomic	Flushing of skin, edema, lack of sweating	Vasoconstriction: cold skin, pallor, cyanosis (dark blue color of skin); excessive sweating; perpetuation of pain (see Chapter 7)
Motor	Paresis, paralysis, hypotonia, muscle atrophy	Spasms, muscle fasciculations and/or fibrillations
Reflexes	Decreased or absent	Normal

Table 11-4   DISTINGUISHING PERIPHERAL FROM CENTRAL NERVOUS SYSTEM DYSFUNCTION

	Peripheral Nervous System	Central Nervous System
Distribution of signs and symptoms	Peripheral nerve pattern	Dermatomal or myotomal pattern
Nerve conduction study	Slowed or blocked conduction; decreased amplitude of recorded potentials	Normal
Muscle tone	If lower motor neuron involvement, hypotonia	If upper motor neuron involvement, hypertonia
Muscle atrophy	Rapid muscle atrophy indicates denervation	Muscle atrophy progresses slowly
Phasic stretch reflexes	Reduced or absent	Hyperactive or normal
Paraspinal sensation and/or paraspinal muscles	Normal	Involved

muscle groups. Orthoses (braces) are frequently used to stabilize weight-bearing joints, thus preventing sprains and strains, and to prevent dropping of the forefoot during gait in cases of paresis or paralysis of the tibialis anterior muscle. Orthoses are also used to prevent deformities that can result from paresis, paralysis, and lack of sensation. The use of electrical stimulation to prevent atrophy of denervated muscles by evoking muscle contractions is controversial because controlled studies have not been performed in humans (Buttress and Herren, 2002).

SUMMARY

Somatic peripheral nerves convey signals between sensory receptors and the central nervous system and between the central nervous system and skeletal muscles. Somatic peripheral nerves consist of axons, connective tissue, and sensory endings. Peripheral nerve lesions produce signs and symptoms in a peripheral nerve distribution. In contrast, spinal region lesions produce signs and symptoms in a myotomal and/or dermatomal distribution. When peripheral nerves are stretched, axons unwrinkle, the connective tissue tubes extend, fascicles glide relative to each other, fascicular plexuses share the loading, and the entire nerve slides relative to surrounding tissues. Normal stretching and shortening of nerves facilitates blood and axoplasm flow, contributing to the health of peripheral nerves. Mononeuropathy results when excessive mechanical stimuli damage peripheral nerves by compromising blood flow and axonal transport, causing edema, eventual thickening of certain connective tissues, leading to myelin damage, development of ectopic foci, and decreased nerve conduction velocity.

Polyneuropathy is symmetrical damage to peripheral nerves. Examples include diabetic polyneuropathy, Guillain-Barré syndrome, and hereditary motor and sensory neuropathy (HMSN). Electrodiagnostic studies are useful for evaluating neuropathy and may be used to distinguish neuropathy from myopathy.

CLINICAL NOTES

Case 1

RV is a 35-year-old man who was brought to the emergency room by a friend 2 days ago. At that time, RV complained of aching, burning pain in his thighs and a feeling of weakness that began 2 days prior to admission. He has no history of trauma. His current condition is as follows:
- He is unable to communicate, so sensation and cognitive functions cannot be tested.
- He is subject to abnormal variations in blood pressure and heart rate.
- He is completely paralyzed. His breathing is maintained by a respirator.
- Nerve conduction velocity is markedly slowed bilaterally in the tested nerves, the median and tibial nerves. Amplitude of recorded potentials is normal.

Question
What is the location of the lesion(s) and probable etiology?

Case 2

A 16-year-old woman was injured 2 days ago when a load of lumber fell from a shelf, pinning her left forearm. The following signs and symptoms are noted on her left side:
- She does not feel pinprick, touch, temperature differences, or vibration on the medial hand, little finger, and medial half of the ring finger.
- Sweating is absent in the same distribution as the sensory loss.
- Radial wrist extension and flexion and finger extension are normal strength on manual muscle tests.
- She is unable to flex the middle and distal phalanges of the fourth and fifth digits, abduct or adduct her fingers, or adduct the hand.

Questions
1. What is the location of the lesion(s)?
2. How could the probable rate of recovery be predicted?

Continued

CLINICAL NOTES

Case 3

A 7-year-old boy has progressive proximal muscle weakness. Clinical examination and electrodiagnostic tests reveal the following:

- Sensation and coordination are within normal limits.
- He falls twice when walking 100 feet.
- He has difficulty coming to standing and climbing stairs.
- Lumbar lordosis is increased.
- Manual muscle tests indicate that shoulder girdle and hip muscles are approximately 50% of normal strength, knee and elbow muscles are about 75% of normal strength, and distal muscles have near-normal strength.
- Velocity of nerve conduction is normal.
- Electromyographic potentials recorded from hip girdle muscles are of small amplitude.

Question

What is the location of the lesion(s) and probable etiology?

REVIEW QUESTIONS

1. What mechanisms allow peripheral nerves to lengthen and shorten without injury?
2. What signs are produced by complete severance of a peripheral nerve?
3. List the trophic changes that occur in denervated tissues.
4. Give an example of a myelinopathy. What part of the nerve is damaged in a myelinopathy? Describe the sequence of events that produce a compression mononeuropathy.
5. Describe an axonopathy.
6. Why is the prognosis for a severed nerve poor?
7. What is multiple mononeuropathy?
8. What are the most common causes of polyneuropathy?
9. Why do the signs and symptoms of polyneuropathy usually appear distally first?
10. How can myelinopathy be distinguished from axonopathy?
11. How can neuropathy be distinguished from myopathy?
12. Classify each of the following signs as resulting from neuronal hyperactivity or hypoactivity: absent reflexes, muscle spasms, lack of sweating, paralysis, muscle fasciculations, and cyanosis of the skin.
13. Sensory loss in a dermatomal pattern, normal NCS, muscle hypertonia, and slowly progressive muscle atrophy that includes the paraspinal muscles are indicative of lesions in what region of the nervous system?

References

Atroshi I, Gummesson C, et al. (1999). Prevalence of carpal tunnel syndrome in a general population [see comments]. Journal of the American Medical Association, 282(2), 153-158.

Buttress S, Herren K (2002). Towards evidence based emergency medicine: Best BETs from the Manchester Royal Infirmary. Electrical stimulation and Bell's palsy. Emergency medicine Journal: EMJ, 19(5), 428.

Chang MH, Liu LH, et al. (2004). Does retrograde axonal atrophy really occur in carpal tunnel syndrome patients with normal forearm conduction velocity? Clinical Neurophysiology, 115(12), 2783-2788.

Chipkin SR, Klugh SA, et al. (2001). Exercise and diabetes. Cardiology Clinics, 19(3), 489-505.

de Krom MC, Knipschild PG, et al. (1992). Carpal tunnel syndrome: Prevalence in the general population. Journal of Clinical Epidemiology, 45(4), 373-376.

Devor M, Seltzer Z (1999). Pathophysiology of damaged nerves in relation to chronic pain. In PD Wall, R Melzack (Eds.), Textbook of Pain. (4th ed.). Edinburgh: Churchill Livingstone.

Dilley A, Lynn B, et al. (2003). Quantitative in vivo studies of median nerve sliding in response to wrist, elbow, shoulder and neck movements. Clinical Biomechanics (Bristol, Avon), 18(10), 899-907.

Durkan JA (1991). A new diagnostic test for carpal tunnel syndrome. Journal of Bone and Joint Surgery (American), 73, 535-538.

England JD, Asbury AK (2004). Peripheral neuropathy. Lancet, 363(9427), 2151-2161.

Franklin GM, Kahn LB, et al. (1990). Sensory neuropathy in non-insulin-dependent diabetes mellitus. The San Luis Valley Diabetes Study. American Journal of Epidemiology, 131(4), 633-643.

Greene DA, Simal AF, et al. (1990). Diabetic neuropathy. Annual Review of Medicine, 41, 303-317.

Herman WH, Kennedy L (2003). Physician perception of neuropathy in a large Type 2 diabetes population (GOAL A1C study) confirms underdiagnosis of neuropathy in everyday clinical practice. 18th International Diabetes Federation Congress, Paris, France.

Johnson EW (1980). Practical electromyography. Baltimore: Williams & Wilkins.

Kasdan M, Lane C, et al. (1993a). Carpal tunnel syndrome: The workup. Patient Care, 27(7), 97-102, 104-108.

Kasdan M, Lane C, et al. (1993b). Carpal tunnel syndrome: Management techniques. Patient Care, 27(7), 111-112, 115, 123-126.

Liu X, Eschenfelder S, et al. (2000). Spontaneous activity of axotomized afferent neurons after L5 spinal nerve injury in rats. Pain, 84(2-3), 309-318.

MacDonald BK, Cockerell OC, et al. (2000). The incidence and lifetime prevalence of neurological disorders in a prospective community-based study in the UK. Brain, 123(Pt 4), 665-676.

Maji D (2004). Prevention of microvascular and macrovascular complications in diabetes mellitus. Journal of the Indian Medical Association, 102(8), 426, 428, 430 passim.

Millesi H, Zoch G, et al. (1995). Mechanical properties of peripheral nerves. Clinical Orthopaedics and Related Research, (314), 76-83.

Nee RJ, Butler D (2003). Nerves. In G Kolt, L Snyder-Mackler, et al. (Eds.), Physical Therapies in Sport and Exercise: Principles and Practice. New York: Churchill-Livingstone.

Olaleye D, Perkins BA, et al. (2001). Evaluation of three screening tests and a risk assessment model for diagnosing peripheral neuropathy in the diabetes clinic. Diabetes Research and Clinical Practice, 54(2), 115-128.

Rempel D, Dahlin L, et al. (1999). Pathophysiology of nerve compression syndromes: Response of peripheral nerves to loading. Journal of Bone and Joint Surgery. American Volume, 81(11), 1600-1610.

Rempel DM, Diao E (2004). Entrapment neuropathies: Pathophysiology and pathogenesis. Journal of Electromyography and Kinesiology, 14(1), 71-75.

Richardson JK (2002). The clinical identification of peripheral neuropathy among older persons. Archives of Physical Medicine and Rehabilitation, 83(11), 1553-1558.

Richardson JK, Sandman D, et al. (2001). A focused exercise regimen improves clinical measures of balance in patients with peripheral neuropathy. Archives of Physical Medicine and Rehabilitation, 82(2), 205-209.

Rosenstock L (1996). National Occupational Research Agenda (NORA) Priority Research Areas, Hyattsville, MD: National Center for Health Statistics.

Sunderland S (1990). The anatomy and physiology of nerve injury. Muscle Nerve, 13(9), 771-784.

vanMeeteren NL, Brakkee JH, et al. (1997). Exercise training improves functional recovery and motor nerve conduction velocity after sciatic nerve crush lesion in the rat. Archives of Physical Medicine and Rehabilitation, 78(1), 70-77.

Williams FH, Johns JS, et al. (2005). Neuromuscular rehabilitation and electrodiagnosis. 1. Mononeuropathy. Archives of Physical Medicine and Rehabilitation, 86(1 Pt 2), 3-10.

Wright TW, Glowczewskie F, Jr., et al. (2001). Ulnar nerve excursion and strain at the elbow and wrist associated with upper extremity motion. Journal of Hand Surgery, 26(4), 655-662.

Suggested Readings

Hankey GJ, Wardlaw JM (2002). Diseases of the peripheral nerve: Mononeuropathies. Clinical Neurology. (pp. 579-656). New York: Demos Medical Publishing.

Richardson EP, Girolami UD (1995). General reactions of peripheral nerve to disease: Metabolic and nutritional neuropathies. In Pathology of the Peripheral Nerve. (pp. 8-21, 78-93). Philadelphia: Saunders.

12 Spinal Region

Laurie Lundy-Ekman,
PhD, PT

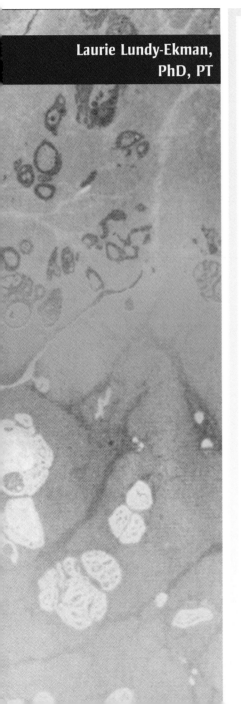

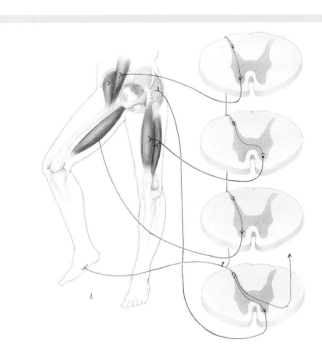

Five years ago, I had an accident. I recall the doctor saying afterwards: "You have a spinal cord injury, a thoracic 7 lesion, but you can manage yourself in the future."

The last part was most important, since I have two children. What the doctor didn't tell me was how to achieve independence and how to return to a normal life. I am a physical therapist, and my specialty was in treating the neurologic problems of children. I am a pioneer in this field in the Netherlands, and for the past 25 years I have worked with handicapped children in their daily situations.

I left the rehabilitation center after 9 months of therapy and training. It could have been earlier, but my home was not ready for my return. Some things needed to be adapted and made accessible to me from my wheelchair. I have a car that my work paid to have adapted for hand control. I can organize all the daily things in life for me and my children. We are a good team.

Now, I had to work for a new life for myself. Because of my profession and my specialty, I was able to return to my job after only about 6 months. Part of my job involved my own physical therapy practice, and the other part was working as an instructor/senior tutor for children with cerebral palsy. Due to my injury, I sold my physical therapy practice and began teaching, from my wheelchair, at a physical therapy school. In this surrounding, nobody noticed the wheelchair; I was just myself.

Now it has been 5 years and sometimes I think to myself: "What is different?" I can do all the things I want and enjoy. I cannot walk, and sometimes I have a lot of pain. Once I spilled hot tea on my stomach and burned myself quite severely without realizing it until later. Because I lack sensation in my abdomen and legs, I did not become aware of the burn until I saw blisters on my skin. But I am happy in my wheelchair and I am happy with my son (18) and my daughter (16). The doctor was right. It is a hard and long way to come, but it is possible.

Last year, while visiting the United States, I learned how to catheterize my bladder while remaining sitting in my wheelchair. This was very important to my independence. Now I can go anywhere and not need special equipment. This year I went to the United States for my work and was driving a car on the interstate. I thought to myself, "It really is true; you can do almost anything if you have friends and your own desires." When I use the terms *impairment, disability,* and handicap, I can say that I am not handicapped.

I use no medications. I can deal with the spasticity very well, since for 25 years in my profession I worked with spasticity in other people. I control the spasticity by using slow stretch, correct foot and leg positioning, prolonged positions, and making sure to empty my bladder on schedule. My professional knowledge helped me a lot, but on the other hand I am now a patient and sometimes need the guidance of professionals.

—*Tineke Dirks*

ANATOMY OF THE SPINAL REGION

The spinal region includes all neural structures contained within the vertebrae: spinal cord, dorsal and ventral roots, spinal nerves, and meninges (Figure 12-1). Lateral enlargements of the cord at the cervical and lumbosacral levels accommodate the neurons for upper and lower limb innervation. The spinal cord is continuous with the medulla and ends at the L1-L2 intervertebral space in adults (Figure 12-2). Inferior to the end of the spinal cord is the filum terminale, a bundle of connective tissue and glia that connects the end of the cord to the coccyx. Because the spinal cord is not present below the L1 vertebral level, long roots are required for axons from the termination of the cord to exit the lumbosacral vertebral column. These long roots form the cauda equina within the lower vertebral canal (Figure 12-3).

Vertical grooves mark the external spinal cord. The anterior cord has a deep median fissure, and the posterior

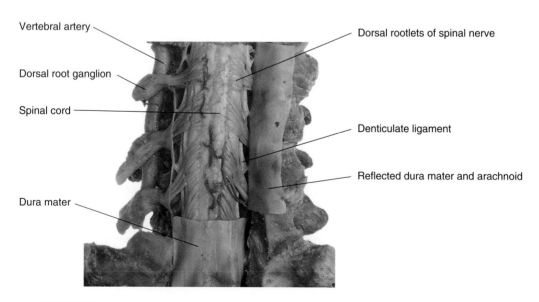

FIGURE 12-1
Posterior view of part of the cervical spinal region. Vertebral arches have been removed, and part of the dura and arachnoid have been reflected. *(From Abrahams PH, Marks SC, et al. (2003). McMinn's Color Atlas of Human Anatomy. (5th ed., p. 104). Philadelphia: Mosby.)*

Spinal cord

Vertebral column and spinal nerve levels

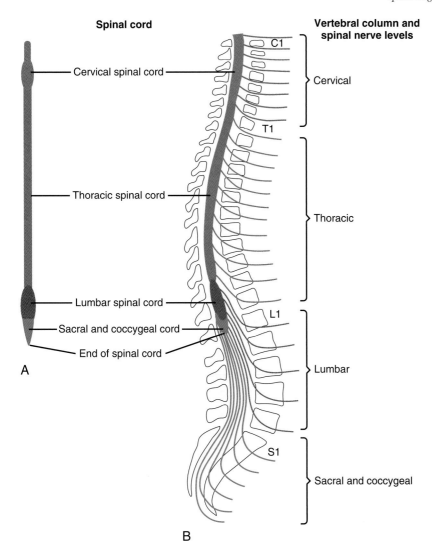

Cervical spinal cord

Thoracic spinal cord

Lumbar spinal cord

Sacral and coccygeal cord

End of spinal cord

A

C1

Cervical

T1

Thoracic

L1

Lumbar

S1

Sacral and coccygeal

B

FIGURE 12-2
Relationship of spinal cord segments to the vertebral column. **A,** Anterior view of the spinal cord. **B,** Spinal cord segment levels (neurologic levels) are indicated on the left. Vertebral levels and spinal nerves are indicated on the right. Spinal nerves are named for the vertebral level that they exit the vertebral canal. The spinal cord ends at the L2 vertebral level. Because the spinal cord is significantly shorter than the vertebral column, only at C1 and C2 are the spinal cord segment levels and vertebral levels the same level. The L2-S5 nerve roots travel downward below the end of the spinal cord before exiting the vertebral canal. This collection of nerve roots inferior to the spinal cord within the bony canal is the cauda equina.

cord has a shallow median sulcus. The anterior cord also has two anterolateral sulci, where nerve rootlets emerge from the cord. The posterior cord has two posterolateral sulci, where nerve rootlets enter the cord.

Ventral and Dorsal Roots

Axons sending information to the periphery (motor) leave the anterolateral cord in small groups called *rootlets.* Ventral rootlets from a single segment coalesce to form a **ventral root.** The **dorsal root** contains sensory axons bringing information into the spinal cord and enters the posterolateral spinal cord via rootlets. Unlike the ventral

roots, each dorsal root has a **dorsal root ganglion** located outside the spinal cord. The dorsal root ganglion contains the cell bodies of sensory neurons. Where sensory axons enter the spinal cord, the large-diameter fibers, transmitting proprioceptive and touch information, are located medially, and the small-diameter fibers, transmitting pain and temperature information, are located laterally (Figure 12-4).

The dorsal and ventral roots join briefly to form a **spinal nerve.** The spinal nerve is a mixed nerve because it contains both sensory and motor axons. Spinal nerves are located in the intervertebral foramen.

The ventral root contains motor axons. The dorsal root contains sensory neurons. The somas of sensory neurons are found in the dorsal root ganglion. The spinal nerve consists of all sensory and motor axons connecting with a single segment of the cord.

Segments of the Spinal Cord

A striking and significant feature of the spinal cord is **segmental organization.** Each segment of the cord is connected to a specific region of the body by axons traveling through a pair of spinal nerves. The connections of nerve rootlets to the exterior of the cord indicate the segments (Figure 12-5). Segments are identified by the same designation as their corresponding spinal nerves. For example, the term *L4 spinal segment* refers to the section of the cord whose spinal nerve traverses the L4 intervertebral foramen. However, within the cord, the distinct segments are not evident because the cord consists of continuous vertical columns extending from the brain to the cord termination.

Spinal Nerves and Rami

Spinal nerves are unique in carrying all of the motor and sensory axons of a single spinal segment. In the cervical region, spinal nerves are found above the corresponding vertebra, except for the eighth spinal nerve, which emerges between the C7 and T1 vertebrae. In the remainder of the cord, spinal nerves lie below the corresponding vertebra. The spinal nerve innervation of muscles in the upper and lower limbs is summarized in Tables 12-1 and 12-2.

After a brief transit through the intervertebral foramen, the spinal nerve splits into two rami; this division marks the end of the spinal region and the beginning of the peripheral nervous system. The dorsal rami innervate the paravertebral muscles, posterior parts of the vertebrae, and overlying cutaneous areas. The ventral rami innervate the skeletal, muscular, and cutaneous areas of the limbs and of the anterior and lateral trunk. Both rami are mixed nerves.

A segment of the spinal cord is connected to a specific region of the body by a pair of spinal nerves.

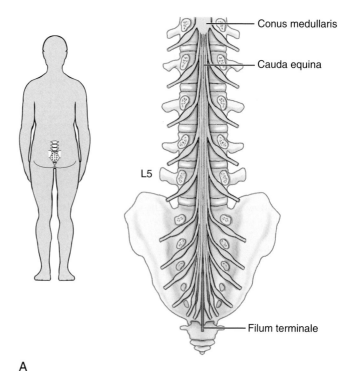

Conus medullaris

Cauda equina

L5

Filum terminale

FIGURE 12-3

Cauda equina. **A,** Dorsal view of the cauda equina in relationship to the vertebral column. Note the end of the spinal cord (conus medullaris) at the L1-L2 intervertebral space.

A

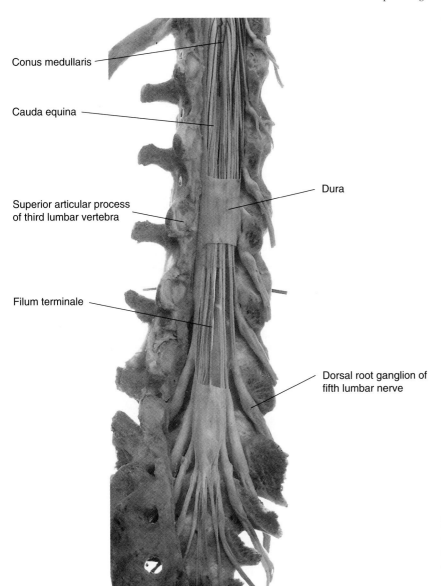

Conus medullaris

Cauda equina

Superior articular process
of third lumbar vertebra

Filum terminale

Dura

Dorsal root ganglion of
fifth lumbar nerve

B

FIGURE 12-3, cont'd
B, Vertebral arches and part of the
meninges have been removed to
reveal the cauda equina. (**B** *from
Abrahams PH, Marks SC, et al.
(2003). McMinn's Color Atlas of
Human Anatomy. (5th ed., p. 107).
Philadelphia: Mosby.)*

Internal Structure of the Spinal Cord

The internal structure of the spinal cord can be observed
in horizontal sections. Throughout the spinal cord, white
matter surrounds the gray matter. White matter contains the axons connecting various levels of the cord and
linking the cord with the brain. Axons that begin and
end within the spinal cord are called **propriospinal.** The

propriospinal axons are adjacent to the gray matter. Cells
with long axons connecting the spinal cord with the
brain are **tract cells.** The dorsal and lateral columns of
white matter contain axons of tract cells, transmitting
sensory information upward to the brain. The lateral and
anterior white matter contains axons of upper motor
neurons, conveying information descending from the
brain to interneurons and lower motor neurons. Specific

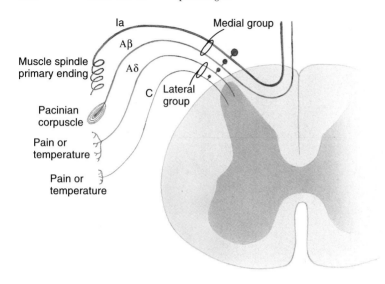

FIGURE 12-4

In the dorsal root entry zone, axons conveying information from touch and proprioceptive receptors enter the cord medially, while axons carrying information about painful stimuli and temperature enter the cord laterally.

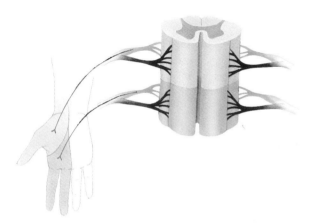

FIGURE 12-5

Two segments of the spinal cord. The axons traveling through the rootlets, roots, and spinal nerves connect a spinal segment with a specific part of the body. The axons shown are sensory axons, conveying information from the C6 and C7 dermatomes through the dorsal root into the C6 and C7 spinal cord segments. Red indicates motor rootlets and roots.

- Dorsal horn
- Lateral horn
- Ventral horn

The **dorsal horn** is primarily sensory, containing endings and collaterals of first-order sensory neurons, interneurons, and dendrites and somas of tract cells. For example, the somas of second-order neurons in the spinothalamic pathway are in the dorsal horn (see Chapter 6). The **lateral horn** (present only at T1-L2 spinal segments) contains the cell bodies of preganglionic sympathetic neurons. A region analogous to the lateral horn in the S2-S4 spinal segments includes the preganglionic parasympathetic cell bodies. Preganglionic autonomic neurons are efferent neurons. Both sympathetic and parasympathetic preganglionic neurons exit the cord via the ventral root. The **ventral horn** is primarily cell bodies of lower motor neurons whose axons exit the spinal cord via the ventral root.

tracts have been discussed in Chapters 6-10. The propriospinal axons and tracts in the spinal cord are illustrated in Figure 12-6.

The central part of the cord is marked by a distinctive *H*-shaped pattern of gray matter (Figure 12-7). Lateral sections of spinal gray matter are divided into three regions called *horns:*

The dorsal horn processes sensory information, the lateral horn processes autonomic information, and the ventral horn processes motor information.

Much of the gray matter is composed of spinal interneurons, cells with their somas in the gray matter that act upon other cells within the cord. Spinal interneurons include cells that remain entirely within the gray matter and also cells whose axons travel in white matter to different levels of the cord.

Table 12-1   SPINAL NERVE INNERVATION OF UPPER-LIMB MUSCLES

C2	C3	C4	C5	C6	C7	C8	T1
Sternocleidomastoid							
Trapezius							
	Levator scapulae						
	Diaphragm						
		Rhomboids (major and minor)					
		Supraspinatus					
			Serratus anterior				
			Biceps				
			Brachialis				
			Deltoid				
			Pectoralis major—clavicular head				
			Supinator				
				Pronator teres			
				Latissimus dorsi			
					Triceps		
				Long extensors of wrist and fingers			
				Pectoralis major—sternal head			
					Long flexors of wrist and fingers		
						Hand intrinsics	

Table 12-2   SPINAL NERVE INNERVATION OF LOWER LIMB MUSCLES

L2	L3	L4	L5	S1	S2	S3
Iliopsoas						
Adductors						
	Quadriceps femoris					
		Tibialis anterior				
		Tibialis posterior				
		Gluteus medius, minimus, tensor fasciae latae				
			Gluteus maximus			
			Hamstrings			
			Extensor digitorum longus			
			Extensor hallucis longus			
			Peroneus (longus and brevis)			
				Triceps surae		
					Foot intrinsics	

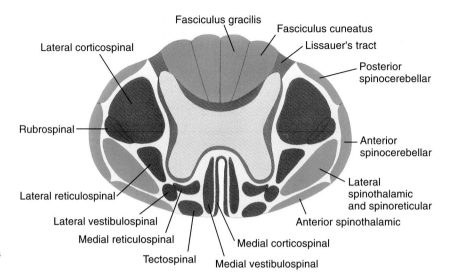

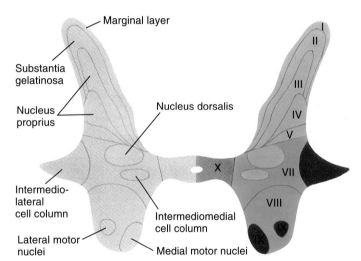

FIGURE 12-6
White matter of the spinal cord. The propriospinal fibers are indicated in purple, the sensory tracts in blue, and the motor tracts in red.

FIGURE 12-7
Gray matter of lower thoracic spinal cord. Named regions are indicated on the left, and Rexed's laminae are indicated on the right. Lamina VI is present in the segments of the spinal cord that innervate the limbs and is not present between T4 and L2. The correspondence between Rexed's laminae and the named areas is inconsistent. For example, some authors include laminae III-VI in the nucleus proprius.

Rexed's Laminae

Spinal gray matter has been classified into 10 histologic regions called *Rexed's laminae;* these regions are illustrated in Figure 12-7. In the dorsal horn, laminae I-VI are numbered from dorsal to ventral. Lamina VII includes the intermediolateral horn and part of the ventral horn. In the ventral horn, locations of laminae VII-IX vary, depending on the level of the cord. Lamina X is the central region of gray matter.

Laminae I and II, called the *marginal layer* and *substantia gelatinosa,* respectively, process information about noxious stimuli. Laminae III and IV, together known as

the *nucleus proprius,* process proprioceptive and two-point discrimination information.* Lamina V cells process information about noxious stimuli and information from the viscera. Lamina VI cells process proprioceptive information. Lamina VII includes the nucleus dorsalis, or Clarke's column, extending from T1-L3 and the intermediolateral horn. The nucleus dorsalis receives proprioceptive information, and its axons relay unconscious

*The correspondence between Rexed's laminae and some of the named spinal cord areas is controversial. For example, some authors include laminae III-VI in the nucleus proprius.

proprioceptive information to the cerebellum. The intermediolateral horn contains somas of autonomic efferents. Lamina VIII cells connect with the contralateral cord and the brain. Lamina IX contains cell bodies of lower motor neurons, whose axons travel through a ventral root, a spinal nerve, and then a peripheral nerve to innervate skeletal muscles. Lamina X consists of axons crossing to the opposite side of the cord.

> Rexed's laminae are 10 histologic and functionally specific regions in the spinal cord gray matter.

Meninges

The meninges, layers of connective tissue surrounding the spinal cord, are continuous with the meninges surrounding the brain. The pia mater closely adheres to the spinal cord surface, the arachnoid is separated from the pia by cerebrospinal fluid in the subarachnoid space, and the dura is the tough, outer layer. Between the arachnoid and dura is the subdural space, and the epidural space separates the dura from the vertebrae.

MOVEMENTS OF THE CENTRAL NERVOUS SYSTEM WITHIN THE VERTEBRAL COLUMN

The static and dynamic deformations of the vertebral column and movements of the limbs are directly transmitted to spinal cord, nerve roots, and spinal nerves via the meninges. Because the meninges surrounding the spinal cord are anchored to the skull and to the vertebrae, flexion of the vertebral column stretches the spinal cord and the spinal nerves. The nervous system connective tissue is continuous, so stretching the sciatic and tibial nerves by flexion of the hip joint, extension of the knee, and dorsiflexion of the ankle generates tension in the lumbosacral trunk and the spinal cord (Harrison et al. 1999). The lumbosacral roots are stretched when hip flexion produces anterior movement of the cauda equina (Hirabayashi et al. 2002).

You can demonstrate the continuity of neural connective tissue by comparing your ability to fully extend your knee in different sitting postures. First, sit upright with your thighs fully supported and extend one knee while your foot is plantarflexed. Second, flex your lumbar and thoracic spine, place your hands behind your head and flex your neck, dorsiflex your foot, and then extend your

knee. The decrease in knee extension in the slumped position is probably the result of tension in the neural structures, created by stretch of the meninges and peripheral nerve connective tissue (Butler, 2000; Laessoe and Voigt, 2004). Normally, when the vertebrae change position, the spinal cord slides up or down in the vertebral canal, unfolds or folds, repositions, and stretches (Harrison et al. 1999). The dentate ligaments (see Figure 12-1) exert forces on the pia to maintain the position of the spinal cord in the center of the vertebral canal and in the center of the subarachnoid space (Harrison et al., 1999).

Extension of the spine reduces the stretch of CNS structures. Flexion of any part of the vertebral column can produce longitudinal stretch of the entire spinal cord and nerve roots. As the neck flexes from a neutral posture to full flexion, the anterior cervical cord elongates 6% of its initial length and the posterior cervical cord lengthens 10%. Within the vertebral canal, the upper cord moves inferiorly and the lower cord moves superiorly, again with larger movements on the posterior surface (Yuan et al., 1998). During flexion, unfolding produces 70% of the total change in length and elastic deformation produces 30% (Harrison et al., 1999). Axial rotation of the vertebral column stretches nerve roots on the contralateral side (Harrison et al., 1999).

Nerve roots and spinal nerves are protected from excessive mechanical loads by (1) occupying 23%-50% of the space available within the intervertebral foramina (Min et al., 2005), (2) cushioning by fat, and (3) dural sleeves surrounding the nerve roots within the intervertebral foramen.

Although physiologic motions do not significantly change the vertebral canal space in people with normal vertebral canals (Nuckley et al., 2002), extending the neck increases the intervertebral foramen pressure at all cervical levels, and neck flexion only increases intervertebral foramen pressure at the C5 and C7 nerve root levels (Farmer and Wisneski,1994). Therefore, neck extension increases cervical nerve root signs and symptoms.

FUNCTIONS OF THE SPINAL CORD

Segments of the spinal cord exchange information with other spinal cord segments, with peripheral nerves, and with the brain. Tracts convey this information, yet spinal cord functions are far more complex than a simple conduit. Only for one type of information does the spinal cord serve as a simple conduit: axons carrying touch and proprioceptive information enter the dorsal column and project to the medulla without synapsing. All other tracts conveying information in the spinal cord synapse in the cord, and thus their information is subject to processing and modification within the cord.

For example, after one hammers a thumb, the pain signals can be modified by rubbing the thumb and/or by activity of the descending pain inhibition pathways (see Chapter 7). The pain information is modified within the spinal cord by signals from large-diameter sensory afferents and by signals in the descending tracts, both of which decrease the frequency of signals in slow pain pathways. Similarly, the information conveyed by an axon in a descending tract to a lower motor neuron is only one of many influences on that lower motor neuron (see Chapter 9). The origins and functions of the tracts in the spinal cord are listed in Table 12-3.

Classification of Spinal Interneurons

In most textbooks, spinal interneurons are considered only in the context of reflexes. To study interneurons, experimenters have often disconnected the spinal cord from the brain, stimulated only one type of afferent neuron, and then recorded from interneurons. These experiments led to the concept of reflexes as an invariant coupling of input and output, with discrete spinal circuits dedicated to each reflex. Voluntary movement was considered to be entirely separate from reflexes. Although reductionism may be required to simplify the system for experiments, interneurons do not normally function with isolated inputs. Subsequent research has demonstrated the following:

- Natural stimuli simultaneously excite a variety of receptor types. For example, flexing a joint stimulates

Table 12-3 ORIGINS AND FUNCTIONS OF TRACTS OF THE SPINAL CORD

Tract	Origin	Function
Dorsal column/medial lemniscus	Peripheral receptors; first-order neuron synapses in medulla	Conveys information about discriminative touch and conscious proprioception
Spinothalamic	Dorsal horn of spinal cord	Conveys discriminative information about pain and temperature
Spinolimbic, spinomesencephalic, spinoreticular	Dorsal horn of spinal cord	Nonlocalized perception of pain; arousal, reflexive, motivational, and analgesic responses to nociception
Spinocerebellar	High-fidelity paths originate in peripheral receptors; first-order neurons synapse in nucleus dorsalis or medulla	Conveys unconscious proprioceptive information
	Internal feedback tracts originate in the dorsal horn of the spinal cord	Conveys information about activity in descending activating pathways and spinal interneurons
Lateral corticospinal	Supplementary motor, premotor, and primary motor cerebral cortex	Fractionation of movement, particularly of hand movements
Medial corticospinal	Supplementary motor, premotor, and primary motor cerebral cortex	Control of neck, shoulder, and trunk muscles
Tectospinal	Superior colliculus of midbrain	Reflexive movement of head toward sounds or visual moving objects
Rubrospinal	Red nucleus of midbrain	Facilitates contralateral upper limb flexors
Medial reticulospinal	Pontine reticular formation	Facilitates postural muscles and limb extensors
Lateral reticulospinal	Medullary reticular formation	Facilitates flexor muscle motor neurons, and inhibits extensor motor neurons
Medial vestibulospinal	Vestibular nuclei in medulla and pons	Adjusts activity in neck and upper back muscles
Lateral vestibulospinal	Vestibular nuclei in medulla and pons	Ipsilaterally facilitates lower motor neurons to extensors; inhibits lower motor neurons to flexors
Ceruleospinal	Locus ceruleus in brainstem	Enhances the activity of interneurons and motor neurons in spinal cord
Raphespinal	Raphe nucleus in brainstem	Same as ceruleospinal

muscle spindles, Golgi tendon organs, joint stretch and pressure receptors, and cutaneous stretch and pressure receptors.

- Afferent and descending information converges on the same spinal interneurons.
- Reflexes and voluntary control act together to produce goal-oriented movements. Reflexes are not hardwired but depend upon the environmental context and the task.

By integrating volleys of peripheral, ascending, and descending inputs, spinal circuitry provides the following:

- Modulation of sensory information
- Coordination of movement patterns
- Autonomic regulation

In this text, interneurons are categorized by function.* Modulation of sensory information was covered in Chapter 7 and will not be considered here. The other mechanisms will be discussed individually for simplicity; however, recall that none of these mechanisms act in isolation.

SPINAL CORD MOTOR COORDINATION

Interneuronal circuits integrate the activity from all sources and then adjust the output of lower motor neurons. Thus interneurons coordinate activity in all the muscles when a limb moves.

What determines whether a single alpha motor neuron will fire? The summation of activity at 20,000 to 50,000 synapses determines whether an alpha motor neuron will fire. These synapses provide information from the following:

- Ia, Ib, and II afferents
- Interneurons
- Descending tracts, including the medial, lateral, and nonspecific activation pathways

In normal movement, motor activity elicited by descending commands can be modified by afferent input. The contribution of interneurons to this modification is illustrated in Figure 12-8.

Alternatively, descending commands can also modify the motor activity elicited by afferent input. Jendrassik's

*HISTORICAL NOTE: Until recently, spinal interneurons were categorized according to the earliest discovery of associated afferents. Thus, interneurons activated by type Ia spindle afferents are often called type Ia inhibitory interneurons, despite subsequent findings that these interneurons are also strongly influenced by other afferents and by descending tracts.

maneuver provides a demonstration of the effect of descending influences on alpha motor neurons. The maneuver consists of voluntary contraction of certain muscles during reflex testing of other muscles. For example, subjects hook their flexed fingers together, and

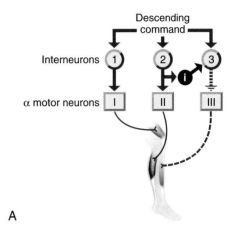

A

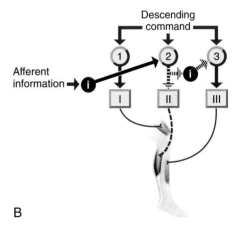

B

FIGURE 12-8
Modification of the action of descending commands by afferent information. At the bottom of both **A** and **B** are three muscles in the lower limb. Solid lines indicate active axons. Dotted lines indicate inactive axons. **A,** Descending commands stimulate all three interneurons (1, 2, and 3). A collateral of interneuron 2 excites an interneuron (black) that inhibits interneuron 3. As a result, alpha motor neurons I and II fire, and III is silent. **B,** Afferent input excites an interneuron (black) that inhibits interneuron 2. As a result, alpha motor neurons I and III fire, and II is silent. *(Modified from McCrea DA (1994). Can sense be made of spinal interneuron circuits? In P Cordo and S Harnad (Eds.), Movement Control. (pp. 31-41). Cambridge, England: Cambridge University Press.)*

then pull isometrically against their own resistance; this activity facilitates the quadriceps deep tendon reflex by producing a generalized increase in spinal interneuron activity. In Jendrassik's maneuver, activity in descending activating tracts contributes to increasing the general level of excitation in the cord.

The following pattern generating, reflexive, and inhibitory circuits are examples of connections that use interneuron activity to shape motor output.

Stepping Pattern Generators

Stepping pattern generators are adaptable neural networks that produce rhythmic output (see Chapter 9). Stepping pattern generators (SPGs) contribute to stepping by activating lower motor neurons, eliciting alternating flexion and extension at the hips and knees. In humans, SPGs are normally activated when the person voluntarily sends signals from the brain to the SPGs in the spinal cord to initiate walking. SPG neurons are activated in sequence (Figure 12-9, *A*). At specific times in the sequence, signals from branches of SPG neurons activate lower motor neurons innervating flexor muscles. At other times in the sequence, lower motor neurons to extensor muscles are activated. Thus spinal SPG activity elicits repetitive, rhythmic, alternating flexion and extension movements of the hips and knees. Each of the lower limbs has a dedicated SPG. The reciprocal movements of the lower limbs during walking are coordinated by signals conveyed in the anterior commissure of the spinal cord (Lanuza et al., 2004).

The processing of proprioceptive information in the SPG produces a biomechanical snapshot at a specific time. When a person is walking or running, information from all of the activated proprioceptors is processed to create a proprioceptive image of time and space. The SPG computes the exact position of the limb, the status of muscle contractions, and the relationship of the limb to the environment. The somatosensory information affecting SPG function is shown in Figure 12-9, *B*. Thus SPGs interpret somatosensory input within the context of a task and the environment, then predict and program the appropriate actions (Edgerton et al., 2004). For example, the proprioceptive input from the stretched iliopsoas at the end of stance phase triggers initiation of swing phase (Stecina et al., 2005).

SPG output is adapted to the task, the environment, and the stage of the walking cycle. Walking requires different SPG output than running. If you step off a sidewalk onto sand, your SPGs alter their output to adapt your stepping movements to the changed environment. The effect of somatosensation on SPG activity

depends upon the stage of the step cycle. For example, during the flexor phase of walking, input from flexor muscle GTOs facilitates motor neurons to flexor muscles, and during extensor phase the same input inhibits motor neurons to flexor muscles (Quevedo et al., 2000). Another

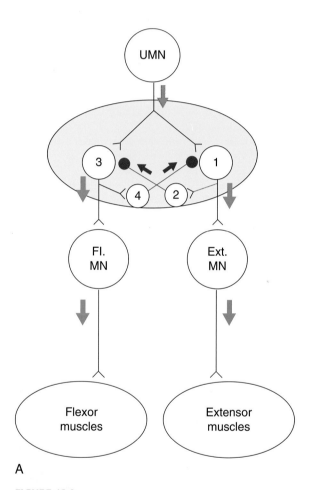

A

FIGURE 12-9

A simplified conceptual model of a stepping pattern generator (SPG). **A,** Only the motor pathways are shown. The SPG is represented by the neurons within the large oval. Firing of the upper motor neuron (UMN) initiates cycles of activity in the SPG. SPG neuron 1 activates extensor motor neurons that signal extensor muscles to contract. Collaterals from neuron 1 synapse with an inhibitory interneuon (neuron 2), inhibiting neuron 3. When the interneuron fatigues, neuron 3 begins firing, activating flexor motor neurons that signal flexor muscles to contract. Collaterals from neuron 3 synapse with an inhibitory interneuron (neuron 4) inhibiting neuron 1. When this interneuron fatigues, neuron 1 resumes firing.

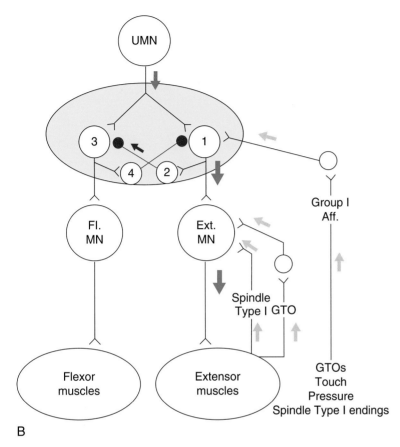

B

FIGURE 12-9, cont'd

B, The sensory pathways have been added to the right side of the illustration. Neural activity during stance phase is indicated by arrows. Sensory information from the muscle spindle Type I endings and the Golgi tendon organs (GTOs) feeds back to the extensor motor neurons. The pathway from the GTO to the extensor motor neuron pool involves an interneuron (IN). Type I afferents convey information from muscle spindle type I endings, Golgi tendon organs, and touch and pressure receptors to adjust activity in the SPG. During stance phase, GTO input facilitates the extensor motor neurons. Similar sensory pathways are present on the left (flexor) side but have been omitted to simplify the diagram. *(Developed from models in Lam T, Pearson K (2002). The role of proprioceptive feedback in the regulation and adaptation of locomotor activity. In S Gandevia, U Proske, et al. (Eds.), Sensorimotor Control of Movement and Posture. Kluwer Academic/Plenum Publishers: New York, and from Quevedo J, Fedirchuk B, et al. (2000). Group I disynaptic excitation of cat hindlimb flexor and bifunctional motoneurones during fictive locomotion. Journal of Physiology, 525(Pt 2), 549-564.)*

example is the modification of the withdrawal reflex elicited during gait (Figure 12-10).

When a person is walking, electrical stimulation to a single point on the foot produces different responses depending upon the phase of the gait cycle. If the stimulus occurs at the onset of swing phase, tibialis anterior activity increases. If the stimulus occurs at the end of swing phase, tibialis anterior activity decreases and antagonist muscle activity increases (Duysens et al., 2004). This response reversal adapts the ongoing activity of the stepping pattern generators to the task and environment. At the start of swing phase, dorsiflexion is required to clear the foot. However, at the end of swing phase, increasing tibialis anterior contraction would prevent appropriate positioning of the foot for weight bearing. Plantarflexion during late swing would result in faster whole foot contact with the ground (Duysens et al., 2004).

Human SPGs are normally activated when a person initiates walking by sending signals from the brain to the spinal cord. However, after spinal cord injury, SPGs can be activated by artificial stimulation. When the spinal cord is completely severed, the brain cannot communicate with the cord below the level of the lesion. Therefore, a complete thoracic lesion causes paralysis of voluntary movements of the lower limbs. However, a lumbar spinal cord isolated from the brain is still capable of generating near-normal reciprocal lower limb movements similar to walking. Patients with complete spinal cord injuries can experience steppinglike movements of the lower limbs following nonpatterned electrical stimulation of the posterior lumbar spinal cord. Minassian et al. (2004) electrically stimulated the lumbar spinal cord in people with complete spinal cord lesions, using an electrode on the surface of the dura mater. During stimulation, an electromyogram (EMG, recording of the electrical activity produced by muscle fibers) and lower limb joint movement were recorded. The electrical stimulation elicited rhythmic steplike EMG activity and flexion-extension movements of the lower limbs

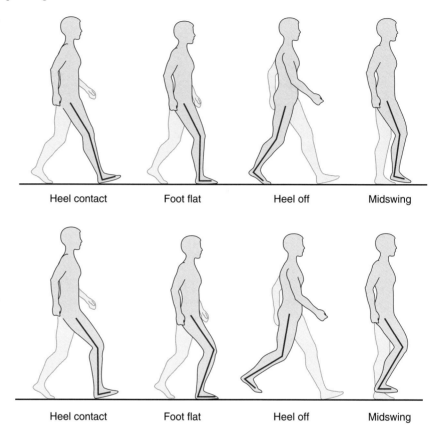

FIGURE 12-10

The withdrawal reflex induces changes in joint angles during walking. **A,** Normal hip, knee, and ankle joint angles at four points during the gait cycle. **B,** Joint angle changes induced by electrically stimulating the mid-medial sole of the foot. Maximal increases in joint angles occurred when stimulation occurred during the swing phase. During swing, the response to electrical stimulation increased the average maximal hip flexion by 9°, knee flexion by 20°, and dorsiflexion by 4°. *(Modified from Spaich EG, Arendt-Nielsen L, et al. (2004). Modulation of lower limb withdrawal reflexes during gait: A topographical study. Journal of Neurophysiology, 91(1), 258-266.)*

Heel contact   Foot flat   Heel off   Midswing

Heel contact   Foot flat   Heel off   Midswing

(Figure 12-11). However, without additional neural control, the alternating flexion/extension elicited by SPG activity is inadequate to produce walking. Postural control, cortical control of dorsiflexion (Capaday et al. 1999), and afferent information to adapt movements to the environment and task are also essential for normal human walking. See Burke et al. (2001) for a review of the structure of stepping pattern generators.

Sensory input strongly influences the output of stepping pattern generators in people with spinal cord lesions. When subjects with minimal or no sensory or voluntary motor function below the level of the injury are manually assisted in walking on a treadmill, their lower motor neuron output is modulated by sensory input. Despite the lack of upper motor neuron input to lower motor neurons, information about hip joint position, cutaneous stimulation, and contralateral limb position contribute to patterns of lower motor neuron activity (Harkema et al., 1997). Sensory input from bilateral alternate leg movements amplifies induced locomotor-type activity of the lower limbs in people

with complete spinal cord injuries, indicating that the spinal cord is able to coordinate lower limb walking movements despite being deprived of information from the brain (Kawashima et al., 2005).

Reflexes

Except for the monosynaptic phasic stretch reflex, spinal reflexes involve interneurons. The phasic and tonic stretch reflexes, reciprocal inhibition, and withdrawal reflexes were introduced as spinal region reflexes in Chapter 9. In this chapter the focus is on the capacity of interneuronal circuits to generate complex movements. This is demonstrated by the **withdrawal reflex.** Afferent information from skin, muscles, and/or joints can elicit a variety of withdrawal movements. Each withdrawal movement is specific for most effectively removing the stimulated area away from the provocation. For example, if one steps on a tack, the involved lower limb flexes to remove the foot from the stimulus. However, if a bee stings the inside of one's calf, the lower limb abducts. The specificity of the movement pattern is

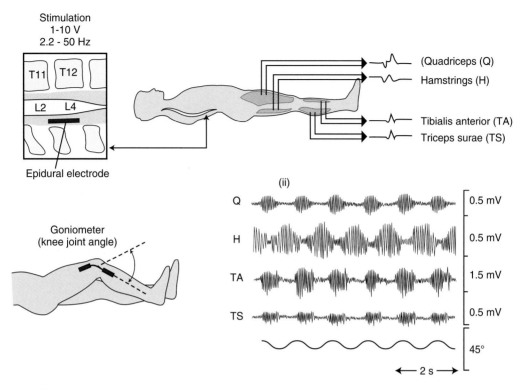

FIGURE 12-11

In a patient with complete spinal cord injury, electrical stimulation of the posterior spinal roots elicits stepping-like movements. **A,** A stimulating electrode has been implanted inside the T11 and T12 vertebra, outside the dura at the L2-L4 spinal cord levels. The patient is supine during the electrical stimulation. **B,** Epidural electrical stimulation at a rate of 31 Hz produces rhythmic EMG activity in the quadriceps (Q), hamstrings (H), tibialis anterior (TA), and triceps surae (TS). The EMG activity produces alternating knee flexion and extension (knee movement = KM). *(Modified from Minassian K, Jilge B, et al. (2004). Stepping-like movements in humans with complete spinal cord injury induced by epidural stimulation of the lumbar cord: Electromyographic study of compound muscle action potentials. Spinal Cord, 42(7), 401-416.)*

referred to as local sign, indicating that the response depends on the site of stimulation. Because the muscles removing the part from the stimulation are usually not innervated by the same cord segment that received the afferent input, the information is relayed to other cord segments by collaterals of the primary afferent and by interneurons. In an intact nervous system, the stimulation must be quite strong to evoke a powerful withdrawal reflex. If one is standing when one lower limb is abruptly withdrawn, another interneuronal circuit quickly adjusts the muscle activity in the stance limb to prevent falling; this is the **crossed extension reflex.** The withdrawal and the associated crossed extension reflexes are illustrated in Figure 12-12.

Inhibitory Circuits

Interneurons in inhibitory circuits also contribute to spinal cord motor coordination. Inhibitory interneurons provide the following:

- Reciprocal inhibition
- Recurrent inhibition

Reciprocal Inhibition

Reciprocal inhibition decreases activity in an antagonist when an agonist is active, allowing the agonist to act unopposed. When agonists are voluntarily recruited, the reciprocal inhibition interneurons prevent unwanted activity in the antagonists (Figure 12-13). Thus,

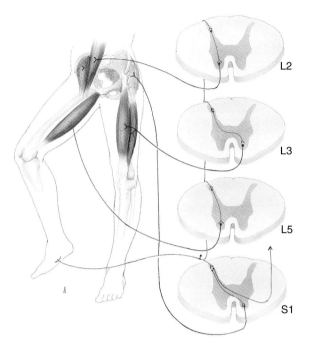

FIGURE 12-12
Withdrawal reflex in the right leg, and crossed extension reflex in the left leg. The interaction of several spinal cord segments is required to produce the coordinated muscle action.

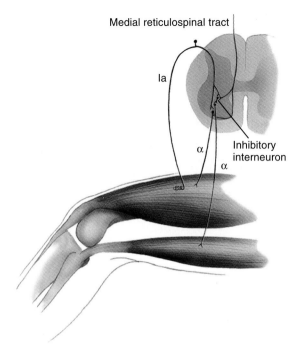

FIGURE 12-13
Reciprocal inhibition. For simplicity, only the medial reticulospinal input to an alpha motor neuron activating fibers in the quadriceps and to a reciprocal inhibition interneuron inhibiting an alpha motor neuron to fibers in the semitendinosus muscle are shown.

reciprocal inhibition separates muscles into agonists and antagonists. For efficient motor control, collaterals of descending pathways activate reciprocal inhibitory interneurons simultaneously with excitation of selected lower motor neurons.

Type Ia, cutaneous, and joint afferents, other interneurons, and cortico-, rubro-, and vestibulospinal tracts provide input to reciprocal inhibition interneurons (see review in McCrea, 1994). Reciprocal inhibition occurs with afferent input as well as during voluntary movement. For example, during a quadriceps stretch reflex, reciprocal inhibition interneurons inhibit the hamstrings. Occasionally, reciprocal inhibition is suppressed to allow cocontraction of antagonists. This occurs in people with intact nervous systems when they are anxious, anticipate unpredictable movement disturbances, or are learning new movements.

Recurrent Inhibition

Recurrent inhibition has effects opposite to reciprocal inhibition: inhibition of agonists and synergists, with disinhibition of antagonists (Figure 12-14). **Renshaw cells,** interneurons that produce recurrent inhibition, are stimulated by a recurrent collateral branch from the alpha motor neuron. A recurrent collateral branch is a side branch of an axon that turns back toward its own cell body. Renshaw cells inhibit the same alpha motor neuron that gives rise to the collateral and also inhibit alpha motor neurons of synergists. Renshaw cells focus motor activity, thus isolating desired motor activity from gross activation (Chalmers and Knutzen, 2004). Loss of descending influence on Renshaw cell activity may cause difficulty in achieving fine-motor control.

Reciprocal inhibition decreases antagonist opposition to the action of agonist muscles. Recurrent inhibition focuses motor activity.

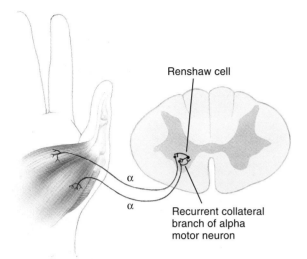

Renshaw cell

α

α

Recurrent collateral
branch of alpha
motor neuron

FIGURE 12-14

Recurrent inhibition. The recurrent collateral branch of the
alpha motor neuron stimulates the Renshaw cell. The Renshaw
cell inhibits agonists and synergists and facilitates antagonists.
For simplicity, the antagonist facilitation is not shown.

SPINAL CONTROL OF PELVIC ORGAN FUNCTION

The sacral spinal cord contains centers for the control of
urination, bowel function, and sexual function. In a
normal infant, when the bladder is empty, the sympathetic efferents from T11-L2 levels inhibit contraction
of the bladder wall and maintain contraction of the internal sphincter (Figure 12-15, *A*). When the bladder fills,
proprioceptors sense the stretching of the bladder wall,
impulses regarding fullness of the bladder are transmitted to the reflex center in the sacral cord, and efferent
impulses initiate voiding. Parasympathetic impulses
stimulate bladder wall contraction and open the internal
sphincter; somatic efferents (S2-S4) open the external
sphincter (Figure 12-15, *B*). Thus, **reflexive bladder
function,** which is normal in infants, requires the
following:

- Afferents
- T11-L2 and S2-S4 cord levels
- Somatic, sympathetic, and parasympathetic efferents

Even when voluntary control of voiding is achieved,
bladder filling remains primarily an involuntary process,
controlled by sympathetic signals that induce relaxation
of the bladder wall and contraction of the internal
sphincter. For voluntary control of voiding, three central

nervous system urination centers are essential. The
centers are located in the frontal cortex, pons, and sacral
spinal cord. When the bladder is filling, the frontal
cortex urination center inhibits the pontine urination
center, to prevent the pons from signaling the sacral
urination center to empty the bladder. If the bladder is
full but circumstances are not appropriate for urination,
the frontal lobe urination center signals corticospinal
neurons to lower motor neurons that control pelvic floor
muscle contraction. Contraction of the levator ani
compresses the bladder neck, thus assisting the external
sphincter in preventing urination (Madersbacher,
2004).

When the bladder is full and conditions are appropriate, the frontal cortex initiates voiding by disinhibition
of the pontine urination center. The pontine urination
center then signals "GO" to the sacral spinal cord urination center, which sends signals via parasympathetic
neurons to stimulate contraction of the bladder wall and
relax the internal sphincter (Figure 12-16). Simultaneously, signals from the pontine center to the spinal cord
facilitate neurons that inhibit the external sphincter and
inhibit pelvic floor muscles; together, these actions
empty the bladder (Madersbacher, 2004). See Box 12-1,
which summarizes neural control of the bladder.

Bowel control is similar to bladder control. The signal
to empty the bowels is stimulation of stretch receptors
in the wall of the rectum. Afferent fibers transmit the
information to the lumbar and sacral cord, the information is conveyed to the brain, and, if appropriate, the
efferent signal is sent to relax the sphincters.

The lower spinal cord is also vital for sexual function.
Erection of the penis or clitoris is controlled by parasympathetic fibers from S2-S4 spinal cord levels, and ejaculation is elicited by sympathetic nerves originating
in L1-L2 and the pudendal nerve with cell bodies in
S2-S4.

Reflexive functions of the bladder, bowels, and male sexual
organ require intact afferents, lumbar and sacral cord segments, and somatic and autonomic efferents. Voluntary
control of these functions requires intact neural pathways
between the organ and the cerebral cortex.

EFFECTS OF SEGMENTAL AND TRACT LESIONS IN THE SPINAL REGION

A lesion in the spinal region may interfere with the
following:

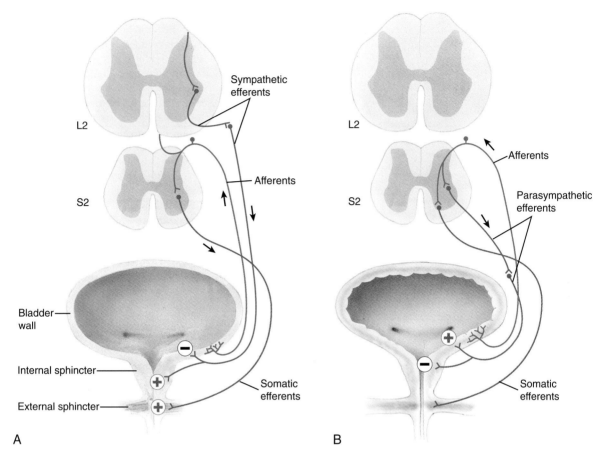

FIGURE 12-15
Reflexive control of the bladder. **A,** Bladder is filling. Afferents convey information regarding stretch of the bladder wall to the spinal cord. Signals in sympathetic efferents maintain relaxation of the bladder wall and constriction of the internal sphincter. Somatic efferent signals elicit contraction of the external sphincter. **B,** When the bladder is full, reflexive voiding is initiated by signals in the parasympathetic efferents, producing contraction of the bladder wall and relaxation of the internal sphincter. Decreased somatic efferent activity produces relaxation of the external sphincter. Plus signs (+) indicate facilitation, and minus signs (−) indicate inhibition.

- Segmental function
- Vertical tract function
- Both segmental and vertical tract function

Segmental Function

Segmental function is the function of a spinal cord segment. Segmental lesions interfere with neural function only at the level of the lesion. For example, complete severance of the C5 dorsal root (roots are considered within the spinal region, although not in the spinal cord) would prevent sensory information from the C5 derma-tome, myotome, and sclerotome from reaching the spinal cord.

Vertical Tract Function

Vertical tracts convey ascending and descending information. Lesions interrupting the vertical tracts result in a loss of function below the level of the lesion. A complete lesion prevents sensory information from below the lesion from ascending to higher levels of the central nervous system and prevents descending signals from reaching levels of the spinal cord below the lesion.

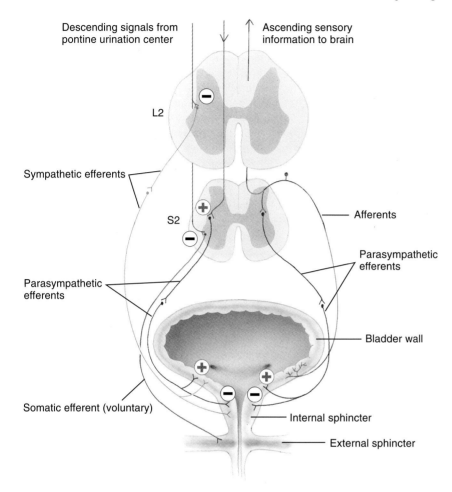

Descending signals from pontine urination center

Ascending sensory information to brain

L2

Sympathetic efferents

S2

Afferents

Parasympathetic efferents

Parasympathetic efferents

Bladder wall

Somatic efferent (voluntary)

Internal sphincter

External sphincter

FIGURE 12-16
Neural control of the bladder. Efferents and descending signals from the brain are indicated on the left side of the illustration. Ascending sensory neurons, afferents, and a reflexive connection between afferents and parasympathetic efferents are shown on the right.

BOX 12-1 NEURAL CONTROL OF THE BLADDER

To Allow Bladder Filling
From sacral spinal cord urination center:
- **Sympathetic signals** *relax the bladder wall and constrict internal sphincter*
- **Somatic signals** *constrict external sphincter*
- **Frontal cortex** *inhibits the pontine urination center, to prevent bladder wall from contracting until voiding is socially appropriate*

If the urge to void is powerful but circumstances are inappropriate, **corticospinal signals** *to lower motor neurons elicit contraction of pelvic floor muscles to reinforce the contraction of the external sphincter*

To Empty Bladder
- **Frontal cortex** *releases the pontine urination center from inhibition*
- **Pontine urination center** *provides the "GO" signal to the sacral spinal cord for emptying the bladder; the signals from the pons facilitate sacral spinal cord parasympathetic activity and inhibit sympathetic activity*
- *From sacral spinal cord urination center: parasympathetic signals elicit contraction of the bladder wall and relax the internal sphincter*

Segmental and Vertical Tract Function

Spinal region lesions may cause both segmental and tract signs. A lesion at the C5 level on the right that involves the right dorsal quadrant would prevent discriminative touch and conscious proprioception from the right side of the body below C5 from reaching the brain (tract signs), and the sensory information from the C5 dermatome, myotome, and sclerotome would be lost (segmental signs).

Signs of Segmental Dysfunction

A focal lesion involving a single level of the spinal cord, the dorsal or ventral roots, or a spinal nerve results in segmental signs due to interruption of pathways. At the level of the lesion, sensory, motor, and/or reflexive changes occur. In Figure 12-17, the effects of a C5 spinal nerve lesion are contrasted with the effects of a C5 hemisection of the spinal cord. Autonomic signs are difficult to detect with a lesion at a single level because of the overlapping distribution of autonomic fibers from adjacent cord segments.

A lesion of the dorsal root, spinal nerve, or dorsal horn interferes with sensory function in a spinal segment, causing abnormal sensations or loss of sensation in a dermatomal distribution. For example, a dorsal root can be avulsed from the cervical spinal cord by extreme traction on the upper limb. If avulsion occurs at C5, the spinal cord is deprived of sensory information from the C5 dermatome, myotome (proprioceptive and muscle pain information), and sclerotome innervated by that dorsal root.

A lesion of the ventral horn, ventral root, or spinal nerve interferes with lower motor neuron function. Signs of lower motor neuron dysfunction include flaccid weakness, atrophy, fibrillation, and fasciculation. If lower motor neuron signs occur in a myotomal pattern (see Chapter 9), the lesion is in the spinal region. A myotome includes paraspinal muscles, so signs of paraspinal involvement help differentiate spinal region from peripheral nerve lesions. Reflexes are absent if either the motor or sensory fibers contributing to the reflex circuit are damaged.

Segmental signs include abnormal or lost sensation in a dermatomal distribution and/or lower motor neuron signs in a myotomal distribution.

Signs of Vertical Tract Dysfunction

Lesions interrupting the vertical tracts result in loss of communication to and/or from the spinal levels below the lesion. Therefore, all signs of damage to the vertical tracts occur below the level of the lesion. Ascending tract (sensory information) signs are ipsilateral if the dorsal column is interrupted and contralateral if the spinothalamic tracts are involved because the dorsal columns remain ipsilateral throughout the cord, while the spinothalamic tracts cross the midline within a few levels of where the information enters the cord. Autonomic signs may include problems with regulation of blood pressure, sweating, and bladder and bowel control.

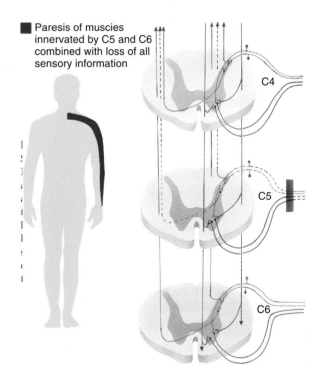

Paresis of muscles innervated by C5 and C6 combined with loss of all sensory information

C4

C5

C6

FIGURE 12-17
Spinal region lesions: segmental signs versus vertical tract signs. Dotted lines indicate neural pathways that have been interrupted and do not convey information. **A,** The lesion interrupts all axons in the left C5 spinal nerve. This produces loss of sensation from the C5 dermatome and weakness of the biceps and brachioradialis, partially innervated by the C5 spinal nerve. The biceps and brachioradialis are not paralyzed because C6 also supplies these muscles. Thus the losses are limited to only part of the left arm. The entire remainder of the nervous system functions normally.

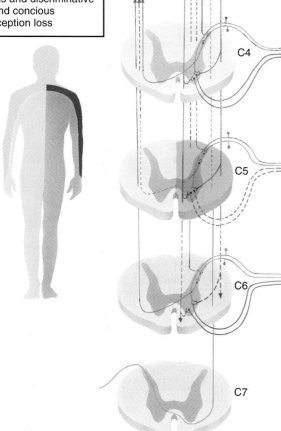

Analgesia and loss
of discriminative
temperature sensation

Paralysis combined
with loss of all sensory
information

Paralysis and discriminative
touch and concious
proprioception loss

C4

C5

C6

C7

FIGURE 12-17, cont'd
B, In contrast, the hemisection of the cord at
C5 produces the following conditions below
the C5 level: paralysis on the left side, loss of
discriminative touch and conscious proprioceptive
information from the left side, and analgesia and
loss of discriminative temperature sensation from
the right side. In addition, the segmental losses are
the same as in lesion **A.**

Descending tract (upper motor neuron) signs include
paralysis, hyperreflexia, and muscle hypertonia; if the
lateral corticospinal tract is interrupted, Babinski's sign
(see Chapter 9) is present. Deep tendon reflex testing
(biceps, triceps, patellar, and tendo calcaneus [see Chapter
7]) may help to distinguish between upper motor neuron
and lower motor neuron involvement: hyperreflexia indicates upper motor neuron, and hyporeflexia or areflexia
may indicate lower motor neuron involvement. However,
hyporeflexia or areflexia may also occur with damage to
type Ia afferents.

An incomplete bilateral lesion at the C5 level limited
to the dorsal columns would prevent ascending conscious
proprioceptive and discriminative touch information
from reaching the brain. Thus a person with a spinal
cord tumor that damaged the dorsal columns at C5
would not be aware of the location of light touch or
passive joint movement below the C5 level but would
be able to distinguish between sharp and dull stimuli,
locations of pinprick, and among different temperatures.
Information in the descending pathways would also be
intact, although coordination would be somewhat

impaired because of the lack of conscious proprioceptive information.

Differentiating Spinal Region From Peripheral Region Lesions

Peripheral region lesions produce deficits in the distribution of a peripheral nerve. Peripheral nerve lesions cause:

- Altered or lost sensation in a peripheral nerve distribution
- Decrease or loss of muscle power in a peripheral nerve distribution
- No vertical tract signs

Spinal region segmental signs occur when nerve roots and/or spinal nerves are compromised. Segmental signs include:

- Altered or lost sensation in a dermatome
- Decreased or lost muscle power in a myotome
- Decreased or lost phasic stretch reflex

Spinal region vertical tract signs include:

- Altered or lost sensation below the level of the lesion
- Altered or lost descending control of blood pressure, pelvic viscera, and thermoregulation

Upper motor neuron signs include:

- Decrease or loss of muscle power
- Hyperreflexia
- Muscle hyperstiffness
- If the lateral corticospinal tract is involved, positive Babinski's sign and clonus

SPINAL REGION SYNDROMES

Syndromes are a collection of signs and symptoms that do not indicate a specific etiology. The following syndromes usually result from tumors or trauma (Figure 12-18):

- Anterior cord syndrome (Figure 12-18, *A*) interrupts ascending spinothalamic tracts and descending motor tracts and damages the somas of lower motor neurons. Thus anterior cord syndrome interferes with pain and temperature sensation and with motor control. Because tracts conveying proprioception and discriminative touch information are located in the posterior cord, these functions are spared.
- Central cord syndrome (Figure 12-18, *B*) usually occurs at the cervical level. If the lesion is small, loss of pain and temperature information occurs at the level of the lesion because spinothalamic fibers crossing the midline are interrupted. Larger lesions addi-

tionally impair upper limb motor function, due to the medial location of upper limb fibers in the lateral corticospinal tracts.

- Brown-Séquard syndrome (Figure 12-18, *C*) results from a hemisection of the cord. Segmental losses are ipsilateral and include loss of lower motor neurons and all sensations. Below the level of the lesion, voluntary motor control, conscious proprioception, and discriminative touch are lost ipsilaterally; pain and temperature sensation are lost contralaterally. This syndrome is also illustrated and explained in Figure 12-17, *B*.
- Cauda equina syndrome (Figure 12-18, *D*) indicates damage to the lumbar and or sacral spinal roots, causing sensory impairment and flaccid paresis or paralysis of lower limb muscles, bladder, and bowels. Muscle hypertonia and hyperreflexia do not occur because the upper motor neurons are intact. See Box 12-2, on cauda equina syndrome.
- **Tethered cord syndrome** (not illustrated). During development, the vertebral column grows longer than the spinal cord (see Chapter 5). Infrequently, the spinal cord becomes attached to surrounding structures during early development. Scar tissue, a fatty mass (lipoma), or abnormal development can lead to tethering of the spinal cord. As the vertebral column elongates, the tethered spinal cord becomes stretched. Stretch injury damages the spinal cord and/or cauda equina (Henderson et al., 2005). The consequences of a tethered spinal cord include low back and lower limb pain, difficulty walking, excessive lordosis, scoliosis, problems with bowel and/or bladder control, and foot deformities. Lower motor neuron signs (weakness, flaccidity) occur if the anterior cauda equina is stretched. Upper motor neuron signs (abnormal reflexes, paresis, and changes in skeletal muscles) occur if the spinal cord is excessively stretched. Often, abnormal signs on the lower back indicate a tethered cord: an unusually located dimple, a tuft of hair, a hemangioma (tangle of blood vessels), or the bulge of a fatty mass. Tethered cord is often associated with myelomeningocele at the L4, L5, or S1 level. In severe cases, surgery may be indicated to untether the cord.

> Syndromes are a collection of signs and symptoms that occur together. Spinal cord syndromes indicate the location of a lesion but do not signify etiology. Thus, an anterior cord syndrome could be caused by trauma, loss of blood supply, or other pathology.

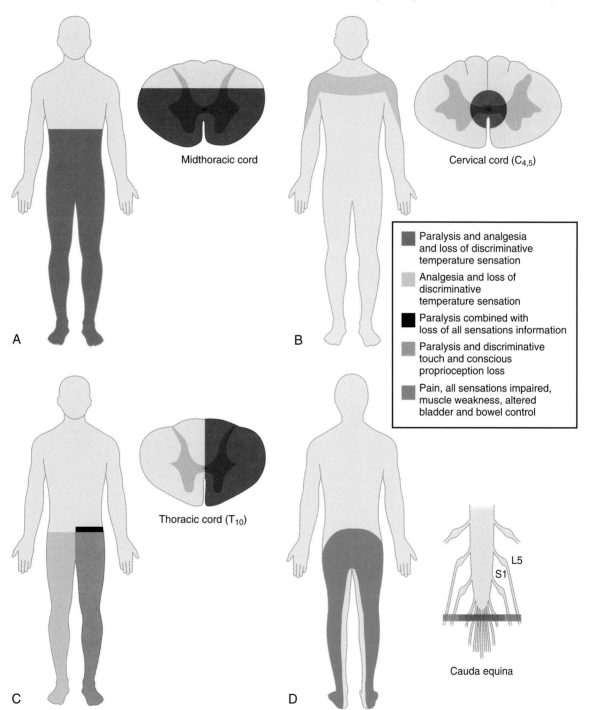

FIGURE 12-18
Spinal cord syndromes: **A,** Anterior. **B,** Central. **C,** Brown-Séquard. **D,** Cauda equina. The cauda equina syndrome shown affects nerve roots L5-S5, causing paralysis of the foot and toe dorsiflexors and plantarflexors, and the bladder and anal sphincters.

BOX 12-2   CAUDA EQUINA SYNDROME

Pathology

Compression and/or irritation of nerve roots below the L2 vertebral level

Etiology

Decreased space in the vertebral canal below L2. Common causes include: herniated disk (may be secondary to narrowing of the vertebral canal and/or long history of heavier than normal loading of the lumbar spine due to work and/or recreation), vertebral fracture, and tumor. 90% of lumbar disk herniations occur at L4-L5 or L5-S1.

Speed of Onset

Usually acute (develops in less than 24 hours); rarely subacute or chronic

Signs and Symptoms

Consciousness

Normal

Communication and Memory

Normal

Sensory

Low back pain and sciatica aggravated by Valsalva maneuver and by sitting; relieved by lying down

Decreased sensation; extent of decreased sensation depends upon the level of the cauda equina affected. The "saddle area" (part of the body that would be in contact with the saddle on a horse; innervated by S2-S5) is usually affected

Autonomic

Retention or incontinence of urine and/or stool

Impotence

Motor

Paresis or paralysis; distribution depends upon the nerve roots affected

Reflexes

Decreased or lost reflexes that involve the impaired nerve roots

Region Affected

Spinal region lumbosacral nerve roots; the lesion does not directly affect the spinal cord

Demographics

Rare

Incidence

Cauda equina syndrome: 3.4 per 1,000,000 people (Podner, 2006)

Operated disk cases: between 1% and 10% (Chang et al., 2000)

Prevalence

9 per 100,000 people (Podner, 2006)

Prognosis

Markedly improves with surgical decompression. Without surgery, greater chance of persistent problems with bladder function, severe motor deficits, pain, and sexual dysfunction (Shapiro, 2000). Recovery correlates with function at initial consult: if patient is ambulatory, likely to continue to be ambulatory; if able to walk with assistance, has 50% chance of independent walking post-surgery; if unable to walk, unlikely to walk after surgery (Della-Guistina, 1999). Recovery is gradual, ranging from months up to five 5 years (Ahn et al., 2000)

Red Flag

Low back pain and/or sciatica combined with bladder or bowel retention or incontinence requires emergency medical referral because cauda equina syndrome may progress to paraplegia and/or to permanent problems with bladder and/or bowel control

EFFECTS OF SPINAL REGION DYSFUNCTION ON PELVIC ORGAN FUNCTION

Control of bladder, bowel, and sexual function depends on the level of cord damage. Lesions above the sacral level of the cord produce signs similar to upper motor neuron lesions. Lesions in the S2-S4 spinal cord levels, the afferents, and/or the parasympathetic efferents produce signs similar to lower motor neuron lesions.

Complete lesions that damage any part of the reflexive bladder emptying circuit—that is, levels S2-S4—or the afferents or parasympathetic efferents—produce a flaccid, paralyzed bladder (Figure 12-19, *A*). The flaccid, paralyzed bladder overfills with urine, and when the bladder cannot stretch any further, urine dribbles out.

In contrast, complete lesions above the sacral cord interrupt descending axons that normally control bladder function but do not interrupt sacral level reflexive control of the bladder. This results in a hypertonic, hyperreflexive bladder with reduced bladder capacity (Figure 12-19,

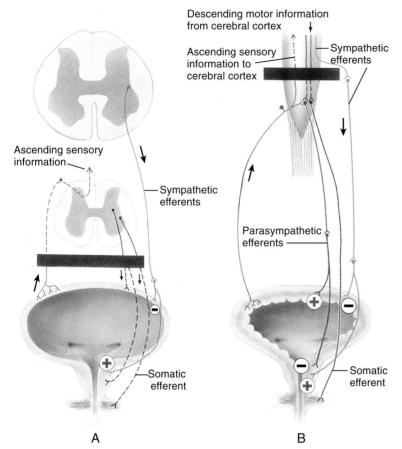

Descending motor information
from cerebral cortex

Sympathetic
efferents

Ascending sensory
information to
cerebral cortex

Ascending sensory
information

Sympathetic
efferents

Parasympathetic
efferents

Somatic
efferent

Somatic
efferent

A

B

FIGURE 12-19

Bladder dysfunction after spinal region injury. Dotted lines indicate neural pathways that have been interrupted and do not convey information. **A,** Flaccid bladder due to a complete lesion of the cauda equina. All neural connections with the bladder are severed, except the sympathetic efferents. A complete lesion of spinal cord levels S2-S4 would also produce a flaccid bladder, owing to interruption of the reflexive bladder emptying circuit. **B,** Hypertonic bladder caused by a complete lesion above the S2 level. Communication between the brain and the sacral level parasympathetic neurons controlling the bladder are interrupted, preventing voluntary control. The reflexive connections between the bladder and spinal cord are intact, so reflexive emptying of the bladder can occur.

B). Because the reflex circuit for bladder emptying is intact, reflexive emptying may occur automatically whenever the bladder is stretched; or, if the sphincter is also hypertonic, flow of urine is functionally obstructed and the kidneys can be damaged (Aslan and Kogan, 2002).

Bowel control and sexual organ function are similarly affected by spinal cord lesions because the parasympathetic reflexive connections for these organs are also located at levels S2-S4. The person with a spinal cord lesion above the sacral cord is unaware of rectal stretch and has no voluntary control of sphincters, yet rectal stretch can elicit reflexive emptying of the lower bowel because the reflexive lower bowel emptying circuit is intact. If the bowel emptying reflex circuit is interrupted by a lesion of S2-S4 or the parasympathetic connections with S2-S4, the parasympathetic influence on peristalsis and reflex emptying of the bowels is lost.

Reflexive sexual erection can occur if the sacral cord is intact. In some men with complete spinal lesions above the lumbar level in whom the lumbosacral cord is intact, ejaculation can be elicited reflexively because sympathetic axons from the L1 and L2 levels and somatic nerves from the S2-S4 levels control ejaculation. Fertile women with spinal cord lesions can conceive and often have a normal pregnancy, but they frequently require cesarean delivery.

Complete lesions above the sacral cord interfere with the transmission of sensory information from the pelvic organs to the brain and with descending control of pelvic organ function. Complete sacral spinal cord, afferent neuron, or parasympathetic lesions interfere with reflexive control of the pelvic organs.

TRAUMATIC SPINAL CORD INJURY

Traumatic injuries to the spinal cord are usually caused by motor vehicle accidents, sports injuries, falls, or penetrating wounds. The first three types of injuries typically do not sever the cord. Instead, damage is due to crush, hemorrhage, edema, and infarction. Penetrating wounds, by a knife or a bullet, directly sever neurons in the cord.

Immediately after a traumatic injury to the spinal cord, cord functions below the lesion are depressed or lost. This condition, known as **spinal shock,** is due to interruption of descending tracts that supply tonic facilitation to the spinal cord neurons. During spinal shock, the following are lost or impaired:
- Somatic reflexes, including stretch reflexes, withdrawal reflexes, and crossed extension reflexes are lost.
- Autonomic reflexes, including smooth muscle tone and reflexive emptying of the bladder and bowels, are lost or impaired.

- Autonomic regulation of blood pressure is impaired, resulting in hypotension.
- Control of sweating and piloerection is lost.

Several weeks after the injury, most people experience some recovery of function in the cord, leading to return of reflex activity below the lesion. In some people, spinal neurons become excessively excitable, resulting in stretch reflex hyperreflexia (see Chapter 9). The hyperreflexia develops as neuroplasticity produces new synapses in the reflex pathway (Ditunno et al., 2004).

Damage to the cervical cord results in **tetraplegia** (quadriplegia), with impairment of arm, trunk, lower limb, and pelvic organ function. People with lesions above the C4 level cannot breathe independently, because the phrenic nerve (C3-C5) innervates the diaphragm and thoracic nerves innervate the intercostal and abdominal muscles. **Paraplegia** results from damage to the cord below the cervical level, sparing arm function. Function of the trunk, lower limbs, and pelvic organs in paraplegia depends on the level of the lesion. Table 12-4 lists the motor capabilities and sensations mediated by each spinal cord level.

Table 12-4 FUNCTIONAL ABILITIES ASSOCIATED WITH COMPLETE SPINAL CORD LESIONS AT VARIOUS LEVELS

Level of Lesion	Motor Capability*	Intact Sensation
Above C4	Facial, pharyngeal, laryngeal movements	Neck and head (cranial nerves from face; C2: posterior head, upper neck; C3: lower neck)
C4	Scapular elevation, adduction	
C5	Deltoids, elbow flexion (biceps is innervated by C5 and C6)	Lateral upper arm
C6	Pectoralis major, radial wrist extensors, serratus anterior	Lateral forearm and lateral hand
C7	Triceps (C7, C8), latissimus dorsi	Middle finger
C8	Flexor digitorum muscles	Medial hand
T1	Finger abduction	Medial forearm
T1-T6	Erector spinae above the injury	T2: medial upper arm; T3-T6: torso
T7-T12	Abdominal muscles above the injury	T7-T12: torso (T10: level of umbilicus)
L1	Psoas	Anterior upper thigh
L2	Iliacus	Anterior thigh, below L1
L3	Quadriceps (L3, L4)	Anterior knee
L4	Tibialis anterior	Medial leg
L5	Extensor hallucis longus	Lateral leg, dorsum of foot
S1	Peroneus longus and brevis, triceps surae, hamstrings, gluteus maximus	Posterior calf and lateral foot
S2	—	Posterior thigh
S3	—	Ring surrounding S4-S5
S4-S5	Voluntary anal contraction	Ring surrounding anus

*Each additional level adds functions to the capabilities of the higher levels. Muscles listed may be only partially innervated at the level indicated. Thus the quadriceps usually has some voluntary activity if the L3 level is intact; however, the action is weak unless the L4 level is also intact.

Abnormal Interneuron Activity in Chronic Spinal Cord Injury

Chronic spinal cord injury is the period after recovery from spinal shock when the neurologic deficit is stable, neither progressing nor improving. (See Box 12-3, on chronic spinal cord injury.) This period can last for decades.

In chronic spinal cord injury, two abnormalities occur in interneuron activity below the level of the lesion:

- Inhibitory interneuron response to type Ia afferent activity is diminished.
- Transmission from cutaneous afferents to motor neurons is facilitated.

The first change correlates with hyperreflexia, and the second change occurs because of the loss of descending inhibition by the reticulospinal tracts. The reticulospinal tracts normally inhibit interneurons that produce the withdrawal reflex. Without this inhibition, an exaggerated withdrawal reflex occurs in response to normally innocuous stimuli in some people with spinal cord injuries (Mayer, 1997). For example, light touch on the thigh may trigger a withdrawal reflex of the entire lower limb. Additional changes secondary to spinal cord injury include loss of lower motor neurons and changes in mechanical properties of muscle fibers: atrophy of muscle fibers, fibrosis, and alteration of contractile properties toward tonic muscle characteristics.

Classification of Spinal Cord Injuries

Spinal cord injuries are classified according to two criteria (American Spinal Injury Association, 2002):

- Whether the injury is complete or incomplete
- The neurologic level of injury

A **complete injury** is defined as lack of sensory and motor function in the lowest sacral segment. An **incomplete injury** is defined as preservation of sensory and/or motor function in the lowest sacral segment.

The **neurologic level** is the most caudal level with normal sensory and motor function bilaterally. However, motor function may be impaired at a level different from

---

BOX 12-3   CHRONIC SPINAL CORD INJURY

Pathology
Crush, hemorrhage, edema, and/or infarction

Etiology
Trauma

Speed of Onset
Acute

Signs and Symptoms
Consciousness
Normal
Communication and Memory
Normal
Sensory
Depends on what part of the spinal cord is damaged. In a complete spinal cord lesion, all sensation is lost below the level of the lesion.
Autonomic
Depends on what part of the spinal cord is damaged. In a complete spinal cord lesion, all descending autonomic regulation is lost below the level of the lesion, including voluntary bladder and bowel control; and, if the lesion is above T6, autonomic dysreflexia, poor thermoregulation, and orthostatic hypotension may occur.
Motor
Depends on what part of the spinal cord is damaged. In a complete spinal cord lesion, all voluntary motor control is lost below the level of the lesion.

Region Affected
Spinal region

Demographics
4:1 ratio of males to females; 80% of injuries occur between the ages of 16 and 45 years
Incidence
4 per 100,000 population people per year (Jackson et al., 2004)
Lifetime Prevalence
0.1 per 1000 population people (MacDonald et al., 2000)

Prognosis
Currently no functional regeneration of neurons in the central nervous system occurs in humans. Neurologic recovery, if it occurs, is rapid initially (hours to weeks) as the edema and hemorrhage resolve. People with incomplete spinal cord injuries have much better recovery of function than people with complete spinal cord injuries. Once the lesion is stable (no more bleeding, infarction, edema), the neurologic deficit does not change. People with spinal cord injuries may live a normal life span.

sensory function, and the losses may be asymmetrical. In these cases, up to four different neurologic segments may be described in a single patient: right sensory, left sensory, right motor, and left motor.

Determination of Neurologic Levels

The American Spinal Injury Association (ASIA) has developed a standardized assessment for evaluating

neurologic level in spinal cord injury. The ASIA classification form is presented in Figure 12-20. Key sensory points (28 bilateral points) are tested with a safety pin to determine the person's ability to distinguish sharp from dull, and with light touches with cotton to determine the ability to localize light touch. In addition, testing of deep pressure and of position sense in the index fingers and great toes is recommended. Key muscles are

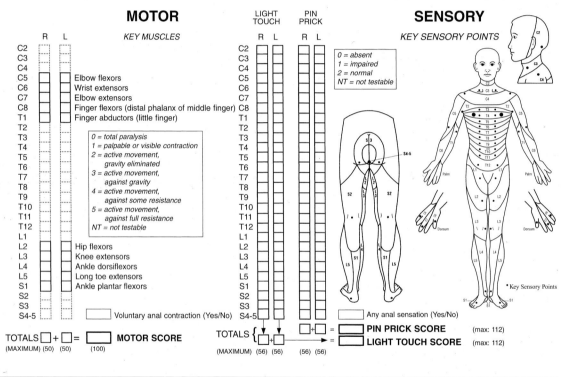

STANDARD NEUROLOGICAL CLASSIFICATION OF SPINAL CORD INJURY

FIGURE 12-20

American Spinal Injury Association classification of spinal cord injury. Motor scores are recorded on the left half of the form. Scoring criteria are listed in the large box. The two columns, headed by the letters R (right) and L (left), are for recording the scores of the listed muscles. To the left of the columns is a list of the segments of the spinal cord. Sensory scores are recorded on the right half of the form. Scoring criteria are listed in the small box. The areas of impaired or absent sensation can be indicated on the dermatome diagrams. At the bottom of the motor and sensory sections are small boxes for totaling motor and sensory scores. The neurologic level is recorded at the bottom of the form, according to the criteria listed there. *(Courtesy American Spinal Injury Association International, Atlanta.)*

tested on the right and left sides of the body. Scoring criteria for each test are listed on the form.

Autonomic Dysfunction in Spinal Cord Injury

During spinal shock, neural control of the pelvic organs is depressed. Therefore, the bladder and bowel walls are atonic, allowing overfilling of these viscera, and overflow leaking occurs (see Figure 12-19, *A*). Overfilling and overflow leaking can be avoided by establishing a regular bladder and bowel emptying routine. After recovery from spinal shock, a complete lesion above the sacral level usually allows some reflexive functioning of the pelvic organs, but voluntary control is not possible, and the person is deprived of conscious awareness of the state of the pelvic organs.

Complete lesions at higher levels of the spinal cord cause more serious abnormalities of autonomic regulation because more segments of the cord are free from descending sympathetic control. Loss of descending sympathetic control due to lesions above T6 results in three dysfunctions:

- Autonomic dysreflexia
- Poor thermoregulation (body temperature regulation)
- Orthostatic hypotension

Autonomic Dysreflexia

Autonomic dysreflexia (also called *mass reflex*) is excessive activity of the sympathetic nervous system, elicited by noxious stimuli below the lesion. Often the precipitating stimulus is overstretching of the bladder or rectum. Collaterals from tract neurons conveying signals regarding noxious input facilitate sympathetic neurons. Normally this facilitation is balanced by inhibitory signals from the brain. Lesions above the T6 level prevent most of the spinal cord from receiving signals from the brain that inhibit sympathetic activity. The excessive sympathetic response is characterized by an abrupt increase in blood pressure and a pounding headache. In addition, flushing of the skin and profuse sweating occur above the level of the lesion. The sudden spike in blood pressure may be life threatening.

Poor Thermoregulation

Poor thermoregulation may interfere with the ability to maintain homeostasis. Normally, body temperature regulation is achieved by descending sympathetic innervation. In spinal cord injury, reflexive sweating below the lesion may be intact; however, interruption of sympathetic pathways prevents thermoregulatory sweating (response to increased ambient temperature) below the level of injury. To compensate, excessive sweating may occur above the level of the lesion. People with complete lesions above the T6 level should avoid exposure to high ambient temperatures because of the risk of heat stroke. The signs of heat stroke are high body temperature, rapid pulse, and dry, flushed skin. These signs indicate a medical emergency because untreated heat stroke can cause permanent brain damage or convulsions and death. In cold weather, hypothermia is a risk because the person with a complete lesion above T6 has lost descending control of blood vessels and the ability to shiver below the lesion. The signs of hypothermia include irritability, mental confusion, hallucinations, lethargy, clumsiness, slow respiration, and slowing of the heartbeat.

Orthostatic Hypotension

Orthostatic hypotension is an extreme fall in blood pressure on assuming an upright position. In people with spinal cord injury, this results from the loss of sympathetic vasoconstriction combined with loss of muscle-pumping action for blood return. Figure 12-21 summarizes the autonomic dysfunctions associated with various levels of spinal cord injury.

Prognosis and Treatment in Spinal Cord Injury

Unlike axons in the peripheral nervous system, severed axons in the adult spinal cord fail to functionally regenerate. The barriers to regeneration include inhibitory molecules on oligodendrocytes, impenetrable glial scars, and decreased rate of growth (compared to embryonic neurons) in mature neurons (Bradbury et al., 2000). However, some of the functional losses after spinal cord injury are not due to the original trauma but are instead due to secondary changes: bleeding, edema, ischemia, pain, and inflammation.

People with incomplete paraplegia have the highest rate of recovery during the first 3 months post injury, with relatively small gains after 3 months. The contrast between functional recovery in complete versus incomplete paraplegia at 1 year post injury is striking. Table 12-5 summarizes ambulation prognosis for people with paraplegia.

Tooth et al. (2003) describe the expected functional outcomes (mobility, self-care, communication, and home management), prevention of complications, and rehabilitation techniques appropriate for the various levels of spinal cord injury. Typical complications after spinal cord injury include urinary tract infection, spasticity, chills and fever, decubiti, autonomic dysreflexia, contractures, heterotropic ossification, and pneumonia (McKinley et al., 2002). Upright posture can provide

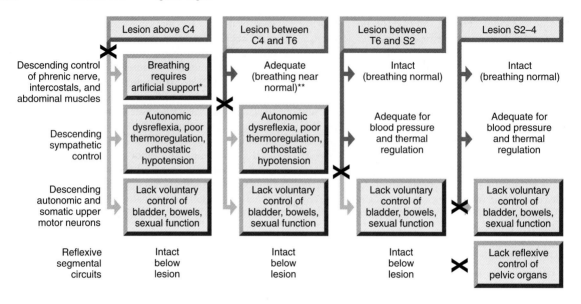

* Ventilator or phrenic nerve stimulator dependent; may learn to breathe using glossopharyngeal technique for short periods.
** Abdominal muscles and lower intercostal muscles do not receive descending control.

FIGURE 12-21
Autonomic dysfunctions associated with various levels of spinal cord injury.

Table 12-5   PERCENTAGE OF PEOPLE WITH DIFFERING ASIA* SCORES ABLE TO WALK AT TIME OF DISCHARGE FROM HOSPITAL

ASIA Impairment Scale Score at Admission	Able to Walk at Time of Discharge
A: Complete. No motor or sensory function is preserved in the sacral segments S4-S5	6%
B: Incomplete. Sensory but not motor function is preserved below the neurologic level and includes the sacral segments S4-S5	23%
C: Incomplete. Motor function is preserved below the neurologic level, and more than ½ of key muscles below the neurologic level have a muscle grade less than 3	50%
D: Incomplete. Motor function is preserved below the neurologic level, and at least half of key muscles below the neurologic level have a muscle grade of 3 or more	89%

*ASIA Impairment Scale from the American Spinal Injury Association. Data on walking ability at discharge from Morganti et al. (2005).

some protection against urinary tract infection and pneumonia; mobility can help avoid contractures and decubiti. Currently strengthening and range of motion exercises, mobility and activities of daily living training, adaptive equipment, and environmental modifications are commonly used in spinal cord injury rehabilitation.

In addition to the commonly used techniques, body-weight-support gait training (BWS-GT) has also been shown to be effective for gait training in people with incomplete spinal cord injury. The patient wears a harness, attached overhead, that supports some of the body weight, and walks on a treadmill with a therapist's assistance for lower limb placement. Wernig et al. (1999) reported the effects of BWS-GT in 44 patients with incomplete spinal cord injury. Prior to training, all but six of the patients used a wheelchair. After completing the training, 38 patients were able to walk using only a walker or a cane. The improvements were maintained at follow-up 0.5-6.5 years after discharge.

Functional electrical stimulation (FES) to restore movement in people with spinal cord injuries is currently primarily an experimental technique, but advances in technology, including combining FES with BWS-GT systems, offer promise for future treatment (Hesse et al., 2004). In humans with long-term degenerated muscle secondary to spinal cord injury, FES training for several years reverses long-term atrophy and does not induce additional damage of myofibers (Carraro et al., 2005).

SPECIFIC DISORDERS AFFECTING SPINAL REGION FUNCTION

Other disorders in addition to traumatic spinal cord injury interfere with spinal region function. These include developmental disorders, lesions of dorsal and ventral nerve roots, multiple sclerosis, and lesions that cause compression in the spinal cord.

Developmental Disorders

Meningomyelocele

Outcomes of meningomyelocele, a developmental defect arising from failure of the inferior neuropore to close (see Chapter 5), are roughly equivalent to spinal cord injury in later life. If the lesion is in the lower lumbar spinal cord, anterior thigh muscles may be functional and sensation intact in the overlying skin, with the remainder of the lower limbs nonmoving and insensitive to sensory stimulation and with no voluntary or reflexive control of the pelvic organs. If the lesion is below S1, bladder and bowel reflexive (as well as voluntary) control is absent because the sacral cord contains the connections for these reflexes, but skeletal muscle control is intact throughout the body and dermatomes are intact above the S2 level.

Spastic Cerebral Palsy

Cerebral palsy is a motor disorder that develops in utero or during infancy. Spastic cerebral palsy is characterized by muscle hyperstiffness and phasic stretch hyperreflexia. The hyperreflexia resulting from overexcitation of local reflex circuits can be inhibited by surgically cutting selected dorsal rootlets, thus decreasing the sensory input to the reflex circuit. Thus, to alleviate lower limb hyperreflexia in children with spastic cerebral palsy, selected

dorsal rootlets are sometimes surgically severed (**dorsal rhizotomy**). Dorsal rhizotomy reduces hyperreflexia by interrupting the afferent limb of the stretch reflex. Each rootlet is electrically stimulated, and only rootlets that contribute to abnormal muscle activity are cut. Dorsal rhizotomy is typically performed at the L2-L5 level. The goals of the surgery are to improve motor function or to make bathing, positioning, and dressing easier. However, motor control remains abnormal following the surgery, and intensive physical therapy is required to maximize benefits from the surgery (McLaughlin et al., 2002). Careful evaluation of the child's potential for improved function is vital prior to the surgery.

Lesions of Dorsal and Ventral Nerve Roots

Lesion of a nerve root is termed **radiculopathy**; however, this term is also often used clinically to refer to damage of a spinal nerve. Mechanical irritation or infection of a dorsal root produces pain in the innervated dermatome and also in the muscles innervated by the spinal cord segment. Mechanical irritation can be produced by a herniated intervertebral disk, a tumor, or a dislocated fracture. However, herniated vertebral disks do not always cause symptoms; Maus (2002) reports that people with herniated disks may be asymptomatic. When a dorsal root is irritated, coughing or sneezing often aggravates the pain.

Other conditions affecting the spinal nerve roots include infections, avulsions, and severance. A common infection of the somas in the dorsal root is varicella zoster, also called *herpes zoster* or *shingles* (see Chapter 7). Avulsion or complete severance of the dorsal root causes loss of sensation in the dermatome. Traumatic avulsion of the C5 and C6 motor nerve roots causes **Erb's paralysis**. This paralysis is the result of forceful separation of the head and shoulder. Birth trauma, produced by traction pulling the head away from the shoulder, and motorcycle accidents in which a person lands on a shoulder often cause Erb's paralysis. Shoulder abduction, external rotation, and elbow flexion are lost, producing the characteristic "waiter's tip" position of the upper limb. The biceps and brachioradialis stretch reflexes are lost.

Klumpke's paralysis, due to avulsion of the motor roots of C8 and T1, results in paralysis and atrophy of the hand intrinsic muscles and the long flexors and extensors of the fingers. The precipitating injury is traction on the abducted arm. A complete severance of a ventral root deprives the muscles in its myotome of motor innervation, resulting in muscle atrophy and fibrillation.

Lesions of Dorsal Root Ganglia

Dorsal root ganglia (DRG), located within the intervertebral foramina, are more sensitive to mechanical damage than the proximal or distal axons of primary nociceptive afferents. DRG compression induces alterations in the production of neuropeptides, receptors (including NMDA receptors), and ion channels in the primary nociceptive afferents. The DRG develop ectopic foci that generate action potentials in response to mechanical stimulation (Song, 2003). Normally action potentials are only generated at the axon hillock (tract and interneurons) or near the receptor (sensory neurons). DRG-generated action potentials are perceived as pain in the distribution of the peripheral axon, resulting in severe hyperalgesia. An example is **sciatica,** pain radiating from the low back and down the lower limb along the path of the sciatic nerve (Govind, 2004). If DRG compression causes sciatica, the pain may be incapacitating. If the nerve roots or peripheral axons are compressed, the pain is less intense. Sciatica may be accompanied by numbness, weakness, and/or tingling sensations. Sciatica is a symptom typically caused by compression of dorsal roots and/or dorsal root ganglia by a herniated disk, spinal stenosis, spondylolisthesis (anterior slipping of one vertebral relative to another), or piriformis syndrome. In piriformis syndrome, the muscle compresses the sciatic nerve.

Multiple Sclerosis

Multiple sclerosis is characterized by random, multifocal demyelination limited to the central nervous system (see Chapter 2). Signs and symptoms of multiple sclerosis are exceptionally variable because the demyelination can occur in a wide variety of locations, and the extent of each lesion also varies. Sensory complaints may include numbness, paresthesias, and **Lhermitte's sign.** Lhermitte's sign is the radiation of a sensation like electrical shock down the back or limbs, elicited by neck flexion. Frequently multiple sclerosis of the spinal cord produces asymmetrical weakness due to plaques interfering with the descending motor tracts and ataxia of the lower limbs due to interruption of conduction in the dorsal columns.

Transverse Myelitis

Transverse myelitis is a rare immune disorder that damages a limited part of the spinal cord. This produces bilateral signs and/or symptoms including weakness; dermatomal sensory signs; upper motor neuron signs; and bladder, bowel, and sexual dysfunction, depending upon the location of the lesion. Transverse myelitis progressively worsens following onset, for up to 3 weeks. The cause may be multiple sclerosis, multisystemic disease, or idiopathic. Recovery usually begins within 6 months. Good recovery occurs in about $1/3$ of cases; another $1/3$ have moderate permanent disability, and $1/3$ have severe disabilities (Kaplin et al., 2005).

Compression in the Spinal Region

Pressure in the spinal region or restriction of blood flow due to compression can cause any of the following symptoms: pain (usually constant), sensory changes, weakness, paralysis, hypertonia, ataxia, and impaired bladder and/or bowel function. The clinical presentation depends on the location of the lesion. Gradual onset, progressive worsening, no history of trauma, and the combination of segmental and vertical tract signs indicate the possibility of a spinal region tumor, cervical spondylosis, or syringomyelia.

Spinal Region Tumors. Tumors outside the dura mater or in the subarachnoid space may compress the spinal cord, nerve roots, spinal nerve, or their blood supply. Tumors can also occur within the spinal cord, resulting in pressure on neurons and vascular supply from within the cord. Pain, aggravated by coughing or sneezing, is the most common initial symptom. Tumors can produce segmental and/or vertical tract signs, depending on their location.

Myelopathy Due to Cervical Spondylosis. Myelopathy is a disorder of the spinal cord. Cervical spondylosis is degeneration of the cervical vertebrae and disks that produces narrowing of the vertebral canal and intervertebral foramina. This narrowing causes increased stretch and shear forces on the spinal cord and nerve roots, damaging glia and neurons (see Henderson et al., 2005 for mechanisms). Gray matter is particularly susceptible to stretch injury. This results in the following:

- Neck and upper limb pain and stiffness
- In some cases, a myotomal pattern of weakness and/or a dermatomal pattern of sensory loss occurs, usually in a C5 and/or C6 segmental distribution
- In some cases, numbness and paresthesias of the feet
- Lower-limb paresis and muscle hyperstiffness
- Babinski's sign

The neck and upper limb pain are segmental signs, caused by irritation of nerve roots. The lower limb signs are vertical tract signs produced by compression of ascending and descending tracts in their course through the lower cervical vertebral canal. The incidence of cervical spondylosis is 2 cases per 100,000 people per year, with a prevalence of 0.4 per 1000 people (MacDonald et al., 2000). Recent research indicates that most cases of cervical spondylosis benefit from surgical intervention (Grundmeyer et al., 2000).

Vertebral Canal Stenosis. Stenosis is the narrowing of the vertebral canal (Figure 12-22), compressing the neural and vascular structures. Stenosis is usually a degenerative disorder caused by bone growth, facet hypertrophy, bulging disks, and hypertrophy of the ligamentum flavum.

Cervical stenosis causes radiating upper limb pain with numbness and paresthesia in a dermatomal distribution. Less often, patients have loss of muscle power in a myotomal distribution. Signs and symptoms of cervical cord compression include loss of proprioception, clumsiness secondary to loss of proprioception, upper motor neuron signs, and problems with bowel and bladder control. Figure 12-23 shows spinal cord compression in a patient with multilevel cervical spinal stenosis.

Lumbar Stenosis. **Lumbar stenosis** produces lower limb and lower back pain that is aggravated by walking and improves with rest. If the stenosis is severe, compression of spinal nerve roots and/or the cauda equina cause additional signs and symptoms. In severe stenosis, paresis, clumsiness, falling, foot drop during gait, numbness, tingling, and/or a heavy, tired feeling in the lower limbs may occur. Flexing the lumbar spine often relieves these signs and symptoms.

Syringomyelia. Syringomyelia is a rare, progressive disorder, most frequently occurring in people 35-45 years of age. A syrinx, or fluid-filled cavity, develops in the spinal cord, almost always in the cervical region. Syringomyelia is usually congenital but can be secondary to trauma or tumors. The accumulation of cerebrospinal fluid in the syrinx causes increased pressure inside the spinal cord, expanding the cavity and compressing the adjacent nerve fibers. Segmental signs occur in the upper

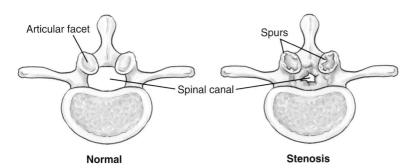

Normal   **Stenosis**

FIGURE 12-22

Spinal stenosis. Narrowing of the spinal canal and intervertebral foramina compresses the spinal cord and/or spinal nerve roots.

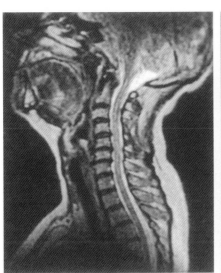
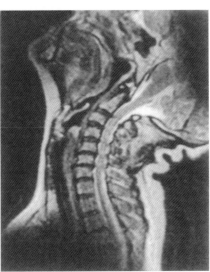

A   B

FIGURE 12-23

Magnetic resonance imaging of multilevel cervical spinal stenosis in neck neutral position (**A**) and extension (**B**). *(From Vitaz TW, Shields CB, et al. (2004). Dynamic weight-bearing cervical magnetic resonance imaging: Technical review and preliminary results. Southern Medical Journal, 97(5), 456-461.)*

limbs, including loss of sensitivity to pain and temperature stimuli, due to interruption of axons crossing the midline in the anterior white commissure; paresis; and muscle atrophy. The sensory loss is often distributed like a cape draped over the shoulders (see Figure 12-18, *B*). Upper motor neuron signs in the lower limbs include paresis, muscle hyperstiffness, phasic stretch hyperreflexia, and loss of bowel and bladder control.

RED FLAGS FOR THE SPINAL REGION

Signs and symptoms that indicate a spinal cord lesion:
- Bilateral alteration or loss of somatosensation
- Incoordination, caused by inadequate somatosensory information to the cerebellum. Confirm that the loss is somatosensory and not cerebellar or vestibular by findings of impaired proprioception, vibration, and two-point discrimination.
- Upper motor neuron signs: decreased muscle power, hyperreflexia, muscle hyperstiffness, Babinski's sign, and clonus
  Signs and symptoms that indicate a possible cauda equina lesion:
- Difficulty with urination/defecation
- Decreased or lost sensation in the saddle area
- Low back pain
- Unilateral or bilateral sciatica
- Lower limb paresis and sensory deficits
- Decreased or lost lower limb reflexes
In cauda equina syndrome, there are no upper motor neuron signs because the lesion is inferior to the end of the spinal cord and thus only affects nerve roots. Sudden onset of cauda equina syndrome is a medical emergency requiring immediate referral.

Signs and symptoms that indicate intermittent claudication, a vascular disorder:
- Cramping in the calf or foot while walking or exercising that disappears after a brief rest
- Decreased pulse in the lower limb
- Cyanosis (bluish color of the skin due to deoxygenated hemoglobin in blood vessels near the surface of the skin)

SUMMARY

Lesions of the spinal cord produce segmental and/or vertical tract signs. Segmental signs include the following:
- Sensory changes: impaired sensations, paresthesias, and dysesthesias, in a dermatomal distribution.
- Lower motor neuron signs (paresis or paralysis, atrophy, cramps) in a myotomal distribution.
- If dorsal nerve roots are involved, increasing intra-abdominal pressure by straining, sneezing, or coughing may produce sharp, radiating pain.
  Common vertical tract signs include the following:
- Sensory changes: decreased or lost sensation below the level of the lesion
- Autonomic signs: decreased or lost voluntary control of pelvic organs, autonomic dysreflexia, poor thermoregulation, and/or orthostatic hypotension
- Upper motor neuron lesion signs: muscle hyperstiffness, paresis, phasic stretch hyperreflexia, Babinski's sign

CLINICAL NOTES

Case 1

PE is a 17-year-old woman. She fractured the C7 vertebra in a diving accident 2 months ago. The fracture is stable. Current findings are as follows:
- Sensation is intact (pinprick, temperature, conscious proprioception, and discriminative touch) in her head, neck, and lateral upper limbs.
- She has no sensation in the medial upper limbs, the trunk below the sternal angle, and the lower limbs.
- All head and shoulder movements are normal strength except shoulder extension.
- Elbow flexion and radial wrist extensors are normal strength.
- The remaining upper limb, trunk, and lower limb muscles have no trace of voluntary movement.
- Babinski's sign is present bilaterally.
  Without adaptive equipment, PE is unable to care for herself. Using adaptive equipment, she is able to eat, dress, and groom independently. She uses a wheelchair. She cannot voluntarily control her bladder or bowels.

CLINICAL NOTES

Questions

1. Is the lesion in the dorsal or ventral root or in the spinal cord?
2. What neurologic level is the lesion? Note: The neurologic level in a spinal cord injury is the most caudal level with *normal* sensory and motor function bilaterally. Refer to Table 12-4 to determine the neurologic level. Is the lesion complete or incomplete?

Case 2

BD is a 16-year-old adolescent. He sustained a spinal cord injury 2 months ago in a fall from a bicycle. Current findings are as follows:

- Pinprick and temperature sensation are impaired, as indicated in Figure 12-24. All other sensations are fully intact.
- Manual muscle test scores are also indicated in Figure 12-24.

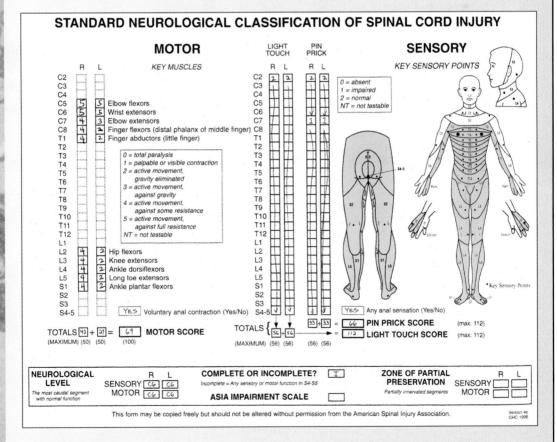

FIGURE 12-24

Motor and sensory test results for Case 2. *(Form courtesy American Spinal Injury Association International, Atlanta.)*

Continued

CLINICAL NOTES

- Babinski's sign is present bilaterally.
- He is independent in all activities. He is able to walk 30 meters using an ankle-foot orthosis on his left leg and a cane.

Questions

1. What level is the cord lesion? Is the lesion complete, or does the pattern indicate a spinal cord syndrome?
2. Why is this patient independent, while the patient in Case 1 requires adaptive equipment, a wheelchair, and maximal assistance on stairs?

Case 3

VK is a 30-year-old man. He plays recreational sports 4 days a week and is a highly competitive soccer player. Two years ago he noted temporary weakness in his left lower leg, which gradually resolved without consultation or treatment. His primary complaint now is inability to control his right foot. He first noted poor kicking skills 3 weeks ago. Sensation and motor control are normal except in the right lower limb. The following deficits are observed in the right lower limb:

- Discriminative touch, vibration sense, and position sense are impaired throughout.
- Pain and temperature sensations are intact.
- Movement is ataxic. Gait deficits: dragging of toes on the ground during swing phase of walking (foot drop), poor placement of the foot on the ground, weight bearing on the right lower limb only half the time spent weight bearing on the left lower limb.
- Gluteals, hamstrings, and all muscles originating below the knee are weak, less than half the strength of the homologous muscles on the left.

Questions

1. Why are pain and temperature sensations intact bilaterally?
2. Where is the lesion?
3. What is the probable etiology?

Case 4

EV is a 62-year-old woman. She reports constant burning pain radiating down the back of her left leg into her foot. When she coughs or sneezes, sharp, stabbing pains become excruciating. The pain began as a backache 3 months ago. Pain intensity has been consistently increasing. Following are the results of testing:

- Sensation is intact in the right lower limb.
- Sensory testing results for the left lower limb are shown in Table 12-6.

Table 12-6   SENSORY TESTING RESULTS FOR LEFT LOWER LIMB FOR CASE 4

Spinal Level	Discriminative Touch	Joint Kinesthesia	Pinprick	Warm	Cold
L4	2	Knee 2	2	2	2
L5	2	Ankle 1	2	2	2
S1	0	Ankle 1	0	0	0
S2	0	—	1	1	1
S3	0	—	1	1	1
S4	2	—	2	2	2
S5	2	—	2	2	2

Scoring: 2, intact; 1, impaired; 0, absent.

CLINICAL NOTES

- Strength is within the normal limits in all limbs.
- Ankle deep tendon reflex is absent on the left side.

Questions

1. Where is the lesion?
2. What is the probable etiology?
3. Why is discriminative touch more affected than pain and temperature sensations?

Case 5

A 48-year-old woman has a 5-year history of intermittent low back pain. She is otherwise healthy. Yesterday she had abrupt onset of severe pain in the perineal and sacral region and intermittent shooting pain down the back of her right lower limb, exacerbated by sitting and coughing. Two hours later she developed increased urinary frequency and a sensation of being unable to fully empty her bladder. Defecation frequency also increased.

   Somatosensation: Decreased light touch and pinprick in perineal and sacral region. Somatosensation intact throughout rest of body. With the patient in the supine position, shooting pain is elicited in the posterior right leg when the therapist lifts the patient's leg to 30° of hip flexion with the knee straight. The same maneuver flexing the left hip to 70° does not elicit pain. Normally this test, the straight leg raise, does not elicit pain with hip flexion to 70°.

   Autonomic: Increased frequency of urination and defecation; abnormal sensation of inability to completely empty bladder.

   Motor: Weak contraction of anal sphincter. MMT (manual muscle test) grade is 5 throughout both lower limbs

Questions

1. Where is the lesion?
2. What is the probable etiology?
3. After the examination, what is the next step with this patient?

REVIEW QUESTIONS

1. What is a spinal nerve?
2. What is the difference between a ventral root and a ventral primary ramus?
3. What is a spinal segment?
4. What is the function of the dorsal horn?
5. Which of Rexed's laminae is also known as the substantia gelatinosa?
6. Are reflexes and voluntary motor control entirely separate systems?
7. What is the function of reciprocal inhibition?
8. How is voluntary voiding of urine controlled?
9. What are the differences in signs between segmental and vertical tract lesions?
10. List the four adult-onset spinal region syndromes, and draw spinal cord cross sections that illustrate the location of the lesion in each syndrome.
11. Why are cord functions below the lesion depressed or lost immediately after a spinal cord injury?
12. Why do some people with spinal cord injuries have exaggerated withdrawal reflexes?
13. What is an incomplete spinal cord injury? Give two examples of syndromes that may result from incomplete spinal cord injury.
14. List the three conditions that arise when the spinal cord below the T6 level is deprived of descending sympathetic innervation.

References

Ahn UM, Ahn NU, et al. (2000). Cauda equina syndrome secondary to lumbar disc herniation: A meta-analysis of surgical outcomes. Spine, 25(12), 1515-1522.

ASIA, American Spinal Injury Association. (2002). International Standards for Neurological Classification of Spinal Cord Injury. Available at http://www.asiaspinalinjury.org/home/index.html

Aslan AR, Kogan BA (2002). Conservative management in neurogenic bladder dysfunction. Current Opinion in Urology, 12(6), 473-477.

Bradbury EJ, McMahon SB, et al. (2000). Keeping in touch: Sensory neurone regeneration in the CNS. Trends in Pharmacological Sciences, 21(10), 389-394.

Burke RE, Degtyarenko AM, et al. (2001). Patterns of locomotor drive to motoneurons and last-order interneurons: Clues to the structure of the CPG. Journal of Neurophysiology, 86(1), 447-462.

Butler D (2000). The Sensitive Nervous System. Adelaide: Nocigroup Publications.

Capaday C, Lavoie BA, et al. (1999). Studies on the corticospinal control of human walking. I. Responses to focal transcranial magnetic stimulation of the motor cortex. Journal of Neurophysiology, 81(1), 129-139.

Carraro U, Rossini K, et al. (2005). Muscle fiber regeneration in human permanent lower motoneuron denervation: Relevance to safety and effectiveness of FES-training, which induces muscle recovery in SCI subjects. Artificial Organs, 29(3), 187-191.

Chalmers GR, Knutzen KM (2004). Recurrent inhibition in the soleus motor pool of elderly and young adults. Electromyography and Clinical Neurophysiology, 44(7), 413-421.

Della-Giustina DA (1999). Emergency department evaluation and treatment of back pain. Emergency Medicine Clinics of North America, 17(4), 877-893, vi-vii.

Ditunno JF, Little JW, et al. (2004). Spinal shock revisited: A four-phase model. Spinal Cord, 42(7), 383-395.

Duysens J, Bastiaanse CM, et al. (2004). Gait acts as a gate for reflexes from the foot. Canadian Journal of Physiolology and Pharmacology, 82(8-9): 715-722.

Edgerton VR, Tillakaratne NJ, et al. (2004). Plasticity of the spinal neural circuitry after injury. Annual Review of Neuroscience, 27, 145-167.

Farmer JC, Wisneski RJ (1994). Cervical spine nerve root compression. An analysis of neuroforaminal pressures with varying head and arm positions. Spine, 19(16), 1850-1855.

Govind J (2004). Lumbar radicular pain. Australian Family Physician, 33(6), 409-412.

Grundmeyer RW, Garber JE, et al. (2000). Spinal spondylosis and disc disease. In RW Evans, DS Baskin, et al. (Eds.), Prognosis of Neurological Disorders. (2nd ed., pp. 119-151). New York: Oxford University Press.

Harkema SJ, Hurley SL, et al. (1997). Human lumbosacral spinal cord interprets loading during stepping. Journal of Neurophysiology. 77(2):797-811.

Harrison DE, Cailliet R, et al. (1999). A review of biomechanics of the central nervous system—Part II: Spinal cord strains from postural loads. Journal of Manipulative and Physiological Therapeutics, 22(5), 322-332.

Henderson FC, Geddes JF, et al. (2005). Stretch-associated injury in cervical spondylotic myelopathy: New concept and review. Neurosurgery, 56(5), 1101-1113; discussion 1101-1113.

Hesse S, Werner C, et al. (2004). Electromechanical gait training with functional electrical stimulation: Case studies in spinal cord injury. Spinal Cord, 42(6), 346-352.

Hirabayashi Y, Igarashi T, et al. (2002). Mechanical effects of leg position on vertebral structures examined by magnetic resonance imaging. Regional Anesthesia and Pain Medicine, 27(4), 429-432.

Jackson AB, Dijkers M, et al. (2004). A demographic profile of new traumatic spinal cord injuries: Change and stability over 30 years. Archives of Physical Medicine and Rehabilitation, 85(11), 1740-1748.

Kaplin AI, Krishnan C, et al. (2005). Diagnosis and management of acute myelopathies. Neurologist, 11(1), 2-18.

Kawashima N, Nozaki D, et al. (2005). Alternate leg movement amplifies locomotor-like muscle activity in spinal cord injured persons. Journal of Neurophysiology, 93(2): 777-785.

Laessoe U, Voigt M (2004). Modification of stretch tolerance in a stooping position. Scandinavian Journal of Medicine & Science in Sports, 14(4), 239-244.

Lam T, Pearson K (2002). The role of proprioceptive feedback in the regulation and adaptation of locomotor activity. In S Gandevia, U Proske, et al. (Eds.), Sensorimotor Control of Movement and Posture. Kluwer Academic/Plenum Publishers: New York.

Lanuza GM, Gosgnach S, et al. (2004). Genetic identification of spinal interneurons that coordinate left-right locomotor activity necessary for walking movements. Neuron, 42(3), 375-386.

MacDonald BK, Cockerel OC, et al. (2000). The incidence and lifetime prevalence of neurological disorders in a prospective community-based study in the UK. Brain, 123(Pt 4), 665-676.

Madersbacher H (2004). Neurourology and pelvic floor dysfunction. Minerva Ginecologica, 56(4), 303-309.

Maus TP (2002). Imaging of the spine and nerve roots. Physical Medicine and Rehabilitation Clinics of North America, 13(3), 487-544, vi.

Mayer NH (1997). Clinicophysiologic concepts of spasticity and motor dysfunction in adults with an upper motoneuron lesion. Muscle & Nerve (Suppl 6), S1-S13.

McCrea DA (1994). Can sense be made of spinal interneuron circuits? In P Cordo and S Harnad (Eds.), Movement Control. (pp. 31-41). Cambridge, England: Cambridge University Press.

McKinley WO, Gittler MS, et al. (2002). Spinal cord injury medicine. 2. Medical complications after spinal cord injury: Identification and management. Archives of Physical Medicine and Rehabilitation, 83(3 Suppl 1), S58-S64, S90-S98.

McLaughlin J, Bjornson K, et al. (2002). Selective dorsal rhizotomy: Meta-analysis of three randomized controlled trials. Developmental Medicine and Child Neurology, 44(1), 17-25.

Min JH, Kang SH, et al. (2005). Anatomic analysis of the transforaminal ligament in the lumbar intervertebral foramen. Neurosurgery, 57(1 Suppl), 37-41; discussion 37-41.

Minassian K, Jilge B, et al. (2004). Stepping-like movements in humans with complete spinal cord injury induced by epidural stimulation of the lumbar cord: Electromyographic study of compound muscle action potentials. Spinal Cord, 42(7), 401-416.

Morganti B, Scivoletto G, et al. (2005). Walking index for spinal cord injury (WISCI): Criterion validation. Spinal Cord, 43(1), 27-33.

Nuckley DJ, Konodi MA, et al. (2002). Neural space integrity of the lower cervical spine: Effect of normal range of motion. Spine, 27(6), 587-595.

Podnar S. (2006). Epidemiology of cauda equina and conus medullaris lesions. Muscle and Nerve, epub ahead of print.

Quevedo J, Fedirchuk B, et al. (2000). Group I disynaptic excitation of cat hindlimb flexor and bifunctional motoneurones during fictive locomotion. Journal of Physiology, 525(Pt 2), 549-564.

Shapiro S (2000). Medical realities of cauda equina syndrome secondary to lumbar disc herniation. Spine, 25(3), 348-351; discussion 352.

Song XJ, Vizcarra C, et al. (2003). Hyperalgesia and neural excitability following injuries to central and peripheral branches of axons and somata of dorsal root ganglion neurons. Journal of Neurophysiology, 89(4), 2185-2193.

Spaich EG, Arendt-Nielsen L, et al. (2004). Modulation of lower limb withdrawal reflexes during gait: A topographical study. Journal of Neurophysiology, 91(1), 258-266.

Stecina K, Quevedo J, et al. (2005) Parallel reflex pathways from flexor muscle afferents evoking resetting and flexion enhancement during fictive locomotion and scratch in the cat. Journal of Physiology, 569(Pt 1):275-290.

Tooth L, McKenna K, et al. (2003). Rehabilitation outcomes in traumatic spinal cord injury in Australia: Functional status, length of stay and discharge setting. Spinal Cord, 41(4), 220-230.

Vitaz TW, Shields CB, et al. (2004). Dynamic weight-bearing cervical magnetic resonance imaging: Technical review and preliminary results. Southern Medical Journal, 97(5), 456-461.

Wernig A, Nanassy A, et al. (1999). Laufband (treadmill) therapy in incomplete paraplegia and tetraplegia. Journal of Neurotrauma, 16(8), 719-726.

Yuan Q, Dougherty L, et al. (1998). In vivo human cervical spinal cord deformation and displacement in flexion. Spine, 23(15), 1677-1683.

13 Cranial Nerves

Laurie Lundy-Ekman, PhD, PT

I'm 25 years old. A few years ago, I swam in very cold water on a Saturday. The next day, the right side of my tongue and mouth had a coated feeling, and by that evening my lips were twitching ever so slightly. Monday, my right eyelids were occasionally twitching uncontrollably. Tuesday morning I had only 25% to 50% control over my right eyelid and facial muscles; I could only get three quarters of a smile. Wednesday morning I had 0% to 5% control of the right facial muscles. I couldn't close my right eye. I felt like I had Novocain in the right side of my face, except that I had sensation in the affected area. It was scary. The physician performed a nerve conduction velocity test, eye blink reflex tests, and needle electromyography to determine the status of the nerve. The disorder was diagnosed as Bell's palsy.

—*Darren Larson*

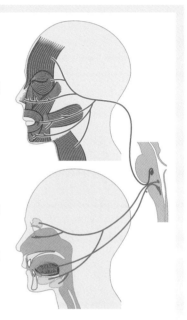

INTRODUCTION

Cranial nerves exchange information between the peripheral and central nervous systems. Twelve pairs of these nerves emanate from the surface of the brain and innervate structures of the head and neck. Cranial nerve X (the vagus) innervates thoracic and abdominal viscera in addition to structures in the head and neck. Axons and receptors of the cranial nerves outside the skull are part of the peripheral nervous system and are myelinated by Schwann cells. Two cranial nerves, the olfactory and optic nerves, are entirely within the skull and have no peripheral component. The olfactory and optic nerves are myelinated by oligodendroglia and therefore can be affected by diseases that affect oligodendroglia, including multiple sclerosis.

Like peripheral nerves connected to the spinal cord, cranial nerves serve sensory, motor, and autonomic functions. Generally, cell bodies for cranial nerves are located similarly to the cell bodies that contribute axons to peripheral nerves that connect with the spinal cord. Cell bodies of sensory neurons in cranial nerves are usually in ganglia outside of the brainstem (the exception: neurons that convey proprioceptive information from the face have cell bodies inside the brainstem). Motor cell bodies are located in nuclei inside the brainstem.

Cranial nerves differ from spinal nerves in specialization. Some cranial nerves are only motor, others only sensory, and some are both sensory and motor. The cranial nerve fibers that innervate muscles of the head and neck are lower motor neurons. As in the spinal cord, these lower motor neurons are influenced by input from upper motor neurons and sensory afferent fibers. Several cranial nerves have unique functions not shared by any other nerves, such as conveying visual, auditory, or vestibular information.

Cranial nerves have four functions:
- Supply motor innervation to muscles of the face, eyes, tongue, jaw, and two neck muscles (sternocleidomastoid and trapezius)
- Transmit somatosensory information from the skin and muscles of the face and the temporomandibular joint
- Transmit special sensory information related to visual, auditory, vestibular, gustatory, olfactory, and visceral sensations
- Provide parasympathetic regulation of pupil size, curvature of the lens of the eye, heart rate, blood pressure, breathing, and digestion

All cranial nerve connections to the brain are visible on the inferior brain (Figure 13-1) except cranial nerve IV, which emerges from the posterior midbrain. Cranial nerve names, primary functions, and connections to the brain are listed in Table 13-1.

CRANIAL NERVE I: OLFACTORY

The **olfactory nerve** is sensory, conducting information from nasal chemoreceptors to the olfactory bulb. Signals

Table 13-1   CRANIAL NERVES

Number	Name	Function	Connection to Brain
I	Olfactory	Smell	Inferior frontal lobe
II	Optic	Vision	Diencephalon
III	Oculomotor	Moves eye up, down, medially; raises upper eyelid; constricts pupil; adjusts the shape of the lens of the eye	Midbrain (anterior)
IV	Trochlear	Moves eye medially and down	Midbrain (posterior)
V	Trigeminal	Facial sensation, chewing, sensation from temporomandibular joint	Pons (lateral)
VI	Abducens	Abducts eye	Between pons and medulla
VII	Facial	Facial expression, closes eye, tears, salivation, taste	Between pons and medulla
VIII	Vestibulocochlear	Sensation of head position relative to gravity and head movement; hearing	Between pons and medulla
IX	Glossopharyngeal	Swallowing, salivation, taste	Medulla
X	Vagus	Regulates viscera, swallowing, speech, taste	Medulla
XI	Accessory	Elevates shoulders, turns head	Spinal cord and medulla
XII	Hypoglossal	Moves tongue	Medulla

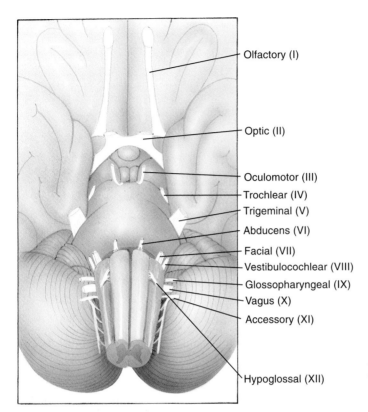

Olfactory (I)

Optic (II)

Oculomotor (III)
Trochlear (IV)
Trigeminal (V)
Abducens (VI)
Facial (VII)
Vestibulocochlear (VIII)
Glossopharyngeal (IX)
Vagus (X)
Accessory (XI)

Hypoglossal (XII)

FIGURE 13-1
Inferior view of the brain, showing cranial nerve connections with the brain. The connection of the trochlear nerve is on the posterior brainstem, inferior to the colliculi.

from the olfactory bulb travel in the olfactory tract to the medial temporal lobe of the cerebrum. The sense of smell is dependent on olfactory nerve function. Much of the information attributed to taste is olfactory because information from taste buds is limited to chemoreceptors for salty, sweet, sour, and bitter tastes.

CRANIAL NERVE II: OPTIC

The **optic nerve** is sensory, transmitting visual information from the retina to the **lateral geniculate body** of the thalamus and to nuclei in the midbrain (Figure 13-2). The retina is the inner layer of the posterior eye, formed by photosensitive cells. Light striking the retina is converted into neural signals by the photosensitive cells. Axons from neurons in the retina travel in the optic nerve, through the optic chiasm, and in the optic tract before synapsing in the lateral geniculate body. The lateral geniculate body is a relay along a pathway to the primary visual cortex. This pathway projects to areas involved in the analysis and conscious awareness of visual

information. The central processing of visual signals will be discussed in Chapter 15.

The visual signals sent to the midbrain are involved in reflexive responses of the pupil, awareness of light and dark, and orienting the head and eyes. Reflexes involving cranial nerves are listed in Table 13-2.

CRANIAL NERVES III, IV, AND VI: OCULOMOTOR, TROCHLEAR, AND ABDUCENS

The **oculomotor, trochlear,** and **abducens nerves** are primarily motor, containing lower motor neuron axons innervating the six extraocular muscles that move the eye (Figure 13-3) and control reflexive constriction of the pupil.

Control of Eye Movement

The extraocular muscles include four straight (rectus) muscles and two oblique muscles. The rectus muscles

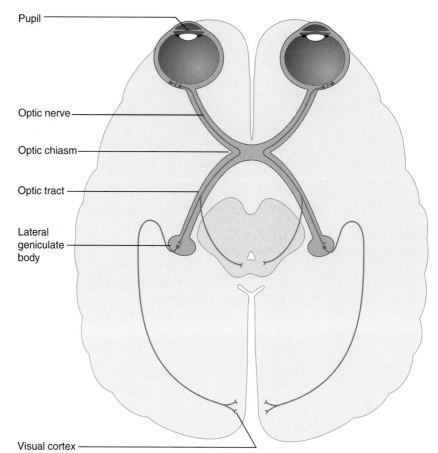

Pupil

Optic nerve

Optic chiasm

Optic tract

Lateral geniculate body

Visual cortex

FIGURE 13-2
The optic nerve projects from the retina to the midbrain and to the lateral geniculate. Reflex connections in the midbrain control the constriction of the pupil and reflexive eye movements. Visual information relayed by the lateral geniculate to the visual cortex provides conscious vision.

Table 13-2   CRANIAL NERVE REFLEXES

Reflex	Description of Reflex	Afferent Neurons	Efferent Neurons
Pupillary	Pupil of eye constricts when light is shined into eye	Optic	Oculomotor
Consensual	Pupil of eye constricts when light is shined into other eye	Optic	Oculomotor
Accommodation	Lens of eye adjusts to focus light on the retina, pupil constricts, and pupils move medially when viewing an object at close range	Optic	Oculomotor
Masseter	When masseter is tapped with a reflex hammer, the muscle contracts	Trigeminal	Trigeminal
Corneal (blink)	When the cornea is touched, the eyelids close	Trigeminal	Facial
Gag	Touching of pharynx elicits contraction of pharyngeal muscles	Glossopharyngeal	Vagus
Swallowing	Food touching entrance of pharynx elicits movement of the soft palate and contraction of pharyngeal muscles	Glossopharyngeal	Vagus

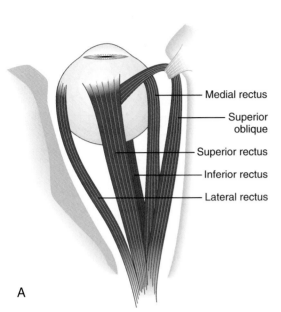

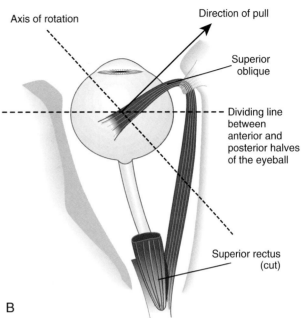

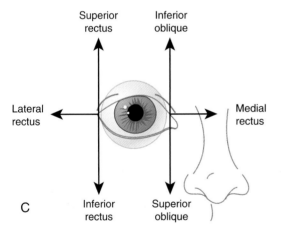

FIGURE 13-3

Left eye and extraocular muscles. **A,** Superior view. **B,** The action of the superior oblique muscle. When the eye is directed straightforward or abducted, contraction of the superior oblique muscle rotates the eye around the axis of the pupil. When the eye is adducted, contraction of the superior oblique muscle moves the pupil downward *(not shown).* **C,** Movements of the right eye by the extraocular muscles. The lateral rectus abducts the eye, and the medial rectus adducts the eye. When the eye is adducted, the superior oblique moves the eye downward and the inferior oblique moves the eye upward. These actions of the oblique muscles occur because of the angle of muscle pull and because the obliques attach to the posterior half of the eyeball (see part **B** for attachment of superior oblique). When the eye is abducted, the superior rectus moves the eye upward and the inferior rectus moves the eye downward.

attach to the anterior half of the eyeball. The lateral rectus moves the eye laterally, and the medial rectus moves the eye medially; thus, these muscles form a pair controlling horizontal eye movement. With the eyes looking straight forward, the actions of the superior and inferior rectus are primarily elevation and depression of the eye, respectively. The two oblique muscles attach to the posterior half of the eyeball (see Figure 13-3, *B*). If the eye is abducted, the obliques primarily rotate the eye. When the eye is adducted, the superior oblique muscle depresses the eye, and the inferior oblique muscle

elevates it (see Figure 13-3, *C*). Cranial nerve supply to the extraocular muscles is shown in Figure 13-4.

Cranial nerve III, the oculomotor nerve, has cell bodies located in the oculomotor nucleus that control the superior, inferior, and medial rectus, the inferior oblique, and the levator palpebrae superioris muscles. These muscles move the eye upward, downward, and medially; rotate the eye around the axis of the pupil; and assist in elevating the upper eyelid. The upper eyelid is also elevated by the sympathetically innervated superior tarsal muscle (see Figure 8-8).

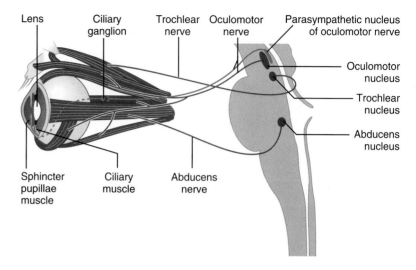

FIGURE 13-4
The innervation of extraocular and intraocular eye muscles. CN, cranial nerve. The red nuclei and axons are motor; the green are autonomic.

Cranial Nerve	Muscle	Movement
III: oculomotor	Levator palpebrae superioris	Lifts eyelid
	Superior rectus	Pupil up
	Medial rectus	Pupil medial
	Inferior rectus	Pupil down
	Inferior oblique	If eye adducted, pupil up; if eye abducted, rotates eye
	Pupillary sphincter	Constricts pupil
	Ciliary	Increases curvature of lens of eye
IV: trochlear	Superior oblique	If eye adducted, pupil down and in; if eye abducted, rotates eye
VI: abducens	Lateral rectus	Pupil lateral

Cranial nerve IV, the trochlear nerve, has cell bodies located in the trochlear nucleus in the midbrain and is the only cranial nerve to emerge from the dorsal brainstem, below the inferior colliculus. The trochlear nerve controls the superior oblique muscle, which rotates the eye or, if the eye is adducted, depresses the pupil.

Cranial nerve VI, the abducens nerve, has cell bodies located in the abducens nucleus in the pontine tegmentum. The abducens nerve controls the lateral rectus muscle, which moves the eye laterally.

Coordination of Eye Movements

Coordination of the two eyes is maintained via synergistic action of the eye muscles. For instance, to look toward the right, the abducens nerve activates the lateral rectus

to move the right eye laterally, while the oculomotor nerve activates the medial rectus to move the left eye medially. This coordination requires connections among the cranial nerve nuclei that control eye movements. Signals conveyed by a brainstem tract, the **medial longitudinal fasciculus,** coordinate head and eye movements by providing bilateral connections among vestibular, oculomotor, and spinal accessory nerve nuclei in the brainstem (Figure 13-5). The medial longitudinal fasciculus is discussed further in Chapter 15.

Eye and head movements are coordinated by signals in the medial longitudinal fasciculus.

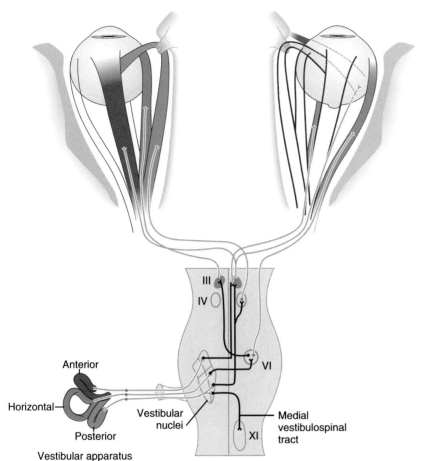

Anterior

Horizontal

Posterior

Vestibular apparatus

III

IV

VI

Vestibular nuclei

XI

Medial vestibulospinal tract

FIGURE 13-5

Axons in the medial longitudinal fasciculus *(brown)* connect the oculomotor, trochlear, abducens, vestibular, and accessory nerve nuclei. Signals conveyed in this tract coordinate head and eye movements.

Parasympathetic Fibers of Cranial Nerve III

In addition to the voluntary control of eye movements, cranial nerve III is involved in reflexive constriction of the pupil and the muscles controlling the lens of the eye. The oculomotor nerve contains parasympathetic fibers with their cell bodies in the parasympathetic nucleus of the oculomotor nerve (also called the *Edinger-Westphal nucleus*). The preganglionic parasympathetic fibers synapse with postganglionic fibers behind the eyeball in the ciliary ganglion. The parasympathetic connections innervate the intrinsic muscles of the eye: the pupillary sphincter and the ciliary muscle. When the pupillary sphincter constricts, the amount of light reaching the retina is decreased. When viewing objects closer than 20 cm, the ciliary muscle contracts, increasing the curvature of the lens. This action, called *accommodation,* increases refraction of light rays so that the focal point will be maintained on the retina.

Pupillary, Consensual, and Accommodation Reflexes

The pupillary, consensual, and accommodation reflexes involve the optic and oculomotor nerves (Figures 13-6 and 13-7). The optic nerve is the afferent (i.e., sensory) limb of these reflexes, while the oculomotor nerve provides the efferent (i.e., motor) limb. The pupillary and consensual reflexes are elicited by the same stimulus: shining a bright light into one eye. The pupillary reflex is pupil constriction in the eye directly stimulated by the bright light. Consensual reflex is constriction of the pupil in the other eye.

The pathways for the pupillary and consensual reflexes consist of neurons that sequentially connect the following:

- The retina to the pretectal nucleus in the midbrain
- The pretectal nucleus to the parasympathetic nuclei of the oculomotor nerve

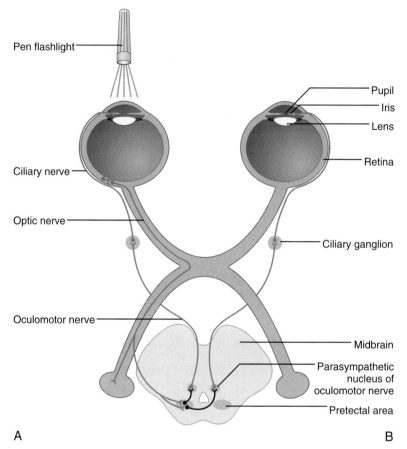

Pen flashlight

Pupil

Iris

Lens

Retina

Ciliary nerve

Optic nerve

Ciliary ganglion

Oculomotor nerve

Midbrain

Parasympathetic nucleus of oculomotor nerve

Pretectal area

A

B

FIGURE 13-6

Eye reflexes. Both the pupillary and consensual reflexes are responses to bright light shined into one eye. Light shined into the left eye elicits reflexive constriction of both pupils. The optic nerve conveys information from the retina to the pretectal area. Interneurons from the pretectal area synapse in the parasympathetic nucleus of the oculomotor nerve. Efferents travel in the oculomotor nerve and then the ciliary nerve. **A,** The pupillary reflex is produced by ipsilateral neural connections. **B,** The consensual reflex, constriction of the opposite pupil, is elicited by the neuron connecting the left pretectal area with the right parasympathetic nucleus of the oculomotor nerve.

- The parasympathetic nuclei of the oculomotor nerve to the ciliary ganglion
- The ciliary ganglion to the pupillary sphincter

> The size of the pupil and the shape of the lens of the eye are reflexively controlled by afferents in the optic nerve and parasympathetic efferents in the oculomotor nerve.

The accommodation reflex consists of adjustments to view a near object: the pupils constrict, eyes converge (adduct), and the lens becomes more convex. This reflex requires activation of the visual cortex and an area in the frontal lobe of the cerebral cortex—the frontal eye field. The circuitry is shown in Figure 13-7.

CRANIAL NERVE V: TRIGEMINAL

The **trigeminal nerve** is a mixed nerve containing both sensory and motor fibers. The sensory fibers transmit information from the face and temporomandibular joint. The motor fibers innervate the muscles of mastication. The trigeminal nerve is named for its three branches: ophthalmic, maxillary, and mandibular (Figure 13-8, *A*). All three branches convey somatosensory signals; the **mandibular branch** also contains lower motor neuron axons to the muscles used in chewing. Pathways carrying information from the trigeminal nerve are illustrated in Figure 13-8, *B*.

Cell bodies of the neurons carrying sensory information for **discriminative touch** are found in the trigeminal ganglion. The central axons synapse in the **main sensory nucleus** in the pons. Second-order neurons cross the midline and project to the ventral posteromedial

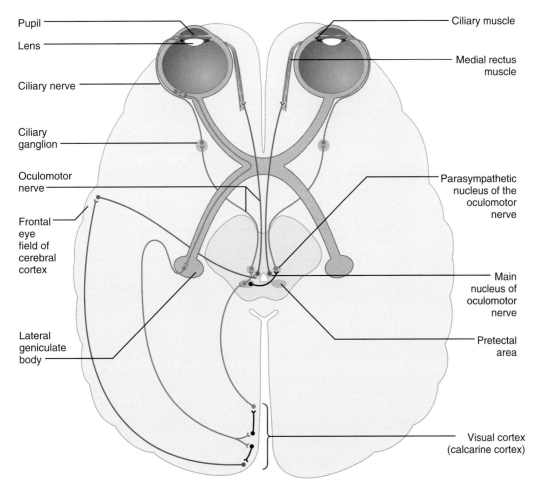

Pupil
Lens
Ciliary nerve
Ciliary ganglion
Oculomotor nerve
Frontal eye field of cerebral cortex
Lateral geniculate body

Ciliary muscle
Medial rectus muscle
Parasympathetic nucleus of the oculomotor nerve
Main nucleus of oculomotor nerve
Pretectal area
Visual cortex (calcarine cortex)

FIGURE 13-7

Accommodation is a change in curvature of the lens, contraction of the pupil, and position of the eyes in response to viewing a near object. The afferent limb is the retinogeniculocalcarine pathway. The efferent limb to control the curvature of the lens and to contract the pupil is from the visual cortex to nuclei in the midbrain, then via parasympathetic neurons to the ciliary muscle. The efferent limb to move the pupils toward the midline is from the visual cortex to the frontal eye fields, then to the main oculomotor nucleus, then the oculomotor nerve, which controls contraction of the medial rectus muscles.

nucleus of the thalamus. Third-order neurons then project to the somatosensory cortex, where discriminative touch signals are consciously recognized.

Proprioceptive information from the muscles of mastication and extraocular muscles is transmitted ipsilaterally by axons of cranial nerve V to the **mesencephalic nucleus** in the midbrain. The primary neuron cell bodies are found inside the brainstem, in the mesencephalic nucleus rather than the trigeminal ganglion. This location for sensory cell bodies is atypical because

the usual location of primary neuron cell bodies is cranial nerve or dorsal root ganglia outside the brainstem or spinal cord. Central branches of mesencephalic tract neurons project to the reticular formation. The pathways from the reticular formation to conscious awareness are not known. Collaterals of proprioceptive fibers project to the trigeminal motor nucleus (reflex connections) and to the cerebellum (motor coordination).

The cell bodies of nociceptive ($A\delta$ and C) fibers are in the trigeminal ganglion. The central axons of $A\delta$

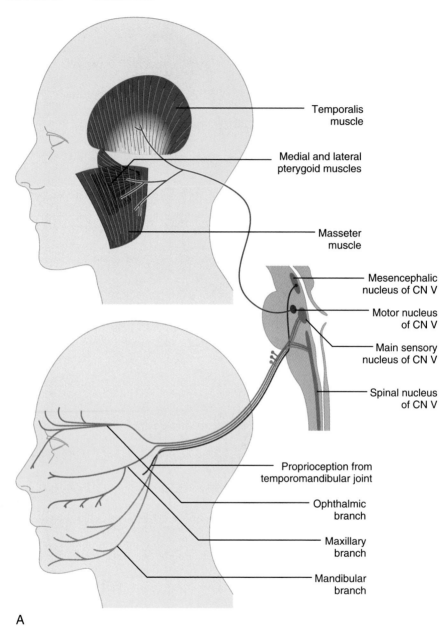

Temporalis
muscle

Medial and lateral
pterygoid muscles

Masseter
muscle

Mesencephalic
nucleus of CN V

Motor nucleus
of CN V

Main sensory
nucleus of CN V

Spinal nucleus
of CN V

Proprioception from
temporomandibular joint

Ophthalmic
branch

Maxillary
branch

Mandibular
branch

A

FIGURE 13-8
Trigeminal nerve. **A,** Distribution to skin of the face, temporomandibular joint, and muscles of mastication.

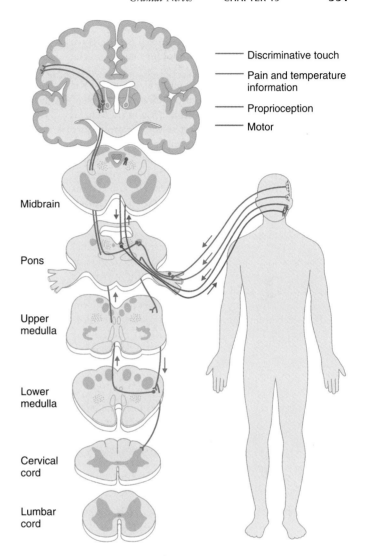

	Discriminative touch
	Pain and temperature information
	Proprioception
	Motor

Midbrain

Pons

Upper medulla

Lower medulla

Cervical cord

Lumbar cord

B

Sensation	Primary Neuron Cell Body	First Synapse	Second Synapse	Termination
Discriminative touch	Trigeminal ganglion	Main sensory nucleus	Ventral posteromedial nucleus of thalamus	Somatosensory cortex
Proprioception	Mesencephalic nucleus	Reticular formation	Unknown	Unknown
Fast pain	Trigeminal ganglion	Spinal trigeminal nucleus	Ventral posteromedial nucleus of thalamus	Somatosensory cortex
Slow pain	Trigeminal ganglion	Reticular formation	Reticular formation and intralaminar nuclei	Limbic system and throughout cortex

FIGURE 13-8, cont'd

B, Pathways conveying somatosensory information from the face and motor signals to the muscles involved in chewing.

neurons enter the pons, then descend as the spinal tract of the trigeminal nerve into the cervical spinal cord. These neurons synapse with second-order neurons in the **spinal trigeminal nucleus.** Axons of second-order neurons transmitting fast pain information cross the midline and ascend to the ventral posteromedial nucleus of the thalamus. Third-order neurons arise in the ventral posteromedial nucleus and project to the somatosensory cortex. Slow pain information travels in the **trigemino-reticulothalamic pathway.** C fibers from the trigeminal nerve synapse in the reticular formation. Projection neurons end in the intralaminar nuclei. The projections from the intralaminar nuclei are similar to the spino-limbic pathways, with projections to many areas of cortex.

Reflex actions are also mediated by the trigeminal nerve. Ophthalmic fibers of the trigeminal nerve provide the afferent limb of the *corneal (blink) reflex.* When the cornea is touched, information is relayed to the spinal trigeminal nucleus via the trigeminal nerve. From the spinal trigeminal nucleus, interneurons convey the information bilaterally to the facial nerve (VII) nuclei. The facial nerve then reflexively activates muscles to close eyelids of both eyes. Another reflex, the *masseter reflex,* relies entirely on trigeminal nerve connections. When a light downward tap is delivered to the chin, a monosynaptic stretch reflex closing the jaw occurs. The afferent information from the muscle spindles and the efferent signals to the muscles both travel in the trigeminal nerve. The synapse is in the motor trigeminal nucleus.

> Somatosensory information from the face is conveyed by the trigeminal nerve and distributed to the three trigeminal nuclei: mesencephalic (proprioceptive), main sensory (discriminative touch), and spinal (fast pain and temperature). Slow pain information projects to the reticular formation.

CRANIAL NERVE VII: FACIAL

The **facial nerve** (Figure 13-9) is a mixed nerve containing both sensory and motor fibers. The sensory fibers transmit touch, pain, and pressure information from the tongue, pharynx, and skin near the ear canal and information from the chemoreceptors located in the taste buds of the anterior tongue to the solitary nucleus.

Motor innervation by the facial nerve includes the muscles that close the eyes, move the lips, and produce

facial expressions. The facial nerve provides the efferent limb of the corneal reflex. The trigeminal nerve provides the afferent information from the cornea, and the facial nerve activates eyelid closure. Cell bodies for the motor fibers are in the motor nucleus of the facial nerve. The facial nerve also innervates salivary, nasal, and lacrimal (tear-producing) glands. Cell bodies for the preganglionic parasympathetic neurons that innervate the glands are all located in the superior salivary nucleus of the medulla.

> The facial nerve innervates the muscles of facial expression and most glands in the head; it also conveys sensory information from the oral region.

CRANIAL NERVE VIII: VESTIBULOCOCHLEAR

Cranial nerve VIII, the **vestibulocochlear nerve,** is a sensory nerve with two distinct branches. The vestibular branch transmits information related to head position and head movement. The cochlear branch transmits information related to hearing. The peripheral receptors for these functions are located in the inner ear, in a structure called the labyrinth. The **labyrinth** consists of the vestibular apparatus and the cochlea (Figure 13-10). The vestibular apparatus and the functions of the vestibular system are discussed in Chapter 15. The cochlear nerve and the structures essential for processing auditory information are discussed in subsequent sections.

Cochlea

The **cochlea** is a snail shell–shaped organ formed by a spiraling, fluid-filled tube (Figure 13-11, *A*). A basilar membrane extends almost the full length of the cochlea, dividing the cochlea into upper and lower chambers. The basilar membrane consists of fibers oriented across the width of the cochlea. The upper chamber (scala vestibuli) is further divided by a membrane that separates the **cochlear duct** from the remainder of the upper chamber. Within the cochlear duct, resting on the basilar membrane, is the **organ of Corti,** the organ of hearing. The organ of Corti is composed of receptor cells (hair cells), supporting cells, a tectorial membrane, and the terminals of the cochlear branch of cranial nerve VIII (Figure 13-11, *B*). The tips of the hairs of the hair cells are embedded in the overlying tectorial membrane.

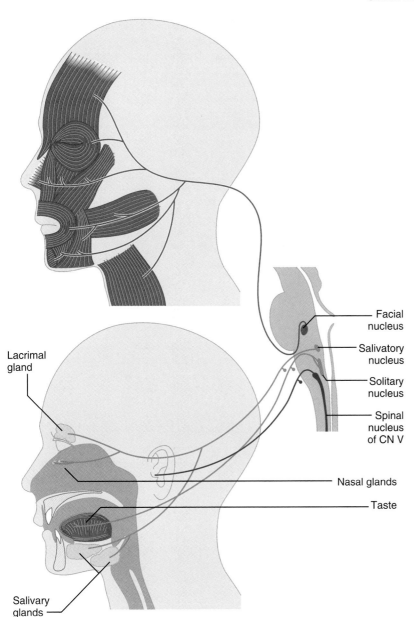

Lacrimal
gland

Facial
nucleus

Salivatory
nucleus

Solitary
nucleus

Spinal
nucleus
of CN V

Nasal glands

Taste

Salivary
glands

FIGURE 13-9

Facial nerve, supplying innervation to
the muscles of facial expression and
most glands in the head. Facial nerve
also transmits sensory information from
skin near the ear canal and from the
tongue and pharynx.

Converting Sound to Neural Signals

Sound is converted to neural signals by a sequence of
mechanical actions. The tympanic membrane (eardrum),
small bones called *ossicles,* and a membrane at the opening
of the upper chamber of the cochlea are connected in
series. When sound waves enter the external ear, the
vibration of the tympanic membrane moves the ossicles.
The ossicles in turn vibrate the membrane at the opening
of the upper chamber, moving the fluid contained in the
upper chamber. This moves the fluid inside the cochlea,
vibrating the basilar membrane and its attached hair
cells. Because the tips of the hair cells are embedded in
the tectorial membrane, movement of the hair cells

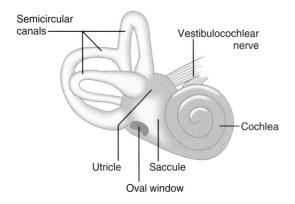

FIGURE 13-10
The vestibulocochlear nerve and the labyrinth of the inner ear.

bends the hairs. This bending results in excitation of the hair cell and stimulation of the cochlear nerve endings (Figure 13-12). The neural signals travel in the cochlear nerve to the cochlear nuclei, located at the junction of the medulla and the pons.

> The organ of Corti converts mechanical energy into neural signals conveyed by the cochlear nerve.

The shape of the basilar membrane is important in coding the frequency of sounds. Because the basilar membrane is narrowest near the middle ear and widest at the free end, the fibers at the free end of the basilar membrane are longer than the fibers at the attached end.

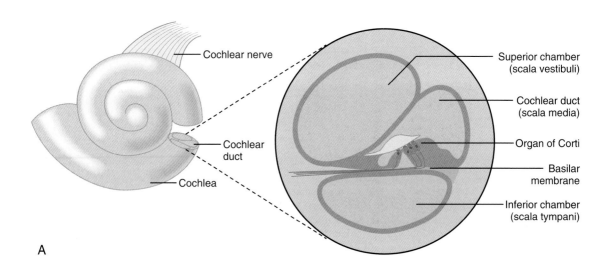

A

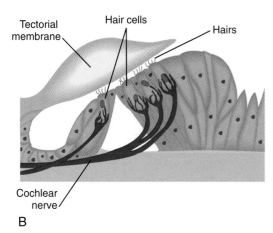

B

FIGURE 13-11
A, Cochlea with a small section cut away and enlarged to show the fluid-filled spaces inside and the organ of Corti. **B,** Organ of Corti.

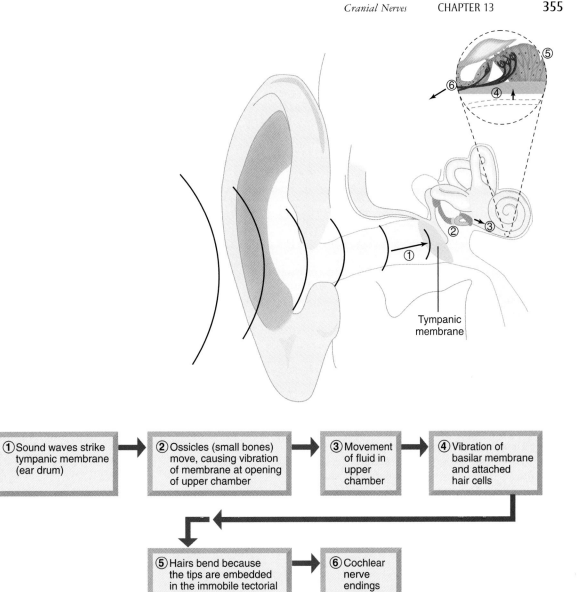

FIGURE 13-12
The conversion of sound waves into neural signals.

The longer fibers vibrate at a lower frequency than the shorter fibers. A low-frequency (low-pitched) sound will cause the longer fibers at the free end to vibrate more than the fibers at the attached end of the membrane. When the free end of the basilar membrane vibrates, the resulting neural signals are eventually perceived as low-pitched sounds.

Auditory Function Within the Central Nervous System

Auditory information
- Orients the head and eyes toward sounds
- Increases the activity level throughout the central nervous system
- Provides conscious awareness and recognition of sounds

For auditory information to be used for any of these functions, signals are first processed by the cochlear nuclei. From the cochlear nuclei, auditory information is transmitted to three structures (Figure 13-13):
- Reticular formation
- Inferior colliculus (directly and via the superior olive)
- Medial geniculate body

The reticular formation connections account for the activating effect of sounds on the entire central nervous system. For example, loud sounds can rouse a person from sleep. The inferior colliculus integrates auditory information from both ears to detect the location of sounds. When the location information is conveyed to the superior colliculus, neural activity in the superior colliculus elicits movement of the eyes and face toward the sound. The **medial geniculate body** serves as a thalamic relay station for auditory information to the primary auditory cortex, where sounds reach conscious awareness. The routing of auditory information is illustrated in Figure 13-14.

Three cortical areas are dedicated to processing auditory information. The primary auditory cortex is the site of conscious awareness of the intensity of sounds. An adjacent cortical area, the auditory association cortex, compares sounds with memories of other sounds, then

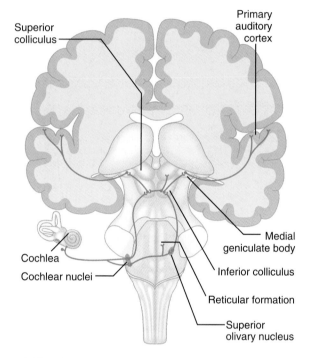

FIGURE 13-13
Pathway for auditory information from the cochlea to the cochlear nuclei, then to the reticular formation, inferior colliculus, and medial geniculate. The superior olivary nucleus relays information from the cochlear nuclei to the inferior colliculus. Information from the medial geniculate projects to the primary auditory cortex.

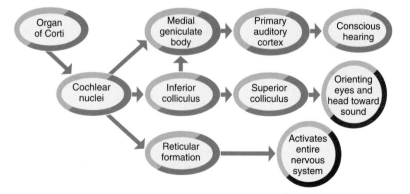

FIGURE 13-14
Flow of signals from the hearing apparatus (organ of Corti) to the outcomes of hearing: conscious hearing, orientation toward sound, and increased general arousal level.

categorizes the sounds as language, music, or noise. Comprehension of spoken language occurs in yet another cortical area, called *Wernicke's area.* These cortical areas are discussed further in Chapters 16 and 17.

CRANIAL NERVE IX: GLOSSOPHARYNGEAL

The **glossopharyngeal nerve** is a mixed nerve containing both sensory and motor fibers. The sensory fibers transmit somatosensation from the soft palate and pharynx and information from chemoreceptors in the posterior tongue (Figure 13-15). The motor component innervates a pharyngeal muscle and the parotid salivary gland.

Glossopharyngeal sensory fibers contribute the afferent limb of the gag reflex, which can be activated by touching the pharynx with a cotton-tipped swab. The information is conveyed to the spinal nucleus located in the dorsal medulla, then by interneurons to the nucleus ambiguus located in the lateral medulla. Cranial nerve X (see subsequent section) then provides the efferent signals, causing the pharyngeal muscles to contract.

> The primary function of the glossopharyngeal nerve is to convey somatosensory information from the soft palate and pharynx.

CRANIAL NERVE X: VAGUS

The **vagus nerve** provides afferent and efferent innervation of the larynx, pharynx, and viscera (Figure 13-16). Cell bodies of the visceral afferent fibers are located in the inferior nucleus of the vagus, outside the brainstem. Cell bodies of the efferent fibers are in the nucleus ambiguus and the dorsal efferent nucleus of the vagus, both in the medulla.

Vagal parasympathetic fibers, both afferent and efferent, are extensively distributed to the larynx, pharynx, trachea, lungs, heart, gastrointestinal tract (except the lower large intestine), pancreas, gallbladder, and liver. These far-reaching connections allow the vagus to decrease heart rate, constrict the bronchi, affect speech production, and increase digestive activity. The motor function of the vagus nerve can be tested by eliciting the gag reflex, discussed in the previous section.

CRANIAL NERVE XI: ACCESSORY

The **accessory nerve** is motor, providing innervation to the trapezius and sternocleidomastoid muscles. The accessory nerve (Figure 13-17) originates in the spinal accessory nucleus in the upper cervical cord, travels upward through the foramen magnum, and then leaves the skull through the jugular foramen. The cell bodies are in the ventral horn at levels C1 to C4.

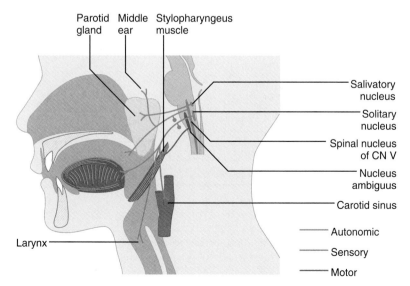

FIGURE 13-15

The glossopharyngeal nerve provides the afferent limb of the gag and swallowing reflexes, supplies taste information, and innervates a salivary gland. The red nucleus and axon are motor; the blue are sensory; the green are autonomic.

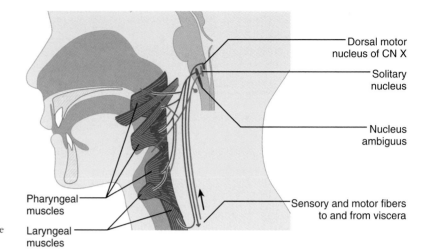

FIGURE 13-16
The vagus nerve regulates viscera, swallowing, and speech and supplies taste information. CN, cranial nerve.

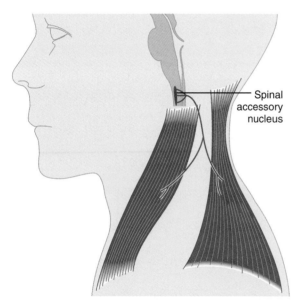

FIGURE 13-17
The accessory nerve innervates the sternocleidomastoid and trapezius muscles.

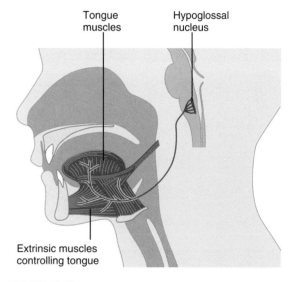

FIGURE 13-18
The hypoglossal nerve innervates muscles of the tongue.

CRANIAL NERVE XII: HYPOGLOSSAL

The **hypoglossal nerve** is motor, providing innervation to the intrinsic and extrinsic muscles of the ipsilateral tongue (Figure 13-18). Cell bodies are located in the hypoglossal nucleus of the medulla. Activity of the hypoglossal nerve is controlled by both voluntary and reflexive neural circuits.

CRANIAL NERVES INVOLVED IN SWALLOWING AND SPEAKING

Swallowing

Swallowing involves three stages: **oral, pharyngeal/laryngeal,** and **esophageal.** Table 13-3 indicates the participation of the cranial nerves in each stage.

Table 13-3   PHASES OF SWALLOWING

Stage	Description	Cranial Nerve
Oral	Food in mouth, lips close	VII
	Jaw, cheek, and tongue movements manipulate food	V, VII, XII
	Tongue moves food to pharynx entrance	XII
	Larynx closes	X
	Swallow reflex triggered	IX
Pharyngeal/laryngeal	Food moves into pharynx	IX
	Soft palate rises to block food from nasal cavity	X
	Epiglottis covers trachea to prevent food from entering lungs	X
	Peristalsis moves food to entrance of esophagus, sphincter opens, food moves into esophagus	X
Esophageal	Peristalsis moves food into stomach	X

Speaking

Speaking requires cortical control, which will be discussed in Chapter 16. At the cranial nerve level, sounds generated by the larynx (cranial nerve X) are articulated by the soft palate (cranial nerve X), lips (cranial nerve VII), jaws (cranial nerve V), and tongue (cranial nerve XII).

Cranial nerves I and II (olfactory and optic) convey information into the cerebrum. Cranial nerves III, IV, and VI (oculomotor, trochlear, and abducens) have nuclei in the pons and midbrain and control eye and upper eyelid movements. Cranial nerve III also constricts the pupil and adjusts the shape of the lens. Cranial nerves V and VII (trigeminal and facial) have nuclei throughout the brainstem and provide somatosensory and motor innervation of the face and muscles of mastication. Cranial nerve VII also innervates lacrimal, nasal, and salivary glands. The nuclei of cranial nerve VIII (vestibulocochlear) are located in the pons and medulla and provide information regarding head position relative to gravity, head movement, and sound. Cranial nerves IX, X, XI, and XII (glossopharyngeal, vagus, accessory, and hypoglossal, respectively) have nuclei in the medulla and spinal cord and provide sensory and motor innervation of the mouth, tongue, pharynx, and larynx; autonomic innervation to salivary glands and viscera; and motor innervation of the sternocleidomastoid and trapezius muscles.

SYSTEMS CONTROLLING CRANIAL NERVE LOWER MOTOR NEURONS

Cranial nerves III-VII and IX-XII contain lower motor neuron fibers. The activity of the motor fibers in cranial nerves is controlled via descending inputs from voluntary and limbic structures of the brainstem and cerebrum and also via local reflex mechanisms.

Descending Control of Motor Cranial Nerves

Like the lower motor neurons in the spinal cord, the cranial nerve efferents receive descending regulation by the corticofugal tracts and the limbic system. Thus, their activity can be affected by voluntary, emotional, or as mentioned previously for individual nerves, by reflexive pathways. Descending limbic pathways are separate from the corticobulbar tracts (Holstege, 1991).

An example of the dissociation of limbic and voluntary controlled movements is the facial nerve activity that produces a spontaneous smile, a result of limbic innervation and an expression of true emotion, versus an insincere smile that is produced voluntarily and can usually be detected. The facial expressions associated with powerful emotions are difficult to suppress voluntarily, but the same expressions may be difficult to produce intentionally.

Similarly, eye movements can be voluntarily controlled, or the eyes may be automatically drawn toward or avoid disturbing sights. Speaking is mainly voluntary but can occur automatically in highly emotional contexts. In some instances in which brain damage interferes with voluntary speech, the ability of the limbic system to produce emotionally charged words, such as profanity, may be preserved. Extreme emotions, by activating limbic pathways that influence motor activity, can interfere with the ability to eat and speak.

DISORDERS AFFECTING CRANIAL NERVE FUNCTION

Olfactory Nerve

Lesions of the olfactory nerve can result in an inability to smell. However, smoking or excessive nasal mucus may also interfere with the function of the olfactory nerve.

Optic Nerve

A complete interruption of the optic nerve results in ipsilateral blindness and loss of the pupillary light reflex. The pupillary light reflex is pupil constriction in response to a light shining into the client's eye. Loss of the pupillary light reflex may also occur with a lesion of cranial nerve III because the oculomotor nerve is the efferent limb of the reflex. Lesions at other sites in the visual pathway can also cause blindness (see Chapter 15).

Oculomotor Nerve

A complete lesion of the oculomotor nerve causes the following deficits (Figure 13-19):
- Ptosis (drooping of the eyelid), owing to paralysis of the voluntary muscle fibers that elevate the eyelid. The autonomic muscle fibers may be able to keep the eyelid partially elevated.
- The ipsilateral eye looks outward and down because the actions of the lateral rectus and the superior oblique muscles are unopposed.
- **Diplopia** (double vision), owing to the difference in position of the eyes. Because the eyes do not look in the same direction, the light rays from objects do not

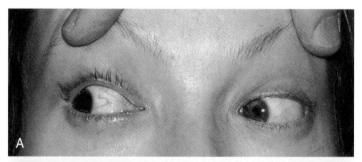
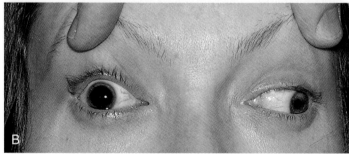
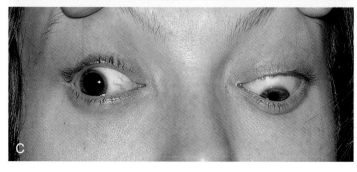

FIGURE 13-19
Weakness of the extraocular muscles due to a lesion involving the right oculomotor nerve (cranial nerve III). **A,** Complete ptosis of the right eye (inability to open eye). **B,** With the eyelids held open, on lateral gaze to the left, the right eye does not adduct. The unopposed pull of the lateral rectus (due to paresis of the medial rectus) abducts the right eye. The pupil is dilated and unresponsive to light. **C,** On looking downward, the vessels in the white part of the right eye show that the right eye is rotated clockwise by the intact superior oblique. *(From Parsons M, Johnson M (2001). Neurology: Diagnosis in Color. St. Louis: Mosby.)*

fall on corresponding areas of both retinas, producing double vision.

- Deficits in moving the ipsilateral eye medially, downward, and upward.
- Loss of pupillary reflex and consensual response to light.
- Loss of constriction of the pupil in response to focusing on a near object.

The signs of an oculomotor nerve lesion are illustrated in Figure 13-20, *A.* The eye movement deficits seen in an oculomotor nerve lesion must be differentiated from the asymmetrical eye movements that occur with upper motor neuron lesions or medial longitudinal fasciculus lesions. The reflexes producing pupillary constriction will be spared in upper motor neuron or medial longitudinal fasciculus lesions. Either of these disorders will be accompanied by more extensive brainstem or cerebral signs and symptoms (see Chapter 14).

Trochlear Nerve

A lesion of the trochlear nerve prevents activation of the superior oblique muscle, so the ipsilateral eye cannot look downward and inward (Figure 13-20, *B*). People with lesions of the trochlear nerve complain of double vision, difficulty reading, and visual problems when descending stairs. Other possible causes of eye movement asymmetry must be ruled out, as discussed for the oculomotor nerve.

Trigeminal Nerve

A complete severance of a branch of the trigeminal nerve results in anesthesia of the area supplied by the ophthalmic, maxillary, or mandibular branch. If the ophthalmic division is affected, the afferent limb of the blink reflex will be interrupted, preventing blinking in response to touch stimulation of the cornea. If the mandibular branch is completely severed, the jaw will deviate toward the involved side when the mouth is opened, and the masseter reflex will be lost.

Trigeminal Neuralgia

Trigeminal neuralgia (also known as *tic douloureux*) is a dysfunction of the trigeminal nerve, producing severe, sharp, stabbing pain in the distribution of one or more branches of the trigeminal nerve (Box 13-1). Several etiologies have been proposed:

- A peripheral lesion leading to segmental demyelination of the nerve, ephaptic transmission, and subsequent secondary changes in the spinal trigeminal nucleus (van Bijsterveld, 2005).

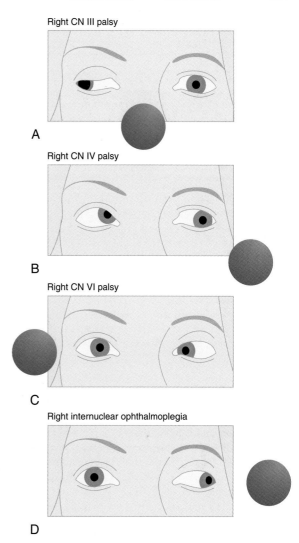

FIGURE 13-20

Lesions affecting eye movements. The ball is positioned in each panel to illustrate an impaired direction of gaze. The ball is distant from the eyes. All lesions are on the right side. Movements of the left eye are normal. **A,** Oculomotor nerve palsy. The right eye is abducted because of weakness of the medial rectus, the right eyelid droops, and the pupil is dilated. **B,** Trochlear nerve palsy. The right eye adducts but is elevated owing to weakness of the superior oblique muscle. **C,** Abducens nerve palsy. The right eye does not abduct because the lateral rectus muscle is weak. **D,** Internuclear ophthalmoplegia. The lesion affects the right medial longitudinal fasciculus, interrupting signals from the abducens nucleus to the oculomotor nucleus. The right eye does not adduct on voluntary gaze. However, the right eye does adduct during convergence eye movements (not illustrated) because different neural connections are involved in convergence eye movements.

BOX 13-1   TRIGEMINAL NEURALGIA (TIC DOULOUREUX)

Pathology
Unknown

Etiology
Unknown; hypotheses include segmental demyelination with subsequent changes in the spinal trigeminal nucleus, damage of trigeminal root ganglia, and compression of the nerve branch by a blood vessel

Speed of Onset
Abrupt

Signs and Symptoms
Weakness is greater than sensory signs
Consciousness
Normal
Communication and Memory
Normal
Sensory
Normal except for sharp, severe pains that last less than 2 minutes, usually only in one branch of the trigeminal nerve distribution and typically triggered by chewing, talking, brushing the teeth, or shaving

Autonomic
Normal
Motor
Normal

Region Affected
Peripheral part of cranial nerve V; may also involve spinal nucleus of cranial nerve V

Demographics
Women are 1.5 times more likely than men to have trigeminal neuralgia; mean age at onset is 55 years
Incidence
8 cases per 100,000 population people per year
Lifetime Prevalence
0.7 cases per 1000 population (MacDonald et al., 2000)

Prognosis
Variable; may resolve spontaneously after a few bouts, may recur, or may require medication or surgery to decompress the nerve

---

- Hyperexcitability of damaged fibers in the trigeminal root ganglia, leading to spontaneous neuronal firing (Rappaport and Devor, 1994)
- Pressure of a blood vessel on the nerve

The pain is triggered by stimuli that are normally not noxious, such as eating, talking, or touching the face. The pain begins and ends abruptly, lasts less than 2 minutes, and is not associated with sensory loss. Trigeminal neuralgia can be treated effectively by drugs or surgery (Mauskop, 1993).

Abducens Nerve

A complete lesion of the abducens nerve will cause the eye to look inward because the paralysis of the lateral rectus muscle leaves the pull of the medial rectus muscle unopposed. A person with this lesion will be unable to voluntarily abduct the eye and will have double vision (Figure 13-20, *C*). Other causes of asymmetrical eye movements must be ruled out, as discussed regarding the oculomotor nerve.

Medial Longitudinal Fasciculus

A lesion affecting the medial longitudinal fasciculus produces **internuclear ophthalmoplegia** (INO), by interrupting the signals from the abducens nucleus to the

oculomotor nucleus. Normally, when a person voluntarily moves his or her eyes in a horizontal direction, an area in the frontal lobe sends signals via an area in the pons to the abducens nucleus. In turn, the abducens nucleus sends signals to the ipsilateral lateral rectus muscle and to the contralateral oculomotor nucleus. The oculomotor nucleus sends signals to the medial rectus muscle via the oculomotor nerve. Therefore, when the connection between the abducens nucleus and the oculomotor nucleus is interrupted, the eye contralateral to the lesion moves normally but the eye ipsilateral to the lesion cannot adduct past the midline when the fellow eye moves laterally (Figure 13-20, *D* and Figure 13-21).

Facial Nerve

A lesion of the facial nerve causes paralysis or paresis of the ipsilateral muscles of facial expression. This causes one side of the face to droop and prevents the person from being able to completely close the ipsilateral eye. Unilateral facial palsy can result from a lesion of the cranial nerve VII nucleus or from a lesion of the axons of cranial nerve VII. If the lesion involves the axons, the disorder is called **Bell's palsy** (Figure 13-22; Box 13-2).

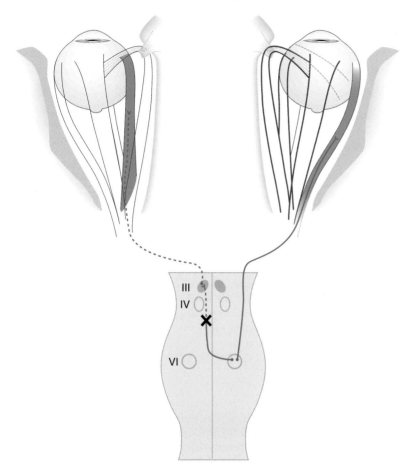

FIGURE 13-21

Mechanism of internuclear ophthalmoplegia. The indicated lesion of the medial longitudinal fasciculus prevents abducens nucleus signals from reaching the contralateral oculomotor nucleus. When the person attempts to voluntarily look to the left, the right eye does not adduct.

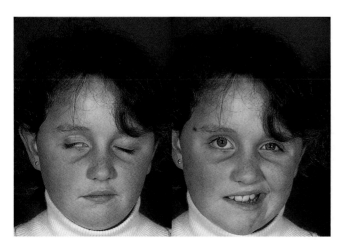

FIGURE 13-22

Right Bell's palsy, paralysis of the muscles innervated by the facial nerve. *(From Perkin GD (2002) Mosby's Color Atlas and Text of Neurology, (2ⁿᵈ ed.). Edinburgh: Mosby.)*

BOX 13-2 BELL'S PALSY

Pathology

Paralysis of the muscles innervated by the facial nerve (cranial nerve VII) on one side of the face

Etiology

Unknown; hypotheses include viral infection or immune disorder causing swelling of facial nerve within the temporal bone, resulting in compression and ischemia of the nerve

Speed of Onset

Acute

Signs and Symptoms

Weakness is greater than sensory signs

Consciousness

Normal

Communication and Memory

Normal

Sensory

Normal

Autonomic

In severe cases, salivation and production of tears may be affected

Motor

Paresis or paralysis of entire half of face, including frontalis and orbicularis oculi muscles; in severe cases, the ipsilateral eye cannot be closed

Region Affected

Peripheral part of cranial nerve VII

Demographics

Men and women affected equally; usually affects older adults

Incidence

25 cases per 100,000 people population per year (Hankey and Wardlaw, 2002)

Prognosis

Eighty percent recover neural control of facial muscles within 2 months; recovery depends on severity of damage, which can be assessed by nerve conduction velocity and electromyography; paresis is typically followed by complete recovery; outcome after complete paralysis varies from complete recovery to permanent paralysis

---

Both the facial and vestibular nerves are affected in **Ramsay-Hunt syndrome.** The syndrome, caused by varicella zoster infection, usually consists of acute facial paralysis accompanied by ear pain and blisters on the external ear. In some cases, blisters in the mouth and problems with balance, gaze stability, vertigo, hearing, and **tinnitus** (the sensation of ringing, hissing, or buzzing sounds) may also occur.

Vestibulocochlear Nerve and Disorders of the Auditory System

Deafness usually results from disorders affecting peripheral structures of the auditory system: the cochlea, the organ of Corti within the cochlea, or the cochlear branch of the vestibulocochlear nerve. Loss of hearing in one ear interferes with the ability to locate sounds, because normally the timing of input from each ear is compared to locate sounds in space. Deafness due to peripheral disorders is classified as either conductive or sensorineural deafness.

Conductive deafness occurs when transmission of vibrations is prevented in the outer or middle ear. The common causes of conductive deafness are excessive wax in the outer ear canal or otitis media (inflammation in the middle ear). In otitis media, movement of the ossicles is restricted by thick fluid in the middle ear.

Sensorineural deafness, due to damage of the receptor cells or the cochlear nerve, is less common than conductive deafness. The usual causes are ototoxic drugs, Ménière's disease (see discussion of vestibular disorders in Chapter 15), and acoustic neuroma. Ototoxic drugs have a poisoning effect on auditory structures, damaging cranial nerve VIII and/or the hearing and vestibular organs. An acoustic neuroma is a benign tumor of myelin cells surrounding cranial nerve VIII within the cranium. An acoustic neuroma causes a slow, progressive, unilateral loss of hearing. Tinnitus and problems with balance occur frequently. As the acoustic neuroma grows, additional cranial nerves are compressed, producing facial palsy (cranial nerve VII) and decreased sensation from the face (cranial nerve V). Very large tumors may interfere with the functions of cranial nerves VI-XII. Acoustic tumors are usually removed surgically.

Disorders within the central nervous system rarely cause deafness because auditory information projects bilaterally in the brainstem and cerebrum. Thus, small lesions in the brainstem typically do not interfere with the ability to hear. In the cerebral cortex, each primary auditory cortex receives auditory information from both ears, so that hearing remains fairly normal when one primary auditory cortex is damaged. If the primary auditory cortex is destroyed on one side, the only loss is the ability to consciously identify the location of sounds, because conscious location of sound is accomplished by comparing the time lag between auditory information reaching the cortex on one side versus the time required for auditory information to reach the opposite cortex.

A complete lesion of the cochlear branch of cranial nerve VIII causes unilateral deafness. Vestibular dysfunctions are discussed in Chapter 15.

Glossopharyngeal Nerve

A complete lesion of cranial nerve IX interrupts the afferent limb of both the gag reflex and the swallowing reflex (cranial nerve X provides the efferent limb for both reflexes). Salivation is also decreased.

Vagus Nerve

A complete lesion of the vagus nerve results in difficulty speaking and swallowing, poor digestion due to decreased digestive enzymes and decreased peristalsis, asymmetrical elevation of the palate, and hoarseness.

Accessory Nerve

A complete lesion of the accessory nerve paralyzes the ipsilateral sternocleidomastoid and trapezius muscles. Upper motor neuron lesions, in contrast, cause paresis rather than paralysis because cortical innervation is bilateral, and the muscles become hypertonic rather than hypotonic.

Hypoglossal Nerve

A complete lesion of the hypoglossal nerve causes atrophy of the ipsilateral tongue. When a person with this lesion is asked to stick out the tongue, the tongue protrudes ipsilaterally rather than in the midline. The problems with tongue control result in difficulty speaking and swallowing.

Dysphagia

Difficulty swallowing is **dysphagia**. Frequent choking, lack of awareness of food in one side of the mouth, or food coming out of the nose may indicate dysfunctions of cranial nerves V, VII, IX, X, or XII. Upper motor neuron lesions may also cause swallowing dysfunctions.

Dysarthria

Poor control of the speech muscles is **dysarthria**. In dysarthria, only vocal speech is affected, that is, motor production of sounds. People with dysarthria can understand spoken language, write, and read. Lower motor neuron involvement of cranial nerves V, VII, X, or XII can cause dysarthria. Dysarthria can also result from upper motor neuron lesions or muscle dysfunction.

TESTING CRANIAL NERVES

Standard tests are used to assess cranial nerve function. Table 13-4 lists the cranial nerve tests and the effects of lesions of individual cranial nerves.

SUMMARY

The cranial nerves innervate the head, neck, and viscera. Cranial nerves I and II are part of the central nervous system and convey olfactory and visual information. Cranial nerves III-XII continue into the periphery. Cranial nerves III, IV, and VI innervate eye muscles. Cranial nerve V conveys somatosensory information from the face and mouth and motor signals to the muscles of mastication. Cranial nerve VII innervates the muscles of facial expression, salivary glands and taste receptors. Cranial nerve VIII conveys auditory and vestibular information. The last four cranial nerves innervate the mouth, neck, and viscera. Cranial nerve IX carries information from the tongue and larynx. Cranial nerve X is motor to the palate, pharynx, larynx, heart, and glands and afferent for visceral sensations. Cranial nerve XI is motor to the sternocleidomastoid and trapezius muscles. Cranial nerve XII is motor to the tongue. Because these nerves are frequently damaged by trauma or disease, knowing their functions and the disorders that affect the cranial nerves is essential for clinical practice.

Table 13-4 CRANIAL NERVE TESTS

Nerve	Test	Normal Response	Cranial Nerve Lesion	Differentiate From
Olfactory	Patient closes eyes, closes one nostril, then smells coffee or cloves.	Patient identifies substance.	Lack of ability to smell; however, mucus or smoking may interfere with the ability to smell.	
Optic	With patient's left eye covered, patient looks into examiner's eye. Examiner covers his or her own right eye. Examiner tells patient, "Keep looking into my eye. I'm testing what you can see at the edges of your vision. Say 'now' when you see my finger." Examiner positions finger midway between patient's eye and examiner's own eye, just beyond edge of examiner's own peripheral vision. Examiner moves the finger slowly toward the visual center until patient reports seeing the finger. Then test patient's right eye.	Patient reports seeing finger.	If optic nerve is completely interrupted, patient is ipsilaterally blind.	Lesions at other sites in the visual pathway also interfere with vision (see Chapter 15).
	Shine light into patient's eye. Observe pupil (pupillary reflex).	Pupil constricts (cranial nerve III provides the reflex efferent limb).	Response is slow or absent.	Lesion in the pretectal area or parasympathetic nuclei of the oculomotor nerve. Other brainstem signs (see Chapter 14) will accompany either of these lesions.

Table 13-4   CRANIAL NERVE TESTS—cont'd

Nerve	Test	Normal Response	Cranial Nerve Lesion	Differentiate From
Oculomotor	Ask patient to look straight ahead. Examine the height of the space between upper and lower eyelids and the position of eyelids relative to the iris and pupil. Then ask the patient to look upward without moving the head.	The position of the eyelids is symmetrical, and the upper eyelid covers the upper iris, superior to the pupil. The upper eyelid retracts with upward gaze.	The height of the space between the eyelids is asymmetrical, and the drooping eyelid (ptosis) does not retract with upward gaze. This finding indicates an oculomotor nerve lesion. Additional signs of oculomotor nerve lesion include dilated pupil, lateral and downward deviation of the eye when attempting to look forward, and diplopia.	The height of the space between the eyelids is asymmetrical, yet the drooping eyelid retracts with upward gaze. This finding indicates a lesion involving the sympathetic innervation of the head. Additional signs of such a lesion include absence of sweating and redness of one side of the face and constriction of the pupil (Horner's syndrome).
	Observe position of patient's eyes with patient looking forward.	Both eyes appear to look in the same direction; no nystagmus (involuntary back-and-forth movements of the eyes).	Ipsilateral eye looks outward and down (pulled by unopposed lateral rectus and superior oblique). Patient reports double vision.	
	Observe size of pupil in room light.	Moderate size.	Dilated pupil.	Extremely small pupil: sympathetic dysfunction (Horner's syndrome—see Chapter 8).
	Patient's eyes follow examiner's finger, moving eyes up, down, and in (testing superior, medial, and inferior rectus muscles).	Eyes move symmetrically and smoothly.	Deficits in adduction, depression, or elevation of the eye.	Asymmetrical eye movements; due to upper motor neuron or medial longitudinal fasciculus lesion.

Continued

Table 13-4 CRANIAL NERVE TESTS—cont'd

Nerve	Test	Normal Response	Cranial Nerve Lesion	Differentiate From
	Patient's eye follows examiner's finger to about 50° adduction, then up (testing inferior oblique muscle).	Eye follows finger movement.	Unable to adduct and elevate eye.	Asymmetrical eye movements; due to upper motor neuron or medial longitudinal fasciculus lesion.
	Dim the room lights, then shine light into patient's eye (pupillary reflex and consensual response to light).	Constriction of pupils (requires cranial nerve II for afferent limb of reflex).	Pupil unchanged.	Lesion in the pretectal area or parasympathetic nuclei of the oculomotor nerve. Other brainstem signs (see Chapter 14) will accompany either of these lesions.
	Patient looks at examiner's finger, then examiner's nose. Observe pupillary response to near and far objects.	Near object: constriction. Far object: dilation.	Pupil unchanged.	
	Convergence. Convergence is adduction of the eyes. Ask patient to look at the tip of a pen as it is slowly moved from about 2 feet away toward the patient's nose.	Both eyes are directed toward the pen tip until the pen is within 10 cm (4 inches) of the nose.	Only one eye moves toward the midline; the other eye moves outward.	Asymmetrical eye movements due to upper motor neuron lesion.
Trochlear	Patient's eye follows examiner's finger to about 50° adduction, then down (testing superior oblique muscle).	Eye moves in, then down.	Deficit in looking inferomedially. Patient reports double vision and difficulty reading, descending stairs.	Asymmetrical eye movements; due to upper motor neuron or medial longitudinal fasciculus lesion.

Table 13-4   CRANIAL NERVE TESTS—cont'd

Nerve	Test	Normal Response	Cranial Nerve Lesion	Differentiate From
Trigeminal	With patient's eyes closed, use light touch and pin to assess facial sensation in three areas: forehead, cheek, chin.	Distinguishes between sharp and dull and can localize stimulus.	Anesthesia in affected area; or patient reports severe pain in trigeminal branch distribution (trigeminal neuralgia, a severe neuropathic pain).	
	Touch outer cornea with a wisp of cotton (corneal reflex).	Eye blinks (requires efferent limb via cranial nerve VII).	Eye does not close (because response is bilateral, can stimulate other eye to determine if absence of reflex is due to problem with afferent or efferent limb).	
	Manual muscle test: jaw opening and closing strength.	Jaw opens strongly and symmetrically. Jaw closes strongly. Palpate the masseter muscles while patient clenches the teeth, then relaxes.	Unilateral damage: jaw deviates toward weak side.	
	Tap downward on patient's chin with reflex hammer.	Masseter contracts, elevating chin.	Lost or decreased reflex.	Hyperreflexia; due to upper motor neuron lesion.
Abducens	Observe position of eyes with patient looking forward.	Both eyes appear to look in same direction; no nystagmus.	One eye looks inward (pulled by unopposed medial rectus); patient reports double vision.	

Continued

Table 13-4 CRANIAL NERVE TESTS—cont'd

Nerve	Test	Normal Response	Cranial Nerve Lesion	Differentiate From
	Patient follows examiner's finger to look laterally.	Eye moves laterally.	Deficit of abduction.	Asymmetrical eye movements; due to upper motor neuron or medial longitudinal fasciculus lesion.
Facial	Facial movements: raise eyebrows, close eyes, smile, puff cheeks.	Able to perform requested movements.	Paralysis or paresis, with upper and lower face equally involved: cranial nerve VII nucleus or Bell's palsy. Bell's palsy affects axons of facial nerve, preventing patient from completely closing ipsilateral eye.	A corticospinal lesion interfering with signals to cranial nerve VII spares the frontalis and orbicularis oculi muscles and causes paresis of the lower face.
Vestibulocochlear	Vestibular function (see Chapter 15).			
	Auditory function: examiner rubs fingers together near patient's ear; performance can be compared with examiner's own hearing.	Patient reports hearing the stimulus equally in each ear.	Difference in acuity of patient's ears or in patient's and examiner's ability to hear should be investigated further.	
	Auditory function: hold vibrating tuning fork on mastoid bone; when patient no longer hears it, move tuning fork into the air about 1 inch from ear canal.	Patient hears through air after cannot hear through bone.	Patient hears through air after cannot hear through bone, but volume is reduced for both air and bone conduction (sensorineural hearing loss).	Hearing longer through bone indicates conduction loss; due to auditory canal or middle ear lesion.

Table 13-4   CRANIAL NERVE TESTS—cont'd

Nerve	Test	Normal Response	Cranial Nerve Lesion	Differentiate From
Glossopharyngeal	Touch soft palate with cotton swab (gag reflex).	Gagging and symmetrical elevation of soft palate; requires cranial nerve X efferents.	Lack of gag reflex, or asymmetrical elevation of soft palate.	
Vagus	Patient opens mouth and says "ah." Examiner observes soft palate.	Elevation of soft palate.	Asymmetrical elevation of soft palate; hoarseness.	
Accessory	Manual muscle test: sternocleidomastoid and upper trapezius.	Normal strength.	Paralysis or paresis.	Upper motor neuron lesion: paresis with hypertonia; bilateral cortical innervation prevents complete paralysis.
Hypoglossal	Patient protrudes tongue.	Tongue protrudes in midline.	Protruded tongue deviates to the side of the lesion, and ipsilateral tongue atrophies.	
	Patient pushes tongue into cheek. On outside of cheek, examiner pushes against the tongue.	Tongue able to resist moderate force.	Force of tongue easily overcome by examiner's pressure.	

CLINICAL NOTES

Case 1

RF is a 62-year-old man who was involved in a car accident 5 days ago. He sustained fractures of the skull, both femurs, and the right tibia. He complains of double vision.
- Consciousness, cognition, language, memory, and somatosensation are normal.
- All autonomic functions, including pupillary and accommodation reflexes, are normal.
- Motor function is normal except for an inability to look downward and inward with the right eye. All other eye movements, including the ability to look medially and laterally with the right eye, are normal. When asked, he says he has been having trouble reading since the accident.

Question

What is the most likely location of the lesion?

Continued

CLINICAL NOTES

Case 2

AK, a 46-year-old engineer, is complaining of double vision. She cannot read or drive unless she closes one eye. The following are findings on the cranial nerve examination:

- Olfaction, vision, facial sensation, control of the muscles of facial expression, mastication, hearing, equilibrium, gag and swallowing reflexes, and contraction of the sternocleidomastoid, trapezius, and tongue muscles are normal.
- When AK is instructed to look straight ahead, her right eye looks outward and down.
- AK cannot look in, down, or up with her right eye.
- AK can only open the right eyelid halfway.
- No pupillary reflex or consensual response occurs when a flashlight is shined into her right eye, nor does the pupil constrict when she focuses on an object 6 inches from her right eye.

Questions
1. Is this an upper motor neuron lesion? Why or why not?
2. Where is the lesion?

Case 3

MR awoke with an inability to move the left side of his face. His neurologic examination was normal, including facial sensation and control of the muscles of mastication and the tongue, except for the following:

- Drooping of the left side of the face.
- Complete lack of movement of the muscles of facial expression on the left. Examples include MR's inability to voluntarily smile, pucker his lips, or raise his eyebrow on the left side. Emotional facial expressions were also absent; when he smiled with the right side of his lips, the left half of his lips did not move.
- Inability to close his left eye.

Question
What is the most likely location of the lesion?

REVIEW QUESTIONS

1. How are the eyes voluntarily moved to follow an examiner's finger to the right and then look up? Include both muscle and cranial nerve activity in the answer.
2. Which cranial nerve provides efferents for the pupillary reflex?
3. Which cranial nerve provides efferents to the tongue muscles?
4. Which cranial nerve provides afferents for the gag reflex?
5. Which cranial nerve provides control of the muscles of facial expression?
6. Which cranial nerve provides somatosensation from the face?
7. Diagram the accommodation reflex.
8. What is the function of the organ of Corti?
9. Why is there a difference between an authentic smile and a false smile?
10. Which cranial nerves are required for swallowing?
11. Lesions of what structures could cause double vision?

References

Hankey GJ, Wardlaw JM. (2002). Clinical Neurology. New York: Demos Medical Publishing.

Holstege G (1991). Descending motor pathways and the spinal motor system: Limbic and non-limbic components. Progress in Brain Research, 87, 307-421.

MacDonald BK, Cockerell OC, et al. (2000). The incidence and lifetime prevalence of neurological disorders in a prospective community-based study in the UK [see comments]. Brain, 123(Pt 4), 665-676.

Mauskop A (1993). Trigeminal neuralgia (tic douloureaux). Journal of Pain Symptom Management, 8(3), 148-154.

Rappaport AH, Devor M (1994). Trigeminal neuralgia: The role of self-sustaining discharge in the trigeminal ganglion. Pain, 56, 127-138.

van Bijsterveld OP, Kruize AA, et al. (2005). Central nervous system mechanisms in Sjogren's syndrome. British Journal of Ophthalmology, 87; 128-130.

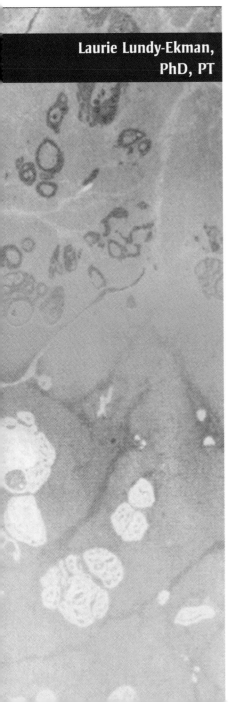

14 Brainstem Region

Laurie Lundy-Ekman,
PhD, PT

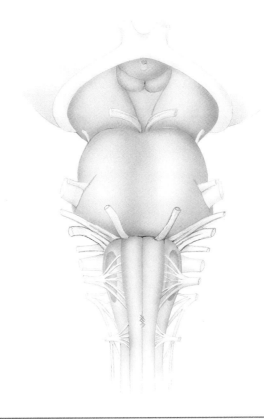

INTRODUCTION

The brainstem is superior to the spinal cord and inferior to the cerebrum, with the cerebellum appended posteriorly. From inferior to superior, the parts of the brainstem are the medulla, pons, and midbrain (Figure 14-1). The locations of cranial nerve nuclei in the brainstem are shown in Figure 14-2.

ANATOMY OF THE BRAINSTEM

Vertical Tracts in the Brainstem

Sensory, autonomic, and motor vertical tracts travel through the brainstem, just as in the spinal cord. The sensory tracts conveying information from the spinal cord to the brain, and the motor tracts conveying signals from the cortex to the brainstem and spinal cord, have been discussed in Chapters 6-10. Some of these tracts continue through the brainstem without alteration. For these tracts, the brainstem acts as a conduit. Other vertical tracts leave the brainstem or synapse in brainstem nuclei. Modifications of the vertical tracts in the brainstem are summarized in Table 14-1 and illustrated in Figure 14-3.

Vertical tracts that originate in the brainstem and project to the spinal cord are the tecto-, rubro-, reticulo-, vestibulo-, ceruleo-, and raphespinal. The origins and functions of these tracts are discussed in Chapter 9.

Longitudinal Sections of the Brainstem

The brainstem is divided longitudinally into two sections: the basilar section and the tegmentum. Throughout the brainstem, the basilar section is located anteriorly and contains predominantly motor system structures (see Chapter 9):

- Descending axons from the cerebral cortex: corticospinal, corticobulbar, corticopontine, and corticoreticular tracts
- Motor nuclei: the substantia nigra, pontine nuclei, and inferior olive
- Pontocerebellar axons

The tegmentum, located posteriorly, includes the following:

- The reticular formation, which adjusts the general level of activity throughout the nervous system
- Sensory nuclei and ascending sensory tracts (see Chapters 6 and 7)
- Cranial nerve nuclei (discussed later in this chapter)
- The medial longitudinal fasciculus, a tract that coordinates eye and head movements

In addition to basilar and tegmentum sections, the midbrain has an additional longitudinal section, posterior to the tegmentum, called the *tectum.* The tectum includes structures involved in reflexive control of

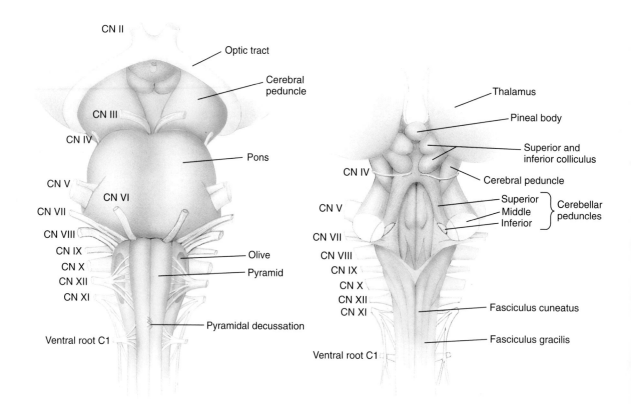

FIGURE 14-1
Anterior and posterior views of the brainstem.

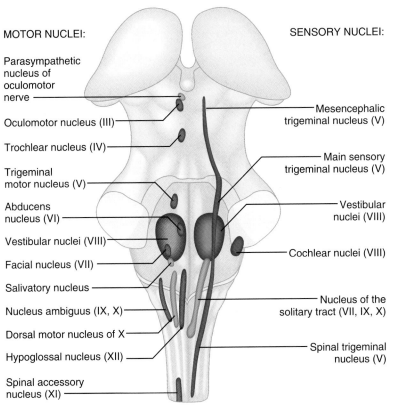

MOTOR NUCLEI:

Parasympathetic nucleus of oculomotor nerve

Oculomotor nucleus (III)

Trochlear nucleus (IV)

Trigeminal motor nucleus (V)

Abducens nucleus (VI)

Vestibular nuclei (VIII)

Facial nucleus (VII)

Salivatory nucleus

Nucleus ambiguus (IX, X)

Dorsal motor nucleus of X

Hypoglossal nucleus (XII)

Spinal accessory nucleus (XI)

SENSORY NUCLEI:

Mesencephalic trigeminal nucleus (V)

Main sensory trigeminal nucleus (V)

Vestibular nuclei (VIII)

Cochlear nuclei (VIII)

Nucleus of the solitary tract (VII, IX, X)

Spinal trigeminal nucleus (V)

FIGURE 14-2

The locations of cranial nerve nuclei in the brainstem. Motor nuclei are indicated on the left in red, and sensory nuclei are indicated on the right in blue. Autonomic nuclei that are the source of efferents are indicated on the left in green, and the autonomic nucleus that receives afferent information is indicated in green on the right.

Table 14-1 VERTICAL TRACTS IN THE BRAINSTEM

Vertical Tract	Modification of Tract in Brainstem
Sensory (Ascending) Tracts	
Spinothalamic	Not modified (tract passes through brainstem without alteration)
Dorsal column	Axons synapse in nucleus gracilis or cuneatus; second-order neurons cross midline to form medial lemniscus
Spinocerebellar	Axons leave brainstem via inferior and superior cerebellar peduncles to enter the cerebellum
Autonomic (Descending) Tracts	
Sympathetic	Not modified (tract passes through brainstem without alteration)
Parasympathetic	Axons synapse with brainstem parasympathetic nuclei or continue through brainstem and cord to the sacral level of spinal cord
Motor (Descending) Tracts	
Corticospinal	Not modified (tract passes through brainstem without alteration)
Corticobulbar	Axons synapse with cranial nerve nuclei in brainstem
Corticopontine	Axons synapse with nuclei in pons
Corticoreticular	Axons synapse within reticular formation

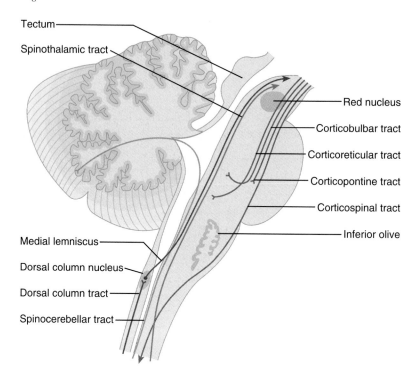

FIGURE 14-3
Vertical tracts in the brainstem. For simplicity, the autonomic tracts are omitted.

intrinsic and extrinsic eye muscles and in movements of the head:

- Pretectal area
- Superior and inferior colliculi

The preceding structures are discussed in the context of their location in the medulla, pons, or midbrain. Because the reticular formation extends vertically throughout the brainstem, it is discussed next.

> The longitudinal sections of the brainstem are the basilar, tegmentum, and in the midbrain, the tectum. The basilar section is primarily motor. The tegmentum is involved in adjusting the general level of neural activity, integrating sensory information, and cranial nerve functions. The tectum regulates eye reflexes and reflexive head movements.

RETICULAR FORMATION

The reticular formation is a complex neural network including the reticular nuclei, their connections, and ascending and descending reticular pathways (Figure 14-4). The reticular formation:

- Integrates sensory and cortical information
- Regulates somatic motor activity, autonomic function, and consciousness
- Modulates nociceptive/pain information

RETICULAR NUCLEI AND THEIR NEUROTRANSMITTERS

Reticular nuclei regulate neural activity throughout the central nervous system. Neurons in each nucleus produce a different neurotransmitter. The transmitters released by the reticular nuclei are all slow acting or neuromodulating, although the same transmitter may be fast acting in other neural subsystems. For example, acetylcholine (ACh) released from a reticular nucleus is slow acting, while ACh released in the peripheral nervous system is fast-acting (Pepeu and Giovannini, 2004). Slow-acting neurotransmitters alter the release of fast-acting neurotransmitters or the response of receptors to fast-acting neurotransmitters. The slow action is achieved by either indirect opening of ion channels or by activating a cascade of intracellular events (see Chapter 3). These slow-acting or neuromodulating neurotransmitters markedly influence activity in other parts of the brain-

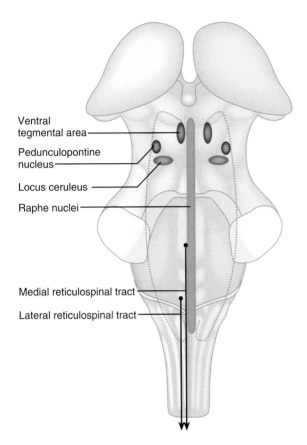

FIGURE 14-4

Reticular formation: reticular nuclei and tracts. Dotted lines indicate the extent of the reticular formation. The reticular nuclei include the ventral tegmental area, pedunculopontine nucleus, locus ceruleus, and raphe nuclei. Two of the upper motor neuron tracts that arise in the reticular formation, the reticulospinal tracts, are shown. The ceruleospinal and raphespinal tracts also arise in the reticular formation (not illustrated). The ascending projections of the reticular nuclei are illustrated in Figure 14-5.

stem and in the cerebrum and cerebellum. Several also influence neural activity in the spinal cord.

Although the reticular nuclei are confined to small regions in the brainstem, their axons project to widespread areas of the brain and, in some cases, to the spinal cord. The major reticular nuclei are as follows:

- Ventral tegmental area
- Pedunculopontine nucleus
- Raphe nuclei
- Locus ceruleus and medial reticular area

Ventral Tegmental Area: Dopamine

Most neurons that produce dopamine are located in the midbrain. Of the two midbrain areas that produce dopamine, only one, the ventral tegmental area (VTA), is part of the reticular formation. The other dopamine-producing area is the substantia nigra, discussed in Chapter 10 as part of the basal ganglia circuit that supplies dopamine to the caudate and putamen. The VTA provides dopamine to cerebral areas important in motivation and in decision making (Figure 14-5, *A*). Activation of the VTA affects the nucleus accumbens, producing feelings of pleasure and reward (Menon and Levitin, 2005; Gardner, 2005). The powerful effect of VTA activity is demonstrated in addiction to amphetamines and cocaine. Both drugs activate the VTA dopamine system. Morphine is habit forming because it inhibits inhibitory inputs to the VTA, thus increasing dopamine release. Excessive VTA activity has been hypothesized to explain certain aspects of schizophrenia, because drugs that block a particular type of dopamine receptor (D$_2$) have antipsychotic effects (Margolis et al., 2006). Schizophrenia is a disorder of perception and thought processes characterized by withdrawal from the outside world.

Pedunculopontine Nucleus: Acetylcholine

The pedunculopontine nucleus is located in the caudal midbrain (Figure 14-5, *B*). Ascending axons from the pedunculopontine nucleus project to the inferior part of the frontal cerebral cortex and the intralaminar nuclei of the thalamus. The pedunculopontine nucleus influences movement via connections with the following (Winn, 2006):

- Globus pallidus and subthalamic nucleus
- Vestibular nuclei
- Reticular areas that give rise to the reticulospinal tracts

In cats that have a lesion separating the brainstem from the cerebrum, electrical stimulation of the pedunculopontine nucleus can induce walking despite the lack of cerebral connection with the spinal cord.

Raphe Nuclei: Serotonin

Most cells that produce serotonin are found along the midline of the brainstem, in the raphe nuclei (Figure 14-5, *C*). The midbrain raphe nuclei project throughout the cerebrum. Serotonin levels also have profound effects on mood. The antidepressant fluoxetine (Prozac) prolongs the availability of serotonin by inhibiting the reuptake of serotonin (Carrasco and Sandner, 2005).

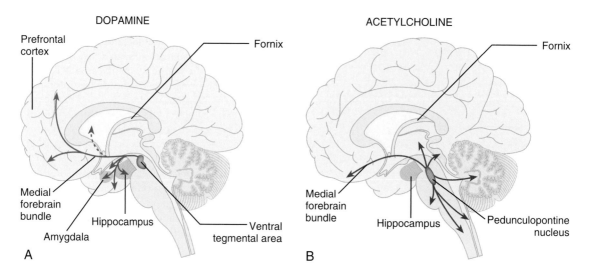

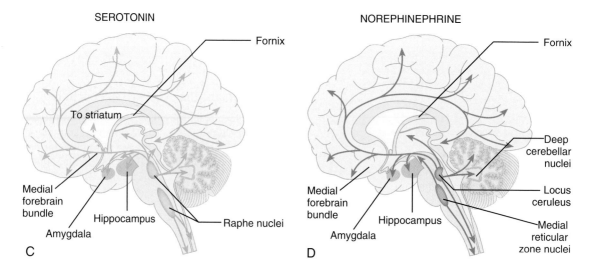

FIGURE 14-5

Reticular nuclei, located in the brainstem, produce neurotransmitters that are slow acting or neuromodulating. The ascending fibers from the reticular nuclei form the ascending reticular activating system, which regulates activity in the cerebral cortex. Descending fibers adjust the general level of activity in the spinal cord. **A,** The ventral tegmental area supplies dopamine to the frontal cortex and limbic areas. **B,** The pedunculopontine nucleus provides ACh to the thalamus, frontal cerebral cortex, brainstem, and cerebellum, and facilitates the reticulospinal tracts. **C,** The raphe nuclei supply serotonin to the thalamus, midbrain tectum, striatum, amygdala, hippocampus, cerebellum, throughout the cerebral cortex, and to the spinal cord (raphespinal tract). **D,** The locus ceruleus and medial reticular zone nuclei provide norepinephrine in a wide distribution similar to the pattern of serotonin distribution. The tracts descending into the spinal cord are the medial reticulospinal and ceruleospinal tracts.

The pontine raphe nuclei modulate neural activity throughout the brainstem and in the cerebellum. The medullary raphe nuclei send axons into the spinal cord to modulate sensory, autonomic, and motor activity (Mason, 2001). Some medullary raphe nuclei are part of the fast-acting neuronal pathway for descending pain inhibition (see Figure 7-11). Ascending pain information stimulates both the periaqueductal gray and the medullary raphe nuclei. In response, axons from the medullary raphe nuclei release serotonin onto interneurons in the dorsal horn that inhibit the transmission of pain information (see Chapter 7). Raphespinal endings in the lateral horn influence the cardiovascular system. Raphespinal endings in the anterior horn provide nonspecific activation of interneurons and lower motor neurons (see Chapter 9).

Locus Ceruleus and Medial Reticular Zone: Norepinephrine

The locus ceruleus and medial reticular zone are the source of most norepinephrine in the central nervous system (Figure 14-5, *D*). Axons from the locus ceruleus project throughout the brain and spinal cord. The locus ceruleus is most active when a person is attentive and is inactive during sleep. Activity of the ascending axons from the locus ceruleus provides the ability to direct attention (Aston-Jones, 2005). Descending axons from the locus ceruleus form the ceruleospinal tract, providing nonspecific activation of interneurons and motor neurons in the spinal cord. Ceruleospinal endings in the dorsal horn provide direct inhibition of spinothalamic neurons conveying pain information.

The medial reticular zone produces both norepinephrine and epinephrine. It regulates autonomic functions—respiratory, visceral, and cardiovascular—by projections to the hypothalamus, brainstem nuclei, and lateral horn of the spinal cord.

> Arousal levels in the cerebrum are influenced by the raphe nuclei, and attention is directed by the locus ceruleus. Descending axons from the locus ceruleus and the raphe nuclei determine the general level of neuronal activity in the spinal cord.

Regulation of Consciousness by the Ascending Reticular Activating System

Consciousness is the awareness of self and surroundings. The consciousness system governs alertness, sleep, and attention. Brainstem components of the consciousness

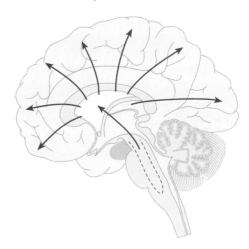

FIGURE 14-6
Ascending reticular activating system. Reticular formation (indicated by the dotted line) cells project to midline and intralaminar nuclei of the thalamus, then axons from these thalamic nuclei project throughout the cerebral cortex. When activated, the ARAS produces arousal of the entire cerebral cortex.

system are the reticular formation and its **ascending reticular activating system** (ARAS; Figure 14-6). The axons of the ARAS project to the cerebral components of the consciousness system: basal forebrain (anterior to the hypothalamus), thalamus, and cerebral cortex (Siegel, 2004). For normal sleep-wake cycles and the ability to direct attention while awake, all brainstem and cerebral components of the consciousness system must be functional.

Sleep, a periodic loss of consciousness, is actively induced by activity of areas within the ascending reticular activating system. The function of sleep is controversial. Current speculation on the role of sleep includes consolidation of memory, particularly memory for motor skills, and adjusting immune activity (Siegel, 2004).

MEDULLA

The medulla is the inferior part of the brainstem, continuous with the spinal cord inferiorly and the pons superiorly.

External Anatomy of the Medulla

Anteriorly, the medulla has two vertical bulges, called *pyramids*. Lateral to the pyramids are two small oval lumps, called *olives* (see Figure 14-1). Cranial nerve XII connects with the medulla between the pyramid and the olive. In a vertical groove lateral to the olive, cranial nerves IX, X, and XI attach to the medulla. The most prominent features of the posterior medulla are the inferior cerebellar peduncle and the widening of the central canal to become a larger space, the fourth ventricle.

Inferior Medulla

The inferior half of the medulla contains a central canal that is continuous with the central canal of the spinal cord. Anteriorly, the pyramids are formed by the descending axons of the corticospinal tract. Most (85%) of the corticospinal axons cross the midline in the pyramidal decussation at the inferior border of the medulla. The spinothalamic tracts maintain an anterolateral position, similar to their location in the cord (Figure 14-7, *B*). The dorsal column tracts synapse in their associated nuclei, the nucleus gracilis and cuneatus. The second-order fibers cross the midline in the decussation of the medial lemniscus, attaining a position posterior to the pyramids before ascending.

In addition to the connections between the spinal cord and cerebrum, the lower medulla also contains cranial nerve structures. The spinal tract and nucleus of the trigeminal nerve are located anterolateral to the nucleus cuneatus and convey pain and temperature information from the face. The medial longitudinal fasciculus, located near the center of the inferior medulla, coordinates eye and head movements via connections between the vestibular nuclei, spinal accessory nucleus, and the nuclei that control eye movements (see Figure 15-3).

> The corticospinal and dorsal column/medial lemniscus pathways cross the midline in the caudal medulla. Thus, these tracts connect the spinal cord with the opposite cerebral cortex. Cranial nerve V fibers conveying pain and temperature synapse in the caudal medulla.

Upper Medulla

In the upper half of the medulla, the central canal widens to form part of the fourth ventricle. Tracts in the rostral medulla maintain approximately the same positions as in the caudal medulla, except that the medial longitudinal fasciculus is located more posteriorly (Figure 14-7, *A*). Most cranial nerve nuclei in the rostral medulla are clustered in the dorsal section; from medial to lateral, the nuclei are the hypoglossal (cranial nerve XII), the dorsal motor nucleus of the vagus (cranial nerve X), the

solitary nucleus (visceral afferents from cranial nerves VII, IX, and X), and the vestibular and cochlear nuclei (cranial nerve VIII). The solitary nucleus receives visceral and taste afferent information. The nucleus ambiguus is the only cranial nerve nucleus in the medulla that is separate from the dorsally located group. The nucleus ambiguus is located more anteriorly and contributes motor fibers to striated muscles in the pharynx, larynx, and upper esophagus via cranial nerves IX and X. Corticobulbar tracts provide cortical input to the nucleus ambiguus and the hypoglossal nucleus. The corticobulbar projections are usually bilateral; however, occasionally the projections to the hypoglossal nucleus are contralateral.

At the junction of the medulla and the pons are the cochlear and vestibular nuclei, which receive auditory and vestibular information via cranial nerve VIII. Auditory information from the cochlea of the inner ear is transmitted to the cochlear nuclei by the cochlear nerve. Head movement and head position relative to gravity are signaled by receptors in the labyrinths of the inner ear (see Chapter 15); the vestibular nerve relays this information to the vestibular nuclei. The medial and lateral vestibulospinal tracts (see Chapter 10) that arise from the vestibular nuclei contribute to the control of postural muscle activity.

Deep to the olive is the inferior olivary nucleus (see Figure 14-7, *A*). Shaped like a wrinkled paper bag, this nucleus receives input from most motor areas of the brain and spinal cord. Axons from the inferior olivary nucleus project to the contralateral cerebellar hemisphere via the olivocerebellar tract. Current theory on the role of the inferior olivary nucleus is that these neurons are important for the perception of time (Xu et al., 2006).

The medulla sends many fibers (spino-, olivo-, vestibulo-, and reticulocerebellar) to the cerebellum via the inferior cerebellar peduncle. Only one fiber tract, the cerebellovestibular tract, sends information from the cerebellum to the medulla.

> The rostral medulla contains nuclei for cranial nerves VII-X and XII. Most of the cranial nerve nuclei are located dorsally. The inferior olive is involved with the perception of time. Vestibular nuclei help regulate head and eye movements and postural activity.

Functions of the Medulla

Medullary neuronal networks coordinate cardiovascular control, breathing, head movement, and swallowing.

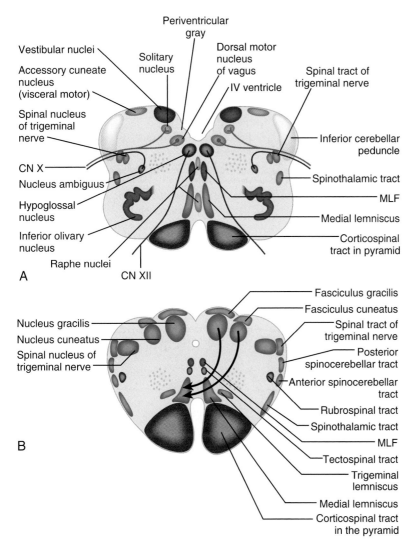

FIGURE 14-7

Horizontal sections of the medulla. Levels of the horizontal sections are indicated on the lateral view of the brainstem. Nuclei are labeled on the left side of each horizontal section. Tracts are labeled on the right side. **A,** Upper medulla. **B,** Inferior medulla. MLF, medial longitudinal fasciculus; CN, cranial nerve. Color coding: red, motor; blue, sensory; purple, motor and sensory or bidirectional; green, autonomic; orange, modulates motor and nociceptive activity in the spinal cord.

These activities are partially executed by cranial nerves with nuclei in the medulla: VII-X and XII. The medullary neuronal networks regulating these functions are normally influenced by cerebral activity. For example, the tonic neck reflexes seen in infants less than 6 months old require reflex circuits in the medulla (see Chapter 10). As the cerebral cortex matures, information from the cortex modulates the activity of the reflex circuit, modifying the reflexive activity.

> The medulla contributes to the control of eye and head movements, coordinates swallowing, and helps regulate cardiovascular, respiratory, and visceral activity.

PONS

The pons is located between the midbrain and medulla. The posterior pons borders on the fourth ventricle. Most vertical tracts continue unchanged through the pons (Figure 14-8, *C* and *D*). Only the corticopontine tracts and some corticobulbar tracts synapse in the pons. The corticopontine tracts synapse on pontine nuclei; then the postsynaptic axons, called *pontocerebellar fibers,* leave the pons to enter the cerebellum via the middle cerebellar peduncle. The corticobulbar tracts synapse with neurons in the trigeminal motor nucleus and the facial nucleus.

The basilar (anterior) section of the pons contains descending tracts (corticospinal, corticobulbar, and corticopontine axons), pontine nuclei, and pontocerebellar axons. The posterior section of the pons, the tegmentum, contains sensory tracts, reticular formation, autonomic pathways, medial longitudinal fasciculus, and nuclei for cranial nerves V-VII. These cranial nerves are involved in the following:
- Processing sensation from the face (cranial nerve V)
- Controlling lateral movement of the eye (cranial nerve VI)
- Control of facial and chewing muscles (cranial nerves VII and V, respectively)

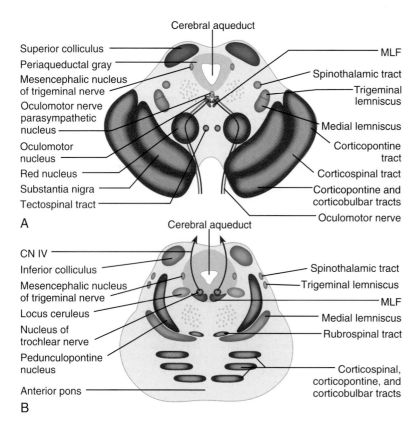

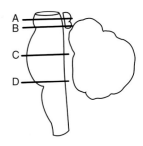

FIGURE 14-8

Horizontal sections of upper midbrain (**A**), junction of pons and midbrain (**B**), upper pons (**C**), and lower pons (**D**). The levels of the horizontal sections are indicated on the lateral view of the brainstem. Nuclei are labeled on the left side of each horizontal section. Tracts are labeled on the right side. MLF, medial longitudinal fasciculus; CN, cranial nerve. Stippled areas are the reticular formation. Color coding: red, motor; blue, sensory; purple, motor and sensory or bidirectional; green, autonomic or, in the case of locus ceruleus, modulates attention in the cerebrum and motor and nociceptive activity in the spinal cord.

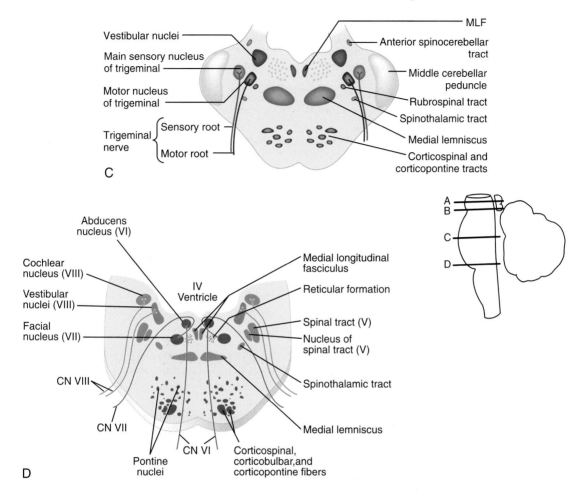

FIGURE 14-8, cont'd

The pons processes motor information from the cerebral cortex and forwards the information to the cerebellum. Pontine cranial nerve nuclei process sensory information from the face (cranial nerve V) and control contraction of muscles involved in facial expression (cranial nerve VII), lateral movement of the eye (cranial nerve VI), and chewing (cranial nerve V).

MIDBRAIN

The uppermost part of the brainstem, the midbrain, connects the diencephalon and the pons. The cerebral aqueduct, a small canal through the midbrain, joins the third and fourth ventricles. The midbrain can be divided into three regions, from anterior to posterior: basis pedunculi, tegmentum, and tectum.

Basis Pedunculi

Anteriorly, the basis pedunculi is formed by the cerebral peduncles (composed of descending tracts from the cerebral cortex) and an adjacent nucleus, the substantia nigra (Figure 14-8, *A*). The substantia nigra is one of the nuclei in the basal ganglia circuit (see Chapter 10). The other basal ganglia nuclei are the caudate, putamen, globus pallidus, pedunculopontine nucleus, and subthalamic nucleus.

Midbrain Tegmentum

The middle region of the midbrain, the tegmentum, contains vertical sensory tracts, the superior cerebellar peduncle, the red nucleus, the pedunculopontine nucleus (Figure 14-8, *B*), and the nuclei of cranial nerves III and IV. Most vertical tracts occupy similar positions as in the pons, except that the spinothalamic tract and medial lemniscus are located more laterally in the midbrain. The superior cerebellar peduncle connects the midbrain with the cerebellum, transmitting primarily efferent information from the cerebellum.

The red nucleus is a sphere of gray matter that receives information from the cerebellum and cerebral cortex and projects to the cerebellum, spinal cord (via rubrospinal tract), and reticular formation. Activity in the rubrospinal tract contributes to upper limb flexion. Pedunculopontine nucleus neurons are part of the basal ganglia circuit and are involved in the initiation and termination of locomotor activity (Winn, 2006).

Anterior to the cerebral aqueduct are the oculomotor complex (nuclei of cranial nerve III) and the nucleus of the trochlear nerve (cranial nerve IV). The oculomotor complex consists of the oculomotor nucleus, supplying efferent somatic fibers to the extraocular muscles innervated by the oculomotor nerve, and the oculomotor parasympathetic (Edinger-Westphal) nucleus, supplying parasympathetic control of the pupillary sphincter and the ciliary muscle. The oculomotor complex is superior to the trochlear nucleus. The trochlear nerve innervates the superior oblique muscle that moves the eye.

Surrounding the cerebral aqueduct is the periaqueductal gray. Involvement of the periaqueductal gray in pain suppression was discussed in Chapter 7. The periaqueductal gray also coordinates somatic and autonomic reactions to pain, threats, and emotions. Activity of the periaqueductal gray results in the fight-or-flight reaction (Misslin, 2003) and in vocalization during laughing and crying (Schulz et al., 2005).

Midbrain Tectum

The posterior region of the midbrain, the tectum, contains the pretectal area and the colliculi. The pretectal area is involved in the pupillary, consensual, and accommodation reflexes of the eye (see Chapter 13). The inferior colliculi relay auditory information from the cochlear nuclei to the superior colliculus and to the medial geniculate body of the thalamus (see Chapter 13). The superior colliculi are involved in reflexive eye and head movements (see Chapter 15).

CEREBELLUM

The cerebellum is discussed briefly in this chapter because cerebellar function is entirely dependent on

input and output connections with the brainstem. Furthermore, the cerebellum and brainstem share the tightly confined space of the posterior fossa, bringing them into a close anatomic relationship. The following list summarizes cerebellar functions:

- Coordination of movement, including fine finger movements, limb and head movements, postural control, and eye movements
- Motor planning
- Cognitive functions, including rapid shifts of attention (Ronning et al., 2005)
- Fibers from the cerebellum synapse with fibers in the reticular formation to achieve their role in directing attention.

In addition to its roles in motor control and motor planning, the cerebellum also contributes to voluntary shifting of attention.

DISORDERS IN THE BRAINSTEM REGION

Evaluating the function of cranial nerves (see Chapter 13) and vertical tracts can localize lesions within the brainstem. A single brainstem lesion may cause a mix of ipsilateral and contralateral signs (see Figure 7-5). The mix of ipsilateral and contralateral signs occurs because cranial nerves supply the ipsilateral face and neck, while many of the vertical tracts cross the midline in the brainstem to supply the contralateral body. Aside from the outcomes of vertical tract and cranial nerve damage, lesions in the brainstem may also interfere with vital functions and consciousness.

Vertical Tract Signs

The lateral corticospinal, dorsal column/medial lemniscus, and spinothalamic tracts connect the spinal cord with the contralateral cerebrum. Lesions of the lateral corticospinal and dorsal column tracts in the brainstem usually cause contralateral signs because these tracts cross the midline in the inferior medulla. The only location where a brainstem lesion would cause ipsilateral corticospinal or dorsal column/medial lemniscus signs would be a lesion of the corticospinal tract or dorsal column nuclei in the inferior medulla. The spinothalamic tract crosses the midline in the spinal cord, so any brainstem lesion that damages the spinothalamic tract causes contralateral signs.

Corticobulbar Lesions

The corticobulbar tracts convey motor signals from the cerebral cortex to cranial nerve nuclei in the brainstem. Thus, neurons with axons in the corticobulbar tract serve as upper motor neurons to the lower motor neurons in cranial nerves V, VII, IX, X, XI, and XII. Although both upper and lower motor neuron lesions cause paresis or paralysis, upper motor neuron lesions are associated with muscle hyperstiffness, while lower motor neuron lesions are associated with hyporeflexia and muscle flaccidity. Corticobulbar projections are bilateral, except to lower motor neurons innervating the muscles of the lower face and sometimes to the hypoglossal nucleus.

Facial Nerve versus Corticobulbar Tract Lesions

A complete lower motor neuron lesion of the facial nerve, cranial nerve VII, prevents commands from reaching all ipsilateral facial muscles. The result is flaccid paralysis of the muscles in the ipsilateral face. A person with a complete facial nerve lesion is completely unable to contract the muscles of facial expression and cannot close the ipsilateral eye. In contrast, unilateral upper motor neuron lesions interrupt voluntary control of contralateral facial muscles in the lower half of the face. The muscles in the upper half of the face are spared because

both the right and left cerebral cortex have projections to lower motor neurons innervating muscles of the forehead and surrounding the eye. Thus, an upper motor neuron lesion that prevents corticobulbar information from the left cerebral cortex from reaching the facial nerve nuclei causes paresis or paralysis of the right lower face, but cerebral control of muscles of the upper face is relatively unaffected. The difference between a lesion of the facial nerve (lower motor neuron lesion) and a corticobulbar lesion (upper motor neuron lesion) is illustrated in Figure 14-9. People with upper motor neuron lesions preventing voluntary control of the contralateral lower face are able to laugh and cry normally because the pathway involved in emotional vocalization is separate from the corticobulbar tract for the same activity (Schulz et al., 2005).

> In the brainstem, lesions cause contralateral vertical tract signs unless the lesion affects the corticospinal tracts or dorsal column nuclei in the inferior medulla. Complete lesions of the facial cranial nerve cause ipsilateral paralysis of the facial muscles, while lesions of the corticobulbar axons to the facial nucleus cause paralysis of the contralateral lower face with sparing of control of the upper face.

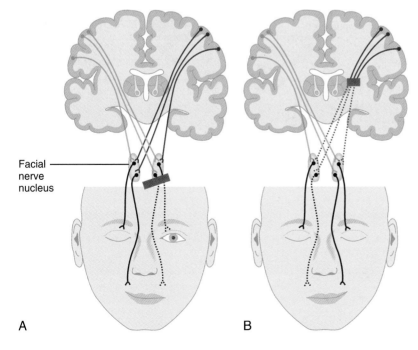

Facial nerve nucleus

A   B

FIGURE 14-9

Lower motor neuron lesion versus upper motor neuron lesion (corticobulbar) affecting the facial nerve. In both **A** and **B**, the person has been requested to close the eyes and smile. Dotted lines indicate axons that, subsequent to the lesions, do not convey information. **A,** With a facial nerve lesion, the lower motor neurons are interrupted, preventing control of the ipsilateral muscles of facial expression. Therefore the person cannot close the eye or contract the muscles that move the lips on the left. **B,** An upper motor neuron lesion prevents information from the left cortex from reaching the facial nerve nuclei. Because the contralateral cortex controls the muscles of the lower face, the person is unable to generate a smile on the right side. However, because the upper face is innervated bilaterally, the person with this upper motor neuron lesion can close both eyes.

Contralateral and Ipsilateral Signs

A single lesion in the upper anteromedial medulla (Figure 14-10, *A*) on the left side can cause paralysis of the right hand and foot, loss of discriminative touch and proprioceptive information on the right side of the body, and paresis of the left side of the tongue. The right hand and foot paralysis is due to interruption of lateral corticospinal tract in the pyramids, superior to the pyramidal decussation where the tract crosses the midline. The contralateral sensory loss occurs because the dorsal column/medial lemniscus tract crosses the midline in the lower medulla. The left tongue paresis occurs following damage to the left hypoglossal nerve. Pain and temperature information is spared because the lateral medulla is undamaged. Additional examples of brainstem lesions are provided in Figure 14-10.

Disorders of Vital Functions

Disruption of vital functions secondary to brainstem damage may cause the heart to stop beating, blood pressure to fluctuate, and/or breathing to cease. Areas in the medulla and pons regulate vital functions.

Four *Ds* of Brainstem Region Dysfunction

Dysphagia, dysarthria, diplopia, and dysmetria are the cardinal signs of brainstem dysfunction. Dysphagia is difficulty in swallowing; dysarthria is difficulty in speaking; diplopia is double vision; and dysmetria is the

FIGURE 14-10

A, Lesions are indicated on the brainstem sections. The charts summarize the structures damaged by the lesion and the results of the damage. Because the corticospinal tract and medial lemniscus are located in the anteromedial medulla and pons, an anteromedial lesion in either the medulla or the pons will damage those tracts. Because the spinothalamic tract, spinal tract and nucleus of cranial nerve V, and vestibular nuclei are located laterally in the medulla and pons, a lateral lesion in either the medulla or pons will damage those structures. A/M, anteromedial lesion; CN, cranial nerve; L, lateral lesion; MLF, medial longitudinal fasciculus.

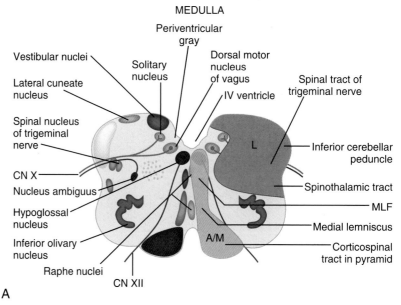

MEDULLA

ANTEROMEDIAL LESIONS		
	Structures involved	*Lesion interferes with*
Either medulla or pons	Corticospinal tract Medial lemniscus	Fractionated movements Discriminative touch and conscious proprioception
Medulla only	Hypoglossal nerve	Tongue movement
Pons only	Medial longitudinal fasciculus between the abducens and oculomotor nucleus	Adduction of eye past midline during lateral gaze

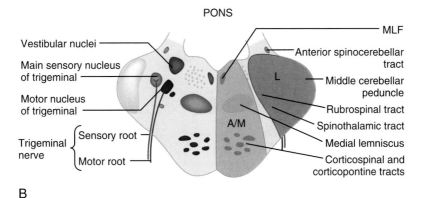

B

	LATERAL LESIONS	
	Structures involved	Lesion interferes with
Either medulla or pons	Spinothalamic tract	Pain and temperature sensation from the body
	Spinal tract and nucleus of CN V (inferior to level of section)	Pain and temperature sensation from the face
	Vestibular nuclei (in upper medulla, lower pons)	Control of posture, head position, and eye movement
Medulla only	Nucleus ambiguus	Swallowing, vocalization
	Inf. cerebellar peduncle	Smoothness of movement
	Descending sympathetic pathway (not shown in illustration)	Sympathetic control of face; causes Horner's syndrome
	Vagus nerve	Digestion, ability to slow heart rate
Pons only	Middle cerebellar peduncle	Smoothness of movement
	Main sensory nucleus of CN V	Discriminative touch information from face; afferent information for corneal reflex
	Motor nucleus trigeminal nerve	Motor to muscles of mastication
	Facial nerve (inferior to the level of section)	Control of muscles of facial expression; efferent information for corneal reflex

FIGURE 14-10, cont'd

B, Refer to part A for lesions in medulla.

Continued

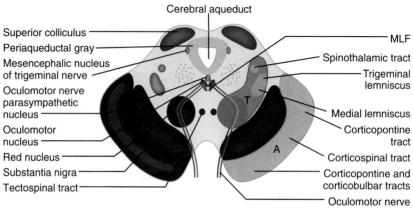

C

ANTERIOR LESIONS		
	Structures involved	*Lesion interferes with*
Midbrain	Corticospinal tract	Control of fractionated movement; face may be involved
	Corticopontine tract	Deficit should cause ataxia, but deficit not visible because hemiparesis or hemiplegia prevents movement
	Corticobulbar tracts	Weakness or paralysis of muscles supplied by cranial motor nerves below the level of the lesion
	Oculomotor nerve	Ability to move eye medially, downward, and upward; also causes drooping upper eyelid, dilated pupil

TEGMENTAL LESIONS		
	Structures involved	*Lesion interferes with*
Midbrain	Oculomotor nerve	Same functions as above
	Medial lemniscus, trigeminal lemniscus, and spinothalamic tract	Discriminative tactile, conscious proprioception, temperature, and pain sensation from face and body
	Superior cerebellar peduncle and red nucleus	Smoothness of movement; causes ataxia, dysdiadochokinesis, and hypotonia

FIGURE 14-10, cont'd

C, A, Anterior lesion; T, tegmental lesion.

inability to control the distance of movements. The first three of these disorders are covered in Chapter 13; dysmetria is discussed in Chapter 10.

Disorders of Consciousness

States of altered consciousness may occur with lesions to either the brainstem or the cerebrum because structures in both regions are required for consciousness. Brainstem damage that affects the reticular formation and/or the axons of the ascending reticular activating system interferes with consciousness. Damage to the cerebrum that interferes with hypothalamic/thalamic activating areas or with the function of the entire cerebral cortex may also impair consciousness. States of altered consciousness are defined in Table 14-2.

A disconnection syndrome, called *locked-in syndrome,* may mimic the signs of impaired consciousness. In locked-in syndrome, consciousness is intact, but damage to upper motor neurons completely prevents the person from voluntarily moving. In some cases, the person is able to voluntarily control eye movements and can communicate by coded eye movements. Figure 14-11 shows a section of medulla from a patient with locked-in syndrome.

The integrity of brainstem function can be assessed with auditory evoked potentials. As in somatosensory evoked potentials, a sense organ is stimulated, and the resulting electrical activity is recorded from electrodes on the scalp. For auditory evoked potentials, a brief burst of tone is presented and the brainstem response is recorded. Auditory evoked potentials are most commonly used to assess brainstem function in comatose patients. Auditory evoked potentials can also be used to evaluate whether the cochlea, cochlea nerve, and auditory nuclei in the brainstem are functioning.

Tumors in the Brainstem Region

Tumors within the cerebellum or brainstem cause increased intracranial pressure. The pressure may cause headache, nausea, vomiting, cranial nerve disorders, or hydrocephalus. If the tumor is within the cerebellum, ataxia commonly occurs.

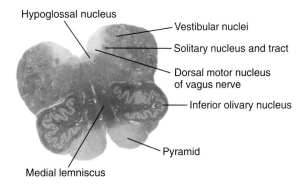

FIGURE 14-11
Section of the medulla from a patient with locked-in syndrome. In this section, the myelin has been stained to appear dark. Normally the medullary pyramids appear dark with this stain, because the corticospinal neurons are normally myelinated. The pale appearance of the medullary pyramids in this section indicates degeneration of the medullary pyramids. The destruction of the corticospinal and other descending pathways produced locked-in syndrome.

Table 14-2   STATES OF ALTERED CONSCIOUSNESS

Coma	Unarousable; no response to strong stimuli such as strong pinching of the Achilles tendon
Stupor	Arousable only by strong stimuli, such as strong pinching of the Achilles tendon
Obtunded	Sleeping more than awake; drowsy and confused when awake
Vegetative state	Complete loss of consciousness, without alteration of vital functions*
Minimally conscious state	Severely altered consciousness with at least one behavioral sign of consciousness. Signs include: following simple commands, gestural or verbal yes/no responses, intelligible speech, and movements or affective behaviors that are not reflexive (Giacino and Kalmar, 2005).
Syncope (fainting)	Brief loss of consciousness due to a drop in blood pressure†
Delirium	Reduced attention, orientation, and perception, associated with confused ideas and agitation

*Vegetative state is distinguished from coma by the following signs: spontaneous eye opening, regular sleep-wake cycles, and normal respiratory patterns.
†Benign syncope results from overactivity of the vagus nerve (vasovagal syncope). Orthostatic hypotension (decreased blood pressure in the upright position) may cause syncope in patients with spinal cord injury or who have experienced prolonged bed rest.

Damage caused by a benign tumor may be extensive because the unyielding bone and dura prevent brain tissue from moving away from the pressure. For example, an acoustic neuroma is a benign tumor of the Schwann cells surrounding the vestibulocochlear nerve. If the surrounding bones did not confine the nerve, the acoustic neuroma could enlarge without compromising function. Unfortunately, bony restriction causes the enlarging tumor to compress the vestibulocochlear nerve, resulting in tinnitus (sensation of ringing or buzzing in the ear) and eventual deafness. If the tumor continues to grow, more and more structures are compressed. The trigeminal and facial nerves will be the next structures compressed by the enlarging tumor, causing loss of sensation from the face and paresis of the facial muscles. Next, cerebellar signs, including ipsilateral limb ataxia, intention tremor, and nystagmus (abnormal eye movements), appear as the pressure builds on the cerebellum. Eventually, brainstem compression interferes with vertical tracts and nuclear functions. Acoustic neuromas affect approximately 1 in 100,000 adults per year (Propp et al., 2006). Acoustic tumors can be surgically removed at any stage of their growth.

Brainstem Region Ischemia

Typically, ischemia in the brainstem region produces an abrupt onset of neurologic symptoms, including dizziness, visual disorders, weakness, incoordination, and somatosensory disorders. Vertebrobasilar artery insufficiency produces transient symptoms of brainstem region ischemia when the neck is extended and rotated.

Strokes that affect the lateral medulla produce Wallenberg's syndrome, also called posterior inferior cerebellar artery syndrome (see Figure 1-20). The syndrome consists of ipsilateral limb ataxia, dysarthria, dysphagia, vertigo (sensation of spinning), **pathologic nystagmus** (abnormal involuntary eye movements), ipsilateral Horner's syndrome, ipsilateral impairment of pain and temperature sensation in the face, and contralateral loss of pain and temperature sensation in the body. The ataxia results from damage to the inferior cerebellar peduncle, dysarthria and dysphagia from damage to the nucleus ambiguus, vertigo and nystagmus from damage to the vestibular nuclei (see Chapter 15), Horner's syndrome from damage to the descending sympathetic pathway, and somatosensory disorders from damage to the spinothalamic tract and the spinal nucleus of the trigeminal nerve (see Figure 14-9, *B*).

SUMMARY

The brainstem contains the origin of most upper motor neurons (excluding corticospinals), axons transmitting somatosensory information, and nuclei for cranial nerves III-X and XII and the reticular formation. The reticular formation is essential for modulation of neural activity throughout the central nervous system. A mnemonic for remembering the effects of brainstem region lesion is the four *D*s: dysphagia, dysarthria, diplopia, and dysmetria.

CLINICAL NOTES

Case 1

PC is a 32-year-old man who was found unconscious at home 4 days ago. He regained consciousness today. The therapist's evaluation reveals the following:

- Lack of pain and temperature sensation on the right side of the body
- Lack of somatosensation on the left side of the face
- Ataxia on the left side of the body
- Paralysis of muscles of facial expression on the left side
- Loss of corneal reflex on the left side

The therapist also notes nystagmus, vertigo, nausea, and vomiting when PC turns his head.

Questions
1. List the structure associated with each loss.
2. Where is the lesion?

CLINICAL NOTES

Case 2

LD, a 78-year-old woman, awoke with an inability to voluntarily move the muscles of facial expression in her right lower face. In the clinic, the following signs are noted:

- Sensation is intact throughout the body and face, and movements of the limbs and trunk are normal.
- Movement of the upper face and the left lower face are normal. She is able to completely close both eyes on request. When she is asked to smile or frown, muscles in the right lower face do not contract. However, when she frowns due to frustration, muscles in the right lower face contract.
- Test results for all cranial nerves other than cranial nerve VII are normal.

Question

Where is the lesion?

Case 3

MZ is 17 years old. He suffered a severe head injury in a car accident 2 months ago. After a month-long hospitalization, MZ has been in a long-term care facility for 4 weeks. Notes in his chart indicate that he is in a vegetative state and is not expected to recover. MZ is completely immobile except for eye movements. His family believes that he is aware and able to communicate with them via eye movements. When the therapist asks him to blink three times, MZ complies. When the therapist asks him to look toward his right, he does. However, MZ does not move any other part of his body on request.

Questions

1. Is MZ's behavior consistent with a vegetative state?
2. If not, what is the condition?

Case 4

RV, a 58-year-old man, was in a meeting when suddenly he lost control of the right side of his body, including his face. He slumped in his chair, and the right side of his face appeared to sag, but he did not lose consciousness. RV complains of double vision. The clinical findings are as follows:

- Somatosensation is intact.
- Movement and strength on the left side of his body are normal. He is able to sit unassisted in a chair with arm and back support but cannot sit unassisted without support. RV is able to voluntarily move his right upper limb at the shoulder and his right lower limb at the hip, but strength is less than half that of the left side. He cannot move any other joints in his limbs on the right.
- All cranial nerves are intact except for the following:
  He is unable to voluntarily move his right lower face.
  He cannot move his left eye medially, downward, or upward.
  He cannot fully open his left eye (left eyelid droops).
  The left pupil is dilated and does not contract in response to light shined into either eye.

Questions

1. List the structures associated with the functional losses.
2. Where is the lesion?

REVIEW QUESTIONS

1. List the vertical tracts that are modified in the brainstem.
2. What are the functions of the reticular formation?
3. List the major reticular nuclei and the slow-acting neurotransmitters produced by these nuclei.
4. Which neurotransmitter produced in the brainstem is important in the cerebral processes of motivation and decision making?
5. How does the pedunculopontine nucleus affect movement?

6. Which medullary nuclei are part of a system that inhibits the transmission of pain information?

7. What is the role of the ascending fibers from the locus ceruleus?

8. For each of the following functions, list the cranial nerve nucleus responsible for the function and the part of the brainstem where the nucleus is located (lower medulla, upper medulla, junction of the medulla and pons, pons, junction of the pons and midbrain, midbrain):
   - Control of voluntary muscles in the pharynx and larynx
   - Integration and transmission of pain information from the face
   - Control of tongue muscles
   - Processing of information about sounds
   - Perception of timing
   - Control of muscles of mastication
   - Contraction of the pupillary sphincter and change in curvature of the lens to focus on near objects

9. Which nuclei in the midbrain are part of the basal ganglia circuit?

10. What are the functions of the cerebellum?

11. Why do brainstem lesions above the inferior medulla cause contralateral loss of discriminative touch information from the body?

12. What midbrain region coordinates somatic and autonomic reactions to pain, threats, and emotions?

13. What tracts convey motor signals from the cerebral cortex to cranial nerve motor nuclei?

14. How can a complete lesion of the facial nerve be differentiated from a lesion affecting the corticobulbar tracts that convey information from the cerebral cortex to the facial nerve nucleus?

15. Would a person with a complete facial nerve lesion on the left side be able to smile involuntarily on the left side of the face? Why or why not?

16. Disorders of consciousness can occur with damage to what brainstem structures?

17. A person who has a complete loss of consciousness combined with normal vital functions is in what state of altered consciousness?

18. Why are space-occupying lesions in the brainstem region, such as benign tumors, so disruptive of brainstem function?

References

Aston-Jones G (2005). Brain structures and receptors involved in alertness. Sleep Medicine, 6 (Suppl 1), S3-S7.

Carrasco JL, Sandner C (2005). Clinical effects of pharmacological variations in selective serotonin reuptake inhibitors: An overview. International Journal of Clinical Practice, 59(12), 1428-1434.

Gardner EL (2005). Endocannabinoid signaling system and brain reward: Emphasis on dopamine. Pharmacology, Biochemistry, and Behavior, 81(2), 263-284.

Giacino JT, Kalmar K (2005). Diagnostic and prognostic guidelines for the vegetative and minimally conscious states. Neuropsychological Rehabilitation, 15(3-4), 166-174.

Margolis EB, Lock H, et al. (2006). Kappa opioids selectively control dopaminergic neurons projecting to the prefrontal cortex. Proceedings of the National Academy of Sciences of the United States of America, 103(8), 2938-2942.

Mason P (2001). Contributions of the medullary raphe and ventromedial reticular region to pain modulation and other homeostatic functions. Annual Review of Neuroscience, 24, 737-777.

Menon V, Levitin DJ (2005). The rewards of music listening: Response and physiological connectivity of the mesolimbic system. Neuroimage, 28(1), 175-184.

Misslin R (2003). The defense system of fear: Behavior and neurocircuitry. Neurophysiologie Clinique, 33(2), 55-66.

Pepeu G, Giovannini MG (2004). Changes in acetylcholine extracellular levels during cognitive processes. Learning & Memory, 11(1), 21-27.

Propp JM, McCarthy BJ, et al. (2006). Descriptive epidemiology of vestibular schwannomas. Neuro-oncology, 8(1), 1-11.

Ronning C, Sundet K, et al. (2005). Persistent cognitive dysfunction secondary to cerebellar injury in patients treated for posterior fossa tumors in childhood. Pediatric Neurosurgery, 41(1), 15-21.

Schulz GM, Varga M, et al. (2005). Functional neuroanatomy of human vocalization: An H215O PET study. Cerebral Cortex, 15(12), 1835-1847.

Siegel J (2004). Brain mechanisms that control sleep and waking. Die Naturwissenschaften, 91(8), 355-365.

Winn P (2006). How best to consider the structure and function of the pedunculopontine tegmental nucleus: Evidence from animal studies. Journal of the Neurological Sciences, 248(1-2), 234-250.

Xu D, Liu T, et al. (2006). Role of the olivo-cerebellar system in timing. Journal of Neuroscience, 26(22), 5990-5995.

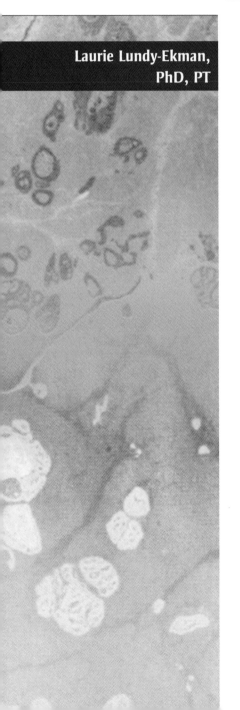

15 Vestibular and Visual Systems

Laurie Lundy-Ekman, PhD, PT

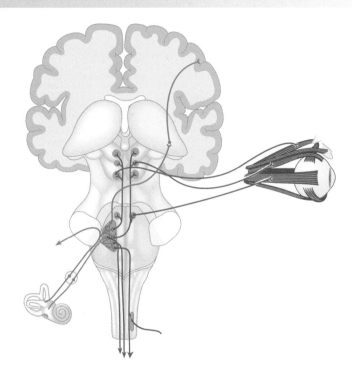

INTRODUCTION

Vestibular receptors and cranial nerve axons in the periphery, vestibular nuclei in the brainstem, and an area of the cerebral cortex are dedicated to vestibular function. The visual system includes specialized neurons in the retina, cranial nerve afferents that are myelinated by oligodendroglia (and thus part of the central nervous system), relay nuclei in the thalamus, visual cortex, and areas of the cerebral cortex and midbrain that direct eye movements. The function of the visual system is partially dependent on the vestibular system because vestibular information contributes to the compensatory eye movements that maintain stability of the visual world when the head moves.

VESTIBULAR SYSTEM

Vestibular information is essential for postural control and for control of eye movements. The vestibular apparatus, located in the inner ear, contains sensory receptors that respond to the position of the head relative to gravity and to head movements. This information is converted into neural signals conveyed by the vestibular nerve to the vestibular nuclei. The vestibular nuclei are located in the brainstem, at the junction of the pons and medulla. Projections from the vestibular nuclei contribute to:

- Sensory information about head movement and head position relative to gravity
- Gaze stabilization (control of eye movements when the head moves)
- Postural adjustments
- Autonomic function and consciousness

Vestibular Apparatus

The vestibular apparatus consists of the bony and membranous labyrinths and the hair cells. The bony labyrinth is a convoluted space within the skull that contains three semicircular canals and two otolithic organs (Figure 15-1). The membranous labyrinth is within the bony labyrinth. The membranous labyrinth is hollow and filled with a fluid called *endolymph.* The receptors inside the membranous labyrinth are hair cells. Bending of the hairs determines the frequency of the signals conveyed by the vestibular nerve (a branch of the vestibulocochlear nerve, cranial nerve VIII).

Semicircular Canals

Receptors in the semicircular canals detect movement of the head by sensing the motion of endolymph. The semicircular canals are three hollow rings arranged perpendicular to each other. Each semicircular canal opens at both ends into the utricle, one of the otolithic organs. Each semicircular canal has a swelling, called the *ampulla,* containing a crista. The crista consists of supporting cells and sensory hair cells. The hairs are embedded in a gelatinous mass, the *cupula.* When the head is stationary, the hair cells fire at a baseline rate. If the head begins to turn, inertia causes the fluid in the canal to lag behind, resulting in bending of the cupula and the hairs of the hair cells (see Figure 15-1, *B*). Bending of the hairs results in an increase or decrease in the baseline rate hair cell firing, depending on the direction of bend. The receptors in semicircular canals are only sensitive to rotational acceleration or deceleration (i.e., speeding up or slowing down rotation of the head).

If the head rotates at a constant speed, the effects of friction gradually cause the endolymph to move at the same speed as the head. When rotation is constant, the hair cells fire at a constant rate. As rotation slows, the cupulae bend in the opposite direction and the excitation level in the vestibular nerves reverses. That is, if the head rotates to the right, during acceleration the right vestibular nerve will fire more frequently than prior to head movement. During deceleration, the right vestibular nerve will fire less frequently than its baseline rate.

Maximum fluid flow in each semicircular canal, and thus maximal change in the frequency of signals generated by bending of the hairs embedded in the cupula, occurs when the head turns on the canal's axis of rotation (Figure 15-2, *A*). Two semicircular canals that have maximal fluid flow during rotation in a single plane form a pair. For example, when the head is flexed 30°, the horizontal canals are parallel to the ground. Rotation of the head in 30° of flexion around the vertical axis maximizes fluid flow in both horizontal canals. The horizontal canals are classified as a pair because maximal fluid flow occurs during movement in a single plane. When the horizontal canals are parallel to the ground, the anterior and posterior canals are vertical.

The anatomic arrangement of the canals, with the semicircular canals oriented at 90° angles to each other, ensures that acceleration or deceleration in a plane of movement that causes maximal fluid flow in a pair of semicircular canals does not stimulate the other semicircular canals. The anterior and posterior semicircular canals are oriented vertically at a 45° angle to the midline. Turning the head 45° to the left and then doing somersaults causes maximal fluid flow in the right anterior canal. This somersault causes no fluid flow in the left anterior canal because the left anterior canal is moving perpendicular to its axis. Because the anterior canals are 90° to each other, there is no plane of movement in which the fluid flow in the anterior canals can be maximized simultaneously. However, the same somersault causes maximal fluid flow in the left posterior canal. Therefore, the right anterior and the left posterior canals are classified as a pair, since movement in a single plane maximizes fluid flow in both (Figure 15-2, *C*). Similarly, the left anterior and the right posterior canals are a pair. The influence of the semicircular canals on eye movements is discussed in the section on vestibulo-ocular reflexes.

Each of the canals in a pair produces reciprocal signals; that is, increased signals from one canal occur simultaneously with decreased signals from its partner. These reciprocal signals are essential for normal vestibular function. If the signals from a pair of semicircular canals are not reciprocal, difficulties with control of posture, abnormal eye movements, and nausea result.

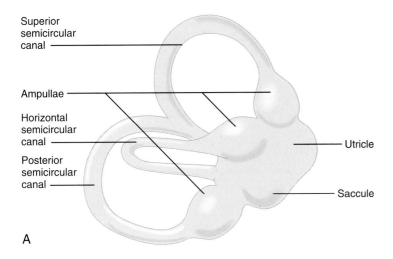

Superior
semicircular
canal

Ampullae

Horizontal
semicircular
canal

Posterior
semicircular
canal

Utricle

Saccule

A

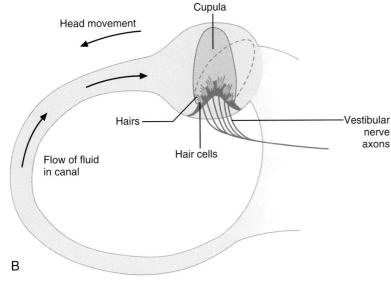

Cupula

Head movement

Hairs

Hair cells

Flow of fluid
in canal

Vestibular
nerve
axons

B

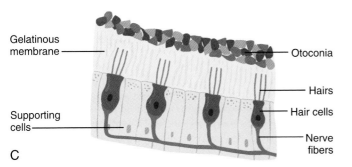

Gelatinous
membrane

Otoconia

Hairs

Hair cells

Supporting
cells

Nerve
fibers

C

FIGURE 15-1

A, The vestibular apparatus consists of the utricle, saccule, and semicircular canals. The three semicircular canals are at right angles to each other. Each semicircular canal has a swelling, the ampulla, which contains a receptor mechanism, the crista. **B,** A section through a semicircular canal showing the crista inside the ampulla. The flow of fluid in the canal, indicated by the arrow, moves the cupula and in turn bends the hair cells. Bending of the hair cells changes the pattern of firing in the vestibular neurons. **C,** Inside the utricle and saccule is a receptor called the macula. In the macula, hairs projecting from hair cells are embedded in a gelatinous material. Atop the gelatinous material are otoconia: small, heavy, sandlike crystals. When the macula is moved into different positions, the weight of the otoconia bends the hairs, stimulating the hair cells and changing the pattern of vestibular neuron firing.

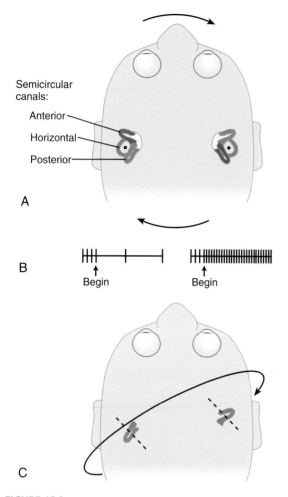

A

B

Begin   Begin

C

Otolithic Organs

The two otolithic organs, the *utricle* and *saccule*, are membranous sacs within the vestibular apparatus. They are not sensitive to rotation but instead respond to head position relative to gravity and to linear acceleration and deceleration. In each of these sacs is a macula, consisting of hair cells enclosed by a gelatinous mass topped by calcium carbonate crystals (see Figure 15-1, *C*). The crystals, called *otoconia*, are more dense than the surrounding fluid and their gelatinous support. Changing the position of the head tilts the macula, and the weight of the otoconia displaces the gelatinous mass, bending the embedded hairs. Bending the hairs stimulates or inhibits the hair cells (depending on the direction of bend), and this determines the frequency of firing of neurons in the vestibular nerve.

The utricular macula is on the floor of the utricle when the head is upright; thus, its orientation is horizontal. The utricular macula responds maximally to head tilts that begin with the head in the upright position, as in bending forward to pick up something off the floor. The saccular macula is oriented vertically. The saccular macula responds maximally when the head moves from a laterally flexed position, as in moving from side-lying to standing. In addition to head position, the utricular maculae also respond to linear acceleration and deceleration. As the head begins to move forward, the otoconia in the utricular macula fall back, bending the hairs and changing the firing rate of hair cells. The resulting impulses are conveyed via the vestibular nerve into the brainstem, signaling head acceleration.

FIGURE 15-2
Axis of rotation of the semicircular canals. The three pairs of canals—horizontal, the right anterior with left posterior, and the left anterior with right posterior—are indicated by colors. **A,** The axes of the horizontal canals are indicated by a dot in the center of each horizontal canal. Rotating the head toward the right as indicated by the arrows causes maximum fluid flow in both horizontal canals. **B,** The graphs indicate vestibular nerve firing. When the head is not moving, the resting discharge rate for both the right and left hair cells is about 90 spikes/second. As the head turns, the hair cells on the side away from the direction of turn hyperpolarize, decreasing vestibular nerve signals on the left side. Simultaneously, the hair cells toward the direction of the turn depolarize, increasing the vestibular nerve signals on the right (side toward the turn). **C,** Only the left posterior and right anterior canals are shown. The axes are indicated by dotted lines. Because their axes are parallel, rotation in one plane (indicated by the arrow) simultaneously causes maximal fluid flow in both canals.

Much of the information from the semicircular canals is used to stabilize vision. That is, the information keeps the eyes on a target when the head turns. Most of the information provided by the otolithic organs affects the spinal cord, adjusting activity in the lower motor neurons to postural muscles.

The information from the semicircular canals and otolithic organs is transmitted by the vestibular nerve to the vestibular nuclei in the medulla and pons and also to the flocculonodular lobe of the cerebellum. Cell bodies of the vestibular primary afferents are in the vestibular ganglion, within the internal auditory canal. The peripheral part of the vestibular system consists of the vestibular apparatus and peripheral part of the vestibular nerve. The central vestibular system is far more extensive.

Central Vestibular System

Four nuclei, six pathways, the vestibulocerebellum, and the vestibular cortex make up the central vestibular system (Figure 15-3). The nuclei are located bilaterally at the junction of the pons and medulla, near the fourth ventricle. The nuclei are the lateral (or Deiter's nuclei), medial, inferior (or spinal), and superior vestibular nuclei. Connections of the vestibular nuclei are shown in Figure 15-4. In addition to vestibular information, the vestibular nuclei receive visual, proprioceptive, tactile, and auditory information. Thus, the vestibular nuclei integrate information from multiple senses. Pathways that convey information from the vestibular nuclei include:

- The medial longitudinal fasciculus (to extraocular nuclei and superior colliculus, influencing eye movements)
- Vestibulospinal tracts (both medial and lateral, to lower motor neurons that influence posture)
- Vestibulocollic pathways (to the nucleus of the spinal accessory nerve, influencing head position)
- Vestibulothalamocortical pathways (providing conscious awareness of head position and movement)
- Vestibulocerebellar pathways (to the vestibulocerebellum)
- Vestibuloautonomic pathways (to the reticular formation, influencing nausea and vomiting)

The first five of these pathways are illustrated in Figure 15-3.

The vestibulocerebellum is the section of the cerebellum that receives vestibular information and influences eye movements and postural muscles (see Figure 10-13). The vestibulocerebellum adjusts the gain of responses to head movement. For example, when maintaining visual fixation on a target while turning the head, the eyes move precisely opposite to the direction of head movement. The gain of the response (the ratio of head movement to eye movement) is 1. The vestibulocerebellum is vital for adaptation to vestibular disorders and to alterations in the postural and balance systems.

Vestibular Role in Motor Control

In addition to providing sensory information about head movement and position, the vestibular system has two roles in motor control: gaze stabilization and postural adjustments (see Figure 15-4). Gaze stabilization operates by the vestibulo-ocular reflex, discussed later in this chapter. Postural adjustments are achieved by reciprocal connections between the vestibular nuclei and the spinal cord, reticular formation, superior colliculus, the

nucleus of cranial nerve XI, and the cerebellum (Figure 15-5).

The **lateral vestibulospinal tract,** originating in the lateral vestibular nucleus, is the primary tract for vestibular influence on lower motor neurons to postural muscles in the limbs and trunk. The **medial vestibulospinal tract,** via projections to the cervical spinal cord, conveys signals that adjust head position to upright according to information signals from the vestibular apparatus. The **medial longitudinal fasciculus** is the neural connection among the vestibular nuclei, the nuclei that control eye movements, the spinal accessory nucleus, and the superior colliculus.

Connections of the Vestibular Nuclei

Rapidly rotating the head, by simply spinning around or by riding a spinning amusement park ride, activates the semicircular canal connections, eliciting the following:

- Altered postural control (leading to leaning or falling)
- Head orientation adjustment
- Eye movement reflexes
- Autonomic changes (nausea, vomiting)
- Changes in consciousness (light-headedness)
- Conscious awareness of head orientation and head movement

In addition to being the source of the vestibulospinal tracts, the vestibular nuclei are linked with areas that affect the corticospinal, reticulospinal, and tectospinal descending tracts. By these connections, the vestibular nuclei strongly influence the posture of the head and body.

Cerebellar connections with the vestibular apparatus, vestibular nuclei, spinal cord, and inferior olive enable the cerebellum to control the gain of the postural adjustments and eye movement reflexes (vestibulo-ocular reflexes, discussed later in the chapter). Thus the magnitude of the reflex responses to changes in position and movement (of the head, body, or external objects) depends on cerebellar processing of vestibular and visual information.

The vestibular nuclei are connected with the nuclei of cranial nerves III, IV, VI, and XI and the superior colliculus via the medial longitudinal fasciculus (see Figure 15-3). This bilateral linkage of certain cranial nerve nuclei is essential for coordinated movements of the eyes and head. For example, the right lateral rectus (cranial nerve VI) and the left medial rectus (cranial nerve III) muscles must contract simultaneously to turn the eyes to the right. Coordination of this movement is

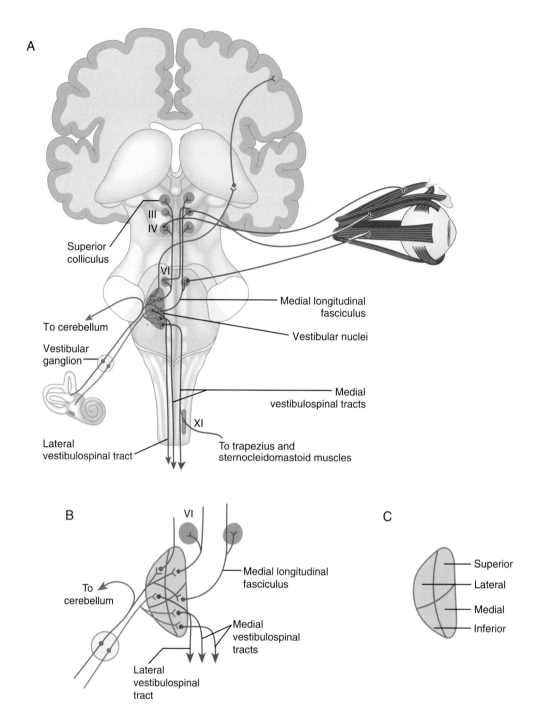

FIGURE 15-3

The vestibular system and the medial longitudinal fasciculus. **A,** Direct connections from the vestibular apparatus to the cerebellum are indicated. The four vestibular nuclei are shown only on the left side. The medial longitudinal fasciculus connects the vestibular nuclei with the nuclei that control eye movements, with the superior colliculus, and with the nucleus of cranial nerve XI (accessory nerve). Note the connection between the left abducens nucleus and the right occulomotor nucleus. The medial and lateral vestibulospinal tracts convey vestibular information to the spinal cord, to adjust activity in postural muscles. Indirect connections from vestibular nuclei to the cerebral cortex via the thalamus (ventroposterolateral nucleus) carry information that contributes to the conscious awareness of head position. **B,** An enlargement of the left vestibular nuclei and their connections. **C,** The vestibular nuclei.

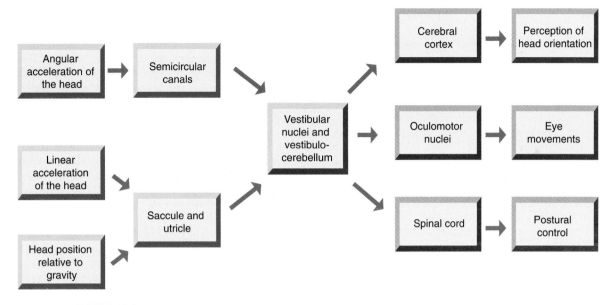

FIGURE 15-4
Flow of information from the vestibular receptors to the outcomes of vestibular input: perception of head movement, movement of the eyes, and postural control.

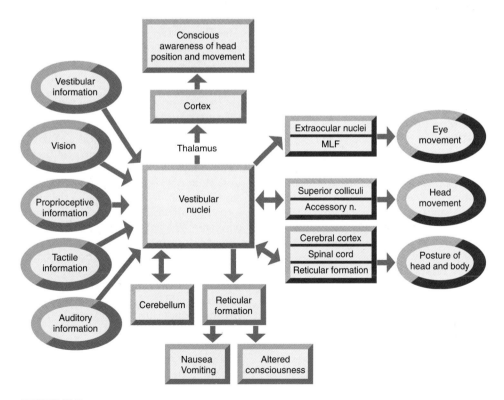

FIGURE 15-5
Connections of the vestibular nuclei. Sensory inputs are shown on the left (in blue), the motor output on the right (in red). Note the wide variety of sensory information feeding into the vestibular nuclei. The vestibular nuclei integrate all types of sensory information that can be used for orientation, not only information from the vestibular receptors. MLF, medial longitudinal fasciculus; n., nerve.

achieved by signals conveyed by the medial longitudinal fasciculus.

The vestibular connections with the reticular formation, in addition to affecting the reticulospinal tracts, affect the autonomic nervous system. Excessive activity of the circuits linking vestibular nuclei and the reticular formation may result in nausea, vomiting, and changes in consciousness. A pathway to the thalamus and then to the cerebral cortex provides conscious awareness of head orientation and movement. Disorders of the vestibular system are discussed later in this chapter.

VISUAL SYSTEM

The visual system provides the following:
- Sight, for the recognition and location of objects
- Eye movement control
- Information used in postural and limb movement control (see Chapter 9)

Sight: Information Conveyed From Retina to Cortex

The visual pathway begins with cells in the retina that convert light into neural signals. The signals are processed within the retina and conveyed to the retinal output cells. Retinal output is conveyed by the axons that travel in the optic nerve, optic chiasm, and optic tract, then synapse in the lateral geniculate nucleus of the thalamus. The optic nerve is the bundle of axons passing from the retina to the optic chiasm. The optic nerves merge at the optic chiasm, where some axons cross the midline. The optic tract conveys visual information from the chiasm to the lateral geniculate.

Postsynaptic neurons travel from the lateral geniculate in the geniculocalcarine tract (optic radiations) to the primary visual cortex. As the optic radiations emerge from the lateral geniculate, they travel in the posterior part of the internal capsule. The primary visual cortex is the region of the cortex that receives direct projections of visual information. Thus, to reach conscious awareness, the neural signals travel to the visual cortex via the retinogeniculocalcarine pathway (Figure 15-6).

The cortical destination of visual information depends on which half of the retina processes the visual information—the nasal retina, nearest the nose, or the temporal retina, nearest the temporal bone. Information from the nasal half of each retina crosses the midline in the optic chiasm and projects to the contralateral visual cortex. Information from the temporal half of each retina

continues ipsilaterally through the optic chiasm and projects to the ipsilateral cortex.

The outcome of the fiber rearrangement in the chiasm is that all visual information from one visual field is delivered to the opposite visual cortex. For example, the right visual field is the part of the environment that people see to the right of their own midline when looking straight ahead. Light from the right visual field strikes the left half of each retina. The left half of the left retina is temporal and projects to the ipsilateral visual cortex. The left half of the right retina is nasal, and its projections cross the midline in the chiasm. Thus, the axons leaving the chiasm in the left optic tract all carry information from the right visual field. Axons of the left optic tract synapse in the left lateral geniculate, and then the information is relayed to the left visual cortex via the geniculocalcarine tract. This results in projection of the right visual field information to the left visual cortex. Similarly, left visual field information is projected to the right visual cortex.

> The retinogeniculocalcarine pathway conveys visual information that reaches conscious awareness. Information from a visual field is conveyed to the contralateral visual cortex.

Processing of Visual Information

Visual information reaching the primary visual cortex stimulates neurons that discriminate the shape, size, or texture of objects. Information conveyed to the adjacent cortical areas, called the *visual association cortex,* is analyzed for colors and motion. From the visual association cortex, the information flows to other areas of the cerebral cortex where the visual information is used to adjust movements or to visually identify objects (see Chapter 16). The stream of visual information that flows dorsally is called the **action stream** because this information is used to direct movement, and the stream of visual information that flows ventrally is called the **perception stream** because this information is used to recognize visual objects (Figure 15-7).

Two areas that process nonconscious visual information are discussed in Chapter 13: the superior colliculus and the pretectal area. Projections from the retina to these areas in the brainstem and to the visual cortex are illustrated in Figure 15-6. The conscious and nonconscious pathways transmitting visual information are summarized in Figure 15-7.

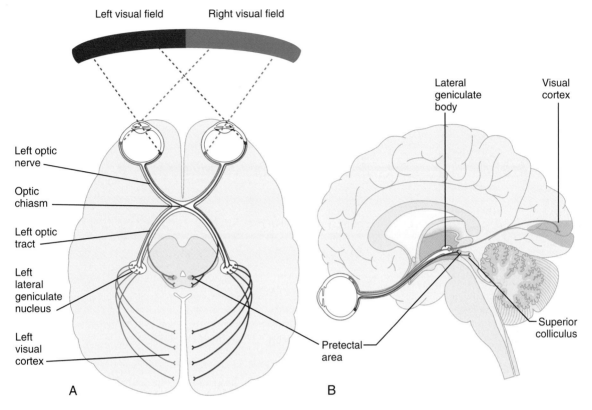

FIGURE 15-6

Visual pathways. **A,** Visual information from the right visual field activates neurons in the left half of the retina of both eyes. Axons from the temporal half of the retina project ipsilaterally to the lateral geniculate body, while axons from the nasal half of the retina cross the midline in the optic chiasm to project to the contralateral lateral geniculate body. Thus all visual information from the right visual field projects to the left lateral geniculate, then through the optic radiations to the left visual cortex. Collaterals from axons in the optic tract to the pretectal area and to the superior colliculus are also shown. **B,** Lateral view of the projections from the retina to the superior colliculus, pretectal area, and lateral geniculate/visual cortex.

Eye Movement System

Normal eye movements require synthesis of information about the following:

- Head movements (vestibular information)
- Visual objects (vision)
- Eye movement and position (proprioceptive information)
- Selection of a visual target (brainstem and cortical areas)

Precise control of eye position is vital for vision because the best visual acuity is available only in a small region of the retina (the fovea) and because binocular perception of an object as a single object requires that the image be received by corresponding points on both retinas. The medial longitudinal fasciculus, reflexes, and cerebral centers achieve this exquisite control of eye position. The superior colliculus coordinates reflexive orienting movements of the eyes and head via the medial longitudinal fasciculus and the tectospinal tract.

Types of Eye Movements

Eye movements have two objectives: keeping the position of the eyes stable during head movements so that the environment does not appear to bounce, and directing the gaze at visual targets. Eye movements are either conjugate or vergence movements. In **conjugate movements,** both eyes move in the same direction. In **vergence movements,** the eyes move toward the midline

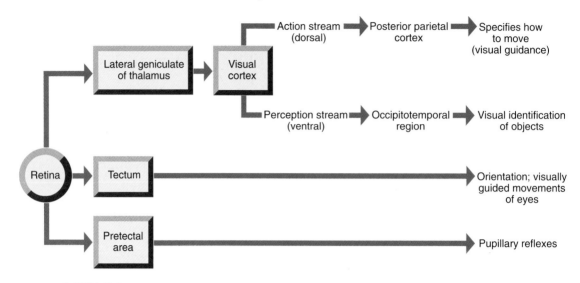

FIGURE 15-7

Flow of visual signals from the retina to the visual cortex, tectum, and pretectal area. Signals arriving in the visual cortex are analyzed and then sent to other areas of the cerebral cortex where directions for movement are created and where objects are recognized visually. Signals arriving in the tectum are used for orientation and eye movement control. Signals arriving in the pretectal area produce pupillary reflexes.

or away from the midline. Vergence movements occur when looking at an object near the eyes or when switching the gaze from a near object to a far object.

Gaze stabilization (also called *visual fixation*) during head movements is achieved by:

- The vestibulo-ocular reflex, the action of vestibular information on eye position during fast movements of the head
- The optokinetic reflex, the use of visual information to stabilize images during slow movements of the head
Direction of gaze is accomplished by:
- **Saccades,** fast eye movements to switch gaze from one object to another. The high-speed eye movements bring new objects into central vision, where details of images are seen.
- **Smooth pursuits,** eye movements that follow a moving object
- Vergence movements, the movement of the eyes toward or away from midline to adjust for different distances between the eyes and the visual target

Vestibulo-ocular Reflexes

Vestibulo-ocular reflexes (VORs) stabilize visual images during head movements. This stabilizing prevents the visual world from appearing to bounce or jump around

when the head moves, especially during walking. Lack of visual image stability can be seen in videotapes when the videographer walks with the camera, as the video-taped objects appear to bounce. Even more disconcerting to the viewer are abrupt swings of the video image, causing the visual objects to jump. Although these visual effects can be entertaining in giant-screen movies of airplanes swooping over canyons, in daily life lack of image stability can be disabling because the ability to use vision for orientation is lost.

Normally, when the head turns to the right, signals from the right horizontal semicircular canal increase and signals from the left horizontal semicircular canal decrease. This information is relayed to the vestibular nuclei for coordination of visual stabilization. Information is sent from the vestibular nuclei to the nuclei of cranial nerves III and VI, activating the rectus muscles that move the eyes to the left and inhibiting the rectus muscles that move the eyes to the right (Figures 15-8 and 15-9).

Similarly, vertical VORs can be elicited by flexion of the head and extension of the head. All VORs move the eyes in the direction opposite to the head movement to maintain stability of the visual field and visual fixation on objects. The effect of stimulation of each semicircular canal on extraocular muscles is illustrated in Figure

15-10. Stimulating a pair of semicircular canals induces eye movements in roughly the same plane as the canals (Brandt and Strupp, 2005).

Sometimes when a person turns the head, the intent is to look in the new direction rather than have the eyes fixate the previous target. To accomplish this, suppression of the VOR is essential. The flocculus of the cerebel-

lum adjusts the gain of the VOR and can completely suppress the VOR when appropriate.

Optokinetic Reflex

The optokinetic reflex adjusts eye position during slow head movements. *Optokinetic* means that the reflex is elicited by moving visual stimuli. When a person is walking, the head moves relative to objects in the environment. The optokinetic system allows the eyes to follow large objects in the visual field. Experimentally, the optokinetic system can be studied by having a person watch a cylinder covered with vertical stripes rotating slowly. A normal response is for the person's eyes to follow a single stripe to the edge of the visual field, and then a saccade moves the eyes to the next stripe. The neurologic control of the optokinetic reflex involves the following structures in sequence: retina, optic tract, pretectal area (in the midbrain; see Figure 13-5), medial vestibular nucleus, and oculomotor nuclei (Delgado-Garcia, 2000) (Figure 15-11).

The influence of optokinetic stimuli on the perception of movement is illustrated by responses to unexpected movement of nearby large objects. For example, a person stopped at a stoplight may misinterpret the sudden movement of a bus in the adjacent lane as the person's car rolling backward. The person hits the brakes, only to realize the car was not moving. This illusion of motion is called *vection*.

Direction of Gaze

Saccades, smooth pursuits, and convergence are eye movements that serve to direct gaze toward selected objects. Brainstem centers control horizontal and vertical eye movements. An area in the pons, the paramedian pontine reticular formation (PPRF), controls voluntary horizontal saccades. The abducens nucleus, as the source of abducens nerve and via connections with the oculomotor nucleus, controls horizontal pursuits and reflexive saccades. The midbrain reticular formation controls vertical eye movements. Cortical centers influencing eye

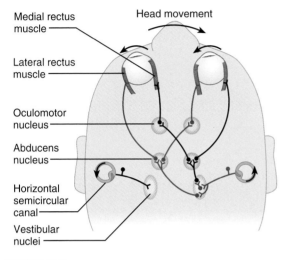

Medial rectus muscle
Head movement
Lateral rectus muscle
Oculomotor nucleus
Abducens nucleus
Horizontal semicircular canal
Vestibular nuclei

FIGURE 15-8
Vestibulo-ocular reflex. When the head is turned to the right, inertia causes the fluid in the horizontal semicircular canals to lag behind the head movement. This bends the cupula in the right semicircular canal in a direction that increases firing in the right vestibular nerve. The cupula in the left semicircular canal bends in a direction that decreases the tonic activity in the left vestibular nerve. Neurons whose activity level increases with this movement are indicated in red. Neurons whose activity level decreases are indicated in black. For simplicity, the connections of the left vestibular nuclei are not shown. Via connections between the vestibular nuclei and the nuclei of cranial nerves III and VI, both eyes move in the direction opposite to the head turn.

Vestibulo-ocular reflex

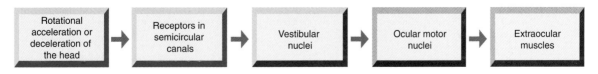

| Rotational acceleration or deceleration of the head | → | Receptors in semicircular canals | → | Vestibular nuclei | → | Ocular motor nuclei | → | Extraocular muscles |

FIGURE 15-9
The generation of the vestibulo-ocular reflex.

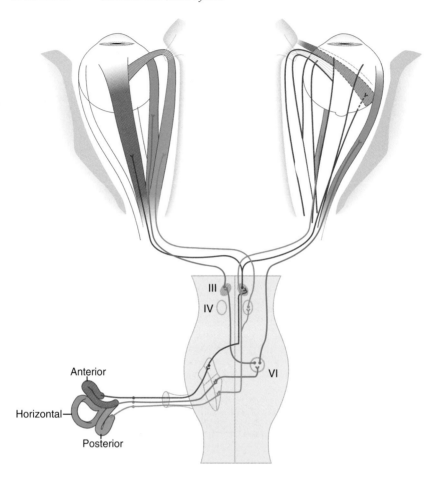

Movement of face	Canal stimulated	1st synapse in vestibular nucleus	2nd synapse in nucleus of:	Muscles activated:	Movement of the eyes
Face tilts down	Anterior	Superior	CN III	Ipsilateral superior rectus Contralateral inferior oblique	Up
Face turns right or left	Horizontal	Medial	CN III, VI	Ipsilateral medial rectus Contralateral lateral rectus	Horizontal
Face tilts up	Posterior	Medial	CN III, IV	Ipsilateral superior oblique Contralateral inferior rectus	Down

FIGURE 15-10

The connections between receptors in the semicircular canals and the nuclei of the nerves to the extraocular muscles are shown. For simplicity, only excitatory connections are shown. The inhibitory connections (not shown) adjust the activity of nerves to antagonistic extraocular muscles so that their activity is inversely proportional to the activity of the agonist muscles.

Optokinetic reflex

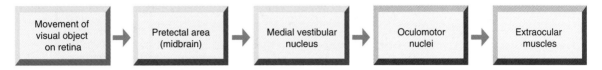

FIGURE 15-11
The generation of the optokinetic reflex.

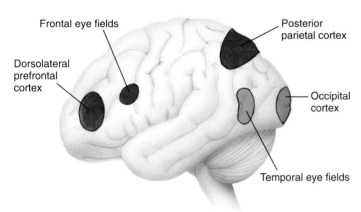

Frontal eye fields

Dorsolateral
prefrontal
cortex

Posterior
parietal cortex

Occipital
cortex

Temporal eye fields

FIGURE 15-12
Areas of the cerebral cortex that direct eye movements. The frontal eye fields control voluntary eye movements. Occipital and temporal regions provide information for pursuit eye movements. The posterior parietal cortex provides spatial information for eye movements. The areas colored blue provide information about the movement of visual objects, essential for optokinetic and smooth pursuit eye movements. The areas colored red are important for saccades. (Note: The occipital eye fields are in the occipital cortex.)

movements include the frontal, occipital, and temporal eye fields (Figure 15-12). The frontal eye fields provide voluntary control of eye movements when a decision is made to look at a particular object. The occipital and temporal eye fields contribute to the ability to visually pursue moving objects (pursuit eye movements). The dorsolateral prefrontal cortex inhibits reflexive eye movements as appropriate. Another area, in the posterior parietal cortex, provides cortical input for smooth pursuit movements.

> The following may influence eye movements:
> • Auditory information (via the superior colliculus)
> • Vestibulo-ocular reflex
> • Visual stimuli
> • Sensory information from extraocular muscles
> • Limbic system (see Chapters 16 and 17) and voluntary control

Saccades quickly switch vision from one object to another. If a person is reading and someone comes into the room, a saccadic eye movement shifts the reader's gaze from the text to the person. For voluntary saccades, the posterior parietal cortex directs visual attention to the stimulus. The posterior parietal cortex signals the superior colliculus, the brainstem center for orientation. The superior colliculus also receives information from the frontal eye fields. The superior colliculus then signals the PPRF and/or the midbrain reticular formation. The PPRF controls voluntary horizontal saccades by activating the abducens nucleus, which then activates the oculomotor nucleus. The midbrain reticular formation controls vertical saccades by activating cranial nerves III and IV (Figure 15-13, *A*). Adjusting the relative levels of activity of the PPRF and midbrain reticular formation controls diagonal saccades.

Saccades can be generated voluntarily (for example, a person decides to look up) and can also be elicited by a variety of stimuli, including visual, tactile, auditory, or nociceptive. For example, a fast-moving object in the peripheral vision elicits reflexive movements of the eyes and head toward the stimulus. The control of reflexive saccades is less complex than control of voluntary saccades. Reflexive horizontal saccades are initiated by the

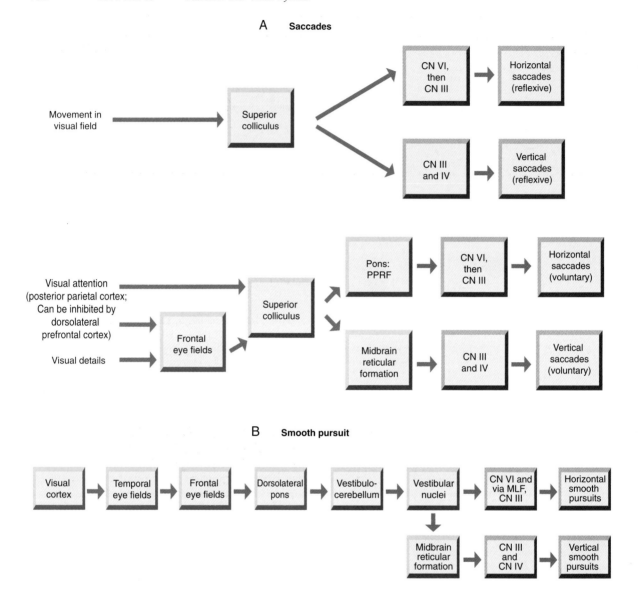

FIGURE 15-13

A, The generation of reflexive and voluntary saccades. **B,** The generation of smooth pursuit eye movements. CN, Cranial nerve; PPRF, paramedian pontine reticular formation.

superior colliculus, then directly signaled to the abducens nucleus, then, via the medial longitudinal fasciculus, to the oculomotor nucleus. Reflexive vertical saccades are signaled directly to the oculomotor and trochlear nuclei. The different actions of the visually guided system, the VOR, and the optokinetic reflex can be

demonstrated by the following task. Extend your arm, and place your index finger about 1.5 feet in front of you. Compare the visual clarity when you move your finger from side to side rapidly versus when the finger is held steady and you move your head rapidly from side to side. Next, keep your head still while you move your finger

Table 15-1   CONTROL OF EYE MOVEMENT

Neural Control System	Purpose	Type of Movement	Origin of Command
Vestibulo-ocular during rapid head movements	To keep the gaze fixed on a target	Reflex conjugate	Vestibular nuclei
Optokinetic	To keep the gaze fixed on a target during slow head movements	Reflex conjugate	Visual cortex
Smooth pursuit	To maintain the gaze on a moving target	Voluntary conjugate	Visual cortex
Saccadic	To rapidly move the eyes to a new target	Voluntary conjugate	Frontal eye fields
Vergence	To align the eyes on a near target	Voluntary disconjugate	Visual cortex

from side to side slowly. Explain the difference in ability to see details.*

Smooth pursuit eye movements are used to follow a moving object. If you watch someone walk across the room, smooth pursuit movements maintain the direction of gaze so that the image is maintained on the fovea. Commands for smooth pursuit movement originate in the visual cortex. In sequence, the signals are transmitted via the temporal eye fields, frontal eye fields, dorsolateral pons, vestibulocerebellum, and then vestibular nuclei to the nucleus of cranial nerve VI (abducens nerve) and/or to the midbrain reticular formation. The nucleus of cranial nerve VI connects with cranial nerve III via the medial longitudinal fasciculus. The activation of cranial nerve VI and part of cranial nerve III activates the appropriate rectus muscles to produce horizontal pursuit movements. The midbrain reticular formation activates ocular motor neurons to produce vertical pursuit movements (see Figure 15-13, *B*). A moving visual stimulus is essential for the production of smooth pursuit movements.

During reading, the pupils are directed toward the midline to allow the image to fall on corresponding areas of the retinas. This convergence is part of the accommodation discussed in Chapter 13. The control of eye movement is summarized in Table 15-1.

Involuntary back-and-forth movements of the eyes, such as occur during or after rapid rotation of the head, are called **nystagmus**. The direction of nystagmus is named according to the direction of saccadic eye movements. Thus, if the fast movements are toward the right, the nystagmus is called right-beating nystagmus.

*The difference in clarity is due to the ability of the nervous system to adjust eye movements based on anticipated head location versus the slower process of adjusting after visual information indicates loss of the target. Thus the difference in the ability to see details results from the rapid adjustments using feed-forward versus the slower process using feedback.

Physiologic nystagmus is a normal response that can be elicited in an intact nervous system by rotational or temperature stimulation of the semicircular canals (see Table 13-4) or by moving the eyes to the extreme horizontal position. Pathologic nystagmus, a sign of nervous system abnormality, is discussed with disorders of the eye movement system.

> The clinical importance of nystagmus (except nystagmus elicited by moving the eyes to the extreme horizontal position) is the evidence that the sensory system perceives head rotation and the eyes are moving to adjust for the perceived rotation.

PERCEPTION: INHIBITORY VISUAL-VESTIBULAR INTERACTION IN THE CEREBRAL CORTEX

During vection, activity in the vestibular cortex is inhibited. Similarly, activation of the vestibular cortex inhibits visual areas of the cortex (Dieterich and Brandt, 2000). Try turning your head and eyes slowly from one side of the room to the other side. Compare the visual detail with that observed when you make the same movement quickly. When the vestibular activity increases, visual details are suppressed.

DISORDERS OF THE VESTIBULAR AND VISUAL SYSTEMS

In either system, disorders may affect the receptors, the cranial nerves, brainstem nuclei, tracts within the central nervous system, or the associated cortical areas. A complete lesion affecting receptors or cranial nerve dedicated to that system produces total ipsilateral loss of sensory input for that system. Thus, a complete peripheral lesion causes ipsilateral loss of vestibular information in the vestibular system. A complete lesion in the retina or optic nerve causes ipsilateral blindness in the visual system. Lesions of these systems within the brain cause more variable outcomes, depending on the location and extent of the lesion.

Disorders of the Vestibular System

The most common symptom of vestibular system dysfunction is vertigo, an illusion of motion. People may falsely perceive movement of themselves or their surroundings. Vertigo occurs with both peripheral and central disorders, and arises from disturbance of spatial orientation in the vestibular cortex. Vestibular disorders may also cause pathologic nystagmus, which is typically more severe in peripheral than in central lesions. However, pathologic nystagmus is fatigable and habituates in most peripheral disorders but does not fatigue or habituate in central disorders. Pathologic nystagmus results from unbalanced inputs to the vestibulo-ocular reflex circuits. Another frequent symptom of vestibular disorders is disequilibrium, a sense of imbalance. Ataxia may occur with vestibular disorders. Vestibular ataxia must be differentiated from cerebellar and from sensory ataxia (see examining the vestibular system later in this chapter). In vestibular lesions, abnormal vestibulospinal, corticospinal, reticulospinal, and tectospinal tract activity causes the disequilibrium and ataxia. Nausea and vomiting may also occur, due to connections that activate the reticular formation.

> Vestibular system lesions cause vertigo, nystagmus, ataxia, and nausea.

When a person moves relative to the environment, or when objects in the environment move, a continuous stream of visual information flows across the retinas. Normally this information is suppressed, and there is no optokinetic effect on equilibrium. However, people with vestibular disorders may experience severe dysequilibrium in these situations. This is illustrated by the "grocery store effect," in which the intensity of optical flow provokes dysequilibrium and disorientation. Walking in a busy mall or walking near traffic can elicit similar effects on equilibrium and orientation. To maintain orientation and control of posture, a person with a vestibular disorder may need to move slowly and devote conscious attention to staying upright.

Common Peripheral Vestibular Disorders

Peripheral vestibular disorders typically cause recurring periods of vertigo, accompanied by more severe nausea than central disorders. Nystagmus always accompanies peripheral vertigo. Because the auditory and vestibular structures are in close proximity in the inner ear, diminished hearing and/or tinnitus are frequently present. No other neurologic findings are associated with peripheral vestibular disorders. Common peripheral vestibular disorders include benign paroxysmal positional vertigo, vestibular neuritis, Ménière's disease (Table 15-2), traumatic injury, and perilymph fistula. Certain drugs may also cause peripheral vestibular damage.

Benign Paroxysmal Positional Vertigo. Benign paroxysmal positional vertigo (BPPV) is an inner ear disorder that causes acute onset of vertigo and nystagmus. The term *benign* indicates not malignant, *paroxysmal* means a sudden onset of a symptom or a disease, and *positional* denotes head position as the provoking stimulus. In BPPV, a rapid change of head position results in vertigo and nystagmus that subsides in less than 2 minutes, even if the provoking head position is sustained. Activities that frequently provoke BPPV include getting into or out of bed, bending over to look under a bed, reaching up to retrieve something from a high shelf ("top shelf vertigo"), and turning over in bed.

Displacement of otoconia from the macula into a semicircular canal is the cause of BPPV. The otoconia may be displaced secondary to trauma or an infection that affects the vestibular apparatus. However, BPPV appears to occur spontaneously in some elderly people. When the head is upright, the otoconia settle in a gravity-dependent position in the posterior semicircular canal. When the head is moved quickly into a provoking position, the otoconia fall to a new position within the canal. Their movement generates an abnormal flow of the endolymph, bending the cupula and initiating unilateral signals in the vestibular nerve. If the provoking head position is maintained, the vertigo fades as the endolymph stops moving. Balance deficits may accompany the vertigo. Frequently the balance disorder outlasts the brief spell of vertigo. The signs and symptoms of BPPV can be provoked using the Hallpike maneuver (Figure 15-14). (See Box 15-1.) A treatment to restore the otoconia to their correct position, the particle repositioning maneuver, begins with the Hallpike maneuver. If the right ear is affected, the Hallpike ends with the head rotated toward the right side. When the vertigo and nystagmus stop, the patient's head is rotated to the left side and the patient turns fully prone. The patient

Table 15-2   COMPARISON OF PERIPHERAL VESTIBULAR DISORDERS

	Benign Paroxysmal Positional Vertigo	Vestibular Neuritis	Ménière's Disease
Etiology	May be otoconia in semicircular canals	Infection	Unknown
Speed of onset	Acute	Acute	Chronic
Duration of typical incident	<2 minutes	Severe symptoms for 2-3 days, gradual improvement over 2 weeks	0.5-24 hours
Prognosis	If untreated, improves in weeks or months; if treated with particle repositioning maneuver, often cured immediately	Improves after 3-4 days	Some patients have only mild hearing loss and a few episodes of vertigo. Most have multiple episodes of vertigo and progressive loss of hearing.
Unique signs	Elicited by change of head position	None	Associated with hearing loss, tinnitus, and feeling of fullness in the ear

---

BOX 15-1   BENIGN PAROXYSMAL POSITIONAL VERTIGO

Pathology

Otoconia freed from macula float into semicircular canal, usually into the posterior semicircular canal; when a quick head movement causes the otoconia to fall to a new gravity-dependent position, the movement of the otoconia produces abnormal fluid flow in the semicircular canal, stimulating the hair cells in the cupula and creating abnormal signals in the vestibular nerve.

Etiology

Often traumatic; may occur after a viral infection that affects the peripheral vestibular system or spontaneously

Speed of Onset

Rapid

Signs and Symptoms

Vertigo lasting less than 2 minutes provoked by moving the head into specific positions

Consciousness

Brief interference with orientation and concentration

Communication and Memory

Normal

Sensory

Normal somatosensation; illusion of environment or self moving

Autonomic

Nausea

Motor

Poor balance and trouble walking (Herdman and Tusa, 2000)

Region Affected

Peripheral nervous system; inner ear

Demographics

Incidence = 0.6% per year

Lifetime prevalence = 2.4%; (von Brevern M, Radtke A, et al. (2006). Epidemiology of benign paroxysmal positional vertigo. A population-based study. Journal of Neurology, Neurosurgery, and Psychiatry. Nov 29; {Epub ahead of print}.)

Incidence tends to increase with age. Oghalai et al., (2000) reported that in a cross-sectional study, 9% of elderly people had unrecognized BPPV.

Prognosis

A double-blind, controlled study demonstrated that 1 week post treatment, 90% of treated patients had full relief of symptoms, versus 27% of patients in the control group (Massoud and Ireland, 1996).

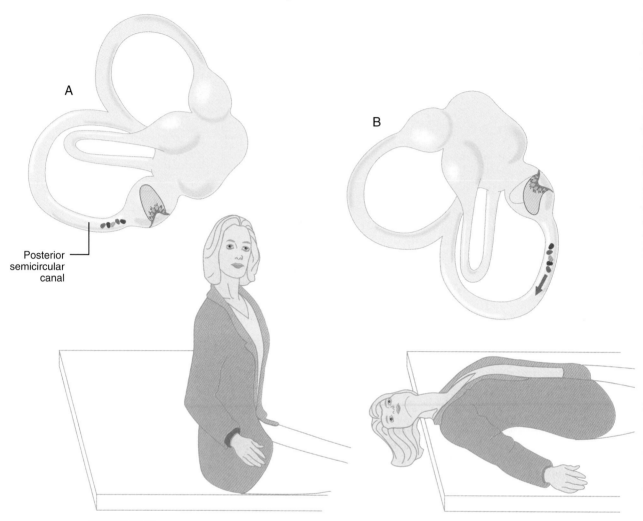

FIGURE 15-14

Canalithiasis and the Hallpike maneuver. In canalithiasis, otoconia are detached from the macula and float freely in a semicircular canal. Most commonly the posterior semicircular canal is affected. **A,** Position of the semicircular canals when a person is sitting with the head turned 45 degrees to the right. Note the otoconia in the posterior canal. **B,** To determine whether otoconia are present in the posterior semicircular canal, the Hallpike maneuver is used. The Hallpike maneuver tests for canalithiasis by provoking maximal movement of the otoconia. The maneuver is performed by turning the person's head 45 degrees to the right (or left), then passively moving the person quickly from a sitting position to a supine position with the head turned and the neck extended 30 degrees. Free-floating otoconia in the posterior semicircular canal fall away from the cupula in response to gravity, creating movement of the endolymph that continues after the head is stationary. The continued movement of the endolymph bends the cupula, producing signals in the vestibular nerve that elicit vertigo and nystagmus. When the endolymph stops moving, the vertigo and nystagmus subside. Thus the Hallpike maneuver tests for canalithiasis by provoking maximal movement of otoconia.

remains in the prone position for 10-15 seconds. Maintaining the head turned toward the left shoulder, the patient is assisted into a sitting position. Prokopakis et al. (2005) report that in 84% of patients, particle repositioning immediately eliminated BPPV, and 92% of patients reported that they were free of vertigo during the follow up period (average follow up was 46 months).

Vestibular Neuritis. Vestibular neuritis is inflammation of the vestibular nerve, usually caused by a virus. Dysequilibrium, spontaneous nystagmus, nausea, and severe vertigo persist up to 3 days. Hearing is unaffected. Caloric testing (see the section on Testing Vestibulo-occular Reflexes in this chapter) shows decreased or absent response on the involved side. During the acute phase, medication may be used to suppress the nausea, vertigo, and vomiting.

Ménière's Disease. Ménière's disease causes a sensation of fullness in the ear, tinnitus (ringing in the ear), severe acute vertigo, nausea, vomiting, and hearing loss. Ménière's disease is associated with abnormal fluid pressure in the inner ear causing expansion of the scala media (the expansion is called *endolymphatic hydrops*), but whether this is a cause of the disease or an effect is unknown. Because different diagnostic criteria are used, the incidence has been reported as ranging from 4.3-150 cases per 100,000 people (Kotimaki, 2003; Schessel et al., 1998). Drugs that suppress vertigo are useful during acute attacks. In extreme cases, the vestibular nerve may be surgically severed to relieve symptoms. Destruction of the labyrinth by injection of drugs that damage the inner ear may also be used to control the nausea and vomiting.

Traumatic Injury. Traumatic injury of the head may cause concussion of the inner ear, fractures of the bone surrounding the vestibular apparatus and nerve, or pressure changes in the inner ear. Any of these injuries can compromise vestibular function.

Perilymph Fistula. Perilymph is the fluid in the space between the bone and the membranous labyrinth in the inner ear. Perilymph fistula occurs when there is an opening between the middle and inner ear, allowing perilymph to leak from the inner ear into the middle ear. This leakage produces the abrupt onset of hearing loss, with tinnitus and vertigo. Most cases are secondary to trauma. Diagnosis requires an incision and endoscopic examination.

Bilateral Lesions of the Vestibular Nerve. Bilateral lesions of the vestibular nerve interfere with reflexive eye movements in response to head movement. People with bilateral vestibular nerve lesions initially complain of oscillopsia. **Oscillopsia** is a subjective sensation of visual objects bouncing when the head is moving. The world seems to bounce up and down as they walk because normal reflexive adjustments for head movement are decreased (decreased VOR). Over time, the nervous system adapts to the change, and people report less difficulty with disorienting movements of the visual field.

Certain antibiotics, specifically gentamicin and streptomycin, may damage both the cochlea and the vestibular apparatus in susceptible people. The effects are typically bilateral. Vertigo is infrequent, while hearing loss, dysequilibrium, and oscillopsia are common.

Central Vestibular Disorders

Central vestibular disorders result from damage to the vestibular nuclei or their connections within the brain. Central disorders typically produce milder symptoms than peripheral disorders. Nystagmus may occur. Vertigo is much less common in central than in peripheral disorders. Lesions that interfere with vestibular nuclei produce signs and symptoms similar to those of unilateral vestibular lesions: nystagmus, vertigo, and dysequilibrium. However, because central lesions are rarely limited to only the vestibular nuclei, central lesions produce additional signs, depending on the involvement of other structures. Any brainstem signs, including sensory and/or motor loss, double vision, Horner's syndrome, clumsiness when the trunk is supported (i.e., sitting or lying down), or dysarthria are indications of a central lesion. Vertigo persisting more than 3 days with mild nausea and vomiting usually indicates a central nervous system dysfunction. Pure vertical positional nystagmus and horizontal or vertical double vision that persists longer than 2 weeks after onset also indicate a central lesion (Solomon, 2000).

Lesions in the vestibulothalamocortical pathway or the vestibular cortex create an abnormal perception of vertical. The vestibular cortex is located in the parieto-insular cortex and receives input from both the semicircular canals and otolithic organs (Slobounov et al., 2006). People with lesions that affect the vestibular system superior to the vestibular nuclei experience head tilt, misidentification of vertical, and lateropulsion. Lateropulsion is pushing toward one side of the body when sitting and/or standing. Lesions of the vestibular cortex may produce lateropulsion (Brandt and Dieterich, 1999). Lateropulsion also occurs in dorsolateral medullary syndrome (Wallenberg's syndrome) via damage to the vestibular nuclei, inferior cerebellar peduncle, or spinocerebellar tracts (Nowak and Topka, 2006).

Central vestibular disorders most commonly result from ischemia or tumors in the brainstem/cerebellar region, cerebellar degeneration, multiple sclerosis, or Arnold-Chiari malformation. Migraine may cause vestibular dysfunction. The diagnosis of migraine-related vestibulopathy is based on vestibular symptoms that do not fit other syndromes, plus a history of migraine, a family history of migraine, and susceptibility to motion sickness and visually evoked vertigo (Cass et al., 1997). Vestibular physical therapy decreases the number of falls and severity of dizziness in people with migraine-related vestibulopathy (Whitney et al., 2000). Table 15-3 lists the signs and symptoms that differentiate peripheral from central vestibular disorders.

Unilateral Vestibular Loss

Unilateral vestibular loss causes problems with posture, eye movement control, and nausea because signals from the damaged side are not correctly balanced with signals from the intact side. A peripheral lesion that interferes with otolithic function on one side causes an imbalance because information from the otoliths on the normal side is not balanced by information from the otoliths on the lesioned side. Acute imbalance in otolithic information affects the vestibulospinal system, producing a tendency to fall toward the side of the lesion. After compensation by the central vestibular system, the direction of falling is variable.

Unilateral semicircular canal lesions are associated with nystagmus and an asymmetrical VOR. The nystagmus beats away from the impaired side and is never vertical. After a few days, central compensation may completely suppress the nystagmus during visual fixation. Unlike resolution of nystagmus, the VOR remains asymmetrical as long as the semicircular canals are impaired (Goebel, 2000).

A central lesion that damages the vestibular nuclei on one side causes unbalanced signals because the vestibular nuclei are operating normally on one side and the signals are decreased or lost from the vestibular nuclei on the damaged side. Unilateral central lesions produce a tendency to fall toward the side of the lesion and nystagmus beating away from the side of the lesion.

A unilateral lesion affecting the otoliths or the vestibular nuclei may produce a complete or partial ocular tilt reaction (Walker and Zee, 2000). The ocular tilt reaction (OTR; Figure 15-15) is a triad of signs consisting of:

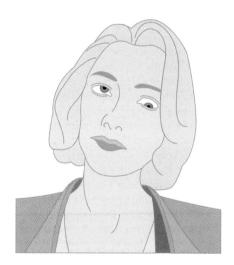

FIGURE 15-15
Ocular tilt reaction. The full ocular tilt reaction consists of a triad of signs: lateral head tilt, skew deviation of the eyes, and ocular rotation. The illustration shows part of the ocular tilt reaction toward the left: left lateral head tilt, left eye looking downward, and right eye looking upward. The rotation of both eyes to the left is not shown.

Table 15-3 DIFFERENTIATING BETWEEN PERIPHERAL AND CENTRAL VESTIBULAR DISORDERS

Symptom	Peripheral Nervous System	Central Nervous System
Nystagmus	Always present; typically unidirectional, not vertical	Frequently present; may be vertical, unidirectional, or multidirectional
Cochlear nerve symptoms	May have tinnitus, decreased hearing	Uncommon
Brainstem region signs	None	May have motor or sensory deficits, Babinski's sign, dysarthria, limb ataxia, or hyperreflexia
Nausea and/or vomiting	Moderate to severe	Mild
Oscillopsia	Mild unless the lesion is bilateral	Severe

- Head tilt
- Ocular torsion
- Skew deviation of the eyes

Head tilt is lateral flexion of the head caused by a misperception of vertical. Due to unbalanced vestibular information, the person perceives true vertical as being tilted. For example, if asked to identify when a lighted rod is upright in a dark room, the person will report that the rod is upright when it is actually tilted. Ocular torsion is the rotation of the eyes around the axis of the pupil. Both eyes rotate downward toward the downward side of the head. Skew deviation of the eyes is the upward direction of one eye combined with downward deviation of the other eye.

Bilateral Vestibular Loss

Bilateral loss of otolith input eliminates a person's internal sense of gravity. Therefore, the person must rely on visual and proprioceptive cues for spatial orientation. This creates difficulty walking in the dark and walking on uneven surfaces. Because no asymmetry of the vestibular information occurs, there is no vertigo (Shepard and Solomon, 2000).

Bilateral loss of semicircular canal input causes failure of the VOR. When the person walks, the world appears to bounce up and down. When the person turns the head, vision is blurry and unstable. This lack of visual stabilization due to lack of the afferent limb of the VOR is oscillopsia. People with chronic vestibular dysfunction often have stiffness of the neck and shoulders. This stiffness may result from attempts to stabilize the head, to lessen vertigo or oscillopsia (Horak and Shupert, 1994).

Disorders of the Visual System

The consequences of damage along the retinogeniculocortical pathway vary according to the location of the lesion (Figure 15-16). Clinically, visual losses are described by referring to the visual field deficit. Interruption of the optic nerve results in total loss of vision in the ipsilateral eye. Damage to fibers in the center of the optic chiasm interrupts the fibers from the nasal half of each retina, resulting in loss of information from both temporal visual fields, called **bitemporal hemianopsia.** A complete lesion of the pathway anywhere posterior to the optic chiasm, in the optic tract, lateral geniculate, or

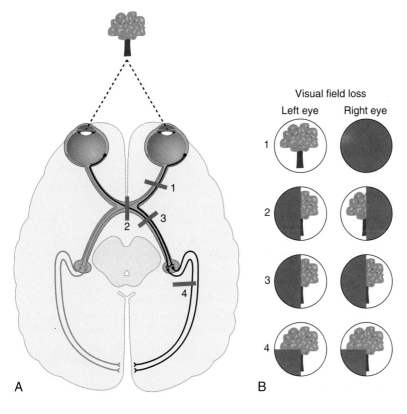

Visual field loss

Left eye   Right eye

FIGURE 15-16
Results of lesions at various locations in the visual system. **A,** Locations of the lesions. **B,** Visual field loss with each lesion. A lesion at location 1, optic nerve, causes loss of vision from the right eye. A lesion at location 2, the middle of the optic chiasm, causes bitemporal hemianopsia, loss of the temporal visual field from both eyes. Any lesion that completely interrupts tracts posterior to the optic chiasm, such as the lesion at location 3, optic tract, causes loss of vision from contralateral visual field of both eyes. An incomplete lesion of tracts posterior to the optic chiasm, as shown at location 4, causes partial loss of vision from the contralateral visual field.

A   B

optic radiations, results in loss of information from the contralateral visual field because all visual information posterior to the chiasm is from the contralateral visual field. This loss of visual information from one hemifield is called **homonymous hemianopsia.**

Following complete, bilateral loss of visual cortex function, some people retain the ability to orient their head position or point to objects, despite being cortically blind. **Cortically blind** means that the person has no awareness of any visual information. The ability of a cortically blind individual to orient or point to visual objects is called blind sight. Blind sight is possible because the ability to vaguely perceive light and dark is retained in the visual system. Blind sight is contingent on intact function of the retina and pathways from the retina to the superior colliculus.

Disorders of the Eye Movement System

Abnormalities of eye movement occur with lesions involving:
- Cranial nerves that control extraocular muscles
- Strength of extraocular muscles
- Medial longitudinal fasciculus
- Vestibular system
- Cerebellum
- Eye fields in the cerebral cortex

Eye movement disorders that result from cranial nerve lesions were discussed in Chapter 13. In addition to the disorders listed in Chapter 13, problems with directing gaze may result from weakness of the extraocular muscles. For example, if the lateral rectus is weak, the position of the pupil in forward gaze will be directed medially. If the disorder is acute, double vision will occur because images of objects will not coincide on the retinas. If the disorder is chronic, the nervous system may suppress the vision from the deviant eye and double vision will be absent. However, with suppression of vision from one eye, the person will lose depth perception.

Difficulty aligning the eyes is called *tropia* or *phoria*. Tropia is a deviation of one eye from forward gaze when both eyes are open. Phoria is a deviation from forward gaze, apparent only when the person is looking forward with one eye (the other eye is covered). The person with a phoria is able to align both eyes accurately when binocular fusion is available. Binocular fusion is the blending of the image from each eye to become a single perception.

A variety of lesions cause abnormal eye movements. If the medial longitudinal fasciculus is affected, eye movements will not be coordinated with each other or

with the movements of the head. Damage to the vestibular system or to the cerebellum can cause pathologic nystagmus, abnormal oscillating eye movements that occur with or without external stimulation. Lesions of the vestibular system or cerebellum may also produce a deficient VOR, leading to inadequate gaze stabilization. Damage to a frontal eye field results in temporary ipsilateral gaze deviation; that is, the eyes look toward the damaged side. Recovery occurs because frontal eye field control of eye movement is controlled bilaterally. Damage to a parieto-occipital eye field causes inadequate pursuit eye movements (Downey and Leigh, 1998). Although the lag of eye movements behind a moving target cannot be seen by an examiner, the disorder is visible because of the compensatory saccades that are required to catch up with a moving object.

MOTION SICKNESS

Motion sickness—the nausea, headache, anxiety, and vomiting sometimes experienced in moving vehicles—is usually caused by a conflict between different types of sensory information (Zajonc and Roland, 2005). For example, when one reads in a car moving at a constant speed, information in central vision and from the vestibular apparatus indicate that one is not moving, yet peripheral vision is reporting movement. Seasickness may be caused by a conflict between visual and vestibular information (Bos et al., 2005). People who are susceptible to motion sickness usually have normal visual and vestibular system function.

EXAMINING THE VESTIBULAR SYSTEM

Differentiation of Dizziness Complaints

Patients reporting dizziness are often describing quite different experiences. The clinician must distinguish among the following:
- Vertigo (illusion of movement)
- Near syncope (feeling of impending faint)
- Dysequilibrium (loss of balance)
- Light-headedness (inability to concentrate)

The differential diagnosis of these conditions is important because the etiology and treatment of each are different. Vertigo indicates vestibular etiology, while the other symptoms typically do not indicate vestibular disorders. Near syncope is commonly caused by cardiovascular disorders. Dysequilibrium results from somatosensory deficits, basal ganglia disorders, cerebellar dysfunction, drug use, complete loss of vestibular function, or tumors in the brainstem/cerebellar region. Lightheadedness is associated with psychological disorders, including affective and anxiety disorders and hyperventilation syndrome. Indications that the disorder is psychological include symptoms unaffected by head movements, lack of ataxia during dizzy spell, and reproduction of symptoms with hyperventilation.

Differential diagnosis of dizziness
- Feeling faint for a few seconds indicates cardiopulmonary disorders
- Feeling lightheaded usually indicates psychologic disorders but may be cardiovascular or hypoglycemic
- Disequilibrium usually indicates neurologic disorders
- Vertigo typically indicates vestibular disorders

When taking a patient's history, often the most accurate information can be elicited by avoiding use of the terms *vertigo* and *dizziness*. Instead, encourage the patient to describe precisely what he or she feels. If prompts are necessary, ask if the patient feels faint, if the surroundings seem to be moving, if the patient feels unsteady, or if the patient is unable to concentrate. The frequencies of specific causes of dizziness are listed in Table 15-4.

Tests of Vestibular Function

If a patient has a vestibular disorder, the most important question to answer is whether the lesion is peripheral or central. The key questions that provide diagnostic information in vestibular disorders are the frequency, duration, severity of symptoms, and the provoking conditions. An examination of the vestibular system includes self-reports in addition to tests of:
- Postural control
- Transitional movements
- Gait
- Coordination
- Sensation (proprioception, vibration, hearing)
- Head position test for benign paroxysmal positional vertigo
- The vestibulo-ocular reflex

The self-report measures are intended to assess the impact of signs and symptoms on daily activities. A typical question is, "Do you feel confident walking in a busy store?"

Table 15-4   FREQUENCY OF SPECIFIC CAUSES OF DIZZINESS

Cause	Frequency (%)*
Peripheral Vestibular	
Benign paroxysmal positional vertigo	16
Inflammation of the inner ear (labyrinthitis)	9
Ménière's disease	5
Other (e.g., ototoxicity)	14
Central Vestibular	
Cerebrovascular	6
Tumor	<1
Other (e.g., multiple sclerosis, migraine)	3
Psychological	
Psychological disorder	11
Hyperventilation	5
Nonvestibular, Nonpsychological	
Presyncope	6
Dysequilibrium	5
Other (e.g., metabolic disorder, anemia)	13
Unknown	13

Data from Kroenke K, Hoffman RM, et al. (2000). How common are various causes of dizziness? A critical review. Southern Medical Journal, 93(2), 160-167.
*The percentages add up to more than 100% because dizziness was attributed to more than one cause in some patients.

Testing Postural Control, Transitional Movements, and Gait

Postural tests can be used to assess vestibular system function (see Table 10-6). However, none of these tests identify the etiology of equilibrium problems. The postural tests are either static or dynamic. Static tests include Romberg's test and stationary posturography. These tests do not evaluate the ability of the subject to prepare for or adapt to challenges to equilibrium. Dynamic tests include tilt boards and dynamic posturography. As discussed in Chapter 10, these tests only assess reactions to externally imposed displacements. The clinical usefulness of stationary posturography (the sensory organization test, discussed in Chapter 10 and illustrated in Figure 10-23) is controversial, because changes on the sensory organization test do not correlate with changes in functional performance nor with dizziness handicap scores (O'Neill et al., 1998; Badke et al., 2005). O'Neill et al. studied people with peripheral vestibular hypofunction and stable symptoms. Posturography scores were compared with gait velocity, Timed Get Up and

Go Test (see Table 15-6 later in this chapter), gait with head rotations, gait with eyes closed, and tandem gait. The researchers concluded that the posturography sensory organization test alone is not useful for assessing balance and function in people with vestibular hypofunction. In contrast to the artificiality of the sensory organization test, the functional reach test (described in Chapter 10) assesses anticipation of internally generated displacements, as typically occur in daily life.

For transitional movements, the patient's ability to move from sitting to standing and from floor to standing is tested. For gait, tests include walking:
- With eyes open and eyes closed
- While turning the head right and left on command
- While moving the head up and down
- Then stopping quickly on command
- Then making a quick pivot turn on command
- While carrying an object
- Up and down stairs
- Over and around objects in an obstacle course
- While answering a question. To administer The Stops Walking When Talking Test, walk with the patient and ask a question. If the patient stops walking to answer the question, walking requires more conscious attention than normal and the patient is at risk for falls (Andersson et al., 2006).

In these gait tests, the clinician assesses symptoms, loss of balance, and/or changes in gait.

Coordination Tests

Tandem walking and the heel-to-shin test examine lower limb coordination. For the heel-to-shin test, the supine patient places the heel on the opposite knee, then slides the heel down to the ankle. To differentiate vestibular from cerebellar and from sensory ataxia, the following criteria are used:
- **Vestibular ataxia** is unique in being gravity dependent. Limb movements are normal when the person is lying down but are ataxic during walking. Stance is more stable with the eyes open than with the eyes closed. In supported sitting, rapid alternating movements (finger or toe tapping, pronation/supination) are normal. Vertigo and nystagmus are associated with vestibular ataxia.
- **Cerebellar ataxia** is evident regardless of whether the person is standing, sitting, or lying down. Difficulty sitting as a result of ataxia may occur. Typically, cerebellar ataxia produces inability to stand with feet together, regardless of whether the eyes are open or closed. Vertigo and nystagmus may be associated with cerebellar ataxia.

- **Sensory ataxia** is characterized by impaired vibratory and position sense, decreased or lost ankle reflexes, and lack of nystagmus and lack of vertigo.

Sensation Testing

Sensation testing is used to localize a lesion. Hearing, proprioception, and vibration are tested. Tests for hearing were discussed in Chapter 13. Impaired hearing associated with vestibular signs and symptoms indicates that a lesion is likely to be located in the periphery. Because impaired proprioception can cause imbalance, proprioception and vibration tests (described in Chapter 7) are used to distinguish between lesions of the conscious proprioception pathways and vestibular lesions.

Head Position Test for Benign Paroxysmal Positional Vertigo

The **Hallpike maneuver** is the most commonly used test for posterior and anterior canal BPPV. The maneuver rapidly inverts the posterior semicircular canal. In people with BPPV, this causes abnormal flow of the endolymph, provoking vertigo and nystagmus. The patient, with knees straight, is sitting on a plinth. The clinician places his or her hands on the sides of the patient's head, then requests that the patient keep the eyes open and to keep looking at the clinician's nose the entire time. The clinician turns the patient's head 45 degrees from the sagittal plane. Then the patient is moved rapidly into a supine position with the head still turned 45 degrees from sagittal and the neck extended about 20 degrees (see Figure 15-14). Vertigo and nystagmus in response to the Hallpike maneuver indicate BPPV. According to El-Kashlan and Telian (2000), the nystagmus evoked in BPPV is characterized by:
- A latency before onset; nystagmus begins several seconds after the movement is completed
- Intensifying then fading
- Lasting 20-30 seconds, even if the patient remains in the provoking position
- Fatigability: with repetition of the provoking position, the vertigo and nystagmus decrease and may disappear

To test for BPPV, the head must be held in the provoking position for at least 30 seconds. Because the posterior semicircular canal is in the most gravity-dependent position when a patient is upright or supine, BPPV most often affects the posterior canal. When the patient is placed in the provoking position, posterior canal BPPV will produce torsional nystagmus with a down-beating vertical component. If the BPPV affects the left ear, the rotary nystagmus is clockwise; if the right ear is affected, the rotation is counterclockwise.

In less than 15% of BPPV cases, the anterior or horizontal semicircular canals are involved (Cakir et al., 2006). Anterior canal involvement produces a torsional nystagmus with an up-beating vertical component (El-Kashlan and Telian, 2000). If the horizontal canal is involved, lateral head turn in the supine position produces a pure horizontal nystagmus.

Testing Vestibulo-ocular Reflexes

The gain of the VOR depends on the frequency of the stimulus. Thus, testing with a frequency of 0.5-5.0 Hz is optimal, because the purpose of the VOR during natural situations is to stabilize gaze while a person is walking and turning the head. The VOR may be tested five ways: (1) by passive, rapid head thrusts, (2) by testing dynamic visual acuity, (3) by using a rotating chair, (4) by caloric testing, and (5) by electronystagmography. The VOR can be tested by passively moving an individual's head and observing the associated eye movements. The passive head turns should be rapid, unpredictable, and small amplitude (10 degrees to 20 degrees). A normal response is stable gaze. If the VOR is decreased or absent, a corrective saccade will be used after the head movement to compensate for loss of the visual target during the head movement.

Dynamic visual acuity tests the patient's ability to read an eye chart while the head is moving. The clinician passively rotates the patient's head at a frequency of 2 Hz, matching the cadence of a metronome to maintain accurate timing. Patients with an intact neural system will have less than one line loss of accuracy during the head movements compared with their acuity when the head is stable. Patients with an abnormal VOR will have a loss of acuity of two or more lines on the eye chart during the head rotation (Walker and Zee, 2000). The three other methods for testing the VOR are performed in vestibular specialty clinics. These tests include the rotating chair test, the caloric test, and electronystagmography.

The VOR can be tested with the individual seated in a rotating chair. With the head in neutral position, when the individual is rotated to the left the eyes will move slowly to the right, as if to maintain fixation on an object in the visual field. When the eyes reach the extreme right, they shift quickly to the left, then resume moving to the right. When the head is rotated to the left, the pursuit eye movements are toward the right, and the saccades are toward the left.

If a person rotates quickly several revolutions to the left, then abruptly stops rotating, the direction of slow and fast eye movements reverses; that is, the eyes repeatedly move slowly to the left and then quickly to the right. This reversal of eye movement is due to the inertia of the fluid continuing to flow in the horizontal canals after the head stops moving. The fluid movement bends the cupulas in the opposite direction to their bend during acceleration, producing the reversal of eye movements. Despite the frequent use of the rotating chair test to evaluate the VOR, this test typically uses frequencies of movement that are too low and too predictable to accurately test the ability of the VOR to compensate for head turning while a person is walking (Leigh and Brandt, 1993).

Another method of testing the VOR is the caloric test. Nontherapist specialists perform this test. A small amount of cold (30°C) or warm (44°C) water is instilled into the ear canal. Nausea and vomiting may result from the vestibular action on autonomic function. In a conscious patient, the mnemonic COWS summarizes the saccadic movements of the eyes: cold opposite, warm same. This indicates that when cold water is instilled, the fast eye movements are toward the opposite side, and when warm water is used the fast eye movements are toward the same side. Caloric stimulation is uniquely valuable in allowing unilateral assessment of the semicircular canal function (primarily the horizontal canal). However, caloric stimulation produces a low frequency of signals in the vestibular nerve, and thus the results of this test do not correlate well with VOR function during natural activities (Leigh and Brandt, 1993).

Electronystagmography (ENG) is a recording of eye movements. Surface electrodes near the eyes detect changes in extraocular muscle electrical potentials during eye movements. ENG can be used to evaluate pursuit and saccadic eye movements as well as nystagmus elicited by changes of head position or by caloric tests. Figure 15-17 illustrates ENG, rotary chair with rotary drum, and caloric testing.

EXAMINING THE VISUAL AND EYE MOVEMENT SYSTEMS

Methods for testing the visual system and convergence were described in Table 13-4. The ability to direct gaze can be tested by three tests that involve observing eye movements when one eye is covered or uncovered: the cover test, the cover-uncover test, and the alternate cover test. The patient is seated and asked to look at a distant

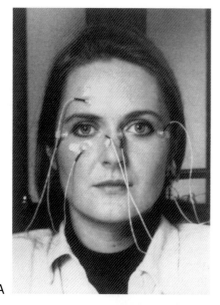

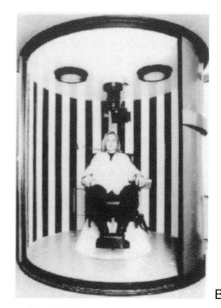

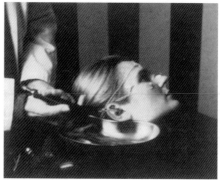

FIGURE 15-17

Electronystagmography (ENG), the recording of involuntary eye movements to evaluate patients with dizziness, vertigo, or balance problems. **A**, Placement of electrodes. **B**, Rotary chair with vertically striped rotary drum. Eye movements can be recorded while the chair is rotating or the surrounding drum is rotating, to distinguish between responses to head rotation or rotating visual stimuli. **C**, Caloric irrigation with ENG. Cool or warm water is placed in the external auditory canal, inducing flow of fluid in the adjacent horizontal semicircular canal. This test isolates the function of one horizontal canal without stimulating the other horizontal canal. *(From Brandt T, Strupp M (2005). General vestibular testing. Clinical Neurophysiology, 116(2), 406-426.)*

object in central vision. To test for tropia, the cover test is used. The clinician covers the patient's left eye. If the right eye remains directed at the target, the response is normal. If the right eye moves to look at the target, the right eye is trophic (Figure 15-18). To test for phoria, the cover-uncover test is used. The left eye is covered for approximately 10 seconds (to prevent fusion), and then uncovered. At the instant the left eye is uncovered, the left eye is observed for any movement. If the left eye does not move, the response is normal. If the left eye moves to look at the target, the left eye is phoric. Another test for phoria is the alternate cover test. In the alternate cover test, the cover is moved from one eye to the other several times. The cover remains over one eye for several

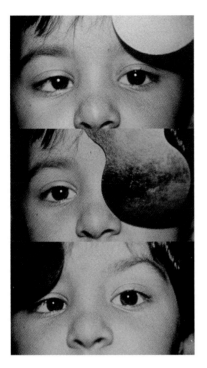

FIGURE 15-18

Cover testing. With both eyes uncovered, the left eye looks forward at the target and the right eye deviates toward the midline. For the cover test, the examiner covers one eye and then the other eye. In this patient, the right tropia corrects temporarily when the left eye is covered. *(From Perkin GD (2002). Mosby's Color Atlas and Text of Neurology. (2nd ed.; p. 13, Figure 1.15). London: Elsevier.)*

seconds, then is quickly moved to cover the other eye. This technique prevents fusion. The eye that is uncovered is observed for movement. If the uncovered eye remains steady, the response is normal. If the uncovered eye moves, the uncovered eye is phoric. The following tests examine eye movements.

Moving a vertically striped piece of cloth across the visual field tests the optokinetic reflex. This should produce pursuit eye movements in the direction of target movement, alternating with rapid eye movements to fixate the next target. The pursuit phase tests ipsilateral parieto-occipital pathways. The saccadic movements test the contralateral frontal lobe.

Asking the patient to move the eyes in response to verbal instructions from the examiner can test voluntary saccades. Damage to the frontal lobe interferes with this movement. To test pursuit eye movements, the patient is asked to keep the head still and follow the clinician's finger in the six directions shown in Figure 13-3, *C*. The eyes should move smoothly and their movements should be well coordinated. Problems with pursuit movements indicate lesions in the parieto-occipital region. The effects of lesions on eye movements are summarized in Table 15-5. Tables 15-6 and 15-7 summarize tests used to examine the vestibular and visual systems. Table 15-8 reviews how to distinguish among four categories of dizziness: feeling faint, feeling light-headed, disequilibrium, and vertigo, and the common causes of each of these symptoms. Type of dizziness, timing of dizziness, and hearing status are critical factors in diagnosing dizziness (Kentala and Rauch, 2003).

Table 15-5   EFFECTS OF LESIONS ON EYE MOVEMENTS

Location of Lesion	Effect on Resting Eye Position	Ability to Voluntarily Direct Eyes Past Midline	Double Vision
Vestibular nerve or vestibular nuclei	Contralateral nystagmus	Normal	No
Frontal eye fields	Both eyes deviated ipsilaterally	Unable to direct eyes past midline contralaterally	No
Pontine paramedian reticular formation	Both eyes deviated contralaterally	Unable to direct eyes past midline ipsilaterally	No
Abducens nucleus	Both eyes deviated contralaterally	Unable to direct eyes past midline ipsilaterally	No
Abducens nerve	Ipsilateral eye deviated medially	Normal	Yes
Medial longitudinal fasciculus	Ipsilateral eye deviated laterally	If the lesion is between the abducens and oculomotor nuclei, unable to adduct the ipsilateral eye past midline	Yes

Table 15-6   EXAMINATION OF THE VESTIBULAR AND EYE MOVEMENT SYSTEMS

Test	Procedure	Interpretation
Subjective Reports		
Rating scales	Patient rates vertigo, oscillopsia, and/or dysequilibrium on a rating scale (0-10) or by marking a line (labeled "no vertigo" at left end and "most severe vertigo imaginable" at right end) to indicate severity of symptoms.	Normal: Rating of zero. Abnormal: Ratings above zero.
Dizziness Handicap Inventory (Jacobson and Newman, 1990)	25-item questionnaire. Patient self-reports the impact of symptoms on everyday activities.	Authors of the study report that a change of more than 17 points in the total score indicates a significant change in self-perceived disability.
Subjective visual vertical	In a completely dark room, patient moves a dimly illuminated bar to vertical.	Normal: Bar aligned within 2 degrees of true vertical. Aligning the bar more than 2 degrees from true vertical usually indicates a unilateral vestibular lesion (Halmagyi and Curthoys, 2000).
Activities-Specific Balance Confidence Scale (Powell and Meyers, 1995)	16 questions. Example: "How confident are you that you will not lose your balance or become unsteady when you walk in a crowded mall where people rapidly walk past you?"	Scored as a percentage, with 100% being completely confident.
Past Pointing Test		
	Patient alternately touches the tip of the examiner's finger then reaches overhead with extended arm. The examiner holds his or her finger directly in front of the patient at about arm's length. Patient makes four attempts with eyes open, then four attempts with eyes closed.	Normal: Patient is able to touch the examiner's fingertip accurately every time. Abnormal: When eyes are closed, patient's finger consistently drifts to one side of the examiner's finger. The side of drift is consistent with both hands. Indicates an acute unilateral vestibular lesion. If performance is equally inaccurate with both eyes open and eyes closed, indicates a cerebellar disorder.
Gait		
Dynamic gait test (Shumway-Cook et al., 1997)	8 tasks. Tests gait at different speeds, with horizontal and vertical head turns, pivot turns, with obstacles, and stairs.	Provides specific commands for the patient and clear scoring criteria. Some of the items and their interpretation follow.
With eyes open and eyes closed	Patient walks with eyes open or closed.	Normal: Little difference in gait whether eyes are open or closed. Abnormal: If gait is worse with eyes closed than with eyes open, this indicates that vision is substituting for impaired somatosensory information. If there is little change in gait regardless of whether vision is available or not, a brainstem or cerebellar lesion is likely.

Table 15-6   EXAMINATION OF THE VESTIBULAR AND EYE MOVEMENT SYSTEMS—cont'd

Test	Procedure	Interpretation
While turning the head right and left on command or while moving the head up and down	Patient responds to commands while continuing to walk.	Tests the ability of the vestibulomotor system to compensate for head movements (vestibulospinal tracts and VOR). A person with a normal vestibular system can perform this task easily. A person with a vestibular lesion will tend to lose balance (due to abnormal input to vestibulospinal tracts) and have difficulty with visual orientation (inadequate VOR).
Stopping quickly on command, making a quick pivot turn on command, or navigating an obstacle course	Patient responds to commands or avoids obstacles while continuing to walk.	Tests the ability to anticipate changes in postural control.
While carrying an object	Patient walks while carrying books or a cup filled with water.	Tests the ability to make adjustments for changes in center of gravity and/or for increased cognitive demands.
Up and down stairs	Patient walks up and down stairs, with and without using railings. The test is made more challenging by having the patient carry an object up and down stairs.	Tests balance ability in a functional task.
Timed Functional Test		
Get Up and Go test	Quick screening of gait speed and control in turning. Patient rises from a chair, walks 3 meters, turns around, walks back to the chair, and sits down. The Timed Get Up and Go test includes timing the test.	Normal: Requires less than 30 seconds. Abnormal: Adults who require more than 30 seconds to complete the test are likely to be dependent in mobility and in activities of daily living.
Positional Testing		
Hallpike maneuver	Patient long sitting (knees extended) on plinth. Examiner asks patient to keep looking at the examiner's nose. Examiner turns patient's head 45 degrees left or right, then quickly moves patient into a supine position with the head still turned 45 degrees and the neck extended 30 degrees.	Tests for benign paroxysmal positional vertigo (BPPV). Normal: No nystagmus or vertigo in the end position. BPPV: After a few seconds, nystagmus and vertigo begin and last 20-30 seconds.
Eye Alignment		
	Examiner observes the position of the patient's eyes while the patient looks straight ahead at a distant object.	Some eye misalignments are severe and can be observed simply by looking at the patient's eyes while the patient looks at a distant object.
Cover test	To test eye alignment using the cover test, cover one of the patient's eyes and observe the other eye for movement.	Normal: Eye that is not covered does not move. Abnormal: Eye that is not covered moves. This indicates a tropia. Tropia may be congenital or acquired. Tropia results from paresis of one or more of the extraocular muscles of one eye or a lesion of cranial nerve III, IV, or VI. Acute tropia causes double vision.

Continued

Table 15-6   EXAMINATION OF THE VESTIBULAR AND EYE MOVEMENT SYSTEMS—cont'd

Test	Procedure	Interpretation
Cover-uncover test	Cover one of the patient's eyes for about 10 seconds. Watch the covered eye for movement as it is quickly uncovered.	Normal: No movement. Abnormal: Eye that is covered then uncovered moves. This is a phoria.
Alternate cover test	The cover is moved from one eye to the other several times. The cover remains over one eye for several seconds, then is quickly moved to cover the other eye.	Movement of an eye when it is uncovered indicates a phoria.
Spontaneous nystagmus	Patient is looking at a distant object straight ahead.	Normal: No movement of the eyes. Abnormal: Involuntary back-and-forth movements of the eyes; indicates a lesion of the vestibular, smooth-pursuit, or optokinetic system, or the cerebellum.
Eye Movement	Note: Test visual fields prior to testing eye movements (see Table 13-4).	
Voluntary saccades	Ask the patient to look in the directions indicated in Figure 13-3, *C*.	Normal: Smooth, conjugate, full-range movements. Assuming normal strength of extraocular muscles, abnormal responses include: 1. Both eyes deviated ipsilaterally; patient unable to direct eyes past midline contralaterally. Indicates acute or subacute lesion of the frontal eye field. Deficit is temporary because the contralateral frontal eye field can compensate. 2. Both eyes deviated contralaterally; patient unable to direct eyes past midline ipsilaterally. Lesion of the pontine paramedian reticular formation. 3. One eye unable to adduct past midline; other eye moves normally. Indicates a lesion of the medial longitudinal fasciculus between abducens and oculomotor nucleus (internuclear ophthalmoplegia; see Chapter 13).
Pursuits	Ask the patient to keep the head still and follow the movement of your finger. Move your finger slowly in the directions indicated in Figure 13-3, *C*.	Normal: Smooth, conjugate eye movements. Abnormal: Nystagmus and/or double vision. Assuming normal-strength extraocular muscles and intact oculomotor neurons, abnormal results indicate a lesion in the parieto-occipital cortex, cerebellum, or brainstem.

Table 15-6 EXAMINATION OF THE VESTIBULAR AND EYE MOVEMENT SYSTEMS—cont'd

Test	Procedure	Interpretation
Convergence	Convergence is adduction of the eyes. Ask the patient to look at the tip of a pen as it is slowly moved from about 2 feet away toward the patient's nose.	Normal: Both eyes are directed toward the pen tip until the pen is within 10 cm (4 inches) of the nose. Abnormal: Only one eye moves toward the midline. The other eye moves outward. Indicates defective perception or central nervous system control of visual fusion, or dysfunction of ocular motor neurons or ocular muscles.
Physiologic nystagmus	Patient looks at a striped moving target (optokinetic nystagmus), undergoes caloric testing, or moves the eyes to an extreme position.	Normal: Back-and-forth eye movements in response to any of these stimuli.
Pathologic nystagmus	Observe eyes when: 1. Patient is looking straight forward with eyes closed. Eyes are closed to eliminate visual fixation.	1. Symmetrical nystagmus usually is congenital. Jerk nystagmus— fast in one direction, slow in the opposite direction—usually indicates a unilateral vestibular lesion.
	2. Patient looks in the directions indicated in Figure 13-3, *C*.	2. If nystagmus occurs only in a single direction, this indicates weakness of an extraocular muscle or a lesion affecting a lower motor neuron. If nystagmus occurs in several directions, this usually indicates a drug effect, but it may indicate a cerebellar or central vestibular disorder. Central nystagmus does not suppress with fixation and may change direction with gaze. Peripheral vestibular nystagmus is inhibited by fixation and also increases in amplitude when gaze is directed toward the direction of nystagmus.
	3. Test for position-evoked nystagmus by using the Hallpike maneuver (see Figure 15-14).	3. Nystagmus and vertigo occur following a latency of a few seconds and last 20-30 seconds.
Optokinetic eye movements	Ask the patient to look at a vertically striped cloth, then move the cloth horizontally.	Normal: The eyes follow a stripe, then make a quick saccade to the next stripe. Abnormal: Problems with slow phase indicate abnormal pursuit mechanisms; problems with fast phase indicate problems with generating saccades.
Dynamic visual acuity	Patient reads Snellen chart while turning head left and right at a 2 Hz frequency.	Normal: Maximum of one line decrease in visual acuity. Bilateral vestibular deficit: Decrease in visual acuity of two or more lines.

Continued

Table 15-6 EXAMINATION OF THE VESTIBULAR AND EYE MOVEMENT SYSTEMS—cont'd

Test	Procedure	Interpretation
VOR to rapid head thrusts	Ask patient to look at examiner's nose. Examiner rotates patient's head passively, rapidly, about 10 degrees to the left and to the right.	Normal: Eyes remain fixed on examiner's nose. Abnormal: Eyes move away from examiner's nose, and a corrective saccade must be used to regain the target. Abnormal response to rapid head thrusts indicates a vestibular disorder.

Table 15-7 TESTS FOR DIFFERENTIAL DIAGNOSIS OF DIZZINESS COMPLAINTS

Tests	Interpretation
Screening	
Hearing test	If hearing is impaired on same side as a vestibular lesion, usually indicates that vestibular lesion is peripheral
Cranial nerves V and VII	Checks for involvement of brainstem or area adjacent to junction of cerebellum and pons
Hyperventilation	If symptoms are reproduced, indicates a psychological component to dizziness
Compare blood pressure supine to blood pressure after supine to stand	Orthostatic hypotension is a drop in blood pressure >20/10 mm Hg for 3 minutes following move from supine to standing
Check for carotid, subclavian bruits	Presence of bruits indicates arterial disease
Proprioception and vibration sense	Impairment of these senses can produce ataxia and dysequilibrium
Laboratory	(See text for descriptions of laboratory tests.)
Caloric irrigation	Tests function of a single horizontal semicircular canal
Rotary chair	Quantifies eye movements in response to rotation; abnormal responses indicate vestibular, brainstem, or cerebellar lesions
Electronystagmography (ENG)	Quantifies nystagmus, pursuits, saccades, optokinetic nystagmus
Dynamic posturography— sensory organization test	Tests ability to maintain balance when visual and somatosensory information is altered; provides no information about site of lesion; clinical usefulness is controversial (See text.)

REHABILITATION IN VESTIBULAR DISORDERS

Rehabilitation does not directly affect central dysfunctions of the vestibular system and is ineffective for active Ménière's disease. However, patients with certain central vestibular disorders may benefit from learning new ways of moving. Rehabilitation is effective for BPPV, unilateral vestibular loss or dysfunction and bilateral vestibular loss, and central vestibular disorders that benefit from movement retraining. Exercises are designed to promote movement retraining, habituation, or substitution to improve function. Movement retraining consists of practicing and modifying movements

as appropriate. Habituation is exposure to positions or movements that produce symptoms, followed by relaxation until the symptoms abate. The provocative stimuli are repeated frequently until the nervous system adapts to the stimuli. Habituation is effective for BPPV and unilateral vestibular loss. Substitution (also called *compensation*) consists of using alternative sensory inputs or motor responses or using predictive/anticipatory strategies. To compensate for bilateral vestibular loss, people learn to substitute visual and somatosensory cues and anticipation for absent or unreliable vestibular information. See Cohen (2006) for a review of recent prospective studies of the effects of therapy on vertigo and balance disorders in patients with dizziness.

Table 15-8 DIZZINESS EVALUATION

Patient's Report	Specific Sign(s)	Likely Diagnosis
Feeling faint for a few seconds	Blurred vision or loss of consciousness when moving from supine to standing	Postural hypotension
	Dizziness, blurred vision, slurred speech, nystagmus, or loss of consciousness during vertebral artery test (patient supine, examiner slowly extends, rotates, and laterally flexes the patient's cervical spine to each side)	Vertebral artery compression
Feeling light-headed	Lasts more than a few minutes	Low blood sugar
	Lasts only a few minutes and is associated with perioral and distal extremity tingling, tunnel vision, chest pain/tightness, and/or anxiety	Hyperventilation
	Provoked by anxiety, affective disorders, or pain	Vasovagal syncope or presyncope
	Provoked ONLY by coming to sitting or standing	Postural hypotension
	Associated with irregular heart rate, paresis, blurred vision and/or confusion	Cardiopulmonary disease
Disequilibrium (Sensation of losing balance without vertigo or feeling faint)	Impaired somatosensation; patient feels more unsteady in the dark than when adequate lighting is available.	Peripheral neuropathy, vitamin B deficiency, or multiple sclerosis
	Ataxia	Vascular disorder, tumor, alcohol abuse, or anticonvulsant drugs
	Impaired vestibulo-ocular reflexes and oscillopsia. Cannot drive, cannot read signs when walking	Nonfunctioning labyrinths Aminoglycosides (streptomycin, gentamicin, etc.) can damage vestibular receptors
	Positive VOR to rapid head thrusts (corrective saccade occurs)	Peripheral vestibular loss
	Negative VOR to rapid head thrusts, perceptual tilt, skew deviation, lateral head/body tilt	If signs are severe, central vestibular loss; if signs are mild, acute vestibular loss
	Abnormal cranial nerve tests, especially II-VIII	Brainstem vascular disorder or tumor or basilar migraine
	Musculoskeletal impairment	Deconditioning, poor postural alignment, multiple sclerosis
	Provoked by transportation	Motion sensitivity
Vertigo (false perception of movement; often associated with pallor, sweating, nausea, vomiting.)	Episode lasts less than 1 minute; positive vertebral compression test in sitting	Arterial compression or cervical facet pathology
	Lasts less than 1 minute; nystagmus with head positional tests	BPPV or central vestibular disorder
	Episode lasts more than 1 minute; continuous symptoms, including persistent disequilibrium, during an episode; symptoms are worst during first 1-2 hours of an episode	Ménière's or migraine
	More than 12 hours of intermittent episodes provoked by head movement	Unilateral vestibular loss (e.g., neuronitis)
	Continuous vertigo with nystagmus, decreased hearing, and tinnitus	Acoustic neuroma
	Continuous vertigo without nystagmus	Systemic disease or drug effect
	Provoked by transportation	Motion sensitivity

Developed from Sloane PD, Coeytaux RR, et al. (2001). Dizziness: State of the science. Annals of Internal Medicine, 134(9 Pt 2), 823-832; Hanley K, O'Dowd T (2002). Symptoms of vertigo in general practice: A prospective study of diagnosis. British Journal of General Practice, 52(483), 809-812; and Chawla N, Olshaker JS (2006). Diagnosis and management of dizziness and vertigo. Medical Clinics of North America, 90(2), 291-304.

SUMMARY

The labyrinth in the inner ear is the peripheral receptor for the vestibular system. Signals from the labyrinth are essential for postural control and the coordination of movements, including eye movements. Vestibular signals contribute to awareness of head orientation and to actively orienting the head and body relative to gravity and to movement.

Visual information from a visual hemifield is processed in the contralateral visual cortex. From the primary visual cortex, the information flows dorsally in the action stream and ventrally in the perception stream. Gaze stabilization is achieved by the vestibulo-ocular and optokinetic reflexes. Direction of gaze is accomplished by saccades, smooth pursuits, and vergence eye movements.

Clinicians must distinguish between peripheral and central vestibular disorders, and recognize a variety of disorders affecting the visual system and eye movement system.

CLINICAL NOTES

Case 1

AJ is a 57-year-old construction worker. In a fall from a scaffolding 1 week ago, he fractured his right temporal bone. He complains of difficulty maintaining his balance, neck and shoulder stiffness, blurred vision, nausea, and a spinning sensation. Clinical observation reveals the following:

- Walking is slow and unsteady, requiring contact with walls or other objects to avoid falling.
- AJ avoids moving his head as much as possible, resulting in a rigid linkage between his trunk and head.
- Nystagmus is continuous, even when his head is stationary. Hearing is impaired on the right side.
- Muscle strength and somatosensation are normal. Vision and eye movements are intact.

Questions
1. Where is the lesion?
2. How can each of AJ's symptoms be explained?

Case 2

BF, a 37-year-old woman, presents with the following signs and symptoms on the right:

- Loss of sensation from the face
- Loss of voluntary movement of the face
- Ataxia of the limbs
- Inability to move the right eye toward the right
- Deafness

In addition, pain and temperature sensations are impaired from the left side of the body, and she has vertigo, nystagmus, and vomiting. The onset of symptoms has been gradual over the last 6 months, but unremitting.

Questions
1. Where is the lesion?
2. What is the most likely etiology?

Case 3

KW is a 27-year-old man who abruptly sustained the following losses 2 days ago:

- The ability to localize pain, temperature, touch, and proprioceptive information from the right side of his body

CLINICAL NOTES

- Voluntary motor control of the right side of his body
- The ability to see objects in his right visual field

Questions

1. What are possible locations of lesions that would explain the visual loss?
2. Given the combination of visual, motor, and somatosensory loss, where is the most likely location of the lesion?

REVIEW QUESTIONS

1. Describe how rotational acceleration of the head stimulates the endings of the vestibular nerve. Describe the mechanism for converting head position relative to gravity into neural signals.
2. What does "each pair of semicircular canals produces reciprocal signals" mean?
3. Name the tracts that use information from the vestibular nuclei to control posture.
4. What tract conveys signals that coordinate eye and head movements?
5. What is the difference between physiologic and pathologic nystagmus?
6. Explain how information from the left visual field reaches the right visual cortex.
7. If a person can see but cannot recognize an object in the left visual field, where is the lesion?
8. Name the sources of information used to direct eye movements.
9. What are the objectives of eye movements?
10. How is the visual world stabilized when the head moves during walking?
11. What is the optokinetic reflex?
12. Why is there a difference in visual clarity between looking at a stationary object while rapidly moving the head and looking at a rapidly moving object with the head stationary?
13. Normally, what happens to the perception of visual details when the head is quickly turned?
14. What symptom is most common in peripheral vestibular disorders?
15. If a person has hearing loss, tinnitus, vertigo, and nystagmus, where is the lesion?
16. What is BPPV?
17. The abrupt onset of dysequilibrium, spontaneous nystagmus, nausea, and severe vertigo, persisting up to 3 days, indicates what disorder?
18. What is oscillopsia?
19. How can peripheral vestibular disorders be distinguished from central vestibular disorders?
20. Describe the ocular tilt reaction.
21. What is the location of a lesion that produces a left homonymous hemianopsia?
22. What is the difference between a phoria and a tropia?
23. How are cerebellar, vestibular, and sensory ataxia differentiated?

References

Andersson AG, Kamwendo K, et al. (2006). How to identify potential fallers in a stroke unit: Validity indexes of 4 test methods. Journal of Rehabilitation Medicine, 38(3), 186-191.

Badke MB, Miedaner JA, et al. (2005). Effects of vestibular and balance rehabilitation on sensory organization and dizziness handicap. Annals of Otology, Rhinology, and Laryngology, 114(1 Pt 1), 48-54.

Bos JE, MacKinnon SN, et al. (2005). Motion sickness symptoms in a ship motion simulator: Effects of inside, outside, and no view. Aviation, Space, and Environmental Medicine, 76(12), 1111-1118.

Brandt T, Dieterich M (1999). The vestibular cortex: Its locations, functions, and disorders. Annals of the New York Academy of Sciences, 871, 293-312.

Brandt T, Strupp M (2005). General vestibular testing. Clinical Neurophysiology, 116(2), 406-426.

Cakir BO, Ercan I, et al. (2006). What is the true incidence of horizontal semicircular canal benign paroxysmal positional vertigo? Otolaryngology—Head and Neck Surgery, 134(3), 451-454.

Cass SP, Furman JM, et al. (1997). Migraine-related vestibulopathy. Annals of Otology, Rhinology, and Laryngology, 106(3), 182-189.

Chawla N, Olshaker JS (2006). Diagnosis and management of dizziness and vertigo. Medical Clinics of North America, 90(2), 291-304.

Cohen HS (2006). Disability and rehabilitation in the dizzy patient. Current Opinion in Neurology, 19(1), 49-54.

Delgado-Garcia, JM (2000). Why move the eyes if we can move the head? Brain Research Bulletin, 52(6), 475-482.

Dietrich M, Brandt T (2000). Brain activation studies on visual-vestibular and ocular motor interaction. Current Opinion in Neurology, 13(1), 13-18.

Downey DL, Leigh RJ (1998). Eye movements: Pathophysiology, examination and clinical importance. Journal of Neuroscience Nursing, 30(1), 15-22.

El-Kashlan HK, Telian SA (2000). Diagnosis and initiating treatment for peripheral system disorders: Imbalance and dizziness with normal hearing. Otolaryngologic Clinics of North America, 33(3), 563-578.

Goebel, JA (2000). Management options for acute versus chronic vertigo. Otolaryngologic Clinics of North America, 33(3), 483-493.

Halmagyi GM, Curthoys IS (2000). Otolith function tests. In SJ Herdman (Ed.), Vestibular Rehabilitation. (2nd ed.). Philadelphia: F.A. Davis.

Hanley K, O'Dowd T (2002). Symptoms of vertigo in general practice: A prospective study of diagnosis. British Journal of General Practice, 52(483), 809-812.

Herdman SJ, Tusa RJ (2000). Assessment and treatment of patients with benign paroxysmal positional vertigo. In SJ Herdman (Ed.), Vestibular Rehabilitation (2nd ed.). Philadelphia: F.A. Davis.

Horak FB, Shupert CL (1994). Role of the vestibular system in postural control. In GP Jacobson, and CW Newman (1990). The development of the Dizziness Handicap Inventory. Archives of Otolaryngology—Head & Neck Surgery, 116(4), 424-427.

Kentala E, Rauch SD (2003). A practical assessment algorithm for diagnosis of dizziness. Otolaryngology—Head and Neck Surgery, 128(1), 54-59.

Kotimaki J (2003). Meniere's disease in Finland. An epidemiological and clinical study on occurrence, clinical picture and policy. International Journal of Circumpolar Health, 62(4), 449-450.

Kroenke K, Hoffman RM, et al. (2000). How common are various causes of dizziness? A critical review. Southern Medical Journal, 93(2), 160-167 [quiz, 168].

Leigh RJ, Brandt T (1993). A reevaluation of the vestibulo-ocular reflex: New ideas of its purpose, properties, neural substrate, and disorders. Neurology, 43, 1288-1295.

Massoud EA, Ireland DJ (1996). Post-treatment instructions in the nonsurgical management of benign paroxysmal positional vertigo. Journal of Otolaryngology, 25(2), 121-125.

Nowak DA, Topka HR (2006). The clinical variability of Wallenberg's syndrome: The anatomical correlate of ipsilateral axial lateropulsion. Journal of Neurology, 253(4), 507-511.

Oghalai JS, Manolidis S, et al. (2000). Unrecognized benign paroxysmal positional vertigo in elderly patients. Otolaryngology—Head and Neck Surgery, 122(5), 630-634.

O'Neill DE, Gill-Body KM, et al. (1998). Posturography changes do not predict functional performance changes. American Journal of Otology, 19(6), 797-803.

Powell LE, Meyers AM (1995). The Activities-specific Balance Confidence (ABC) Scale. Journals of Gerontology. Series A, Biological Sciences and Medical Sciences 50A(1), M28-M34.

Prokopakis EP, Chimona T, et al. (2005). Benign paroxysmal positional vertigo: 10-year experience in treating 592 patients with canalith repositioning procedure. Laryngoscope, 115(9), 1667-71.

Schessel DA, Minor LB, et al. (1998). Meniere's disease and other peripheral vestibular disorders. In CW Cummings, JM Fredrickson, et al. (Eds.). Otolaryngology—Head and Neck surgery. Philadelphia: Mosby, pp. 2672-2705.

Shepard NT, Solomon D (2000). Functional operation of the balance system in daily activities. Otolaryngologic Clinics of North America, 33(3), 455-469.

Shumway-Cook A, Baldwin M, et al. (1997). Predicting the probability for falls in community-dwelling older adults. Physical Therapy, 77(8), 812-819.

Sloane PD, Coeytaux RR, et al. (2001). Dizziness: State of the science. Annals of Internal Medicine, 134(9 Pt 2), 823-832.

Slobounov S, Wu T, et al. (2006). Neural basis subserving the detection of postural instability: An fMRI study. Motor Control, 10(1), 69-89.

Solomon D (2000). Distinguishing and treating causes of central vertigo. Otolaryngologic Clinics of North America, 33(3), 579-601.

Walker MF, Zee DS (2000). Bedside vestibular examination. Otolaryngologic Clinics of North America, 33(3), 495-506.

Whitney SL, Wrisley DM, et al. (2000). Physical therapy for migraine-related vestibulopathy and vestibular dysfunction with history of migraine. Laryngoscope, 110(9), 1528-1534.

Zajonc TP, Roland PS (2005). Vertigo and motion sickness. Part I: Vestibular anatomy and physiology. Ear, Nose, & Throat Journal, 84(9), 581-584.

16 Cerebrum

Laurie Lundy-Ekman, PhD, PT

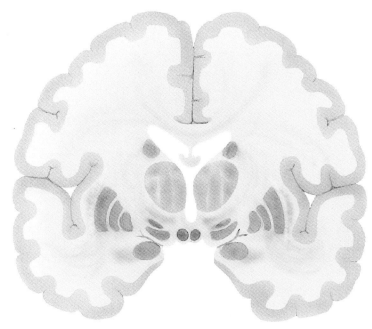

INTRODUCTION

Perception, moving voluntarily, using language and nonverbal communication, understanding spatial relationships, using visual information, making decisions, consciousness, emotions, mind-body interactions, and remembering all rely on systems in the cerebrum. These complex activities require extensive networks of neural connections, some involving brainstem circuits.

The cerebrum consists of the diencephalon and the cerebral hemispheres.* The diencephalon is in the center of the cerebrum, superior to the brainstem, and almost entirely enveloped by the cerebral hemispheres (Figure 16-1). In the intact adult brain, only a small part of the diencephalon is visible: the region between the optic chiasm and the cerebral peduncles, marked by the mamillary bodies. The cerebral hemispheres include both subcortical structures and the cerebral cortex. The subcortical structures include the subcortical white matter, basal ganglia, and amygdala. The cerebral cortex is the gray matter on the external surface of the

*Some authors consider the diencephalon to be part of the brainstem.

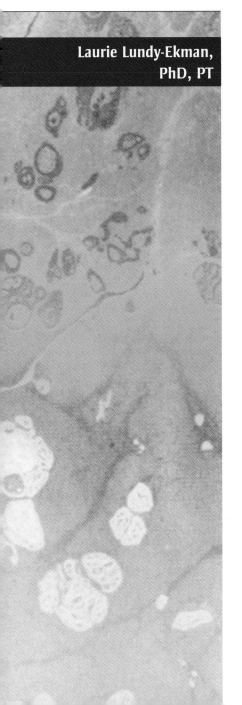

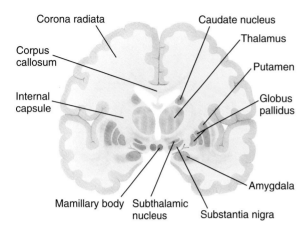

FIGURE 16-1
Cerebrum: diencephalon and cerebral hemispheres.

hemispheres. A collection of diencephalic, subcortical, and cortical structures involved with emotional and some memory functions is the limbic system.

DIENCEPHALON

The diencephalon includes all structures with the term *thalamus* in their names. The thalamus proper, the largest subdivision of the diencephalon, receives information from the basal ganglia, cerebellum, and all sensory systems except olfactory. The thalamus processes the information and then relays the information to specific areas of cerebral cortex. Other areas in the diencephalon are named for their locations relative to the thalamus, not similarities of function. Thus the hypothalamus is inferior and anterior to the thalamus, the epithalamus is superior and posterior to the thalamus, and the subthalamus is directly inferior to the thalamus.

Thalamus

The thalamus is a large, egg-shaped collection of nuclei located bilaterally above the brainstem. A *Y*-shaped sheet of white matter (intramedullary lamina) divides the nuclei of each thalamus into three groups: anterior, medial, and lateral. The lateral group is further subdivided into dorsal and ventral tiers. All nuclei in these groups are named for their location. For example, the ventral anterior nucleus is the most anterior nucleus of the ventral tier.

Additional thalamic nuclei—intralaminar, reticular, and midline—are not included in the three major groups. Intralaminar nuclei are found within the white matter

of the thalamus. The reticular and midline nuclei form thin layers of cells on the lateral and medial surfaces of the thalamus (Figure 16-2).

The thalamus acts as a selective filter for the cerebral cortex, directing attention to important information by regulating the flow of information to the cortex. Thus, overall, the thalamus regulates the activity level of cortical neurons. Individual thalamic nuclei can be classified into three main functional groups:

- Relay nuclei convey information from the sensory systems (except olfactory), the basal ganglia, or the cerebellum to the cerebral cortex.
- Association nuclei process emotional and some memory information or integrate different types of sensation.
- Nonspecific nuclei regulate consciousness, arousal, and attention.

Relay nuclei receive specific information and serve as relay stations by sending the information directly to localized areas of the cerebral cortex. For example, the ventral posteromedial nucleus receives somatosensory information from the face and relays the information to the somatosensory cortex. All relay nuclei are found in the ventral tier of the lateral nuclear group.

Association nuclei connect reciprocally to large areas of the cortex; that is, axons from association nuclei project to the cerebral cortex, and axons from the same cerebral cortical regions project to the association nuclei. Examples include the anterior nucleus, with reciprocal connections to areas of the cortex involved in emotions, and the pulvinar nucleus, reciprocally connecting with parietal, temporal, and occipital cortices. Association nuclei are found in the anterior thalamus, medial thalamus, and dorsal tier of the lateral thalamus.

Nonspecific nuclei receive multiple types of input and project to widespread areas of the cortex. This functional group includes the reticular, midline, and intralaminar nuclei, important in consciousness and arousal. Table 16-1 lists the functions and connections of the thalamic nuclei.

Hypothalamus

The hypothalamus is essential for individual and species survival because the hypothalamus integrates behaviors with visceral functions. For example, small areas in the hypothalamus coordinate eating behavior with digestive activity. Electrical stimulation of these hypothalamic areas causes an animal to search for and ingest food as long as the stimulation is applied. At the same time, peristalsis and blood flow increase throughout the intestine. Bilateral destruction of the areas associated with

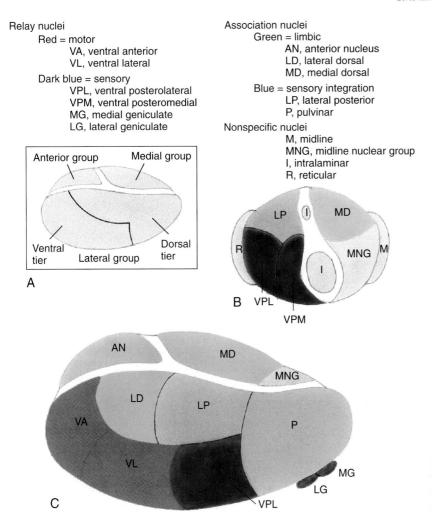

Relay nuclei
  Red = motor
    VA, ventral anterior
    VL, ventral lateral
  Dark blue = sensory
    VPL, ventral posterolateral
    VPM, ventral posteromedial
    MG, medial geniculate
    LG, lateral geniculate

Association nuclei
  Green = limbic
    AN, anterior nucleus
    LD, lateral dorsal
    MD, medial dorsal
  Blue = sensory integration
    LP, lateral posterior
    P, pulvinar
Nonspecific nuclei
    M, midline
    MNG, midline nuclear group
    I, intralaminar
    R, reticular

FIGURE 16-2
Thalamus. **A,** Three major groups of nuclei. **B,** Coronal section through thalamus. **C,** Nuclei of thalamus.

eating behaviors results in refusal of food, causing starvation even when food is readily available. The following functions are orchestrated by the hypothalamus:

- Maintaining homeostasis: adjustment of body temperature, metabolic rate, blood pressure, water intake and excretion, and digestion.
- Eating, reproductive, and defensive behaviors
- Emotional expression of pleasure, rage, fear, and aversion
- Regulation of circadian (daily) rhythms, such as sleep-wake cycles, in concert with other brain regions
- Endocrine regulation of growth, metabolism, and reproductive organs

These functions are carried out by hypothalamic regulation of pituitary gland secretions (hormones) and by efferent neural connections with the cortex (via the thalamus), limbic system, brainstem, and spinal cord (Figure 16-3).

Epithalamus

The major structure of the epithalamus is the pineal gland, an endocrine gland innervated by sympathetic fibers. The pineal gland is believed to help regulate circadian rhythms and influence the secretions of the pituitary gland, adrenals, parathyroids, and islets of Langerhans.

Table 16-1   THALAMIC NUCLEI

Functional Classification	Nuclei	Function	Afferents	Efferents
Relay nuclei	Ventral anterior	Motor	Globus pallidus	Motor planning areas
	Ventral lateral	Motor	Dentate	Motor cortex, motor planning areas
	Ventral posterolateral	Somatic sensation from body	Spinothalamic and medial lemniscus paths	Somatosensory cortex
	Ventral posteromedial	Somatic sensation from face	Sensory nucleus trigeminal nerve	Somatosensory cortex
	Medial geniculate	Hearing	Inferior colliculus	Auditory cortex
	Lateral geniculate	Vision	Optic tract	Visual cortex
Association nuclei	Anterior	Limbic	Reciprocal with limbic cortex	
	Medial dorsal	Limbic	Reciprocal with limbic cortex	
	Lateral dorsal	Limbic	Reciprocal with limbic cortex	
	Lateral posterior	Sensory integration	Reciprocal with parietal cortex	
	Pulvinar	Sensory integration	Reciprocal with parietal, occipital, and temporal cortex	
Nonspecific nuclei	Midline	Limbic	Viscera	Hypothalamus, amygdala, cerebral cortex
	Intralaminar	Limbic, arousal	Ascending reticular system	Widespread areas of cortex
	Reticular	Adjusts thalamic activity	Interconnections with other thalamic nuclei	

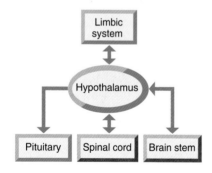

FIGURE 16-3
Interactions of the hypothalamus.

Subthalamus

The subthalamus is located superior to the substantia nigra of the midbrain. Functionally, the subthalamus is part of the basal ganglia circuit, involved in regulating movement. The subthalamus facilitates basal ganglia output nuclei.

SUBCORTICAL STRUCTURES

Subcortical White Matter

All white matter, whether located in the spinal cord or brain, consists of myelinated axons. In the cerebrum, the white matter is deep to the cortex and thus called *subcortical.* Subcortical white matter fibers are classified into three categories, depending on their connections:
- Projection
- Commissural
- Association

Projection Fibers

Projection fibers extend from subcortical structures to the cerebral cortex and from the cerebral cortex to the spinal cord, brainstem, basal ganglia, and thalamus. Almost all projection fibers travel through the internal capsule, a section of white matter bordered by the thalamus posteromedially, the caudate anteromedially, and the lentiform nucleus laterally (Figure 16-4). Like the stems of a bouquet of flowers, the axons of projection

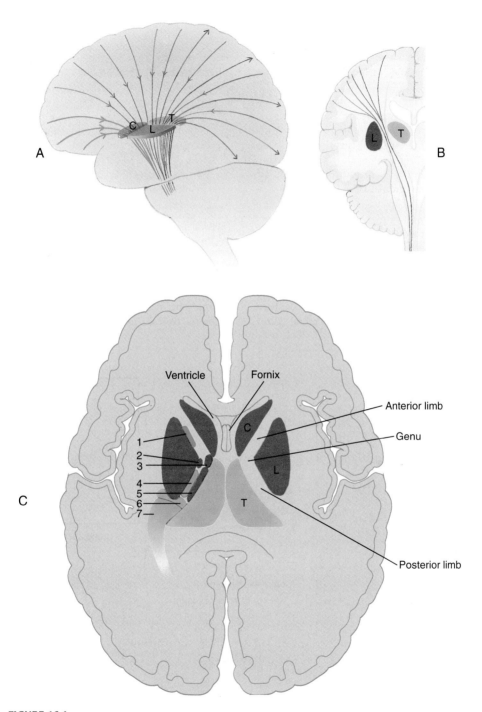

FIGURE 16-4

Internal capsule. Only the fibers projecting beyond the cerebrum are illustrated. Green, frontopontine fibers; red, motor fibers; blue, sensory fibers. **A,** Schematic view of the left internal capsule. The superior parts of the caudate (C) and lenticular (L) nuclei and the thalamus (T) have been removed. **B,** Coronal section showing internal capsule. **C,** Horizontal section. The limbs of the capsule are indicated on the right; the fiber tracts passing through are indicated on the left. The tan areas of the internal capsule on the left contain thalamocortical fibers. Fiber tracts: (1) frontopontine, (2) corticorubral, (3) corticobulbar, (4) ascending sensory, (5) corticospinal, (6) auditory radiation, and (7) optic radiation.

neurons are gathered into a small bundle, the internal capsule. Above the internal capsule, the axons spread apart to form the corona radiata, connecting with all areas of the cerebral cortex.

Regions of the internal capsule are the anterior limb, genu (from the Latin for "knee," indicating a bend), and posterior limb. The anterior limb, lateral to the head of the caudate, contains corticopontine fibers and fibers interconnecting thalamic and cortical limbic areas. The most medial part of the internal capsule, the genu, contains cortical fibers that project to cranial nerve motor nuclei and to the reticular formation. The posterior limb is located between the thalamus and lenticular nucleus, with additional fibers traveling posterior and inferior to the lenticular nucleus (retrolenticular and sublenticular fibers). Corticopontine, corticospinal, and thalamocortical projections comprise the posterior limb. The thalamocortical projections relay somatosensory, visual, auditory, and motor information to the cerebral cortex.

Because axons from so many areas are together in the internal capsule, small lesions in the internal capsule have consequences disproportionate to their size.

Commissural Fibers

Unlike projection fibers connecting cortical and subcortical structures, commissural fibers connect homologous areas of the cerebral hemispheres (Figure 16-5). The largest group of commissural fibers is the corpus callosum, linking many areas of the right and left hemispheres. Fibers of the other two commissures, anterior and posterior, link the right and left temporal lobes.

Association Fibers

Association fibers connect cortical regions within one hemisphere. The short association fibers connect adjacent gyri, while the long association fibers connect lobes within one hemisphere. For example, the cingulum connects frontal, parietal, and temporal lobe cortices.

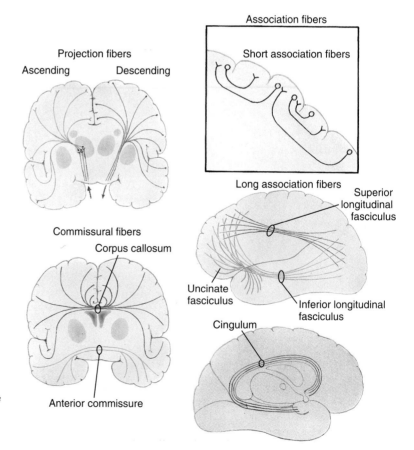

FIGURE 16-5
Types of white matter fibers. (*Modified from Moore JC (1983). Association fibers of cerebrum and commissural fibers. University of Puget Sound: A look at the nervous system from five perspectives. Handout.*)

Additional long association fiber bundles are listed in Table 16-2. Figure 16-5 illustrates the three types of white matter fibers.

Basal Ganglia

As noted in Chapter 10, the basal ganglia are vital for normal motor function. The basal ganglia sequence movements, regulate muscle tone and muscle force, and select and inhibit specific motor synergies. In addition to their motor functions, the basal ganglia are involved in cognitive functions (Cropley et al., 2006), participating in the following:

• Working memory (temporary storage of information while working with that information. For example, recalling the results of previous calculations while performing complex mental arithmetic).
• Sustained attention
• Ability to change behavior as task requirements change
• Motivation

Motivation is centered in the nucleus accumbens, located in the ventral striatum. The ventral striatum is the inferior part of the junction between the caudate and putamen (see Figure 10-1). The nucleus accumbens serves to link motivation and behavior. Specifically, nucleus accumbens activity is essential for the generation of locomotion, and for increasing the frequency of rewarded behaviors (Parkinson et al., 2000).

Table 16-2   SUBCORTICAL WHITE MATTER

Type of Fibers	Examples
Projection	Thalamocortical Corticospinal Corticobulbar
Commissural	Corpus callosum Anterior commissure Posterior commissure
Association	Short association fibers (connect adjacent gyri) Cingulum (connects frontal, parietal, and temporal lobe cortices) Uncinate fasciculus (connects frontal and temporal lobe cortices) Superior longitudinal fasciculus (connects cortex of all lobes) Inferior longitudinal fasciculus (connects temporal and occipital lobes)

CEREBRAL CORTEX

The cerebral cortex is a vast collection of cell bodies, axons, and dendrites covering the surface of the cerebral hemispheres. The most common types of cortical neurons are pyramidal, fusiform, and stellate cells. Pyramidal cells have an apical dendrite that extends toward the surface of the cortex, several basal dendrites extending laterally from the base of the soma, and one axon (Figure 16-6). Although some pyramidal cells have short axons that synapse without leaving the cortex, almost all pyramidal cell axons travel through white matter as projection, commissural, or association fibers. Thus most pyramidal cells are output cells for the cerebral cortex. Fusiform cells are spindle-shaped and are also output cells, projecting mainly to the thalamus. Stellate

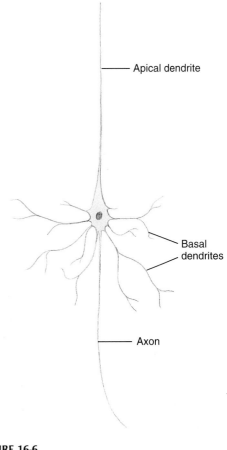

Apical dendrite

Basal dendrites

Axon

FIGURE 16-6
Pyramidal cell.

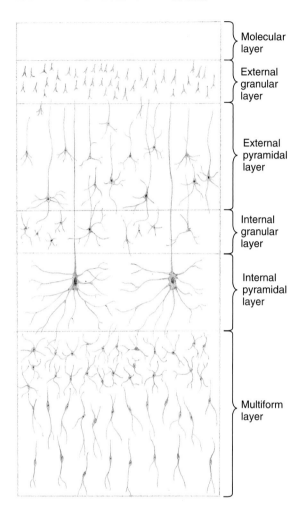

FIGURE 16-7
Layers of the cerebral cortex.

Table 16-3 LAYERS OF THE CEREBRAL CORTEX

Name	Description
I	Molecular layer; mainly axons and dendrites; contains few cells
II	External granular layer; many small pyramidal and stellate cells
III	External pyramidal layer; pyramidal cells
IV	Internal granular layer; mainly stellate cells
V	Internal pyramidal layer; predominantly pyramidal cells, with stellate and other interneurons
VI	Multiform layer; primarily fusiform cells

in these four layers. In 1909, Brodmann published a map of the cortex that distinguished 52 histologic areas (Figure 16-8). Brodmann's areas are commonly used to designate cortical locations.

Mapping of the Cerebral Cortex

People undergoing brain surgery have allowed neurosurgeons to stimulate and record from various areas of the cerebral cortex. During these surgeries, the patients were fully conscious. Some experiments consist of placing recording electrodes on the surface of the brain and then stimulating various parts of the body to determine if the cortical area being recorded responds to the stimulus. For example, when the surgeon touches the patient's fingertip, only a small, specific area of the cortex, located in a consistent position of the cortex among various people, responds.

Other experiments involve mild electrical stimulation of the cortex. In these experiments, the stimulation may elicit movements of a part of the body or cause the patient to recall a particular situation. Imaging techniques can also be used to investigate brain function without invasive procedures. For example, the brain activity when a person is having a conversation can be recorded and analyzed.

Localized Functions of the Cerebral Cortex*

Different areas of the cerebral cortex are specialized to perform a variety of functions. Based on their functions, five categories of cortex have been identified:

*In neuroscience, the term *localization of function* is used to connote that an area contributes to the performance of a specific neural activity. Neural functions are achieved by networks of neurons, not by isolated centers.

(granule) cells are smaller than pyramidal cells, remain within the cortex, and serve as interneurons.

The cerebral cortex contains layers, differentiated by the size and connectivity of the constituent cells. In the olfactory and medial temporal cortex, there are only three layers of cells. In the remainder of the cerebral cortex, six layers of cells are found (Figure 16-7). The six layers, numbered from superficial to deep, are listed in Table 16-3.

This list of cortical layers is a generalization; different areas of the cerebral cortex have distinctive arrangements of cells. For example, although layers II-V can be distinguished in the visual cortex, stellate cells predominate

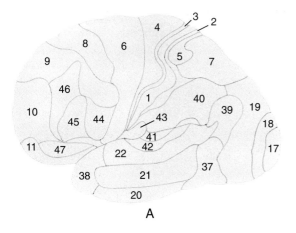

A

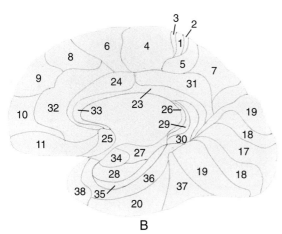

B

- The primary sensory cortex discriminates among different intensities and qualities of sensory information.
- The sensory association cortex performs more complex analysis of sensation.
- The motor planning areas organize movements.
- The primary motor cortex provides descending control of motor output.
- The association cortex controls behavior, interprets sensation, and processes emotions and memories.

Each type of cortex may play a role in response to a stimulus. For example, when one sees a bell, the primary visual cortex discriminates its shape and its brightness from the background. The visual association cortex analyzes the bell's color. The association cortex may recall the name of the object, what sound the bell makes, and specific memories associated with bells. The association cortex also participates in the decision of what to do with the bell. If the decision is to lift the bell, premotor areas plan the movement, and then the primary motor cortex sends commands to neurons in the spinal cord. The flow of cortical activity from the primary sensory cortex to cortical motor output is illustrated in Figure 16-9. Figure 16-9 is a simplified schematic that only applies to movement generated in response to an external stimulus. An equally plausible alternative would begin

←───────────────────────

FIGURE 16-8
Brodmann's areas.

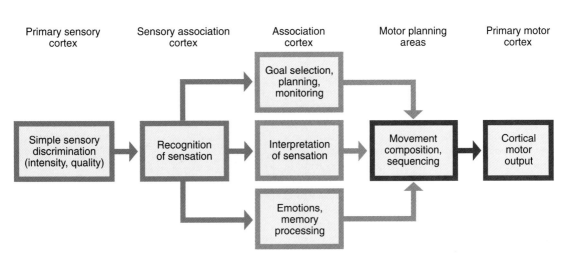

FIGURE 16-9
Flow of cortical information from the primary sensory cortex to motor output.

with a decision in the association cortex leading to movement.

Primary Sensory Areas of the Cerebral Cortex

Primary sensory areas receive sensory information directly from the ventral tier of thalamic nuclei. Each primary sensory area discriminates among different intensities and qualities of one type of input. Thus there are separate primary sensory areas for somatosensory, auditory, visual, and vestibular information. Most primary sensory areas are located within and adjacent to landmark cortical fissures (Figure 16-10). The primary somatosensory cortex is located within the central sulcus and on the adjacent postcentral gyrus. The primary auditory cortex is located in the lateral fissure and on the adjacent superior temporal gyrus. The primary visual cortex is within the calcarine sulcus and on the adjacent gyri. Only the primary vestibular cortex is not close to a landmark fissure; instead, the primary vestibular cortex is posterior to the primary somatosensory cortex.

Primary Somatosensory Cortex. The primary somatosensory cortex receives information from tactile and proprioceptive receptors via a three-neuron pathway: peripheral afferent/dorsal column neuron, medial lemniscus neuron, and thalamocortical neuron. Although crude awareness of somatosensation occurs in the ventral posterolateral and the ventral posteromedial nuclei of the thalamus, neurons in the primary somatosensory cortex identify the location of stimuli and discriminate among various shapes, sizes, and textures of objects. The cortical termination of nociceptive and temperature pathways is more widespread than the discriminative tactile and proprioceptive information and thus is not limited to the primary somatosensory cortex.

Primary Auditory and Primary Vestibular Cortices. The primary auditory cortex receives information from the cochlea of both ears via a pathway that synapses in the inferior colliculus and medial geniculate body before reaching the cortex (see Chapter 13). The primary auditory cortex provides conscious awareness of the intensity of sounds. The primary vestibular cortex receives information regarding head movement and head position relative to gravity by a vestibulothalamocortical pathway (see Chapter 15).

Primary Visual Cortex. Visual information travels to the cortex via a pathway from the retina to the lateral geniculate body of the thalamus, then to the primary visual cortex. Individual neurons in the primary visual cortex are specialized to distinguish between light and dark, various shapes, location of objects, and movement of objects.

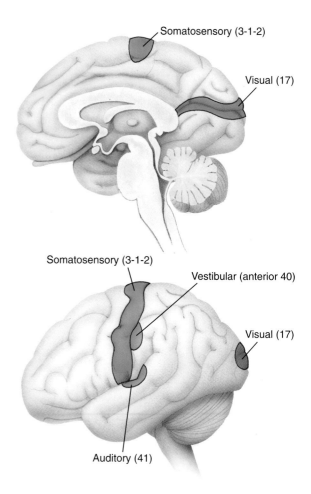

Cortical Area	Function
Primary somatosensory	Discriminates shape, texture, or size of objects
Primary auditory	Conscious discrimination of loudness and pitch of sounds
Primary visual	Distinguishes intensity of light, shape, size, and location of objects
Primary vestibular	Discriminates among head positions and head movements

FIGURE 16-10

Primary sensory areas of the cerebral cortex. Corresponding Brodmann's areas are indicated in parentheses.

Sensory Association Areas

Sensory association areas analyze sensory input from both the thalamus and the primary sensory cortex. Sensory association areas contribute to the analysis of one type of sensory information. For example, if one picks up a pen, the primary somatosensory cortex registers that the object is small, smooth, and cylindrical. The somatosensory association area recognizes the object as a pen, although a different area of the cortex is required to name the object. Somatosensory association areas integrate tactile and proprioceptive information from manipulating an object. Neurons in the somatosensory association area provide stereognosis by somehow comparing somatosensation from the current object with memories of other objects.

The visual association cortex analyzes colors and motion, and its output to the tectum directs visual fixation, the maintenance of an object in central vision. The auditory association cortex compares sounds with memories of other sounds and then categorizes the sounds as language, music, or noise. Sensory association areas are illustrated in Figure 16-11.

Primary Motor Cortex and Motor Planning Areas of the Cerebral Cortex

The primary motor cortex is located in the precentral gyrus, anterior to the central sulcus. The primary motor cortex is the source of most neurons in the corticospinal tract and controls contralateral voluntary movements, particularly the fine movements of the hand and face. Because the primary motor cortex is unique in providing precise control of hand and lower face movements, a much greater proportion of the total area of primary motor cortex is devoted to neurons that control these parts of the body than is devoted to the trunk and proximal limbs, where more gross motor activity is required. The hand, foot, and lower face representations in the motor cortex are entirely contralateral. In contrast, many muscles that tend to be active bilaterally simultaneously—muscles of the back, for example—are controlled by the primary motor cortex on both sides.

The cortical motor planning areas include the following:

- Supplementary motor area
- Premotor area
- Broca's area
- Area corresponding to Broca's area in the opposite hemisphere

Motor Planning Areas. The cortex anterior to the primary motor cortex consists of three areas: supplementary motor area, premotor area, and Broca's area (or, on

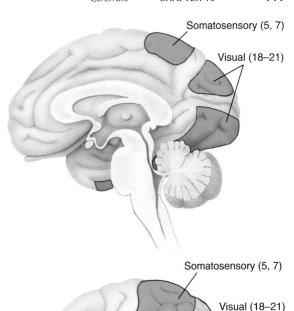

Cortical Area	Function
Somatosensory association	Stereognosis and memory of the tactile and spatial environment
Visual association	Analysis of motion, color; control of visual fixation
Auditory association	Classification of sounds

FIGURE 16-11

Sensory association areas of the cerebral cortex. Corresponding Brodmann's areas are indicated in parentheses.

the contralateral side, the area corresponding to Broca's area). The **supplementary motor cortex,** located anterior to the lower body region of the primary motor cortex, is important for initiation of movement, orientation of the eyes and head, and planning bimanual and sequential movements. The **premotor area,** located anterior to the upper body region of the primary motor cortex, controls trunk and girdle muscles via the medial upper motor neurons. Thus the premotor area stabilizes the shoulders during upper limb tasks and the hips during walking.

Broca's area, inferior to the premotor area and anterior to the face and throat region of the primary motor cortex, is usually in the left hemisphere. Broca's area is responsible for planning movements of the mouth during speech and the grammatical aspects of language. An **area analogous to Broca's area,** in the opposite hemisphere, plans nonverbal communication, including emotional gestures and adjusting the tone of voice. These areas will be considered further in a later section on communication.

Connections of the Motor Areas. Premotor, supplementary motor, and Broca's areas receive information from sensory association areas. Both the primary motor cortex and motor planning areas receive information from the basal ganglia and cerebellum, relayed by the thalamus. The primary motor cortex receives somatosensory information relayed by the thalamus and from the primary somatosensory cortex and motor instructions from the motor planning areas. Cortical motor output, including the corticospinal tracts, corticobulbar tracts, corticopontine tracts, and cortical projections to the putamen, originates in the primary motor and primary somatosensory cortex and motor planning areas (Figure 16-12).

Association Areas of the Cerebral Cortex

Areas of cortex not directly involved with sensation or movement are called the *association cortex.* Three areas of cortex are designated as association cortex (Figure 16-13):

- Dorsolateral prefrontal, the anterior part of the frontal lobe
- Parietotemporal association, at the junction of the parietal, occipital, and temporal lobes
- Limbic, in the anterior temporal lobe and ventromedial prefrontal cortex (including the orbitotemporal cortex; Bechara, 2004).

Enormously complex abilities are localized in the association areas: personality, integration and interpretation of sensations, processing of memory, and generation of emotions. For example, damage to the orbitofrontal cortex can alter personality characteristics, while damage to other cortical areas has little effect on personality. Thus, although the neurophysiology of personality is not understood, personality is said to be local-

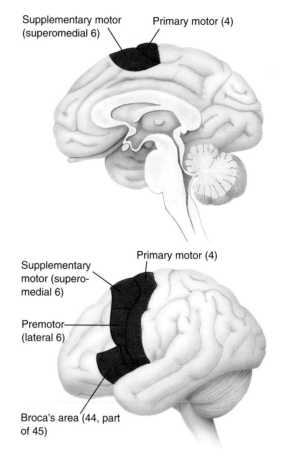

Motor Areas	Function
Primary motor cortex	Voluntarily controlled movements
Premotor area	Control of trunk and girdle muscles, anticipatory postural adjustments
Supplementary motor area	Initiation of movement, orientation planning, bimanual and sequential movements
Broca's area	Motor programming of speech (usually in the left hemisphere only)
Area analogous to Broca's in opposite hemisphere	Planning nonverbal communication (emotional gestures, tone of voice; usually in the right hemisphere)

FIGURE 16-12

Motor areas of the cerebral cortex. Corresponding Brodmann's areas are indicated in parentheses.

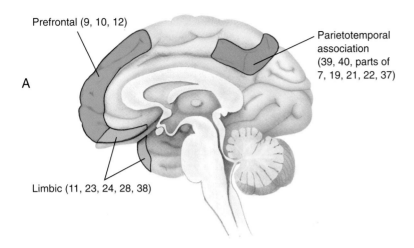

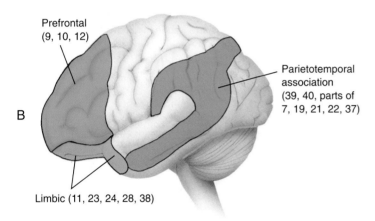

Association Cortex	Function
Prefrontal association	Goal-oriented behavior, self-awareness
Parietotemporal association	Sensory integration, problem solving, understanding language and spacial relationships
Limbic association	Emotion, motivation, personality, processing of memory

FIGURE 16-13
Association areas of the cerebral cortex. **A,** Midsagittal section. **B,** Lateral view.

ized to the orbitofrontal cortex. Similarly, cognitive intelligence, as measured by intelligence tests, and integration and interpretation of sensations are localized in the parietotemporal association areas. Conscious emotions are localized in the limbic association areas.

Dorsolateral Prefrontal Cortex. The dorsolateral prefrontal cortex connects extensively with the sensory association areas in the parietal, occipital, and temporal lobes and with limbic areas. Dorsolateral prefrontal cortex functions include self-awareness and **executive functions** (also called *goal-oriented behavior;* (Salmon

and Collette, 2005). Executive functions include the following:
• Deciding on a goal
• Planning how to accomplish the goal
• Executing a plan
• Monitoring the execution of the plan

Decisions ranging from the trivial to the momentous are made in the prefrontal area; what to wear, whether to buy a new house, and whether to have children are decided in and carried out by instructions from the prefrontal cortex.

Parietotemporal Association Areas. Cognitive intelligence is primarily a function of the parietotemporal association areas, in the posterior parietal and temporal cortices. Here, problem solving and comprehension of communication and of spatial relationships occur. The spatial coordinate system of this area is essential for constructing an image of one's own body and for planning movements.

Limbic Association Area. The third, and final, cortical association area is the limbic association area, located in the anterior temporal lobe and in the ventromedial prefrontal cortex. The ventromedial prefrontal cortex includes the orbitofrontal cortex located above the eyes. The limbic association area connects with areas regulating mood (subjective feelings), affect (observable demeanor), and processing of some types of memory.

LIMBIC SYSTEM

The term *limbic* means "border" and refers to the border between the diencephalon and telencephalon. The term *border* could also be applied to the limbic system's activity as a border region between conscious and nonconscious areas of the brain.

Limbic structures form a ring around the thalamus (Figure 16-14). Although a full consensus on which structures compose the limbic system has not been reached, most authorities include the following areas (Heimer and Van Hoesen, 2006; Herman et al., 2005):

- Hypothalamus
- Anterior and medial nuclei of the thalamus
- Limbic cortex (cingulate gyrus, parahippocampal gyrus, uncus)
- Hippocampus
- Amygdala
- Insula
- Basal forebrain: septal area, preoptic area, nucleus accumbens, and the basal nucleus of Meynert

The hypothalamus and thalamus were described earlier in this chapter. The limbic cortex is a *C*-shaped region of cortex located on the medial hemisphere, consisting of the cingulate gyrus, parahippocampal gyrus, and uncus (a medial protrusion of the parahippocampal gyrus). The hippocampus is named for its fancied resemblance, in coronal section, to the shape of a seahorse. The hippocampus is formed by the gray and white matter of two gyri rolled together in the medial temporal lobe. The amygdala is an almond-shaped collection of nuclei deep to the uncus in the temporal lobe, at the end of the caudate tail. The insula processes information perceived as pain and contributes to the emotional response to pain (Salomons et al., 2004).

In the basal forebrain, the septal area is a region of cortex and nuclei anterior to the anterior commissure, and the preoptic area is anterior to the septal area. The nucleus accumbens (also called *ventral striatum*) is the region where the caudate and putamen blend, and the basal nucleus of Meynert is inferior to the preoptic area.

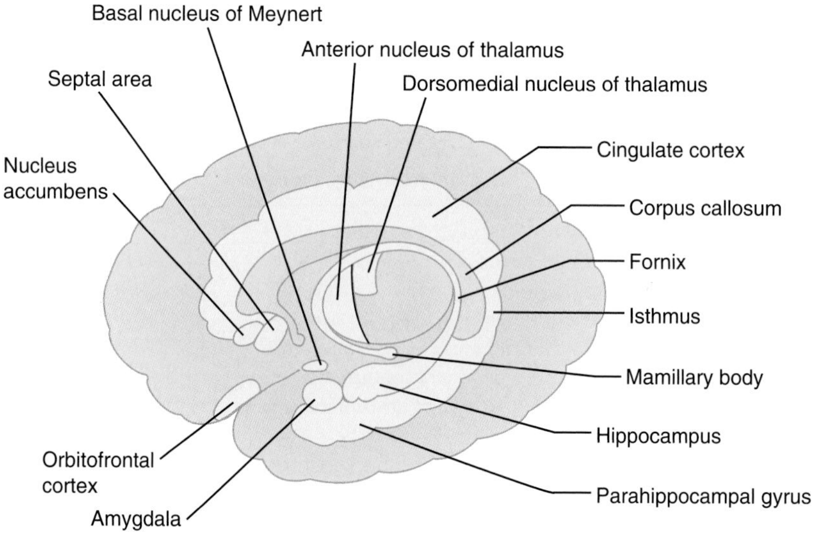

FIGURE 16-14
Limbic areas. Although the insula is part of the limbic system, it is lateral to the section and therefore not shown. The corpus callosum, not part of the limbic system, is labeled for reference.

Basal nucleus of Meynert
Septal area
Nucleus accumbens
Anterior nucleus of thalamus
Dorsomedial nucleus of thalamus
Cingulate cortex
Corpus callosum
Fornix
Isthmus
Mamillary body
Hippocampus
Parahippocampal gyrus
Orbitofrontal cortex
Amygdala

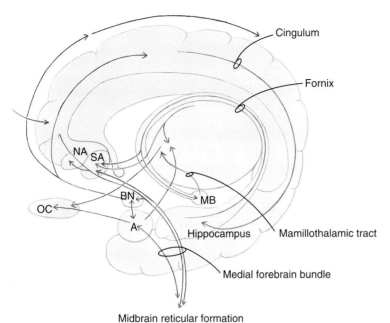

FIGURE 16-15
Connections of the limbic system.
A, Amygdala; OC, orbitofrontal cortex; MB,
mamillary body of the thalamus. All other
areas labeled with initials are parts of the
basal forebrain: NA, nucleus accumbens; SA,
septal area; BN, basal nucleus of Meynert.

Connections of the Limbic System

Connections within the limbic system are extensive. Two major fiber bundles are the fornix and medial forebrain bundle (Figure 16-15). The fornix is an arch-shaped fiber bundle connecting the hippocampus with the mamillary body and anterior nucleus of the thalamus. The medial forebrain bundle connects anterior structures (septal area, nucleus accumbens, amygdala, anterior cingulate gyrus), the hypothalamus, and the midbrain reticular formation. Because the connection between limbic areas and reticular areas of the midbrain are so important in behavior, combining the systems into a reticulolimbic system has been proposed. Additional connections of the limbic system are shown in Figure 16-15. Output from the limbic system travels via autonomic, somatic, reticular, and hormonal pathways. Although the limbic system regulates feeding, drinking, defensive, and reproductive behaviors, in addition to visceral and hormonal functions, only two aspects of limbic function are considered in this text: emotional and memory functions.

Emotional and Memory Functions

These functions use two fairly distinct subsets of limbic structures (Figure 16-16). For emotions, the amygdala, areas in the hypothalamus, septal area, anterior nuclei of the thalamus, anterior limbic cortex, and limbic associa-

tion area are required.* Unlike emotions, which are mediated within the limbic system, memory functions are widely distributed among limbic and nonlimbic areas of the brain. For processing some types of memory, the hippocampus, medial thalamic nuclei, posterior limbic cortex, and basal forebrain are essential.

EMOTIONS AND BEHAVIOR

An emotion is a short-term subjective experience. A mood is a sustained, subjective, ongoing emotional experience. Emotions are mediated within the limbic system, by the amygdala, areas in the hypothalamus, septal area, anterior nuclei of the thalamus, anterior cingulate cortex, and limbic association cortex. The amygdala interprets facial expressions, body language, and social signals, and thus is essential for social behavior (de Gelder, 2006) and is also important for emotional learning (LaBar and Cabeza, 2006). The amygdala receives information from all sensory systems and connects with the orbitofrontal

---

*A highly influential hypothesis of the neural structures involved in emotions was proposed by Papez and became known as the circuit of Papez. Although the hypothesized connections have been confirmed, the circuit is not a major contributor to emotions. Instead, the circuit of Papez contributes to processing some types of memory.

cortex and anterior cingulate gyrus. The anterior cingulate gyrus acts as a conduit between the frontal lobe and other limbic structures. Together the amygdala, orbitofrontal cortex, and anterior cingulate gyrus regulate emotional behaviors and motivation. Figure 16-17 illustrates the areas involved in the production of social behavior.

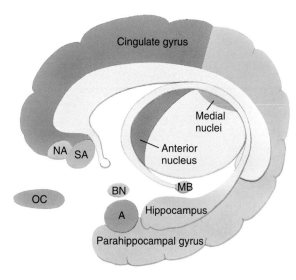

FIGURE 16-16

Sets of limbic structures: emotional and memory. Limbic structures involved in emotions are shown in blue: amygdala, parts of hypothalamus, septal area, anterior nucleus of the thalamus, and anterior limbic cortex. Limbic structures involved in processing memory are shown in green: hippocampus, parahippocampal gyrus, medial thalamic nuclei, posterior limbic cortex, and basal nucleus. Septal area is involved in both emotional and memory functions. Abbreviations are the same as in Figure 16-15.

Emotions color our perceptions and influence our actions. For example, a person vexed by a difficult problem may misinterpret a question about progress in solving the problem as a threat and become angry. The person's facial expressions and abrupt, choppy movements indicating anger are easy to recognize. Immediate responses to a threat include somatic, autonomic, and hormonal changes, including increased muscle tension and heart rate, dilation of the pupils, and cessation of digestion. However, emotions also shape our lives in more subtle ways because emotions signal the nonconscious evaluation of a situation.

Conscious awareness of emotion occurs when information from the amygdala and from the autonomic system reaches the cortex. Emotion is intimately tied to decision making (Bechara et al., 2002). Bechara et al. speculate that part of our decision-making process is imagining consequences and then attending to the resultant emotional signals from the visceral, muscular, and hormonal systems and neurotransmitters. These emotional signals are based on prior experience and provide "gut feelings" about the actions being contemplated. The theory that emotions are crucial for sound judgment is called the **somatic marker hypothesis.** The emotional signals do not make decisions but are considered in the decision process. Emotional and social intelligence, the ability to manage personal and social life, requires the ventromedial prefrontal cortex, amygdala, and insula (Bar-On et al., 2003).

PSYCHOLOGICAL AND SOMATIC INTERACTIONS

Clearly, the conceptual division between the sciences of immunology, endocrinology, and psychology/

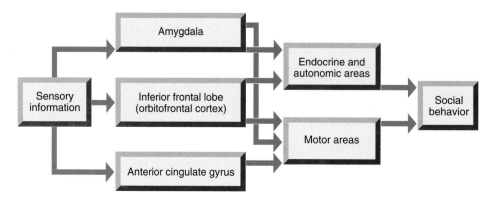

FIGURE 16-17

Social behavior: flow of information from sensory input to motor output.

neuroscience is a historical artifact; the existence of a communicating network of neuropeptides and their receptors provides a link among the body's cellular defense and repair mechanisms, glands, and brain.
—*Candace Pert, (Pert et al., 1985) p. 824s*

Thoughts and emotions influence the functions of all organs. This occurs because of the bidirectional communication between the nervous system and the immune system (Figure 16-18). Neurotransmitters and hormones regulated by the brain modulate immune system cells, and cytokines (chemicals secreted by white blood cells, including tumor necrosis factor and interleukins) regulate the neuroendocrine system. An individual's reaction to experiences can disrupt homeostasis; this is called a *stress response.* When an individual feels threatened, the stress response increases strength and energy to deal with the situation. Three systems create the stress response:

- Somatic nervous system: Motor neuron activity increases muscle tension.
- Autonomic nervous system: Sympathetic activity increases blood flow to muscles and decreases blood flow to the skin, kidneys, and digestive tract.

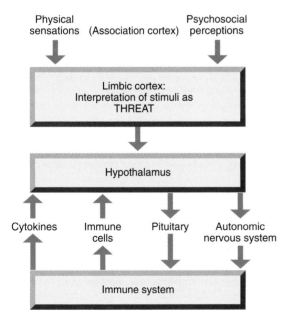

FIGURE 16-18
Chemical signaling between the nervous system and immune system in response to stress. Cytokines are nonantibody proteins that participate in the immune response (e.g., interferons and interleukins).

- Neuroendocrine system: Sympathetic nerve stimulation of the adrenal medulla causes the release of epinephrine into the bloodstream. Epinephrine increases cardiac rate and the strength of cardiac contraction, relaxes intestinal smooth muscle, and increases metabolic rate.

About 5 minutes after the initial response to stress, the hypothalamus stimulates the pituitary to secrete adrenocorticotropic hormone, causing the release of cortisol from adrenal glands. Cortisol mobilizes energy (glucose), suppresses immune responses, and serves as an antiinflammatory agent. As the stress response ends, homeostasis gradually returns. Unfortunately, often the stress response does not terminate because the stress is maintained by circumstances or by the individual's thinking patterns. For example, a social slight that would go unnoticed by one person may cause another person to extensively contemplate why they were snubbed and how they should respond.

Excessive amounts of cortisol are associated with stress-related diseases, including colitis, cardiovascular disorders, and adult-onset diabetes. Excessive cortisol also causes emotional instability and cognitive deficits (Young, 2004).

In healthy married couples, hostile behaviors provoke more severe adverse immunologic changes and slow the rate of healing compared to supportive behaviors. Hostile couples used contempt, criticism, and other negative behaviors during a discussion of conflict-producing marital issues. The healing rate of hostile couples was only 60% of the rate of couples who were mutually supportive during the discussion of marital conflicts (Kiecolt-Glaser et al., 2005).

When the stress response is prolonged, persistent high levels of cortisol continue to suppress immune function. Immune suppression is advantageous for decreasing inflammation and regulating allergic reactions and autoimmune responses. However, chronic stress-induced immune suppression reduces skin resistance to viruses, bacteria and fungi (Dhabhar, 2000). Thus, the effects of the stress response can be beneficial or damaging, depending on the situation and whether the response is prolonged. Figure 16-19 illustrates the consequences of prolonged psychological stress. As noted in the figure, immune cells respond to neurotransmitters, neurohormones, and neuropeptides.

Researchers are also beginning to analyze ways that immune function can be improved. Short-term benefits of hypnotic relaxation have been demonstrated in medical and dental students 3 days prior to an examination. Students who practiced more frequently were more protected from the immune decrement that often

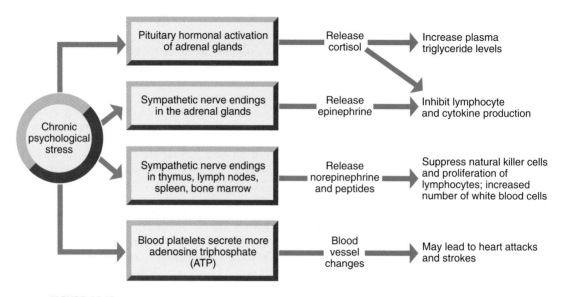

FIGURE 16-19
Effects of prolonged psychological stress on immune and blood-vascular system function.

accompanies acute stress (Kiecolt-Glaser et al., 2001). Thus, cognition, emotions, and immune activity are intertwined. Another component in this complex is how records of new experiences are formed and used to guide subsequent activities. Memory functions involve many more areas of the brain than just limbic structures, as the following section illustrates.

MEMORY

Three memory systems serve distinct types of information. For example, each of the following types of memory is different:

- Remembering feeling elated
- Recalling what happened yesterday
- Knowing how to ride a bicycle

Each type of memory is dependent on different brain regions. Types of memory include emotional (feelings), declarative (facts, events, concepts, locations), and procedural (how-to) (Figure 16-20).

Emotional Memory

Very little is known about the emotional memory system other than that memory for fear involves the amygdala and that damage to either of the other two memory systems does not affect the emotional memory system.

Therefore the emotional memory system will not be considered further.

Declarative Memory

Declarative memory refers to recollections that can be easily verbalized. Declarative memory is also called conscious, explicit, or cognitive memory. Unlike emotional and procedural memory, declarative memory requires attention during recall. Declarative memory has three stages:

- Immediate memory (also called sensory register) lasts only 1 to 2 seconds. Information is processed through primary sensory and sensory association areas of the cortex, but not by the limbic system.
- Short-term memory is brief storage of stimuli that have been recognized. Loss of information occurs within 1 minute unless the material is continually rehearsed.
- Long-term memory is relatively permanent storage of information that has been processed in short-term memory. The conversion of short-term to long-term storage is called *consolidation.*

A probable circuit of neural activity leading to the development of declarative memory is shown in Figure 16-21. In the frontal lobes, voluntary control is exerted over the processing of declarative memory, both in selecting information for storage and accessing stored

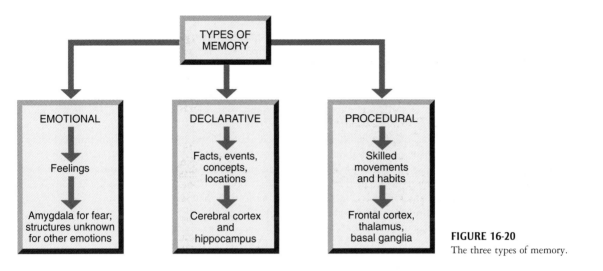

FIGURE 16-20
The three types of memory.

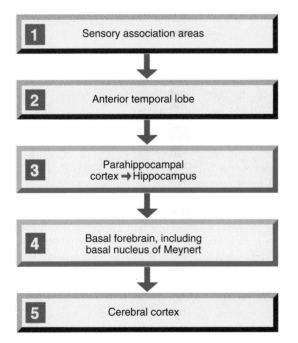

FIGURE 16-21
Formation of declarative memories. Green boxes indicate the contents that are part of the limbic system. Although parts of the limbic system are essential for converting short-term memory into long-term memory, memories are not stored in limbic structures.

information (Blum et al., 2006). Electrical stimulation of the anterior temporal lobe cortex causes people to report that it seems as if a past event or experience was occurring during the stimulation, despite their awareness of actually being in surgery (Penfield, 1958).

A famous case of unintended consequences of a surgery to relieve severe epilepsy contributed significantly to the understanding of memory. The patient, HM, suffered severe, frequent seizures. Because his seizures originated in the medial temporal lobes, which contain the hippocampus, this area of his brain was removed bilaterally. The epilepsy improved, but his memory was permanently damaged. In the 50 years subsequent to the surgery, HM has been unable to remember any new information from 1 year prior to the surgery to the present. He cannot recall text he read minutes ago, nor can he remember people he has met repeatedly subsequent to the operation. Earlier memories are intact, and he is able to learn new skills (Corkin, 2002). These outcomes indicate that the role of the hippocampus is processing memory from short term to long term but that declarative memories are not stored in the hippocampus. Long-term storage is distributed among various cortical areas by the basal nucleus of Meynert.

The mechanism for converting short-term memories to long-term memories is not understood. Short-term memory is assumed to reflect temporary changes in cell membrane excitability. Long-term memory is believed to involve structural changes in neurons. Long-term potentiation (see Chapter 4) is a current proposal for explaining the cellular basis for memory, but more evidence is required to substantiate the hypothesis.

Long-term potentiation consists of persistent enhancement of synaptic transmission following activation of specific receptors by high-frequency stimulation of presynaptic axons (Pfeiffer and Huber, 2006).

Procedural Memory

Procedural memory refers to recall of skills and habits. This type of memory is also called *skill, habit, nonconscious memory,* or *implicit memory.* Implicit memory produces changes in performance without conscious awareness. The distinction between declarative memories and procedural memories can be clarified by recalling memories of riding a bicycle. Declarative memories describe the location, terrain, companions on the ride, the weather, and other features of the ride. Procedural memories are not conscious. Thus if you ask a bicycle rider how they restore the bicycle to upright when the bicycle begins to fall to the left, most will say by leaning right. However, this would make the bicycle tilt further to the left. What the rider actually does is turn the handlebars to the left, restoring the center of gravity between the two wheels. Thus the typical rider accurately performs the effective movement to prevent falling without being conscious of how the fall is prevented.

Practice is required to store procedural memories. Once the skill or habit is learned, less attention is required while performing the task. For example, the initially difficult skill of driving a car in traffic becomes automatic with practice.

For learning motor skills, three learning stages have been identified:
• Cognitive
• Associative
• Autonomous

During the cognitive stage, the beginner is trying to understand the task and find out what works. Often beginners verbally guide their own movements, as seen in people who talk their way through descending stairs with crutches: "First the crutches, then the cast, then the right leg…" During the associative stage, the person refines the movements selected as most effective. Movements are less variable and less dependent on cognition. During the autonomous stage, the movements are automatic, requiring less attention. When movements are automatic, attention can be devoted to having a conversation or other activities while the movements are being executed.

Learning a motor sequence involves the motor and parietal cortex and the striatum (Doyon et al., 2003). The representation of the learned movement sequences appears to be located in supplementary motor area and the putamen/globus pallidus (Poldrack et al., 2005). Motor adaptation, the ability to adjust movements to environmental changes, involves the cerebellum and the parietal and motor cortices (Doyon et al., 2003).

The abilities of HM, the man with both hippocampi removed, illustrate the dissociation of declarative and procedural memories. He is able to learn new motor skills but cannot consciously remember that he has learned them. Thus his procedural memory is intact, despite his total loss of ability to consciously recall having practiced a task. HM's communication abilities are intact because different brain areas are responsible for communication than for procedural memories (MacKay, 2006).

COMMUNICATION

People use both language and nonverbal methods to communicate. In approximately 94% of adults, the cortical areas responsible for understanding language and producing speech are found in the left hemisphere (Wood et al., 2004). Frost et al. (1999), using functional magnetic resonance imaging, demonstrated that language is strongly lateralized in the left hemisphere in both women and men. There is no significant difference between women and men in the side of the brain that processes language. The distinction between language, a communication system based on symbols, and speech, the verbal output, is clinically important because different regions of the brain are responsible for each function.

Comprehension of spoken language occurs in Wernicke's area, a subregion of the left parietotemporal cortex. Broca's area, in the left frontal lobe, provides instructions for language output. These instructions consist of planning the movements to produce speech and providing grammatical function words, such as the articles *a, an,* and *the.* The contributions of the cortical and subcortical areas involved in normal conversation are shown in Figure 16-22.

In contrast to the auditory neural networks used during conversation, reading requires intact vision, visual association areas for visual recognition of the written symbols, plus connections with an intact Wernicke's area for interpreting the symbols. Writing requires motor control of the hand in addition to connections with Wernicke's and Broca's areas. Broca's area provides the grammatical relationship between words when writing, and Wernicke's area provides formulation of language.

Given that the right hemisphere typically does not process language, what do the contralateral areas corre-

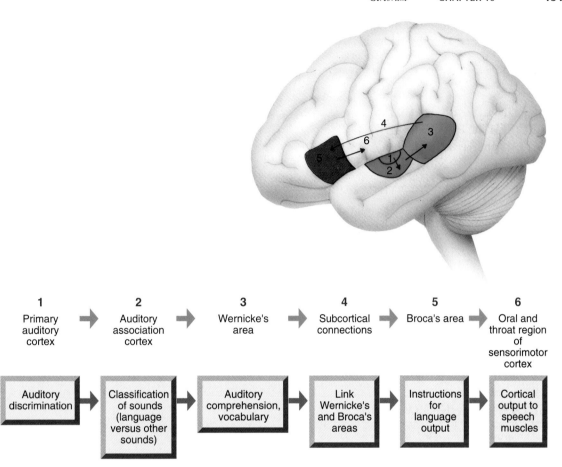

FIGURE 16-22
Flow of information during conversation, from hearing speech to replying.

sponding to Wernicke's and Broca's areas contribute? In most people, activity in these areas of the right hemisphere is associated with nonverbal communication. Gestures, facial expressions, tone of voice, and posture convey meanings in addition to a verbal message. In the right hemisphere, the area corresponding to Wernicke's area is vital for interpreting the nonverbal signals from other people. The right hemisphere area corresponding to Broca's area provides instructions for producing nonverbal communication, including emotional gestures and intonation of speech.

Cerebral Dominance

Traditionally the hemisphere that manages language is called the *dominant hemisphere,* and the hemisphere with less language capacity is considered nondominant.

The hemisphere that is dominant for language is also superior at logic and analytic tasks. This terminology may be misleading because the nondominant hemisphere is superior in understanding and producing nonverbal communication and comprehending spatial relationships.

PERCEPTION

Perception is the interpretation of sensation into meaningful forms. Perception is an active process, requiring interaction among the brain, the body, and the environment. For example, eye movements are essential to visual perception, and manipulating objects improves the ability to recognize objects via tactile input.

Perception involves memory of past experiences, motivation, expectations, selection of sensory information, and active search for pertinent sensory information. The thalamus and many areas of the cerebrum are involved in perception.

COMPREHENSION OF SPATIAL RELATIONSHIPS

The area corresponding to Wernicke's area, located in the right hemisphere, comprehends spatial relationships, providing schemas of the following:

• The body
• The body in relation to its surroundings
• The external world

The body schema, also known as the *body image,* is a mental representation of how the body is anatomically arranged (e.g., with the hand distal to the forearm). Schemas of the self in relation to the surroundings enable us to locate objects in space and to navigate accurately, finding our way within rooms and hallways and outside. Schemas of the external world provide the information necessary to plan a route from one site to another.

USE OF VISUAL INFORMATION

Visual information processed by the visual association cortex flows in two directions: dorsally, in an action stream to the frontal lobe via the posterior parietal cortex, and ventrally, in a perceptual stream to the temporal lobe (Figure 16-23). Information in the action stream is used to adjust limb movements. For example, when a person reaches for a cup, the visual information in the dorsal stream is used to orient the hand and position the fingers appropriately during the reach. In contrast, information in the perceptual stream is used to identify objects, as in recognizing the cup. The two streams operate independently. As noted in Chapter 17, people with damage in the dorsal stream have problems with visually guided movements but no difficulty identifying objects, while people with damage in the ventral stream cannot identify objects by sight but are able to use visual information to adjust their movements.

CONSCIOUSNESS

Waking and sleeping, paying attention, and initiation of action are the province of the consciousness system.

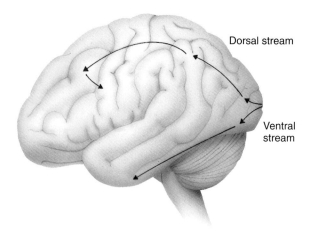

FIGURE 16-23

Use of visual information by the cerebral cortex: the action stream (dorsal) and the perceptual stream (ventral).

Various aspects of consciousness require different subsystems. Aspects of consciousness include the following:

• Generalized arousal level
• Attention
• Selection of object of attention, based on goals
• Motivation and initiation for motor activity and cognition

Each of these aspects of consciousness is associated with activity of specific neurotransmitters produced by brainstem neurons (Zeman, 2001) and delivered to the cerebrum by the reticular activating system (see Chapter 14). The neurotransmitters are serotonin, norepinephrine, acetylcholine, and dopamine. Serotonin is widely distributed throughout the cerebrum and modulates the general level of arousal. Norepinephrine contributes to attention and vigilance via locus ceruleus projections primarily to sensory areas. Acetylcholine activation of the anterior cingulate gyrus (Bentley et al., 2003) contributes to voluntary direction of attention toward an object. Finally, dopamine contributes to the initiation of motor or cognitive actions, based on cognitive activity. Figure 16-24 summarizes the function and distribution of each brainstem neurotransmitter involved in consciousness.

Although the brainstem is the source of neurotransmitters that regulate consciousness, consciousness also requires activity of the thalamus and cerebral cortex. Thus, lesions of the brainstem, thalamus, and/or cerebral cortex may result in the alterations of consciousness listed in Chapter 14.

CONSCIOUSNESS SYSTEMS

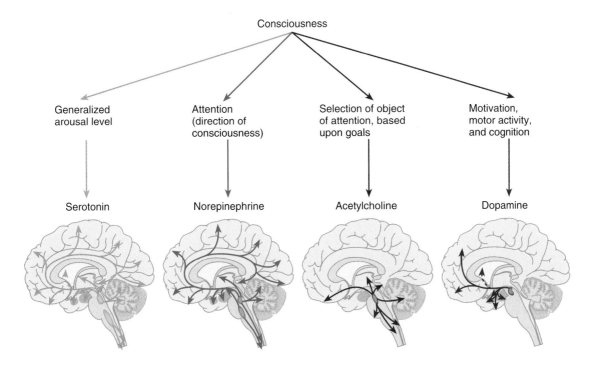

DISTRIBUTION OF NEUROTRANSMITTER

Transmitter		Serotonin	Norepinephrine	Acetylcholine	Dopamine
Origin		Raphe nuclei	Locus ceruleus and medial reticular zone	Pedunculopontine nucleus	Substantia nigra and ventral tegmental area
Limbic	Amygdala				
	Nucleus accumbens, septal area				
Basal forebrain					
Neocortex					
					Frontal only
Thalamus					
Striatum					
Cerebellar cortex					

FIGURE 16-24

The function and distribution of neurotransmitters involved in consciousness. The neurotransmitters are produced in the brainstem and delivered to the cerebrum by the reticular activating system. Colored boxes below each neurotransmitter indicate that the neurotransmitter is distributed to the indicated brain area.

In addition to the general effects indicated above, specific anatomic locations have been proposed for the ability to attend to and orient to stimuli (Vandenberghe et al., 2000). Maintaining attention requires the right frontal and parietal lobes.

Distinct areas of the cerebral cortex are devoted to analyzing sensation, planning and controlling movements, communication, behavioral control, and intellectual activity. Both cortical and subcortical structures are involved in consciousness, emotions, and memory.

SUMMARY

Subcortical structures are involved in the nonconscious regulation of sensory, autonomic, and motor functions.

REVIEW QUESTIONS

1. What neural connections would be lost with lesions of each of the thalamic relay nuclei?
2. Why is compression of or damage to the hypothalamus potentially life-threatening?
3. What signs would follow destruction of the genu region of the internal capsule?
4. What are the five functional categories of the cerebral cortex?
5. Draw a flowchart of the cortical areas activated to comply with the request, "Please pass the salt."
6. How is the stress response produced?
7. What are the effects of excessive, prolonged cortisol secretion?
8. What is the role of the hippocampus in memory?
9. Which structures are important for learning and storing procedural memories?
10. How do we use visual information in the ventral stream?
11. Bob is reading intently when he hears someone call his name. He looks up and begins a conversation with a friend. What brain areas contribute to Bob's ability to maintain his attention while reading, then disengage from reading and shift his attention to his friend?

References

Bar-On R, Tranel D, et al. (2003). Exploring the neurological substrate of emotional and social intelligence. Brain, 126(Pt 8), 1790-1800.

Bechara, A. (2004). The role of emotion in decision-making: Evidence from neurological patients with orbitofrontal damage. Brain and Cognition, 55(1), 30-40.

Bechara A, Tranel D, et al. (2002). The somatic marker hypothesis and decision-making. In F Boller and J Grafman (Eds.), Handbook of Neuropsychology: Frontal Lobes (Vol. 7, 2nd ed., pp. 117-143). Amsterdam: Elsevier.

Bentley P, Vuilleumier P, et al. (2003). Cholinergic enhancement modulates neural correlates of selective attention and emotional processing. Neuroimage, 20(1), 58-70.

Blum S, Hebert AE, et al. (2006). A role for the prefrontal cortex in recall of recent and remote memories. Neuroreport, 17(3), 341-344.

Brodmann K (1909). Vergleichende Lokalisationslehre der Grosshirnrinde in ihren Prinzipien dargestellt auf Grud des Zellenbaues. Leipzig: Barth.

Corkin S (2002). What's new with the amnesic patient H. M.? Nature Reviews. Neuroscience, 3(2), 153-160.

Cropley VL, Fujita M, et al. (2006). Molecular imaging of the dopaminergic system and its association with human cognitive function. Biological Psychiatry, 59(10), 898-907.

de Gelder B (2006). Towards the neurobiology of emotional body language. Nature Reviews. Neuroscience, 7(3), 242-249.

Dhabhar FS (2000). Acute stress enhances while chronic stress suppresses skin immunity. The role of stress hormones and leukocyte trafficking. Annals of the New York Academy of Sciences, 917, 876-893.

Doyon J, Penhune V, et al. (2003). Distinct contribution of the cortico-striatal and cortico-cerebellar systems to motor skill learning. Neuropsychologia, 41(3), 252-262.

Frost JA, Binder JR, et al. (1999). Language processing is strongly left lateralized in both sexes. Evidence from functional MRI [see comments]. Brain, 122(Pt 2), 199-208.

Heimer L, Van Hoesen GW (2006). The limbic lobe and its output channels: Implications for emotional functions and adaptive behavior. Neuroscience and Biobehavioral Reviews, 30(2), 126-147.

Herman J, Ostrander MM, et al. (2005). Limbic system mechanisms of stress regulation: Hypothalamo-pituitary-adrenocortical axis. Progress in Neuro-Psychopharmacology & Biological Psychiatry, 29(8), 1201-1213.

Kiecolt-Glaser JK, Loving TJ, et al. (2005). Hostile marital interactions, proinflammatory cytokine production, and wound healing. Archives of General Psychiatry, 62(12), 1377-1384.

Kiecolt-Glaser JK, Marucha PT, et al. (2001). Hypnosis as a modulator of cellular immune dysregulation during acute stress. Journal of Consulting and Clinical Psychology, 69(4), 674-682.

LaBar KS, Cabeza R (2006). Cognitive neuroscience of emotional memory. Nature Reviews. Neuroscience, 7(1), 54-64.

MacKay DG (2006). Aging, memory, and language in amnesic H.M. Hippocampus, 16(5), 491-494.

Parkinson JA, Willoughby PJ, et al. (2000). Disconnection of the anterior cingulate cortex and nucleus accumbens core impairs pavlovian approach behavior: Further evidence for limbic cortical-ventral striatopallidal systems. Behavior and Neuroscience, 114(1), 42-63.

Penfield W (1958). Functional localization in temporal and deep sylvian areas. Research Publications—Association for Research in Nervous and Mental Disease, 36, 210-226.

Pfeiffer BE, Huber KM (2006). Current advances in local protein synthesis and synaptic plasticity. Journal of Neuroscience, 26(27), 7147-7150.

Pert CB, Ruff MR, et al. (1985). Neuropeptides and their receptors: A psychosomatic network. Journal of Immunology, 135(Suppl 2), 820s-826s.

Poldrack RA, Sabb FW, et al. (2005). The neural correlates of motor skill automaticity. Journal of Neuroscience, 25(22), 5356-5364.

Salmon E, Collette F (2005). Functional imaging of executive functions. Acta Neurologica Belgica, 105(4), 187-196.

Salomons TV, Johnstone T, et al. (2004). Perceived controllability modulates the neural response to pain. Journal of Neuroscience, 24(32), 7199-7203.

Vandenberghe R, Duncan J, et al. (2000). Maintaining and shifting attention within left or right hemifield. Cerebral Cortex, 10(7), 706-713.

Wood AG, Harvey AS, et al. (2004). Language cortex activation in normal children. Neurology, 63(6), 1035-1044.

Young AH (2004). Cortisol in mood disorders. Stress, 7(4), 205-208.

Zeman A (2001). Consciousness. Brain, 124(Pt 7), 1263-1289.

17 Cerebrum: Clinical Applications

Laurie Lundy-Ekman, PhD, PT

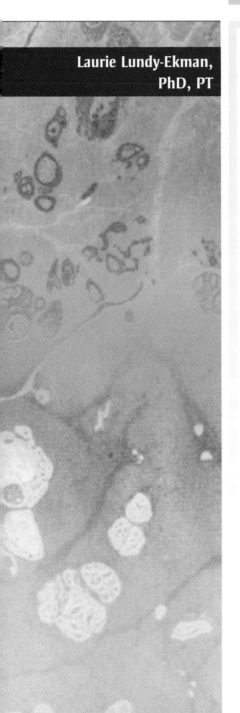

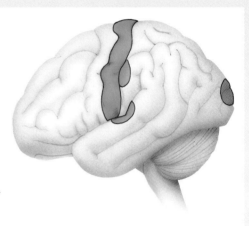

On July 4, almost 2 years ago, I had served a brunch for family and friends. Everything seemed fine. After our guests left, my husband found me collapsed on the floor. I don't remember anything about July that year. An aneurysm burst and took away some parts of my life. I had surgery to repair the aneurysm on July 5 and another surgery on August 3 to insert a shunt. I remember things since the second surgery. I had 3 weeks of rehabilitation in the hospital and then physical and occupational therapy twice a week for almost a year.

Now my movements are still too slow; everything takes me twice as long as before, I can't move my right foot, so I wear a brace to keep from turning my ankle or tripping. I used to bicycle long distances. Now I can't bicycle independently, so I ride a tandem bicycle. I can move my right arm from the wrist up but can't move my right hand. Writing is almost impossible because I was right-handed. I can type on the computer keyboard using my left hand only. Cooking takes me a long time, and I have trouble lifting things out of the oven. I enjoy traveling, but it's hard to get around in other countries. Many places don't have stair railings, and that makes it tough to go up or down stairs. I have minimal problems with language; my mouth works slower, and sometimes I forget parts of what I want to say.

I've made a lot of progress since the aneurysm burst. At first I could barely speak; trying to figure out the words was too difficult. I had to use a wheelchair because my balance was so bad. Now I can walk long distances, and I am completely independent.

In therapy we worked on walking, strengthening, balance, and stretching. I used an electrical stimulator to help contract the muscles that lift the front of the foot up, but that didn't seem to help. I haven't taken any medications for my condition.

—*Jane Lebens*

INTRODUCTION

This chapter begins with disorders of the deep cerebral structures: thalamus, subcortical white matter, and basal ganglia, and then covers dysfunctions of specific areas of the cerebral cortex. The second part considers cerebral functions that involve several areas of cerebral cortex and specific deep cerebral structures. These functions include emotions, memory, communication, spatial understanding, use of visual information, and ability to maintain upright posture. The third part covers diseases and disorders affecting cerebral function. The final section comprises testing of cerebral function.

SITES OF DAMAGE TO CEREBRAL SYSTEMS

Thalamic Injury

Thalamic lesions involving the relay nuclei interrupt ascending pathways, severely compromising or eliminating contralateral sensation. Usually proprioception is most affected. Rarely, a thalamic pain syndrome ensues after damage to the thalamus, producing severe contralateral pain that may occur with or without provoking external stimuli.

Subcortical White Matter Lesions

Occlusion or hemorrhage of arteries supplying the **internal capsule** is common. Because the internal capsule is composed of many projection axons, even a small lesion may have severe consequences. For example, a lesion the size of a nickel could interrupt the posterior limb and adjacent gray matter. This would prevent messages in corticospinal, corticobulbar, corticopontine, corticoreticular, and thalamocortical fibers from reaching their destinations, resulting in the following:

- Contralateral decrease in voluntary movement
- Contralateral decrease in automatic movement control
- Contralateral loss of conscious somatosensation

If the lesion extended more posteriorly, into the retrolenticular and sublenticular part of the capsule, conscious vision from the contralateral visual field would be lost because optic radiation fibers would be interrupted.

Callosotomy

Remarkable outcomes occur when the huge fiber bundle connecting the hemispheres, the **corpus callosum**, is surgically severed. The surgery (callosotomy) is performed in cases of intractable epilepsy when the excessive neuronal activity that characterizes epilepsy cannot be controlled by medication or surgical damage of a single cortical site. Callosotomy is usually successful in preventing excessive firing from spreading from one hemisphere to the other, thus limiting the seizure to one hemisphere. Although people with callosotomies are rarely seen for rehabilitation, because callosotomies are performed infrequently and because recovery is usually spontaneous, the results of callosotomies illustrate the difference in function between the cerebral hemispheres.

Initially, after recovery from the surgery, many people with callosotomies report conflicts between their hands: the left hand will begin a task, and the right hand will interfere with the left hand's activity. A physical therapist working with a person post callosotomy reported to the doctor, "You should have seen Rocky yesterday—one hand was buttoning up his shirt and the other hand was coming along right behind it undoing the buttons!" (Bogen, 1993). Typically, these competitive hand movements resolve with time. Following recovery, compensation occurs, allowing the person with a "split brain" to interact normally in social situations and to perform normally on most traditional neurologic examinations. Specialized tests designed to assess the performance of a single hemisphere are required to demonstrate abnormalities.

The most commonly used specialized tests involve assessment of vision and stereognosis. Results from right-handed people with callosotomies are summarized here. When words are presented briefly to the right visual field, people are able to read the words. However, when words are flashed in the left visual field, people are unable to read them and often report seeing nothing.

For somatosensory tests, people handle objects that are out of sight. For example, when handling a comb in the right hand, a person with a callosotomy is able to name and verbally describe the comb, yet unable to demonstrate using the comb. If the comb is handled by the left hand, the same person is able to demonstrate its use but unable to name it.

Why the great disparity in the abilities of the separated hemispheres? Information presented to the right visual field or right hand projects to the language-dominant left hemisphere, so the person is able to name and describe the word or object. Information from the left visual field or left hand is processed in the right cerebral hemisphere, which excels at comprehending space, manipulating objects, and perceiving shapes. Thus the person is able to manipulate the object appropriately but cannot name or verbally describe the object, because, in most people, the right hemisphere does not process language.

Basal Ganglia Disorders

In contrast to the movement disorders associated with lenticular dysfunction (see Chapter 10), lesions or dysfunctions of the caudate rarely cause motor disorders but instead cause behavioral disturbances. The most common behavioral abnormality secondary to caudate damage is apathy, with loss of initiative, spontaneous thought, and emotional responses (Herrero et al., 2002). Conversely, excessive activity of the circuit connecting the caudate, anterior cingulate cortex, and orbitofrontal cortex is correlated with obsessive-compulsive disorders (Chamberlain et al., 2005). People with obsessive-compulsive disorder have a tendency to perform certain acts repetitively, as in an irresistible urge to wash their hands hundreds of times per day.

DISORDERS OF SPECIFIC AREAS OF THE CEREBRAL CORTEX

Primary Sensory Areas: Loss of Discriminative Sensory Information

Lesions of the primary sensory areas impair the ability to discriminate intensity and quality of stimuli, severely interfering with the capacity to use the sensations. Lesions of the primary somatosensory cortex interfere most with the localization of tactile stimuli and with proprioception. Crude awareness of touch and thermal stimuli is not affected in lesions of the primary somatosensory cortex, since crude awareness occurs in the thalamus. Also, lesions confined to the primary somatosensory cortex do not compromise localization of pain. Pain information is processed in the sensory association cortex, insula, and anterior cingulate cortex rather than the primary somatosensory cortex (Peyron et al., 2000).

Because auditory information has extensive bilateral projections to the cortex, a lesion in the primary auditory cortex only interferes with the ability to localize sounds (see Chapter 13). Lesions in the primary vestibular cortex interfere with conscious awareness of head position and movement. Primary visual cortex lesions cause contralat-

eral homonymous hemianopia (see Chapter 15). The consequences of lesions in primary sensory areas are illustrated in Figure 17-1.

Sensory Association Areas: Agnosia

Agnosia is the general term for the inability to recognize objects when using a specific sense, even though discriminative ability with that sense is intact. The forms of agnosia are as follows:
- Astereognosis
- Visual agnosia
- Auditory agnosia

Astereognosis

The inability to identify objects by touch and manipulation despite intact discriminative somatosensation is astereognosis. A person with astereognosis would be able to describe an object being palpated but not recognize

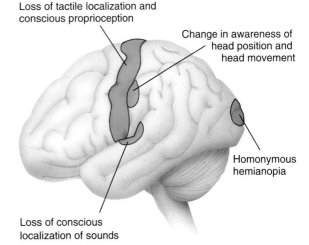

Loss of tactile localization and conscious proprioception

Change in awareness of head position and head movement

Homonymous hemianopia

Loss of conscious localization of sounds

Functional Change	Cortical Area
Loss of tactile localization and conscious proprioception	Primary somatosensory
Loss of localization of sounds	Primary auditory
Homonymous hemianopia	Primary visual
Change in awareness of head postion and movement	Primary vestibular

FIGURE 17-1

Results of lesions in primary sensory areas.

the object by touching and manipulating it. Astereognosis results from lesions in the somatosensory association area. A person with astereognosis affecting the information from one hand may avoid using that hand as a result of perceptual changes if information from the other hand is processed normally.

Visual Agnosia

Similarly, lesions in the visual association area interfere with the ability to recognize objects in the contralateral visual field, although the capacity for visual discrimination remains intact. **Visual agnosia** is the inability to visually recognize objects despite having intact vision. A person with visual agnosia can describe the shape and size of objects using vision but cannot identify the objects visually.

A highly specific type of visual agnosia is prosopagnosia. People with this rare condition are unable to visually identify people's faces, despite being able to correctly interpret emotional facial expressions and being able to visually recognize other items in the environment. Only visual recognition is defective; people can be identified by their voices or by mannerisms. Prosopagnosia is usually associated with bilateral damage to the inferior visual association areas (part of the ventral stream).

Auditory Agnosia

Destruction of the auditory association cortex spares the ability to perceive sound but deprives the person of recognition of sounds. If the lesion destroys the left auditory association cortex, the person is unable to understand speech (see later section). Destruction of the right auditory association cortex interferes with the interpretation of environmental sounds (Kaga et al., 2003). For example, a person cannot distinguish between the sound of a doorbell and the sound of footsteps. The areas of cortex involved in agnosias are illustrated in Figure 17-2.

> Agnosia results from damage to sensory association areas.

Motor Planning Areas: Apraxia, Motor Perseveration, and Broca's Aphasia

Apraxia is the inability to perform a movement or sequence of movements despite intact sensation, automatic motor output, and understanding of the task. Thus persons with apraxia may be unable to touch their nose on request, but then easily scratch their nose if it itches. Apraxia occurs as a result of damage to the premotor or supplementary motor areas (Haaland et al., 2000). A subtype of apraxia, **constructional apraxia**, interferes

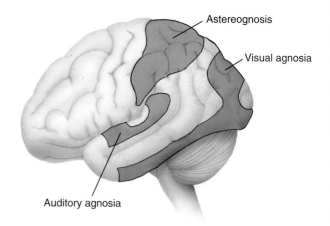

Functional Change	Cortical Area
Astereognosis	Somatosensory association
Visual agnosia	Visual association
Auditory agnosia	Auditory association

FIGURE 17-2
Results of lesions in sensory association areas.

with the ability to comprehend the relationship of parts to the whole. This deficit impairs the ability to draw and to arrange objects correctly in space.

Motor perseveration is the uncontrollable repetition of a movement. For example, a person may continue to lock and unlock the brakes of a wheelchair despite intending to lock the brakes. Motor perseveration is more associated with the amount of neural damage than with damage to a specific site (Ruchinskas and Giuliano, 2003).

Broca's aphasia is difficulty expressing oneself using language or symbols. A person with Broca's aphasia is impaired in both speaking and writing. Broca's aphasia occurs with damage to Broca's area and will be discussed further in a later section.

Primary Motor Cortex: Loss of Movement Fractionation and Dysarthria

Damage to the primary motor cortex is characterized by contralateral paresis and loss of fractionation of movement (see Chapter 9). The worst effects are distal: people with complete destruction of the primary motor cortex cannot voluntarily move their contralateral hand, lower face, and/or foot because movements of these parts of the body are controlled exclusively by the contralateral primary motor cortex.

Dysarthria is a speech disorder resulting from paralysis, incoordination, or spasticity of the muscles used for speaking. Two types of dysarthria can be distinguished: spastic and flaccid. Damage to upper motor neurons causes **spastic dysarthria,** characterized by harsh, awkward speech. In contrast, damage to lower motor neurons (cranial nerves IX, X, and/or XII) produces **flaccid dysarthria,** resulting in breathy, soft, and imprecise speech. In pure dysarthria, only the production of speech is impaired; language generation and comprehension are unaffected. The difficulty is with the mechanics of producing sounds accurately, not with finding words or with grammar. Lesions in areas of cortex that produce motor disorders are illustrated in Figure 17-3.

> The four *As* for remembering cerebral cortex disorders are aphasia, apraxia, agnosia, and astereognosis. These disorders indicate damage to specific areas of the cerebral cortex.

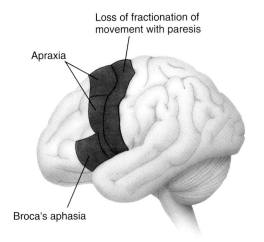

Loss of fractionation of movement with paresis

Apraxia

Broca's aphasia

Functional Change	Motor Areas
Paresis, loss of fine motor control, spastic dysarthria	Primary motor cortex
Apraxia	Premotor area
Apraxia	Supplementary motor area
Broca's aphasia or difficulty producing nonverbal communication	Broca's area in language-dominant hemisphere, or analogous area in opposite hemisphere

FIGURE 17-3
Results of lesions in motor areas of the cerebral cortex.

Dorsolateral Prefrontal Association Cortex: Loss of Executive Functions and Divergent Thinking

Although physical and occupational therapy do not focus on remediation of association cortex deficits, these deficits may have a profound influence on compliance and outcomes. Apathy and lack of goal-directed behavior are typical of people with lesions in the dorsolateral prefrontal area. People with damage to this region have difficulty with executive functions: choosing goals, planning, executing plans, and monitoring the execution of a plan. The lack of initiative may interfere with the ability to live independently and to be employed. In extreme cases, the person may not attend to basic needs, including eating and drinking. The behavior of people with dorsolateral prefrontal damage may be misinterpreted as uncooperative or unmotivated, when actually they have lost the neural capacity to initiate goal-directed action.

Perhaps surprisingly, lesions in the dorsolateral prefrontal cortex have little effect on intelligence as measured by conventional intelligence tests. People with prefrontal damage are able to perform paper-and-pencil problem-solving tasks nearly as well as they were able to prior to the damage. This may be because conventional intelligence tests assess convergent thinking, or the ability to choose one correct response from a list of choices. In people with prefrontal lesions, divergent thinking, the ability to conceive of a variety of possibilities, is impaired (Goel and Vartanian, 2005). For example, if asked to list possible uses of a stick, they perform much worse than people without brain damage. Despite the ability to perform normally on conventional intelligence tests, people with prefrontal lesions function poorly in daily life because they lack goal orientation and behavioral flexibility due to loss of executive functions and limited divergent thinking.

Limbic Association Cortex: Personality and Emotional Changes

Damage to the area of cortex above the eyes (orbitofrontal cortex) leads to inappropriate and risky behavior (Bechara, 2003). People with orbitofrontal lesions have intact intellectual abilities but use poor judgment and have difficulty conforming to social conventions. They have problems with behavioral control, saying and doing things that are socially unacceptable. Their actions are often impulsive, despite their ability to verbally identify their actions as unwise. Minor frustrations may lead to outbursts of physical and verbal aggression. In some cases, the lack of tact, lack of concern for others, and poor judgment can have disastrous consequences, causing violent behavior, damaged relationships, and inability to be employed.

Bechara et al. (2002) report that patients with damage to the orbitofrontal cortex are unable to make sound decisions in an experimental card game. Unlike people with intact nervous systems or patients with brain damage to other areas, patients with lesions in the orbitofrontal cortex showed no elevation of galvanic skin response prior to picking a card from a high-risk deck. Thus a possible explanation of the inappropriate behavior is lack of a sense of risk, that is, no emotional concern about outcomes.

Parietotemporal Association Areas: Problems With Communication, Understanding Space, and Directing Attention

Parietotemporal association areas are specialized for communication and for comprehending space. Damage to this area in the left hemisphere causes a language disturbance called Wernicke's aphasia; damage to the same area in the right hemisphere causes deficits in directing attention, comprehending space, and understanding nonverbal communication. Detailed discussion of these areas and disorders is deferred to a later section. The results of lesions in the association cortex are illustrated in Figure 17-4.

DISORDERS OF EMOTIONS

Understanding of the neural basis of emotions is in its infancy. Only the lateralization of emotions, functions of the amygdala, ventromedial prefrontal cortex, insula, and the neurochemistry of depression currently enjoy widespread consensus.

Changes in emotions and moods may occur with damage to the prefrontal cortex and/or to the temporal lobe. Left prefrontal cortex damage tends to produce unusually severe depression (Demaree et al., 2005). Right prefrontal lesions are often associated with euphoria or indifference. Similarly, people with left temporal lobectomies report increased depression, and people with right temporal lobectomies report increased happiness (Demaree et al., 2005). However, emotions are not completely lateralized. Although decreased activity in the left hemisphere often produces depression, euphoria occurs in some cases, and, rarely, decreased activity in

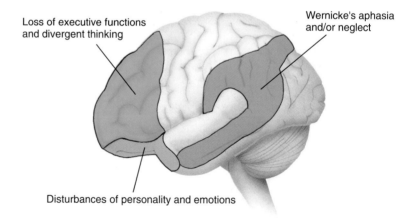

Loss of executive functions and divergent thinking

Wernicke's aphasia and/or neglect

Disturbances of personality and emotions

Functional Change	Association Cortex
Loss of executive functions and divergent thinking	Dorsolateral prefrontal association
Wernicke's aphasia	Parietotemporal association in dominant hemisphere
Neglect and/or difficulty understanding nonverbal communication	Parietotemporal association in nondominant hemisphere
Disturbances of personality and emotions	Limbic association

FIGURE 17-4

Results of lesions in the association cortex.

the right hemisphere produces depression (Canli et al., 1998).

Changes in the expression of emotion may occur following brain lesions. **Emotional lability** (also called *labile affect*) is abnormal, uncontrolled expression of emotions. Abrupt shifts in affect may occur, accompanied by a tendency to laugh and cry easily. For example, a person post brain injury may become enraged remarkably quickly in response to a minor provocation. In some cases the emotion the person is feeling may be incongruous with the emotional expression. For example, the person may be laughing while feeling grief.

In lesions that affect the somatic marker circuitry (amygdala, ventromedial prefrontal cortex, insular cortex), poor judgment and defective social intelligence cause severe problems in social function, employment, interpersonal relationships, and social status. Although executive functions and cognitive intelligence are intact, people with lesions in the somatic marker circuitry fail to learn from their mistakes (Bar-On et al., 2003). This occurs because the brain areas that make social decisions are separate from the areas that make decisions about goals and from areas essential for cognitive intelligence. Social intelligence depends on limbic structures that process emotions, whereas executive functions require the dorsolateral prefrontal cortex and parietal cortex (Carpenter et al., 2000; Collette et al., 2006). Cognitive intelligence requires white matter in the parietal lobe (Gaffan, 2005).

A woman with damage to both amygdalae has been studied extensively due to her inability to mediate emotions (Adolphs et al., 1994). She has difficulty recognizing the emotions conveyed by people's facial expressions, and she makes poor social and personal decisions. Despite these deficits, her memory for facts and events is completely intact. Young et al. (1995) reported a similar case, concluding that the amygdala has a role in social learning and behavior associated with personal interactions.

Damasio (1994) reported that a man with damage to the orbitofrontal cortex (part of the ventromedial prefrontal cortex) was unable to choose between two dates for a return appointment. For nearly half an hour, the man considered the pros and cons of the dates without approaching a conclusion. When told to come on the second date, he quickly accepted the suggestion. According to Damasio, in the absence of emotional cues that some considerations were more important than others and without the sense that the decision was trivial, the man with orbitofrontal damage was unable to make decisions. In other circumstances, that is, driving on icy roads, the same man performed well because he remained calm even when witnessing accidents. Orbitofrontal syndrome, consisting of disinhibition, impulsivity, and emotional lability (Chow, 2000), may also occur after a stroke that deprives the orbitofrontal cortex of blood flow.

Depression, a syndrome of hopelessness and a sense of worthlessness, with aberrant thoughts and behavior, has been linked to neurotransmitter rather than structural abnormalities. People with depression have reduced levels of serotonin metabolites in their cerebrospinal fluid. Drugs that effectively treat depression all increase the effectiveness of serotonin transmission. Tricyclic antidepressants inhibit both norepinephrine and serotonin uptake. Newer antidepressants, such as fluoxetine (Prozac), selectively inhibit serotonin uptake, prolonging the availability of serotonin in synapses.

MEMORY DISORDERS

Amnesia is the loss of long-term memory. Retrograde amnesia involves the loss of memories for events that occurred prior to the trauma or disease that caused the condition. In HM (see Chapter 16), after removal of both hippocampi, past memories are intact, and he cannot remember events occurring after the surgery. This loss of memory for events following the event that caused the amnesia is called anterograde amnesia.

People with amnesia affecting only declarative memory retain the ability to form new preferences, despite lacking cognitive awareness of the preferences. A patient with postencephalitic amnesia was studied to determine whether he would learn to distinguish among different response patterns of staff members. Three staff members consistently provided different responses to his request for special foods: positive, negative, and neutral. When asked whom he would ask for special foods, he indicated the staff member who responded positively to his requests, although he was totally unable to show familiarity with any of the staff members (Damasio et al., 1989). The patient's behavior demonstrated his ability to unconsciously recall the staff member who would provide him with special foods.

The dissociation of declarative and procedural memory is important clinically. People with severe declarative memory deficits following head trauma learn new motor skills, despite their inability to consciously recall having practiced the tasks (Corkin, 2002). Similarly, a patient called Boswell sustained extensive damage to the areas of the brain that process declarative memory (temporal lobes and basal forebrain). He has one of the most severe impairments ever reported for learning of all types of declarative knowledge. Yet Boswell learns motor skills at a normal rate, and retains motor skills as well as people with intact nervous systems (Tranel et al., 1994). Learning of motor skills may proceed even when declarative memory fails.

LANGUAGE DISORDERS

Disorders of language can affect spoken language (**aphasia**), comprehension of written language (**alexia**), and/or the ability to write (**agraphia**). Because aphasia has the most severe impact on communication during treatment, the following discussion focuses on aphasia. The common types of aphasia are Broca's, Wernicke's, conduction, and global.

Broca's aphasia is difficulty expressing oneself using language. The ability to understand language and to control the muscles used in speech for other purposes (swallowing, chewing) are not affected. People with Broca's aphasia may not produce any language output, or they may be able to generate habitual phrases, such as "Hello. How are you?" or make brief meaningful statements, and may be able to produce emotional speech (obscenities, curses) when upset. People with Broca's aphasia are usually aware of their language difficulties and are frustrated by their inability to produce normal language. Usually writing is as impaired as speaking. The ability to understand spoken language and to read is spared. Motor, expressive, and nonfluent aphasia are synonymous with Broca's aphasia.

In **Wernicke's aphasia**, language comprehension is impaired. People with Wernicke's aphasia easily produce spoken sounds, but the output is meaningless. An example of a meaningless phrase repeated by one of my patients is "Wishrab lamislar blagg." For a person with Wernicke's aphasia, listening to other people speak is equally meaningless, despite the ability to hear normally. The inability to produce and understand language may be analogous to when a person with an intact native language encounters an unknown foreign language. Wernicke's aphasia also interferes with the ability to comprehend and produce symbolic movements, as in sign language (Gordon, 2004). Because the ability to comprehend language is lost, people with Wernicke's aphasia have alexia (inability to read) and inability to write meaningful words. Unlike people with Broca's aphasia, people with Wernicke's aphasia often appear to be unaware of the disorder. In mild cases, word substitu-

tion, called *paraphrasia,* is common. For example, a person might say or write "captain of the school" instead of "principal." Synonyms for Wernicke's aphasia are receptive, sensory, or fluent aphasia, although language output is also abnormal.

Conduction aphasia results from damage to the neurons that connect Wernicke's and Broca's areas. In the most severe form, the speech and writing of people with conduction aphasia are meaningless. However, their ability to understand written and spoken language is normal. In mild cases, only paraphrasias occur.

The most severe form of aphasia is **global aphasia,** an inability to use language in any form. People with global aphasia cannot produce understandable speech, comprehend spoken language, speak fluently, read, or write. Global aphasia is usually secondary to a large lesion damaging much of the lateral left cerebrum: Broca's area, Wernicke's area, intervening cortex, the adjacent white matter, caudate, and anterior thalamus. Common types of aphasia are summarized in Table 17-1.

DISORDERS OF NONVERBAL COMMUNICATION

Damage to the right cortex in the area corresponding to Broca's area may cause the person to speak in a monotone, to be unable to effectively communicate nonverbally, and to lack emotional facial expressions and gestures. These consequences are sometimes referred to as **flat affect.** If the area corresponding to Wernicke's is damaged on the right side, the person has difficulty understanding nonverbal communication. Thus the person may be unable to distinguish between hearing "get out of here" spoken jokingly and "GET OUT OF HERE" spoken in anger. As noted earlier, the area corresponding to Wernicke's area is also important for body image and for understanding the relationship between self and the environment. Damage to the area corresponding to Wernicke's area may cause neglect.

NEGLECT

The tendency to behave as if one side of the body and/or one side of space does not exist is called neglect. People with neglect fail to report or respond to stimuli present on the contralesional side. Neglect usually affects the left side of the body because the right parietal area is necessary for directing attention and the area analogous to

Table 17-1   COMMUNICATION DISORDERS

Name	Synonyms	Characteristics	Comprehend Spoken Speech	Speak Fluently	Produce Meaningful Language	Normal Use of Grammatical Words	Read	Write	Structures Involved
Dysarthria	None	Lacks motor control of speech muscles	Yes	No	Yes, although difficult to understand	Yes	Yes	Yes	Lower motor neurons or corticobulbar neurons
Broca's aphasia	Motor, expressive, or nonfluent aphasia	Grammatical omissions and errors, short phrases, effortful speech	Yes	No	Yes, although grammatical words missing	No	Yes	No	Broca's area, usually in left hemisphere
Wernicke's aphasia	Sensory, receptive, or fluent aphasia	Cannot comprehend language; speaks fluently but unintelligibly	No	Yes	No	No	No	No	Wernicke's area, usually in left hemisphere
Conduction aphasia	Disconnection aphasia	Understands language; language output unintelligible	Yes	Yes	No	No	Yes	No	Neurons connecting Wernicke's area with Broca's area
Global aphasia	Total aphasia	Cannot speak fluently; cannot communicate verbally	No	No	No	No	No	No	Wernicke's area, Broca's area, and the intervening cortical and subcortical areas

Wernicke's in the right hemisphere comprehends spatial relationships (Hillis, 2006). In people with left neglect, underactivity of the damaged right-brain attention areas is associated with hyperactivity in left brain attention system (Corbetta et al., 2005). There are two types of neglect: personal and spatial. Aspects of personal neglect include the following:

- Unilateral lack of awareness of sensory stimuli
- Unilateral lack of personal hygiene and grooming
- Unilateral lack of movement of the limbs

Personal neglect results from a failure to direct attention, affecting awareness of one's own body parts. Therefore, personal neglect is also called hemi-inattention. Some people with personal neglect are able to localize light touch and to distinguish between sharp and dull if a stimulus is presented unilaterally but fail to respond to stimulation on one side when both sides of the body are stimulated concurrently. This phenomenon is called *bilateral simultaneous extinction* (see Chapter 7).

A form of denial, **anosognosia,** occurs in some people with severe hemiparesis and personal neglect. People with anosognosia deny their inability to use the paretic limbs, claiming they could clap their hands or climb a ladder. However, when asked what the experimenter would be able to do if he had exactly the same impairments as theirs, people with anosognosia who claimed they could perform the tasks reported that the experimenter would be impaired or unable to do the same task (Marcel and Tegner, 1993).

Spatial neglect is characterized by a unilateral lack of understanding of spatial relationships, resulting in a deranged internal representation of space. In an intriguing investigation of spatial neglect, Bisiach and Luzzatti (1978) asked two people with neglect to describe from memory what they would see looking at the main square in Milan from the steps of the cathedral and then describe the same scene looking across the square at the cathedral. Describing the view from the steps of the cathedral, both people consistently mentioned buildings on the right side of the visualized scene. When asked to mentally change their perspective, imagining looking at the cathedral, both described buildings on the right side and omitted buildings they had described moments earlier. Similarly, one of my patients who had been a successful artist painted the right half of a scene, leaving the left half of the canvas blank. She claimed the painting was finished and appeared perplexed when questioned about the missing parts of the boy in the painting. When I inverted the canvas to show her that the painting was incomplete, she began a new, different painting on the fresh canvas, oblivious to the image on

the left side. Figure 17-5 illustrates aspects of spatial neglect.

Some aspects of neglect are currently unexplained. Bisiach and Berti (1989) have shown that when a person with spatial neglect was asked to copy three figures, he completed both the right and left figures but drew only half of the central figure. Attentional theories of neglect would predict that the person would omit the left figure, not part of the central figure.

Manifestations of spatial neglect include problems with:

- Navigation
- Construction
- Dressing

One aspect of a deficit in understanding spatial relationships is difficulty with finding the correct route to a location. People with spatial neglect may have difficulty finding their way even within a single room. People with spatial neglect may catch part of a wheelchair on an object and continue to try to move forward, unaware of the object interfering with the intended movement. Decreased comprehension of spatial relationships also causes construction apraxia, difficulty with drawing and assembling. Dressing apraxia is difficulty with dressing due to inability to correctly orient clothing to the body.

People with neglect may have only one sign (e.g., lack of awareness of people or objects on their left) or any combination of signs. In most cases, neglect follows damage to the right cortex in the parietal lobe, the superior temporal lobe, or in the area corresponding to Wernicke's area (Hillis, 2006). Thus neglect is a complex phenomenon, with different presentations and diverse causes.

INABILITY TO USE
VISUAL INFORMATION

Visual information is used independently in the ventral and dorsal visual streams (Goodale et al., 2005). The ventral stream is involved with perception and identification of visual objects, and the dorsal stream contributes to actions based on visual input. For example, a woman with damage to the ventral stream was profoundly unable to consciously recognize the shape, orientation, or size of objects, yet she was able to pick up the unrecognized objects using normal approach and anticipatory positioning of her hand and fingers. If she saw a glass of water, she could not identify it using vision. But if she reached for the glass, her hand was oriented correctly and the

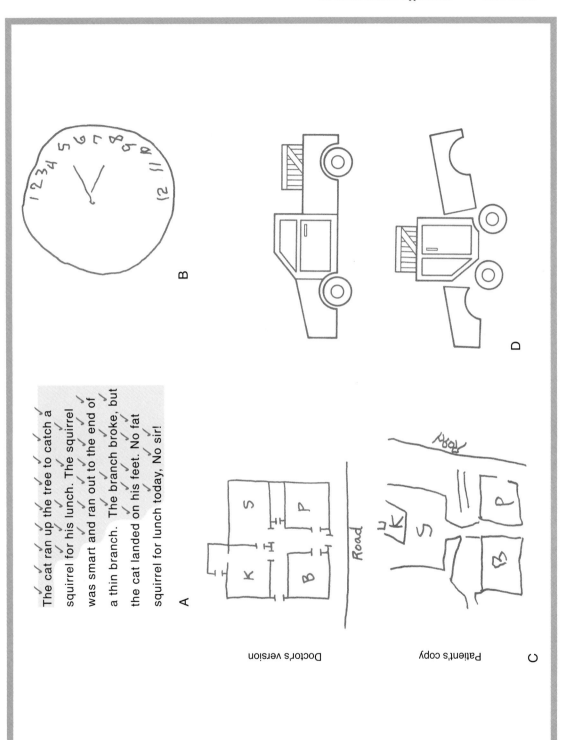

FIGURE 17-5

Signs indicating neglect. **A,** The patient is asked to read a paragraph and misses words on the left side of the text. **B,** When asked to draw a clock, the patient draws a circle yet places all or most of the numbers on the right side for the clock face. **C,** Compare the doctor's version of a house floor plan to the patient's version. **D,** The patient is unable to duplicate a block construction while looking at a model. *(From Haines DE (2006). Fundamental Neuroscience for Basic and Clinical Applications. (3rd ed., p 523). Philadelphia: Churchill Livingstone.)*

space between the thumb and fingers was appropriate to grasp the glass. Thus, despite visual agnosia, use of visual information for controlling movement was normal. The opposite impairment was noted in another woman with damage in the parietal lobe: she was unable to adjust her reach and hand orientation appropriately to the size and shape of objects, yet she was able to describe and identify the objects. Thus, optic ataxia does not affect the ability to consciously perceive visual information.

CONTRAVERSIVE PUSHING

Approximately 10% of people post stroke exhibit the unusual behavior of contraversive pushing. Contraversive pushing is a powerful pushing away from the less paretic side in sitting, during transfers, during standing, and during walking. The patient extends the nonparetic arm and pushes, creating a high risk for falls. People who present with this behavior are extremely resistant to attempts to passively adjust their posture to a symmetrical position. This problem is sometimes called *pusher syndrome.* Contraversive pushing appears to be a response to a specific deficit in sensing postural alignment relative to gravity due to a lesion of the posterior thalamus (Karnath et al., 2005) or secondary to spatial inattention (Lafosse et al., 2005). At 1 week post stroke 63% of patients demonstrated pushing; however, only 21% of those persisted in pushing at 3 months. Motor recovery requires more time in people with contraversive pushing, but they do attain significant motor and functional recovery (Danells et al., 2004). Karnath et al. (2002) report that contraversive pushing has a good prognosis: 6 months after stroke the pathologic pushing is usually resolved.

DISEASES AND DISORDERS AFFECTING CEREBRAL FUNCTION

Loss of Consciousness

At any age, a blow to the head may cause a temporary loss of consciousness. The loss of consciousness results from movement of the cerebral hemispheres relative to the brainstem, causing torque of the brainstem, and from the abrupt increase in intracranial pressure. Consciousness may also be impaired by large, space-occupying lesions of the cerebrum, located in the diencephalon or exerting pressure on the brainstem.

Attention Deficit Hyperactivity Disorder

Difficulty sustaining attention with onset during childhood is called *attention deficit hyperactivity disorder (ADHD).* People with ADHD display developmentally inappropriate inattention and impulsiveness. The etiology has not been established, but recent research implicates abnormal function of circuits linking the prefrontal cortex, striatum, and cerebellum (Castellanos and Acosta, 2002). Imaging studies also show decreases in the size of the anterior corpus callosum, right anterior white matter, and cerebellum (Paule et al., 2000). Girls are more likely to be inattentive than boys (Staller and Faraone, 2006). Boys with ADHD tend to be hyperactive or impulsive. In ADHD, both underdiagnosis and overdiagnosis occur frequently, with the reported incidence ranging from 8%-12% of children (Staller and Faraone, 2006). The disorder may persist in approximately 50% of the cases into adulthood, impairing social, academic, and work capabilities (Asherson, 2005; Okie, 2006).

Autism Spectrum Disorders

Characteristics of autism, Asperger's syndrome, and pervasive developmental disorder include a range of impaired social skills, restricted interests, and repetitive behaviors, as described in Chapter 5. Abnormal anatomy and connectivity of the limbic and striatal social brain systems is found in children and adults with autism spectrum disorders (McAlonan et al., 2005). In people who develop autism, the brain grows abnormally rapidly for the first few years, beginning soon after birth, then the rate of brain development slows. The pattern as well as the pace of brain development is abnormal (Herbert, 2005).

Epilepsy

Epilepsy is characterized by sudden attacks of excessive cortical neuronal discharge interfering with brain function. Involuntary movements, disruption of autonomic regulation, illusions, and hallucinations may occur. Partial seizures affect only a restricted area of the cortex. Generalized seizures affect the entire cortex. The two main types of generalized seizures are absence seizures, identified by brief loss of consciousness without motor manifestations, and tonic-clonic seizures, which begin with tonic contraction of the skeletal muscles followed by alternating contraction and relaxation of muscles. Typically the tonic and clonic phases last about 1 minute each. After the seizure, the person is confused for several minutes and has no memory of the seizure.

The incidence of epilepsy is 46 per 100,000 people per year, and the prevalence is 4 per 1000 (MacDonald et al., 2000). Epileptic seizures are not always medical emergencies.

SEIZURES AS MEDICAL EMERGENCIES

A seizure is a medical emergency if:
- The cause of the seizure is unknown; that is, the person has not been identified as having epilepsy or other seizure disorder
- The person is diabetic, injured, or pregnant
- The seizure lasts longer than 5 minutes, or a second seizure begins after the first
- Consciousness does not return
- The seizure occurred in water

Treatments for epilepsy include drug therapy, brain surgery to remove the neurons most prone to excessive discharge or to interrupt connections between neurons, behavioral adjustments (regular sleep and stress coping strategies), and vagus stimulation. The vagus nerve stimulation consists of attaching pacemaker to the vagus nerve to deliver electrical pulses. The rationale is that vagal visceral afferents project diffusely in the central nervous system, and activation of these pathways has widespread beneficial effects on neuronal excitability (DeGiorgio, 2000).

Disorders of Intellect

Mental retardation, dementia, and dyslexia all reduce the capability for understanding and reasoning. Common causes of mental retardation are trisomy 21 and untreated phenylketonuria.

Trisomy 21

Trisomy 21, also known as *Down syndrome,* is a genetic disorder due to an extra copy of chromosome 21. People with trisomy 21 have round heads, slanted eyes, a fold of skin extending from the nose to the medial end of the eyebrow, and simian creases on the palms of their hands. The weight of the brain and the relative size of the frontal lobes are both reduced compared to normal brains. The prevalence has been reported as 10.3 cases per 10,000 live births (Bell et al., 2003).

Phenylketonuria

Phenylketonuria is an autosomal recessive defect in metabolism resulting in retention of a common amino acid, phenylalanine. The accumulation of phenylalanine results in demyelination and, later, neuronal loss. If the condition is diagnosed in infancy (by blood and urine tests), nervous system damage may be prevented by a diet low in phenylalanine.

Dementia

In contrast to mental retardation, dementia usually occurs late in life. Dementia is generalized mental deterioration, characterized by disorientation and impaired memory, judgment, and intellect. Many different etiologies lead to dementia. Among the most common causes of dementia are multiple infarcts and Alzheimer's disease. Multiple infarcts in the cerebral hemispheres result in focal neurologic signs in addition to deterioration in intellectual function.

Alzheimer's disease causes progressive mental deterioration consisting of memory loss, confusion, and disorientation. Typically symptoms become apparent after age 60, and death follows in 5-10 years. Initially the disease presents with signs of forgetfulness, progressing to an inability to recall words and finally failure to produce and comprehend language. People with Alzheimer's disease become lost easily, and in the late stage they neglect to dress, groom, or feed themselves. Tetewsky (1999) found that Alzheimer's disease is characterized by motion blindness. Motion blindness is inability to interpret the flow of visual information. For example, when a person walks forward, the objects in the visual field flow past the person in a radial pattern. People with Alzheimer's disease are unable to interpret the direction of motion of objects in their visual field. They cannot tell whether objects are moving toward or away from them, or whether they are moving relative to objects (Kavcic et al., 2006). This inability interferes with using visual information to guide self-movement, and may explain the tendency to wander and to become lost. Another difficulty experienced by people with Alzheimer's disease is uncontrollable emotional outbursts that are unrelated to their true emotional state (emotional lability; Lopez et al., 2003).

The cause of cognitive loss in Alzheimer's disease is extracellular accumulation of a soluble amyloid-beta assembly and an abnormal form of tau protein within neurons (Lesne et al., 2006; Spires et al., 2006). The late signs of Alzheimer's disease include severe atrophy of the cerebral cortex, amygdala, and hippocampus. Figure 17-6 compares the neural activity of a normal brain and a brain with Alzheimer's disease.

The age-specific incidence of Alzheimer's disease per person-year between the ages of 65 and 74 years is 1.3%, between the ages of 75 and 84 it is 4.0%, and above the age of 84 it is 7.9% (Tang et al., 2001). Virtually all

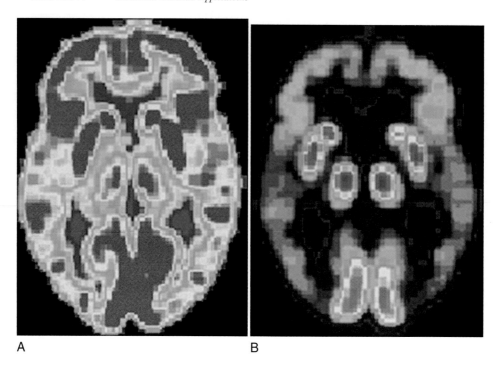

A   B

FIGURE 17-6
PET scans of a normal brain (**A**) and an Alzheimer's brain (**B**). Red and yellow indicate areas of high neural activity; blue and purple represent low neural activity. *(Courtesy Alzheimer's Disease Education and Referral Center, a service of the National Institute on Aging.)*

people with trisomy 21 develop cellular-level changes similar to those in Alzheimer's disease by age 40, although in most cases behavioral changes are not obvious, owing to the prior low level of function. People with trisomy 21 have the trisomy of chromosome 21 in all cells. In contrast, people with Alzheimer's disease have some genetically normal cells and other cells with trisomy 21 (Geller, 1999).

Another type of dementia is **diffuse Lewy body disease.** Lewy bodies are abnormal protein aggregates found in the neurons of the cerebral cortex, brainstem nuclei, and limbic areas. Core signs include progressive cognitive decline, memory impairments, and deficits in attention, executive function, and visuospatial ability. Fluctuating alertness, visual hallucinations, and parkinsonism may also occur (McKeith et al., 2005).

Learning Disabilities

In contrast to the generalized intellectual deficits of mental retardation and dementia, learning disabilities arise from a failure to develop specific types of intelli-

gence. The most common learning disability is dyslexia, a condition of inability to read at a level commensurate with the person's overall intelligence. People with dyslexia have difficulty with reading, writing, and spelling words, yet their conversational and visual abilities are normal. They can interpret visual objects and illustrations without difficulty. Some cases of dyslexia have been traced to abnormalities of a gene on chromosome 6.

Traumatic Brain Injury

A majority of traumatic brain injuries occur in motor vehicle accidents. The impact tends to damage the orbitofrontal, anterior, and inferior temporal regions and to cause diffuse axonal injury. Diffuse axonal injury results from stretch injury to the membrane of an axon. This injury allows excessive calcium influx, producing cytoskeletal collapse that disrupts anterograde axonal transport. Organelles collect at the damaged site, the axon swells at the site of injury, and the axon eventually breaks (Henderson et al., 2005). The distal axon degenerates. Axonal injury primarily affects the basal ganglia, superior cerebellar peduncle, corpus callosum, and midbrain.

Because frontal, temporal, and limbic areas are typically damaged, people show poor judgment, decreased executive functions (planning, initiating, monitoring behavior), memory deficits, slow information processing, attentional disorders, and poor divergent thinking. The inability to effectively use new information results in concrete thinking, inability to appropriately apply rules, and trouble distinguishing relevant from irrelevant information. Due to impaired judgment, people with traumatic brain injury are at significant risk for problems with substance abuse, aggression, and inappropriate sexual behaviors. Even people who sustain relatively minor head injuries often have decreased frustration tolerance, leading to easily aroused anger, and require more time and direction to complete tasks than they needed prior to the injury. Other problematic behaviors secondary to traumatic brain injury may include agitation, emotional lability, lack of self-awareness, lack of empathy, lack of motivation, and inflexibility. Imbalance may also be a persistent problem: physically well-recovered men with traumatic brain injury have impaired balance, agility, and coordination (Rinne et al., 2006).

Even mild traumatic brain injury, called a **concussion,** may have long-term behavioral effects. A concussion is distinguished by a brief loss of consciousness, a transitory posttraumatic amnesia, or a brief period of confusion following head trauma. Following concussion, some people develop post concussion syndrome, a lingering set of disorders that at 1 year post most frequently includes poor cognitive function, difficulty with concentration, and irritability (Sterr et al., 2006). (See Box 17-1.)

BOX 17-1 TRAUMATIC BRAIN INJURY DUE TO BLUNT TRAUMA WITHOUT FRACTURE

Pathology
Diffuse axonal injury; contusion, hemorrhage, swelling, and/or laceration

Etiology
Trauma

Speed of Onset
Acute

Signs and Symptoms
Personality
Decreased goal-directed behavior (executive functions) if dorsolateral prefrontal cortex involved; impulsiveness and other inappropriate behaviors if orbitofrontal cortex damaged; low tolerance for frustration; emotional lability

Consciousness
May be impaired temporarily or for a prolonged period; often have difficulty directing attention (distractibility)

Communication and Memory
Communication usually normal; declarative memory impairments may be temporary or prolonged

Sensory
May be impaired

Autonomic
May have problems with autonomic regulation secondary to damage to or compression of the brainstem and/or hypothalamus

Motor
Perseveration of movements; degree of motor impairment depends on severity of injury

Region Affected
Most frequently affects the anterior frontal and temporal lobes

Demographics
For traumatic brain injury (including open head injury and closed injuries with and without fractures), the incidence is 444 per 100,000 persons; males are 1.6 times as likely as females to suffer traumatic brain injury until age 65 years, when the female rate exceeds the male rate; the highest overall incidence of traumatic brain injury occurs in the <5 year age group (1091 per 100,000), closely followed by the >85 year age group (1026 per 100,000) (Jager et al., 2000)

Prevalence of disability caused by traumatic brain injury 20 per 1000 people (Hirtz et al, 2007)

Prognosis
Severity of injury and age at time of injury determine outcome. Five to seven years after head injury, 24% had died; of the survivors, 19% were severely disabled, 33% were moderately disabled, and 47% had a good recovery (Whitnall et al., 2006). The ratings of disability and recovery were based on the Glasgow Coma Scale—Extended. In addition to duration of amnesia, items include eye opening, verbal responses, and motor responses, with scores ranging from spontaneous to no response. For example, on the eye opening item, the person might open his or her eyes spontaneously, or might not open the eyes in response to a loud voice or a painful stimulus.

Traumatic brain damage in infants is most frequently attributable to accidental falls, but brain damage consequent to most falls is relatively minor. More severe brain injury usually requires greater force than a typical fall, forces that sometimes are generated when an infant is violently shaken. The trauma from shaking is due to the impact of the brain's striking the skull repeatedly. Soon after the incident, cerebral edema may increase the infant's head circumference and cause bulging of the anterior fontanelle. Brain scans show hemorrhage and edema. Survivors may exhibit motor signs similar to those of developmental delay or cerebral palsy and have a pattern of cognitive deficits similar to that seen in adults with traumatic brain injury (Barlow et al., 2005).

Stroke

The neurologic outcome of interruption of blood flow to the cerebrum depends on the etiology, location, and size of the infarct or hemorrhage. Infarcts occur when an embolus or thrombus lodges in a vessel, obstructing blood flow.

Signs and Symptoms of Stroke

The signs and symptoms of stroke depend on the location and size of the lesion; a small insult to the cortex may produce no symptoms, while the same size or a smaller lesion in the brainstem could cause death. Large hemorrhages or edema secondary to large infarcts can cause death regardless of location by compressing vital structures. The following acute neurologic deficits have each been reported to affect more than 25% of people surviving brain infarctions: hemiparesis, ataxia, hemianopia, visual-perceptual deficits, aphasia, dysarthria, sensory deficits, memory deficits, and problems with bladder control. Chapter 18 presents localization of deficits in the context of the vascular supply.

Although hemiplegia and hemisensory deficits resulting from stroke often appear to be unilateral, "uninvolved side" is usually a misnomer. Pai et al. (1994) report that subjects with right hemiparesis who were able to walk independently (some with assistive devices) were able to successfully transfer and maintain their weight to the nonparetic side in only 48% of trials and to the paretic side in only 20% of trials. In patients with chronic hemiplegia who had suffered penetrating brain wounds, Smutok et al. (1989) found that motor function was impaired in the ipsilateral upper limb. Compared to normals, subjects with hemispheric lesions showed decreased grip or pinch strength and poorer finger tapping and pegboard performance ipsilateral to the lesion. See Chapter 9 for possible mechanisms of ipsilateral involvement in cerebrovascular accident.

Recovery From Stroke

In physical and occupational therapy, an ongoing controversy is the long-term effectiveness of compensation, remediation, and motor control approaches to stroke rehabilitation. Compensation approaches emphasize performing tasks using either the paretic limb with an adapted approach or using the nonparetic limb to perform the task. The compensation approaches assume that damaged neural mechanisms cannot be restored, so external aids or environmental supports are used to assist patients in daily activities. For example, the ankle on the paretic side might be braced to allow early ambulation.

Remediation approaches attempt to decrease the severity of the neurologic deficits. Here the assumption is that activation or stimulation of damaged processes will result in change at both the behavioral and neural level. Using the remediation approach, the therapist might use hands-on techniques to inhibit muscle tone and work on a sequence of activities from supine to upright prior to gait training. During gait training, the therapist might move the client's hips.

Motor control approaches emphasize task specificity, that is, practicing the desired task in a specific context. If the goal is independent walking outdoors, walking outdoors is practiced, rather than preparatory activities like standing balance or lateral weight transfers in standing (Dobkin, 2004). Using the motor control approach, the client might walk an obstacle course with the therapist guarding for loss of balance.

Current research indicates that intensive, task-specific therapy produces significantly better motor function, and decreased length of hospital stay, compared with the remediation approach (Langhammer and Stanghelle, 2000). Chan et al. (2006) report that a task-specific program combined with patient self-identification of their own problems in performance produced significantly improved balance, self-care, ability to perform instrumental activities of daily living (laundry, taking public transportation, and cleaning a floor), and integration into the community than a conventional, remediation approach in people an average of 3 to 4 months post stroke.

Tumors

A tumor is a spontaneous abnormal growth of tissue that forms a mass. The signs and symptoms produced by brain tumors are usually due to compression and thus are determined by the location and size of the tumor. Brain tumors frequently cause mild to moderate intermittent headaches. The headaches are aggravated by changes in position or by abrupt increases in intracranial pressure (coughing, sneezing, or straining to empty bowels increases intrathoracic pressure, followed by an increase in aortic pressure that subsequently raises intracranial pressure) and are accompanied by nausea and vomiting.

Tumors that arise in the brain are named for the type of cell involved (see Box 17-2). Most primary central nervous system tumors are derived from glia and therefore are called gliomas. The incidence of primary CNS tumors (both malignant and benign) is 14 per 100,000 people per year, and the lifetime prevalence is 0.7 per 1,000 people (MacDonald et al., 2000). Prognosis depends on the histology, size, and location of the tumor, the age of the patient, and the effectiveness of surgical, chemical, and radiation therapy.

Psychological Disorders

Some psychological disorders are characterized by associated physical symptoms. In somatoform disorders, emotional distress is subconsciously converted into physical symptoms. People with somatoform disorders use their symptoms to avoid emotional conflicts or to manipulate other people. Common symptoms of somatoform disorders include back pain, joint pain, aching of the extremities, trouble walking, muscle weakness, gastrointestinal problems, nonexertional shortness of breath, problems with swallowing, double vision, and blurred vision. Somatoform disorders are distinct from malingering

because no external gain can be identified. In malingering, the person intentionally exaggerates or feigns symptoms for external gain. For example, receiving time off from work, access to drugs, and/or financial incentives may motivate a person who is malingering.

Personality disorders have more pervasive effects on the individual than somatoform disorders. People with personality disorders have inflexible, maladaptive patterns of inner experience and behavior. The three general types are eccentric, acting out, and fearful. People with personality disorders may be prone to rapid mood swings, excessive sensitivity to the judgment of other people, passive resistance to instructions (e.g., "losing" a home exercise program, talking excessively to avoid practicing tasks during therapy), and/or ambiguous complaints.

The treatment by occupational and physical therapists for people with these disorders should focus on improving activities of daily living, work, leisure activities, and physical function. Psychological counseling is outside the scope of occupational and physical therapy practice. Referral of the patient to a mental health professional may be beneficial.

Schizophrenia

Schizophrenia is a group of disorders consisting of disordered thinking, delusions, hallucinations, and social withdrawal. The syndrome involves both anatomic and neurotransmitter abnormalities. The frontal and temporal lobes and the amygdala and hippocampus are smaller in people with schizophrenia than in normals. Abnormalities of the basal ganglia, thalamus, and corpus callosum are also characteristic of schizophrenia (Niznikiewicz et al., 2003). Drugs that block the reuptake of serotonin or that block dopamine receptors reduce symptoms in many people with schizophrenia. Thus abnormality of neurotransmitter regulation may contribute to the symptoms of schizophrenia.

TESTING CEREBRAL FUNCTION

Therapists often briefly assess cerebral function. Part of this assessment may include evaluating the level of consciousness. Normal consciousness requires intact function of the ascending reticular activating system, thalamus, and thalamic projections to the cerebral cortex in addition to the cerebral cortex. Functions that are localized in the cerebral cortex include language, orientation, declarative memory, abstract thought, identification of objects, motor planning, and comprehension of spatial relationships (Table 17-2). Consciousness and

---

BOX 17-2 TYPES OF BRAIN TUMORS

Malignant
- Astrocytoma (from astrocytes; some are benign)
- Glioblastoma multiforme (from glial cells)
- Oligodendroglioma (from oligodendrocytes)
- Ependymoma (from ependymal cells)
- Medulloblastoma (from neuroectodermal cells)
- Lymphoma (from lymphatic tissue)
- Metastatic (commonly arise from lung, skin, kidney, colon, or breast)

Benign
- Meningioma (from arachnoid)
- Adenoma (from epithelial tissue)
- Acoustic neuroma (from Schwann cells)

Table 17-2 EVALUATION OF MENTAL FUNCTION

Function	Test	Interpretation
Consciousness level	Observe the person's interaction with the environment. Levels of consciousness are classified as: *Alert:* Attends to ordinary stimuli *Lethargic:* Tends to lose track of conversations and tasks; falls asleep if little stimulation is provided *Obtunded:* Becomes alert briefly in response to strong stimuli; cannot answer questions meaningfully *Stupor:* Alert only during vigorous stimulation *Coma:* Little or no response to stimulation	Levels of consciousness depend on neural activity in the ascending reticular activating system, thalamus, thalamic projections to the cerebral cortex, and the cerebral cortex.
Language and speech	Evaluate the spontaneous use of words, grammar, and fluency of speech.	Disorders may be caused by any form of aphasia, or by dysarthria. Brain areas involved may be Broca's area, Wernicke's area, connections between Broca's and Wernicke's area, premotor and/or motor cortex, corticobulbar fibers, or motor cranial nerves.
	Comprehension: Ask the person to answer a question similar to the following: "Is my brother's sister a man or a woman?"	Difficulty may be due to receptive aphasia or a hearing disorder. Brain areas involved may include Wernicke's area, or peripheral or central auditory structures.
	Naming: Ask the person to identify objects (pencil, watch, paper clip) and body parts (nose, knee, eye).	If the person can produce automatic social speech (e.g., "Hello, how are you?") but cannot name objects, the difficulty may be due to dysfunction of Wernicke's area (Wernicke's aphasia).
	Reading: Ask the person to read a simple paragraph aloud. Then ask questions about the paragraph.	Assuming the person has intact speech, difficulty may be due to alexia, dyslexia, short-term memory deficit, visual deficit, or illiteracy. Wernicke's area is the site of dysfunction in alexia.
	Writing: Ask the person to write answers to simple questions.	Difficulty may be due to agraphia, visual deficit, impaired motor control of the upper limb, or illiteracy. Wernicke's area is the site of dysfunction in agraphia.

All of the following tests require language abilities. Some, as noted, also require intact speech.

Orientation	Assess the person's orientation to person, place, and time. Questions similar to the following may be used:
	Person
	  What is your name?
	  Where were you born?
	  Are you married?
	Place
	  Where are we now?
	  What city and state are we in?
	Time
	  What time is it?
	  What day of the week is this?
	  What year is this?
		Test assumes intact speech abilities. These questions assess declarative memory. The questions about the person assess long-term memory, and the questions about time and place assess short-term memory. Difficulty with these questions may indicate dysfunction of the hippocampus; a language or speech disorder; or a generalized cortical processing disorder, such as occurs with drug toxicity, psychosis, or extreme anxiety.

Table 17-2   EVALUATION OF MENTAL FUNCTION—cont'd

Function	Test	Interpretation
Declarative memory	*Short-term memory:* Tell the person that you are going to check his or her memory by asking him or her to remember three words for a few minutes. Give the person three unrelated words, and have him or her repeat the words. Then converse about other topics, and after 3 minutes, ask what the three words were. People with intact short-term memory can recall all three words. Examples of words used include *clock, telephone, shoe.* *Recent memory:* Ask the person about activities in the past several days. Examples include: What did you have for breakfast? Who visited you yesterday? *Long-term memory:* Ask the person to name U.S. presidents, about historical events, or about his or her school and work experience.	Test requires speech abilities. Declarative memory problems occur with damage to the hippocampus or with temporary disruptions of cerebral function, as may occur during psychosis, extreme anxiety, or following acute head trauma.
Interpretation of proverbs	Ask the person to explain what a proverb means. For example, "What does 'a rolling stone gathers no moss' mean?"	Test requires speech abilities. A concrete answer, such as "It means that a rock that keeps moving does not grow moss," indicates difficulty with abstract thinking.
Calculation	*Serial 7s:* Ask the person to subtract 7 from 100 and to keep subtracting 7 from each result. Ask the person simple addition, subtraction, multiplication, or division problems. For example, "What is 6×30?"	Test requires speech abilities. Difficulty may indicate problems with maintaining attention, or a problem with abstract thinking.
Stereognosis	Ask the person to close his or her eyes, then place a small object in the person's hand and ask him or her to identify it. Objects may include a paper clip, a key, or a coin.	Test requires speech abilities. Astereognosis indicates damage to the somatosensory association area of the cerebral cortex.
Visual identification	Show the person an object and ask him or her to identify it.	Test requires speech abilities. If the person cannot identify the object visually but can identify the object by touch or another sense, the disorder is visual agnosia. Visual agnosia is caused by damage to the visual association areas in the cerebral cortex of the occipital lobe.
Motor planning	Ask the person to demonstrate hair brushing, using a screwdriver, or buttoning a shirt.	Assuming intact sensation, understanding of the task, and motor control, inability to produce specific movements indicates apraxia. Apraxia usually occurs as a result of damage to the premotor or supplementary motor areas.

Continued

Table 17-2   EVALUATION OF MENTAL FUNCTION—cont'd

Function	Test	Interpretation
Comprehension of spatial relationships	*Activities of daily living:* Observe the person eating a meal; ask him or her to put on an article of clothing; or ask him or her to perform a grooming task or to get into and out of a bed or chair.	Difficulty may indicate motor impairment, neglect, or a generalized decline in cerebral function. Asymmetry of performance usually indicates neglect. Neglect occurs with damage to the area that corresponds to Wernicke's area.
	Ask the person to copy a simple drawing, or to draw a person, a clock, a house, or a flower from memory.	Difficulty may indicate motor impairment, neglect, constructional apraxia, or a generalized decline in cerebral function. Asymmetry of performance usually indicates neglect. Neglect occurs with damage to the area that corresponds to Wernicke's area. If most parts of the drawing are present but not in correct spatial relationship to each other, and if the drawing improves when the subject is copying a model, the deficit is constructional apraxia. In constructional apraxia, the lesion is typically in the parietal or frontal lobe of the language-dominant hemisphere.
	Visual scanning: Ask the person to read a paragraph aloud, or to cross out specific characters in a printed array (e.g., cross out all of the small stars in an array of large and small stars).	Assuming that visual acuity and visual fields are adequate, omission of words or parts of words located on the left side of the paragraph or failing to cross out all of the specified characters on the left side of a visual array indicates visual neglect.
	Body scheme drawing: Give the person a blank piece of paper and ask him or her to draw a person.	Asymmetry in the drawing of a person (such as omitting part of the left side of the body or providing less detail on the left side of the body) indicates neglect associated with damage to the right parietal lobe.
Concept of relationship of body parts	Ask the person to point to a body part on command, or to imitate the examiner in pointing to parts of his or her own body.	Bilateral inaccuracy or failure to point to body parts indicates a specific deficit in conception of the relationship of body parts to the whole body. The lesion is usually in the parietal or the posterior temporal lobe of the left hemisphere.
Orientation to vertical position	Hold a cane vertically, and then move it to a horizontal position. Give the cane to the person and ask him or her to return it to the original position.	If the cane is not vertical, orientation to vertical position is impaired. The lesion may be in the right parietal lobe, in the posterior thalamus, or in the vestibular system.
Ability to attend to bilaterally simultaneous stimulation	*Touch:* Ask the person to say "yes" if he or she feels a touch. Lightly touch both sides of the body simultaneously. If the person says yes, ask where the touch was felt. *Vision:* Show the person two objects, one in the right visual field and one in the left visual field. Ask the person to name the objects.	If the person is able to correctly report touch or visual objects presented to the left of his or her midline, but is unaware of these stimuli when the stimuli are presented bilaterally, the person has sensory extinction, a form of unilateral neglect.

language are assessed first because the other tests, except comprehension of spatial relationships, require that the person be alert and able to understand language. The message that the therapist wants the person to copy a drawing, in order to assess comprehension of spatial relationships, may be conveyed by gestural cues.

Difficulties with certain tests of mental function indicate lesions in specific parts of the cerebral cortex. For example, Broca's aphasia indicates damage to Broca's area. Difficulty with other tests does not implicate any specific part of the cerebral cortex, but instead indicates more generalized dysfunction. The significance of difficulty with each test is listed in Table 17-2, in the "Interpretation" column. For patients with moderate to severe speech and/or language difficulties, consultation with a speech/language pathologist is recommended.

SUMMARY

Functions and lesions of the four lobes of the cerebrum are considered first, followed by a discussion of the parietotemporal cortex and cerebral lesions.

Frontal lobes control motor function, initiation of activity, planning nonverbal communication, goal-oriented behavior, judgment, interpretation of emotion, attention, flexibility in problem solving, social behavior, and motivation. Lesions cause Broca's aphasia (dominant hemisphere), impaired production of nonverbal communication (nondominant hemisphere), and hemiplegia. Dorsolateral lesions interfere with initiation and monitoring of goal-oriented behavior and divergent thinking. Orbitofrontal lesions produce disinhibited behavior, poor judgment, and disturbances of personality and emotions.

Parietal lobes process sensation and provide perception relating to body schema. Parietal lobe lesions may cause contralateral somatosensory loss, hemiplegia, homonymous hemianopia, agnosia, astereognosis, and apraxia (inability to perform purposeful voluntary movements, despite understanding the task and intact motor and sensory function).

Occipital lobes process vision, including spatial relationships of visual objects, analysis of motion and color, and also control visual fixation. Lesions in the primary visual cortex produce homonymous hemianopia. Lesions in the visual association cortex cause visual agnosia. Disorders of the occipital lobe can also cause visual hallucinations or loss of visual fixation.

Temporal lobes process auditory information, classify sounds, and process emotion and memory. Lesions cause loss of localization of sounds, auditory agnosia, impaired long-term memory, and disturbances of personality and emotions.

Parietotemporal association cortex is involved in sensory integration, communication, understanding spatial relationships, and convergent problem solving. Lesions in the left parietotemporal association cortex can produce disorders of language (Wernicke's aphasia). Lesions in the right parietotemporal cortex may cause contralateral neglect, difficulty understanding nonverbal communication, and anosognosia (denial of deficits).

Consciousness, attention, control of movements, motivation, memory, intellect, sensation, perception, communication, all forms of behavior, personality, and emotions all rely on the cerebrum. Cerebral function is diverse and adaptable. Cerebral dysfunction can be devastating, as in severe brain injury or schizophrenia. Cerebral compensation for injury can also be remarkable, as people recover from cerebral injuries and disorders.

CLINICAL NOTES

Case 1

A famous case in the right-to-die debate involved Karen Quinlan. After ingesting a tranquilizer, an analgesic, and alcohol, she suffered cardiopulmonary arrest that permanently damaged her brain. She became the focus of a conflict between doctors intent on keeping her alive and her parents, who requested that she be allowed to die because no hope for recovery existed. A court ordered the doctors to remove her ventilator. However, she continued to breathe without the ventilator and survived in a vegetative state for 9 more years. She never regained consciousness. Although her brain damage was assumed to be in the cerebral cortex, subsequent analysis of her brain showed that the cortex was relatively intact, and that the region with severe damage was the thalamus (Kinney et al., 1994).

Continued

CLINICAL NOTES

Questions

1. Why does thalamic damage interfere with consciousness?
2. What other structures are required for consciousness?

Case 2

HA is a 47-year-old woman who is recovering from surgery to remove a benign tumor in the optic chiasm region. One day post surgery, the therapist arrives to assess the patient. The therapist notes that the patient is unconscious and has no bedcovers, the air conditioning is on full, and fans are placed to blow across the patient's body, yet the temperature of the patient's skin is unusually warm. When the therapist arrives the next day, the patient is warmly covered, the heater is on, and the room temperature is near 90°F, yet the patient's skin temperature is cool.

Questions

1. What is the hospital staff trying to do by manipulating the room temperature?
2. What part of HA's brain is not functioning optimally?

Case 3

KL is a 72-year-old man who has been transferred to rehabilitation 2 weeks after sustaining a cerebrovascular accident on the left side. He complains of weakness of his right limbs and of being unable to button his clothing or tie his shoes. Right hand movements are clumsy. On the right side of his body, KL is unable to localize tactile stimuli or to distinguish between passive flexion and extension of his joints. He is able to correctly report whether he was touched or not and whether a stimulus is sharp or dull.

Question

Where is the lesion?

Case 4

RB is a 19-year-old boy who was rescued, unconscious, after falling from a 40-foot cliff. One day later he regained consciousness. Strength, position sense, touch localization, and two-point discrimination were normal on both sides. RB was easily able to identify unseen objects in his left hand but totally unable to recognize the same objects using his right hand. Although he was right-handed prior to the accident, after the accident he used his left hand whenever possible.

Questions

1. Name the deficit in ability to recognize an object by palpation.
2. Why does RB avoid using his right hand?

Case 5

FS, a 26-year-old schoolteacher, sustained head trauma and multiple femoral fractures in a traffic accident. She was comatose for 3 days. On regaining consciousness, sensation, movement, and her ability to communicate were intact. However, she seemed listless and did not initiate conversations or activities. FS was unable to learn a partial weight-bearing gait, flailing the crutches rather than bearing weight on them. She appeared totally apathetic, even about her situation and her family.

Question

Where is the lesion?

Case 6

BG, a 34-year-old stockbroker, suffered multiple fractures of the frontal skull in a motorcycle accident. After recovery from surgical repair, he was hemiparetic on the right side. Muscle strength on the right expressed as a percentage of strength on the left was as follows: girdle muscles, 80%; elbow/knee, 50%; and distal muscles, 0%. With an

CLINICAL NOTES

ankle-foot orthosis and a cane, he was able to walk with minimal assistance. However, he frequently attempted to walk independently without the cane or orthosis, and he fell each time. He began making tactless comments and became impulsive, frequently grabbing or pushing people and objects. After 3 days in rehabilitation, he left the hospital against medical advice. A friend drove him to work. Within an hour he was fired because of his behavior toward coworkers, and readmitted to the hospital.

Question
Where is the lesion?

Case 7

Critchley (1953) reported a patient who seemed normal but put a tea bag in the teapot, set the pot on the stove, and poured cold water into a cup. She lit a match, put the match to the gas burner, blew out the match, and turned on the gas.

Question
Name the disorder.

Case 8

HM, a 66-year-old man, is 5 days post stroke. He is able to walk using a step-to-gait, with minimal assist for balance. He is unable to voluntarily move his right arm. The right arm is adducted at the shoulder, and the elbow, wrist, and fingers are flexed. His speech is strained, harsh, and slow, and some sounds are produced incorrectly, as in "Ow are oo? I am fime." His ability to produce and understand language and his writing are entirely normal.

Questions
1. Name the communication disorder.
2. Where is the lesion?

Case 9

VM, a 72-year-old woman, was admitted to the hospital with right hemisensory loss, hemiplegia, and communication problems. She greeted visitors with a halting, effortful, and garbled "Hello, how you?" Language output was marred by poor articulation and omission of grammatical function words. She appeared extremely frustrated by her inability to express herself. Her attempts at writing left-handed also showed omission of grammatical function words. She was able to easily follow simple verbal or written commands, indicating intact ability to comprehend language.

Questions
1. Where is the lesion?
2. Name the communication disorder.

Case 10

PD, an 86-year-old man, was referred to physical therapy following a total hip replacement 1 week ago. Two days ago, while his wife was visiting him in the hospital, he abruptly began speaking nonsense in a conversational tone as if he were speaking normally. His speech was a mixture of jargon and English. For example, he insisted, "I get creekons, tallings, and you must uffners." He became agitated when his wife didn't understand him, and he was unable to understand her questions. With hospital staff he continued to speak freely in his mixture of jargon and English. He showed no indication of comprehending spoken or written language, nor any awareness that his language output was defective. Communication was strictly limited to gestures. No other signs or symptoms are evident. In therapy today, he was cooperative if the therapist pantomimed the desired movements. If the therapist tried to instruct him verbally, he became withdrawn and uncooperative.

Questions
1. Name the communication disorder.
2. Where is the lesion?

Continued

CLINICAL NOTES

Case 11

AG, a 68-year-old man, is 2 weeks post–right cerebrovascular accident. In all situations, he ignores the left side of his body and objects and people on his left. He never looks toward the left, does not respond to touch or pinprick on his left side, does not eat food from the left side of a plate, does not move his left limbs, does not shave the left side of his face, nor dress his left side. Last week, two fingers on his left hand were lacerated while caught in his wheelchair spokes. Although the entrapped fingers prevented the wheelchair from moving, AG continued to try to move forward until stopped by the therapist. Gait requires maximal assistance because he does not bear full weight on the left leg and attempts to take steps using only the right leg, dragging the left leg behind. He becomes lost easily and his attempts to copy drawings are distorted because he omits features that should be included on the left side of the drawing.

Questions

1. Name the disorder.
2. What specific subtypes of the disorder does AG have?

Case 12

A 32-year-old man was hit on the side of the head by a baseball 1 week ago. He complains of clumsiness in picking up objects, although he has no difficulty visually identifying objects. When he reaches for objects, he does not orient the position of his hand to the object; for example, when reaching for a pen held by the examiner, he uses a forearm pronated approach regardless of whether the pen is vertical or horizontal. In reaching for a cup, he does not adjust the opening between fingers and thumb to the size of the cup.

Questions

1. What is this condition called?
2. What area(s) of the brain is (are) damaged?

Case 13

HL is a 17-year-old boy who sustained a closed head injury in an auto accident 1 month ago. HL was comatose for 2 weeks. During week 3, he became responsive to simple commands but was mute. Now HL talks, he believes he is at home, and he cannot report the correct year or month despite daily reminders of time and place. He does not initiate any activities unless prompted. HL is frequently verbally and physically aggressive. All limb movements are ataxic and dysmetric. Coming from sit to stand and gait require moderate assistance due to balance impairments, bilateral weakness, and poor coordination.

Question

What areas of the brain are impaired?

REVIEW QUESTIONS

1. What is the most likely location of a lesion in a person with loss of conscious somatosensation and voluntary movement on the left side of the body and face and loss of conscious vision from the left visual field?
2. Define each of the following terms and identify the area of cortex most commonly damaged with each sign: astereognosis, visual agnosia, apraxia, and spastic dysarthria.
3. A person unable to understand nonverbal communication and exhibiting signs of left neglect probably has a lesion where?
4. Is Broca's aphasia an upper motor neuron disorder?

5. What is the difference between dysarthria and aphasia?

6. A 64-year-old woman has right hemiparesis, hemisensory loss, Broca's aphasia, and intact vision. Where is the most likely site for the lesion?

7. When working with a person who has global aphasia, what type of communication is most effective?

8. JH is 2 weeks post stroke. Although she has been in the same hospital room for 10 days, she cannot find the bathroom or the hallway. What is the name for this problem?

References

Adolphs R, Tranel D, et al. (1994). Impaired recognition of emotion in facial expressions following bilateral damage to the human amygdala. Nature, 372(6507), 669-672.

Asherson P (2005). Clinical assessment and treatment of attention deficit hyperactivity disorder in adults. Expert Review of Neurotherapeutics, 5(4), 525-539.

Barlow KM, Thomson E, et al. (2005). Late neurologic and cognitive sequelae of inflicted traumatic brain injury in infancy. Pediatrics, 116(2):e174-85.

Bar-On R, Tranel D, et al. (2003). Exploring the neurological substrate of emotional and social intelligence. Brain, 126(Pt 8), 1790-1800.

Bechara A (2003). Risky business: Emotion, decision-making, and addiction. Journal of Gambling Studies, 19(1), 23-51.

Bechara A, Tranel D, et al. (2002). The somatic marker hypothesis and decision-making. In F Boller and J Grafman (Eds.), Handbook of Neuropsychology: Frontal Lobes (Vol. 7; 2nd ed., pp. 117-143). Amsterdam: Elsevier.

Bell R, Rankin J, et al. (2003). Down's syndrome: occurrence and outcome in the north of England, 1985-1999. Paediatric and Perinatal Epidemiology, 17(1), 33-39.

Bisiach E, Berti A (1989). Unilateral misrepresentation of distributed information: Paradoxes and puzzles. In WJ Brown (Ed.), Neuropsychology of Visual Perception. Hillsdale, NJ: Erlbaum.

Bisiach E, Luzzatti C (1978). Unilateral neglect of representational space. Cortex, 14, 129-133.

Bogen JE (1993). The callosal syndromes. In KM Heilman and E Valenstein (Eds.), Clinical Neuropsychology (pp. 337-407). New York: Oxford University Press.

Canli T, Desmond JE, et al. (1998). Hemispheric asymmetry for emotional stimuli detected with fMRI. Neuroreport, 9(14), 3233-3239.

Carpenter PA, Just MA, et al. (2000). Working memory and executive function: Evidence from neuroimaging. Current Opinion in Neurobiology, 10(2), 195-199.

Castellanos FX, Acosta MT (2002). [Syndrome of attention deficit with hyperactivity as the expression of an organic functional disorder]. Revista de Neurologia, 35(1), 1-11.

Chamberlain, SR, Blackwell AD, et al. (2005). The neuropsychology of obsessive compulsive disorder: The importance of failures in cognitive and behavioural inhibition as candidate endophenotypic markers. Neuroscience and Biobehavioral Reviews, 29(3), 399-419.

Chan, DY, Chan CC, et al. (2006). Motor relearning programme for stroke patients: A randomized controlled trial. Clinical Rehabilitation, 20(3), 191-200.

Chow TW (2000). Personality in frontal lobe disorders. Current Psychiatry Reports, 2(5), 446-451.

Collette F, Hogge M, et al. (2006). Exploration of the neural substrates of executive functioning by functional neuroimaging. Neuroscience, 139(1), 209-221.

Corbetta M, Kincade MJ, et al. (2005). Neural basis and recovery of spatial attention deficits in spatial neglect. Nature Neuroscience, 8(11), 1603-1610.

Corkin S (2002). What's new with the amnesic patient H. M.? Nature Reviews. Neuroscience 3(2), 153-160.

Critchley, M. (1953). The parietal lobes. London: E. Arnold.

Damasio AR (1994). Descartes' Error: Emotion, Reason, and the Human Brain. New York: G. P. Putnam's Sons.

Damasio AR, Tranel D, et al. (1989). Amnesia caused by herpes simplex encephalitis, infarctions in basal forebrain, Alzheimer's disease, and anoxia/ischemia. In F Boller and J Grafman (Eds.), Handbook of Neuropsychology (Vol. 3, pp. 149-166). Amsterdam: Elsevier.

Danells CJ, Black SE, et al. (2004). Poststroke pushing: Natural history and relationship to motor and functional recovery. Stroke, 35(12), 2873-2878.

DeGiorgio CM, et al. (2000). Prospective long-term study of vagus nerve stimulation for the treatment of refractory seizures. Epilepsia, 41(9), 1195-2000.

Demaree HA, Everhart DE, et al. (2005). Brain lateralization of emotional processing: Historical roots and a future incorporating dominance. Behavioral and Cognitive Neuroscience Reviews, 4(1), 3-20.

Dobkin BH (2004). Strategies for stroke rehabilitation. Lancet Neurology, 3(9), 528-536.

Gaffan D (2005). Neuroscience. Widespread cortical networks underlie memory and attention. Science, 309(5744), 2172-2173.

Geller LN, Potter, H. (1999). Chromosome missegregation and trisomy 21 mosaicism in Alzheimer's disease. Neurobiology of Disease, 6(3), 167-179.

Goel V, Vartanian O (2005). Dissociating the roles of right ventral lateral and dorsal lateral prefrontal cortex in generation and maintenance of hypotheses in set-shift problems. Cerebral Cortex, 15(8), 1170-1177.

Goodale MA, Kroliczak G, et al. (2005). Dual routes to action: Contributions of the dorsal and ventral streams to adaptive behavior. Progress in Brain Research, 149, 269-283.

Gordon N (2004). The neurology of sign language. Brain & Development, 26(3), 146-150.

Haaland KY, Harrington DL, et al. (2000). Neural representations of skilled movement. Brain, 123 (Pt 11), 2306-2313.

Henderson FC, Geddes JF, et al. (2005). Stretch-associated injury in cervical spondylotic myelopathy: New concept and review. Neurosurgery, 56(5), 1101-1113; discussion 1101-1113.

Herbert MR (2005). Large brains in autism: The challenge of pervasive abnormality. Neuroscientist, 11(5), 417-440.

Herrero MT, Barcia C, et al. (2002). Functional anatomy of thalamus and basal ganglia. Child's Nervous System, 18(8), 386-404.

Hillis AE (2006). Neurobiology of unilateral spatial neglect. Neuroscientist, 12(2), 153-163.

Hirtz D, Thurman DJ, et al. (2007). How common are the "common" neurologic disorders? Neurology, 68(5): 326-337.

Jager TE, Weiss HB, et al. (2000). Traumatic brain injuries evaluated in U.S. emergency departments, 1992-1994. Academy of Emergency Medicine, 7(2), 134-140.

Kaga K, Kaga M, et al. (2003). Auditory agnosia in children after herpes encephalitis. Acta Oto-Laryngologica, 123(2), 232-235.

Karnath HO, Johannsen L, et al. (2002). Prognosis of contraversive pushing. Journal of Neurology, 249(9), 1250-1253.

Karnath HO, Johannsen L, et al. (2005). Posterior thalamic hemorrhage induces pusher syndrome. Neurology, 64(6), 1014-1019.

Kavcic V, Fernandez R, et al. (2006). Neurophysiological and perceptual correlates of navigational impairment in Alzheimer's disease. Brain, 129(Pt 3), 736-746.

Kinney HC, Korein J, et al. (1994). Neuropathological findings in the brain of Karen Ann Quinlan: The role of the thalamus in the persistent vegetative state [see comments]. New England Journal of Medicine, 330(21), 1469-1475.

Lafosse C, Kerckhofs E, et al. (2005). Contraversive pushing and inattention of the contralesional hemispace. Journal of Clinical and Experimental Neuropsychology, 27(4), 460-484.

Langhammer B, Stanghelle JK (2000). Bobath or motor relearning programme? A comparison of two different approaches of physiotherapy in stroke rehabilitation: A randomized controlled study. Clinical Rehabilitation, 14(4), 361-369.

Lesne S, Koh MT, et al. (2006). A specific amyloid-beta protein assembly in the brain impairs memory. Nature, 440(7082), 352-357.

Lopez OL, Becker JT, et al. (2003). Psychiatric symptoms vary with the severity of dementia in probable Alzheimer's disease. Journal of Neuropsychiatry and Clinical Neurosciences, 15(3), 346-353.

MacDonald BK, Cockerell OC, et al. (2000). The incidence and lifetime prevalence of neurological disorders in a prospective community-based study in the UK. Brain, 123(Pt 4), 665-676.

Marcel AJ, Tegner R (1993). Knowing one's plegia. Conference presentation at 11th European Workshop on Cognitive Neuropsychology. Cited in Bisiach E, and Berti A (1993). Consciousness in dyschiria. In M Gazzaniga (Ed.), The Cognitive Neurosciences. Cambridge: MIT Press.

McAlonan GM, Cheung V, et al. (2005). Mapping the brain in autism. A voxel-based MRI study of volumetric differences and intercorrelations in autism. Brain, 128(Pt 2), 268-276.

McKeith IG, Dickson DW, et al. (2005). Diagnosis and management of dementia with Lewy bodies: Third report of the DLB Consortium. Neurology, 65(12), 1863-1872.

Niznikiewicz M, Kubicki M, et al. (2003). Recent structural and functional imaging findings in schizophrenia. Current Opinion in Psychiatry, 16, 123-147.

Okie S (2006). ADHD in adults. New England Journal of Medicine, 354(25), 2637-2641.

Pai Y-C, Rogers M, et al. (1994). Alterations in weight-transfer capabilities in adults with hemiparesis. Physical Therapy, 74, 647-659.

Paule MG, Rowland AS, et al. (2000). Attention deficit/hyperactivity disorder: Characteristics, interventions and models. Neurotoxicology and Teratology, 22(5), 631-651.

Peyron R, Laurent B, et al. (2000). Functional imaging of brain responses to pain. A review and meta-analysis (2000). Neurophysiologie Clinique, 30(5), 263-288.

Rinne MB, Pasanen ME, et al. (2006). Motor performance in physically well-recovered men with traumatic brain injury. Journal of Rehabilitation Medicine, 38(4), 224-229.

Ruchinskas RA, Giuliano AJ (2003). Motor perseveration in geriatric medical patients. Archives of Clinical Neuropsychology, 18(5), 455-461.

Smutok MA, Grafman J, et al. (1989). Effects of unilateral brain damage on contralateral and ipsilateral upper extremity function in hemiplegia. Physical Therapy, 69, 195-203.

Spires TL, Orne JD, et al. (2006). Region-specific dissociation of neuronal loss and neurofibrillary pathology in a mouse model of tauopathy. American Journal of Pathology, 168(5), 1598-1607.

Staller J, Faraone SV (2006). Attention-deficit hyperactivity disorder in girls: Epidemiology and management. CNS Drugs, 20(2), 107-123.

Sterr A, Herron K, et al. (2006). Are mild head injuries as mild as we think? Neurobehavioral concomitants of chronic post-concussion syndrome. BMC Neurology, 6(1), 7.

Tang MX, Cross P, et al. (2001). Incidence of AD in African-Americans, Caribbean Hispanics, and Caucasians in northern Manhattan. Neurology, 56(1), 49-56.

Tetewsky SJ, Duffy CJ (1999). Visual loss and getting lost in Alzheimer's disease. Neurology, 52(5), 958-965.

Tranel D, Damasio AR, et al. (1994). Sensorimotor skill learning in amnesia: Additional evidence for the neural basis of nondeclarative memory. Learning and Memory, 1(3), 165-179.

Young AW, Aggleton JP, et al. (1995). Face processing impairments after amygdalotomy. Brain, 118, 15-24.

Whitnall L, McMillan TM, et al. (2006). Disability in young people and adults after head injury: 5-7 year follow up of a prospective cohort study. Journal of Neurology, Neurosurgery, and Psychiatry, 77(5), 640-645.

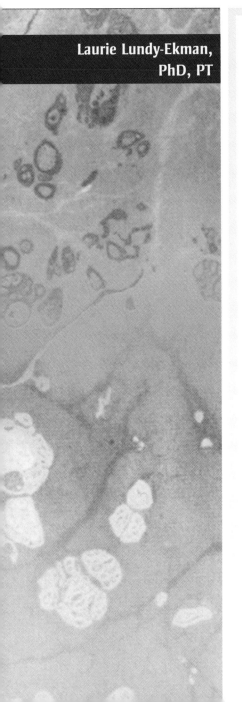

18

Support Systems: Blood Supply and Cerebrospinal Fluid System

Laurie Lundy-Ekman, PhD, PT

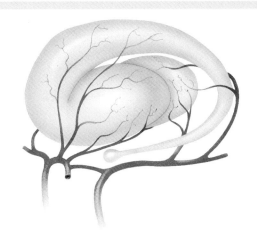

I am a 51-year-old professor of neuroanatomy. I teach physical and occupational therapy students, medical students, dental students, and undergraduates. My particular interest, in both teaching and research, is recovery of function. For 10 years or so, I was doing research on recovery from spinal cord injury using rats, but the money dried up, and I haven't done research in several years.

I have had two strokes. The first stroke was when I was 3 years old. But it was misdiagnosed at the time (they thought I had polio), and I didn't know until my twenties that I had had a stroke. People certainly recover a lot better when they are young. The second stroke occurred when I was 41.

The first signs of this stroke were a very severe headache and (so I am told, since my memory of this time was wiped out) a collapse on my left side due to left hemiparesis. My wife asked me to move my left arm. I said, "My left arm is gone. All I've got is a big hole there." This was the first sign of left side neglect. I had no transient ischemic attacks or other warning signs of impending stroke.

When I was taken into a nearby emergency room, they immediately did a CAT scan, which showed a serious right hemisphere hemorrhage. I think I was also given a lumbar puncture and an angiogram. The physician threw up his hands at the results of the scans and placed me under a no-code order that night.

I had four major effects of the stroke. One, I had a loss of proprioception, which was particularly noticeable. I could never tell where my left arm was without looking. I also had a patchy loss of touch and pain sensation (when starting dialysis, I would feel one needle going in but not the other), but I never got it mapped out. Two, I have left-side hemiparesis. I walk with a quad cane, and my left fingers are tonically flexed so that my left arm is not usable. Three, left-side neglect. At first I would bump into drinking fountains that I just didn't see. This was worst immediately after the stroke, when I missed the first word of every line I read. The neglect has gotten much better over time and is no longer a real problem. Four, I have short-term memory loss. For some reason, the short-term memory loss is worst with food. I can't remember what I eat each day, but otherwise the memory loss doesn't cause me much problem.

All of these problems have improved over time, so that they are no longer the problems they were. This is probably partly because I have learned how to get around them.

I received lots of physical therapy! Intensive PT during recovery right after the stroke (9 weeks inpatient, several months outpatient). Learning how to stand and transfer, as well as how to walk, was the most important. I have also received PT after two fractures—one of the pelvis, and one of the hip. The therapy helped me get going again.

All of the physical therapy was very effective; I couldn't function without it! Working on my own, the best exercise I get is walking as much as possible. I do some other exercises, but not too often.

I take phenobarbital, 400 mL/day, to prevent seizures, but occasionally they happen and I have to increase the dosage. I had one grand mal (generalized tonic-clonic) seizure about 2 years after the stroke, but no subsequent grand mal seizures after being on this medication. I have had a number of minor atonic seizures, most of which caused no problems. My atonic seizures ("drop attacks") hit without any warning—I go along, minding my business, and suddenly find myself on the ground. I am never aware of falling, and I don't know if I lose consciousness, but probably very briefly if so. Most of the time I fall like a rag doll (no muscle tone) and don't hurt myself. As soon as I am aware of being down, I have to figure out how to get up again, which I can't do myself. Fortunately, there has always been someone around to help me up. Only twice have I had serious problems. Once, it hit me as I was getting in the shower, and I fell into the shower door, discovering on the way down that it was not shatterproof glass. I came to, lying in a sea of shards and bleeding profusely. I was lucky my wife was home, or I may not have made it. The other time was last February when I collapsed while walking home from the bus stop one night and fractured my hip. That was nasty, requiring 4 months of hospitalization.

The biggest change due to the stroke was not a physical one but a mental one. I felt very positive, despite the stroke, and felt that life was really good! In addition I discovered new social skills that I never had before and also had wonderfully creative thoughts drop in on me. These changes are described in my book *Life at a Snail's Pace*, published in 1995 by Peanut Butter Publishing in Seattle, Washington.

—*Dr. Roger Harris*

INTRODUCTION

Two fluid systems support the neurons and glial cells of the nervous system: the cerebrospinal fluid (CSF) system and the vascular system. The CSF system includes the ventricles, the meninges, and the CSF. The vascular system includes the arterial supply, veins and venous sinuses, and mechanisms to regulate blood flow.

CEREBROSPINAL FLUID SYSTEM

The CSF system regulates the extracellular milieu and protects the central nervous system. The CSF is formed primarily in the ventricles and then circulates through the ventricles and into the subarachnoid space (between the arachnoid and pia mater) prior to being absorbed into the venous circulation. The CSF supplies water, certain amino acids, and specific ions to the extracellular fluid and probably removes metabolites from the brain. The CSF and extracellular fluid freely communicate in the brain. The meninges and the buoyancy of the fluid provide protection to the brain by absorbing some of the impact when the head is struck (Czosnyka et al., 2004).

Ventricles

The CSF-filled spaces inside the brain form a system of four ventricles (Figure 18-1). The **lateral ventricles** are paired, one in each cerebral hemisphere. The *C*-shaped lateral ventricles consist of a body; an atrium; and anterior, posterior, and inferior horns. The spaces extend into each lobe of the hemispheres. Much of the outside wall of the lateral ventricle is formed by the caudate nucleus, and the tail of the caudate is above the inferior horn. Below the body of the lateral ventricle is the thalamus; above is the corpus callosum. The lateral ventricles connect to each other and to the third ventricle by the interventricular foramina (foramina of Monro).

The **third ventricle** is a narrow slit in the midline of the diencephalon; thus its walls are the thalamus and hypothalamus. An interthalamic adhesion often crosses the center of the third ventricle. A canal through the midbrain, the cerebral aqueduct (aqueduct of Sylvius) connects the third and fourth ventricles.

The **fourth ventricle** is a space posterior to the pons and medulla and anterior to the cerebellum. Inferiorly the fourth ventricle is continuous with the central canal of the spinal cord. The fourth ventricle drains into the subarachnoid space via three small openings: the two

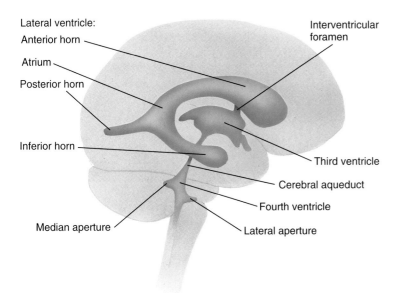

Lateral ventricle:
Anterior horn
Atrium
Posterior horn

Inferior horn

Median aperture

Interventricular foramen

Third ventricle
Cerebral aqueduct
Fourth ventricle
Lateral aperture

A

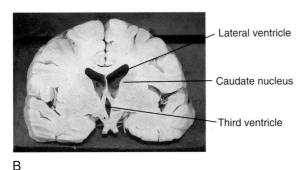

Lateral ventricle

Caudate nucleus

Third ventricle

B

FIGURE 18-1
Ventricles. **A,** Lateral view of the ventricles. **B,** Coronal section of the brain showing the lateral and third ventricles.

lateral foramina (foramina of Luschka) and a midline opening (foramen of Magendie).

Meninges

Three layers of **meninges** cover the brain and spinal cord. From external to internal, the layers are the dura mater, arachnoid, and pia mater. The **dura mater** surrounds the brain and consists of an outer layer firmly bound to the inside of the skull and an inner layer. The inner layer attaches to the arachnoid. The two layers are fused except at the dural sinuses, which are spaces for the collection of venous blood and CSF. The inner layer of dura has two projections: the falx cerebri, separating the cerebral hemispheres, and the tentorium cerebelli, separating the cerebellum from the cerebral hemispheres.

Spinal dura is continuous with the inner layer of brain dura.

The **arachnoid** is a delicate membrane loosely attached to the dura. Projections of arachnoid form arachnoid villi, which pierce the dura and protrude into the venous sinuses. The arachnoid villi allow CSF to flow into the sinuses. Clusters of arachnoid villi form arachnoid granulations (Figure 18-2).

Pia mater, the innermost layer, is tightly apposed to the surfaces of the brain and spinal cord. Arachnoid trabeculae (collagen fibers) connect the arachnoid and pia mater, serving to suspend the brain in the meninges. The subarachnoid space, between the pia and arachnoid, is filled with CSF. Extensions of the pia, the denticulate ligaments, anchor the spinal cord to the dura mater.

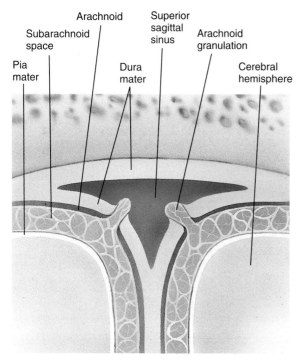

FIGURE 18-2
Coronal section through the skull, meninges, and cerebral hemispheres. This section shows the midline structures near the top of the skull. The three layers of meninges, the superior sagittal sinus, and the arachnoid granulations are indicated.

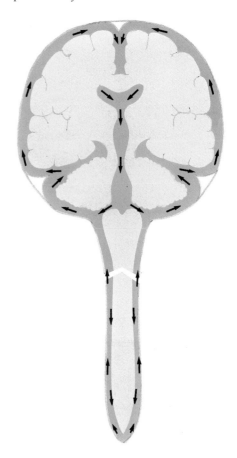

FIGURE 18-3
The flow of CSF from the lateral ventricles, third ventricle, and fourth ventricle into the subarachnoid space surrounding the brain and spinal cord. The CSF is reabsorbed into the venous sinuses.

Formation and Circulation of Cerebrospinal Fluid

Although some CSF is formed by extracellular fluid leaking into the ventricles, choroid plexuses in the ventricles secrete most CSF. A choroid plexus is a network of capillaries embedded in connective tissue and epithelial cells. Through three layers of cells (capillary wall, connective tissue, and epithelium), CSF is formed from blood by filtration, active transport, and facilitated transport of certain substances. These processes result in the formation of a fluid similar to plasma.

The CSF flows from the lateral ventricles into the third ventricle via the interventricular foramina and from the third ventricle into the fourth via the cerebral aqueduct (Figure 18-3). The CSF exits the fourth ventricle through the lateral and medial foramina, entering the subarachnoid space. Within the subarachnoid space, the fluid flows around the spinal cord and brain. Finally the CSF is absorbed through the arachnoid villi,

which project through the dura and into the venous sinuses. In the unidirectional flow of CSF into venous blood, all contents of the CSF (proteins, microorganisms) are included.

Clinical Disorders of the Cerebrospinal Fluid System

Common disorders of the CSF system include epidural and subdural hematomas, hydrocephalus, and meningitis. The hematomas are usually a consequence of trauma. Normally only potential spaces exist between the dura and skull and between the dura and arachnoid. Bleeding into either of these potential spaces can cause separation of the layers, resulting in an epidural or subdural hematoma. **Epidural hematoma** results from arterial bleeding between the skull and dura mater. Most often an epidural hematoma occurs when the middle meningeal artery is torn by a fracture of the temporal or parietal bone. Because arteries bleed rapidly, signs and symptoms develop swiftly. After a blow to the head, the person may have a few hours of normal function and then develop a worsening headache, vomiting, decreasing consciousness, hemiparesis, and Babinski's sign. In contrast, signs and symptoms of **subdural hematoma** gradually worsen over a prolonged period (days to months). Bleeding is slow in subdural hematoma because the hematoma is produced by venous bleeding, where the blood pressure is less than in arteries. The signs and symptoms are similar to those of epidural hematoma, with confusion being more prominent. Both types of hematoma are potentially life threatening because neural tissue is compressed and displaced.

If CSF circulation is blocked, pressure builds in the ventricles, causing **hydrocephalus** (Figure 18-4, *A*). Hydrocephalus is an enlargement of the ventricles. In infants, the cranial bones have not yet fused, so the pressure causes the ventricles, hemispheres, and cranium to expand. Signs of hydrocephalus include disproportionately large head size for age, large anterior fontanel, poor feeding, inactivity, and downward gaze of the eyes (from compression of the oculomotor nerve center; Figure 18-4, *B*). Common causes of congenital hydrocephalus include failure of the fourth ventricle foramina to open, blockage of the cerebral aqueduct, cysts in the fourth ventricle (Dandy-Walker cysts), and the Arnold-Chiari malformation (see Chapter 5). Rarely, hydrocephalus may result from excessive production or inadequate reabsorption of CSF. In older children or adults, because the cranium cannot expand, excessive pressure in the ventricles compresses the nervous tissue, particularly the white matter. This commonly results in gait and balance impairments, incontinence, and headache. Frequently, frontal lobe functions are also involved (i.e., some features of emotions, planning, memory, and intellect). Language, spatial awareness, and declarative memory are spared. In progressive hydrocephalus, a shunt is implanted, usually draining a ventricle into the peritoneum (Figure 18-5). In most cases, the shunts remain in place permanently.

A technique alleged to evaluate and treat the CSF system is craniosacral therapy. Advocates of this therapy claim that CSF production is periodic, with each period of secretion followed by a period during which no CSF is produced. The fluid pressure changes purportedly

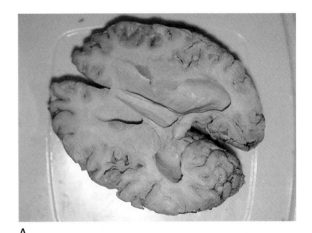

A

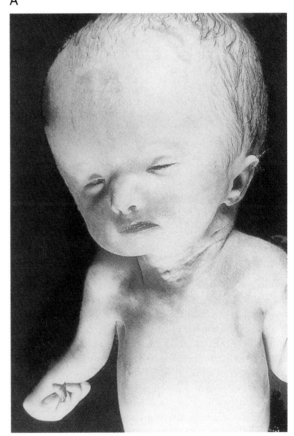

B

FIGURE 18-4

A, Horizontal section showing enlarged ventricles characteristic of hydrocephalus. Note the displacement of white matter by the excessive CSF pressure. **B,** Hydrocephalus. Abnormal accumulation of cerebrospinal fluid expands the ventricles. When hydrocephalus occurs during brain development, the pressure enlarges the skull and fontanelles. (***B** courtesy Children's Hospital Medical Center, Cincinnati, Ohio.*)

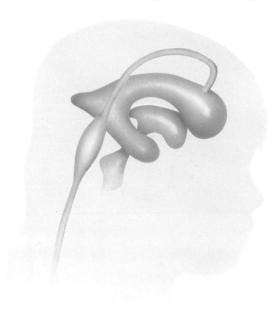

FIGURE 18-5
Placement of a shunt into the lateral ventricle to drain excessive CSF. The swelling in the shunt is the location of a valve that prevents reverse flow of fluid in the shunt.

produce a rhythmical movement of the dura that can be palpated (Upledger and Vredevoogd, 1983). Currently no evidence exists for the existence of craniosacral rhythm (pulselike movement of CSF transmitted to dural mater and to body fascia), and physical therapists' attempts to assess the rhythm have been demonstrated to be unreliable (Rogers et al., 1998; Wirth-Pattullo and Hayes, 1994).

The membranes of the cerebrospinal system may be affected by disease. **Meningitis** is the inflammation of the membranes that surround the brain and/or spinal cord. Signs and symptoms include headache, fever, confusion, vomiting, and neck stiffness. Pain intensifies in the upright position, with head movement, and with sneezing or coughing. Photophobia may accompany meningitis. Bacterial or viral infections can cause the inflammation.

DISORDERS OF VASCULAR SUPPLY

Please review the vascular supply to the nervous system, covered in Chapter 1.

The functional areas of the cerebral cortex are shown with the cerebral arteries in Figure 18-6. Loss of blood supply in a specific area correlates with a specific loss of function. For example, loss of blood supply to Broca's area interferes with expressive speech.

Interrupting the blood flow to a part of the brain usually produces a focal loss of function, except in cases of subarachnoid hemorrhage. The effects of blood flow interruption range from a brief loss of function followed by complete recovery to permanent life-altering impairments and activity limitations to death. Episodes of focal functional loss following vascular incidents are classified according to both the pattern of progression and etiology. The patterns of progression from the time of onset include the following:

- **Transient ischemic attack:** A brief, focal loss of brain function, with full recovery from neurologic deficits within 24 hours. Transient ischemic attacks (TIAs) are believed to be due to ischemia. TIA is a medical emergency despite full recovery because the risk of stroke is high following a TIA (Nguyen-Huynh and Johnston, 2005).
- **Completed stroke:** Neurologic deficits from vascular disorders that persist more than 1 day and are stable (not progressing or improving).
- **Progressive stroke:** Some people with ischemic stroke have deficits that increase intermittently over time. These are believed to be due to repeated emboli (blood clots that formed elsewhere and were transmitted by the blood to a new location) or continued formation of a thrombus (blood clot that stays where it formed).

Types of Stroke

The term *cerebrovascular accident* is synonymous with stroke. Currently some members of the medical community are advocating "brain attack" as a lay term to replace *stroke,* to emphasize that prompt treatment may benefit some people who have strokes, just as prompt treatment is effective for some heart attacks.

Brain infarction occurs when an embolus or thrombus lodges in a vessel, obstructing blood flow. Typically, an **embolus** abruptly deprives an area of blood, resulting in almost immediate onset of deficits. Sometimes the embolus breaks into fragments and is dislodged, resulting in quick resolution of deficits. More commonly,

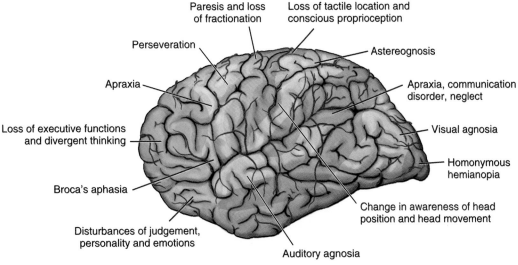

A

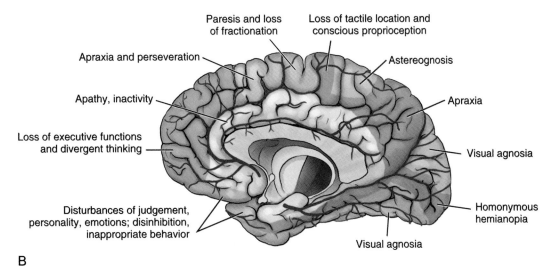

B

FIGURE 18-6
Deficits associated with loss of arterial supply to functional areas of the cerebral cortex. **A,** Lateral cortex.
B, Medial cortex. Compare with Figure 1-22, the cortical territories of the three cerebral arteries: anterior,
middle, and posterior.

residual brain damage is permanent, resulting in prolonged and incomplete functional recovery. The most rapid spontaneous recovery from ischemic stroke occurs during the first and second weeks post stroke. Infarcts cause 80% of strokes. More than 90% of anterior circulation ischemic strokes affect the middle cerebral artery

(Fisher, 1997). The incidence of ischemic stroke affecting each artery is shown in Figure 18-7.

Onset of signs from thrombic ischemia may be abrupt or may worsen over several days. Recovery from a **thrombus** is usually slow, and significant residual disability is common.

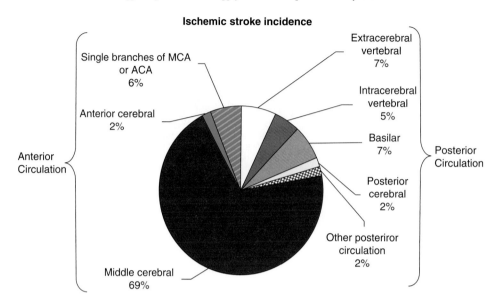

FIGURE 18-7

The incidence of ischemic stroke affecting each cerebral artery. *(Created using data from Fisher M (1997). Anterior circulation ischemia. New Horizons, 5(4), 299-304; Glass TA, Hennessey PM, et al. (2002). Outcome at 30 days in the New England Medical Center posterior circulation registry. Archives of Neurology, 59(3), 369-376; and Graf KJ, Pessin MS, et al. (1997). Proximal intracranial territory posterior circulation infarcts in the New England Medical Center Posterior Circulation Registry. European Neurology, 37(3), 157-168.)*

Obstructions of blood flow in small, deep arteries result in **lacunar infarcts.** Lacunae are small cavities that remain after the necrotic tissue is cleared away (Figure 18-8). Lacunar infarcts occur most often in the basal ganglia, internal capsule, thalamus, and brainstem. Signs of lacunar infarcts develop slowly and are often either purely motor or purely sensory, and good recovery is the norm.

The slow occlusion of an artery has a very different outcome from an abrupt occlusion. For example, if one internal carotid artery is slowly occluded, the anastomotic connections and collateral circulation among the unaffected arteries may be adequate to maintain brain function. Less frequently, an abrupt internal carotid occlusion is fatal due to infarction of the anterior two-thirds of the cerebral hemisphere. The difference in outcome is explained by the time course of occlusion, the location of the occlusion, blood pressure at the time of the occlusion, and individual variation in collateral connections. Gradual occlusion may allow development of increased collateral circulation. Low blood pressure during the occlusion makes adequate perfusion of the brain less likely.

Hemorrhage deprives the downstream vessels of blood, and the extravascular blood exerts pressure on the surrounding brain. Generally, hemorrhagic strokes present with the worst deficits within hours of onset, and then improvement occurs as edema decreases and extravascular blood is removed. Severe hemorrhage within the brain tissue is shown in Figure 18-9.

Subarachnoid hemorrhage Bleeding into the subarachnoid space usually causes sudden, excruciating headache with a brief (a few minutes) loss of consciousness. Unlike other hemorrhages, the initial findings often are not focal. Deficits from subarachnoid hemorrhage are progressive because of continued bleeding or secondary hydrocephalus. Vasospasm and infarction are common sequelae of subarachnoid hemorrhage. Figure 18-10 shows a subarachnoid hemorrhage.

Stroke Signs and Symptoms by Arterial Location

Pathology may involve the main arteries, smaller branches, the capillary network, or arteriovenous formations.

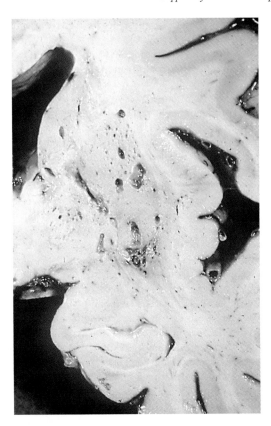

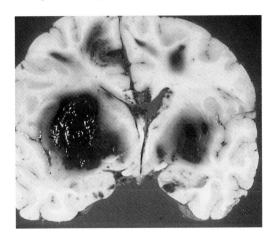

FIGURE 18-9
Multiple hemorrhages within the brain secondary to head trauma. *(Courtesy Dr. Melvin J. Ball.)*

FIGURE 18-8
Coronal section of a cerebral hemisphere, with a lateral ventricle appearing near the top-left corner. The small cavities in the basal ganglia are lacunar infarcts, produced by occlusions of small, deep arteries. *(Courtesy Dr. Melvin J. Ball.)*

Vertebral and Basilar Arteries

Twenty percent of ischemic strokes affect the brainstem/cerebellar region (Savitz and Caplan, 2005). Because the vertebral arteries are subject to shear forces at the atlantoaxial joint, abrupt neck rotation or hyperextension can cause brainstem ischemia. Ernst (2002) reviews published cases of strokes attributable to chiropractic manipulation and maintains that manipulation-induced strokes are underreported. The chief symptom of vertebral artery dissection is pain, usually in the posterior neck or occiput and spreading to the shoulders (Savitz and Caplan, 2005).

In vertebrobasilar-artery ischemia, the most common signs are gait and limb ataxia, limb weakness, oculomotor palsies, and oropharyngeal dysfunction (Savitz and Caplan, 2005). Other signs and symptoms that

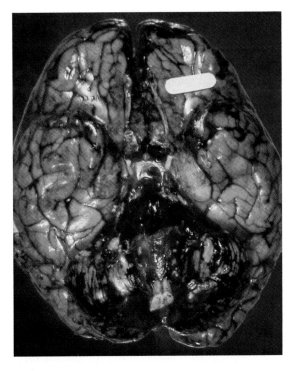

FIGURE 18-10
Subarachnoid hemorrhage is visible as dark areas, most prominent in the brainstem region. *(Courtesy Dr. Melvin J. Ball.)*

frequently occur are loss of vision, double vision, numbness, dizziness, vertigo, headache, and vomiting. Fewer than 1% of patients with vertebrobasilar ischemia have only a single presenting sign or symptom; thus isolated dizziness or brief loss of consciousness is unlikely to be caused by vertebrobasilar ischemia (Savitz and Caplan, 2005).

Emboli in the intracranial vertebral arteries usually cause cerebellar infarction. The most common symptoms in acute cerebellar infarction are dizziness and/or vertigo, inability to sit upright without support, difficulty walking, nausea and vomiting, dysarthria, and headache (Jensen and St. Louis, 2005).

A complete occlusion of the basilar artery causes death due to ischemia of brainstem nuclei and tracts that control vital functions. Partial occlusions of the basilar artery can cause tetraplegia (descending motor tracts), loss of sensation (ascending sensory tracts), coma (reticular activating system), and cranial nerve signs. Severe partial occlusion of the basilar artery causes locked-in syndrome (Savitz and Caplan, 2005), preserving consciousness but preventing voluntary movement below the neck and preventing speech (Smith and Delargy, 2005). Occlusion of a cerebellar artery causes ataxia.

Cerebral Arteries

Occlusion of the cortical branches of the **anterior cerebral artery** results in personality changes (frontal lobe) with contralateral hemiplegia and hemisensory loss. The hemiplegia and hemisensory loss are more severe in the lower limb than in the face and upper limb because the medial sensorimotor cortex and adjacent white matter are affected. Lack of blood supply to the deep branches of the anterior cerebral artery results in motor dysfunction due to damage of the anterior putamen and of frontopontine axons in the internal capsule (Hankey and Wardlaw, 2002).

Occlusion of the cortical branches of the **middle cerebral artery** deprives the optic radiation and the lateral parts of the sensorimotor cortex and adjacent white matter of blood. This produces homonymous hemianopia combined with contralateral hemiplegia and hemisensory loss involving the upper limb and face more than the lower limb because the neurons regulating movement and processing conscious sensation of the upper body are located in the lateral cerebral cortex. Language impairment is common if the lesion is in the language-dominant hemisphere (usually the left hemisphere). Difficulty understanding spatial relationships, neglect, and impairment of nonverbal communication often occur with lesions in the hemisphere that is nondominant for language (usually the right hemisphere) (Hankey and Wardlaw, 2002).

Deep branches of the middle cerebral artery (**striate arteries**) supply the striatum and the genu and limbs of the internal capsule. Loss of blood supply to the deep branches deprives axons passing through the internal capsule, producing contralateral hemiplegia that affects the upper and lower extremities and the face equally. Most ischemic strokes occlude the middle cerebral artery, often producing a stereotypic standing posture on the hemiparetic side: characteristic adduction at the shoulder, flexion at the elbow, and extension throughout the lower limb. Occlusion of the anterior choroidal artery, a branch off the internal carotid, produces contralateral hemiplegia and hemisensory loss with homonymous hemianopia by depriving axons in the posterior internal capsule of blood (Tuzun, 1998).

Occlusion of the midbrain branches of the **posterior cerebral artery** (Hankey and Wardlaw, 2002) can result in contralateral hemiparesis (cerebral peduncle) and eye movement paresis or paralysis, sparing lateral and inferomedial eye movements (oculomotor nerve and its controlling nuclei or descending neurons). Occlusion of the branches to the calcarine cortex result in cortical blindness affecting information from the contralateral visual field (see Chapter 15). Deep branches of the posterior cerebral artery supply much of the diencephalon and hippocampus. Lack of blood flow to the thalamus can cause thalamic syndrome, characterized by severe pain, contralateral hemisensory loss, and flaccid hemiparesis. Vascular compromise of the hippocampus interferes with declarative memory (see Chapter 17). Occlusion of the posterior choroidal branch prevents blood from reaching part of the thalamus and hippocampus (Figure 18-11). Table 18-1 summarizes the common deficits that occur following strokes in specific arteries.

The **watershed area,** the site of anastomoses among the distal branches of cerebral arteries, is vulnerable to ischemia (Figure 18-12). Lack of blood to the watershed region often causes upper limb paresis and paresthesias. Hypotension may result in decreased blood flow in the watershed area, thereby decreasing the effectiveness of the anastomoses (Miklossy, 2003).

> The effects of a stroke depend on the etiology, severity, and location of the stroke.

Disorders of Vascular Formation

Arteriovenous malformations are developmental abnormalities with arteries connected to veins by abnormal,

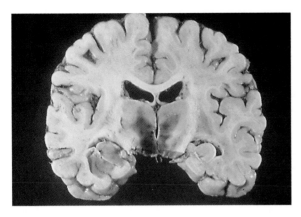

FIGURE 18-11
Occlusion of the posterior choroidal artery, producing necrosis in part of the thalamus. *(Courtesy Dr. Melvin J. Ball.)*

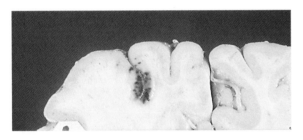

FIGURE 18-12
A coronal section near the top of the skull, showing an infarction in the watershed area. *(Courtesy Dr. Melvin J. Ball.)*

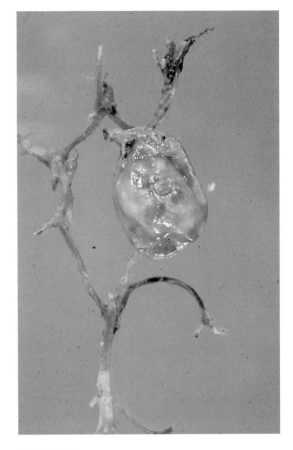

FIGURE 18-13
A large berry aneurysm at the end of the right internal carotid artery. *(Courtesy Dr. Melvin J. Ball.)*

thin-walled vessels larger than capillaries. The malformations usually do not cause signs or symptoms until they rupture; then the bleeding causes dysfunction due to lack of blood to the area the arteries normally supply and due to pressure exerted by the extravascular blood. Rupture of an arteriovenous malformation can cause subdural hematoma, intracerebral hemorrhage, or both, depending on the location of the malformation.

Aneurysm is a dilation of the wall of an artery or vein. These swellings have thin walls that are prone to rupture. Saccular aneurysms are most common, affecting only one side of the vessel wall. A berry aneurysm, a type of saccular aneurysm, is a small sac that protrudes from a cerebral artery and has a thin connection with the artery (Figure 18-13). The hemorrhage resulting from aneurysm rupture may be massive, causing sudden death, or causing a wide variety of signs and symptoms depending on the location and extent of the bleeding. The bleeding

is into the subarachnoid space, producing subdural hematoma.

FLUID DYNAMICS

Blood-Brain Barrier

The blood-brain barrier is a specialized permeability barrier between the capillary endothelium of the central nervous system and the extracellular space. The barrier is formed by tight junctions between the capillary endothelial cells that exclude large molecules (free fatty acids, proteins, specific amino acids). This exclusion is useful for preventing many pathogens from entering the central

Table 18-1   STROKE: COMMON DEFICITS

Type of Deficit	Anterior Cerebral Artery	Middle Cerebral Artery	Posterior Cerebral Artery	Basilar Artery
Somatosensory	Loss of sensation in lower limb	Hemianesthesia affecting face and upper limb more than lower limb	Hemianesthesia	Bilateral sensory loss
Motor	Apraxia; hemiplegia (lower limb more affected than upper limb and face); impaired gait	Face and upper limb more impaired than lower limb; if striate arteries involved, lower limb paresis or paralysis in addition to face and upper limb impairment	Hemiparesis; if lesion near origin of artery, vertical gaze palsy, oculomotor nerve palsy, loss of medial deviation of the eyes with preserved convergence, vertical skew deviation of the eyes	Tetraplegia; abducens nerve palsy (palsy of lateral gaze); locked-in syndrome; oculomotor nerve palsy; decorticate or decerebrate rigidity; paresis or paralysis of muscles of the tongue, lips, palate, pharynx, and larynx
Special senses and autonomic function		Homonymous hemianopia	Homonymous hemianopia; cortical blindness; hallucinations; lack of depth perception; impaired eye movements, except lateral and infero-medial eye movements; visual agnosia	Vertigo, vomiting, nausea, nystagmus
Emotions and behavior	Flat affect; impulsiveness; perseveration; confusion; motor inactivity	If right hemisphere (left hemiplegia): easily distracted, poor judgment, impulsiveness; if left hemisphere phere (right hemiplegia): apraxia, compulsiveness, overly cautious		

Table 18-1 STROKE: COMMON DEFICITS—cont'd

Type of Deficit	Anterior Cerebral Artery	Middle Cerebral Artery	Posterior Cerebral Artery	Basilar Artery
Mentation, language, and memory	Difficulty with divergent thinking	Aphasia if language-dominant hemisphere is affected; difficulty understanding spatial relationships, neglect, impairment of nonverbal communication, dressing apraxia, constructional apraxia if hemisphere that is not language-dominant is affected	Memory loss	Reduced consciousness
Other	Urinary incontinence		Thalamic syndrome (temporary hemiparesis; severe loss of somatosensation; slow pain sensation is preserved; limbs may show vasomotor and/or trophic abnormalities)	Coma; pupil constriction (involvement of descending sympathetic fibers in the pons; however, pupils may be reactive to light)

Derived from Hankey and Wardlaw, 2002.
NOTE: This table indicates possible consequences of lesions involving each of the major arteries. Depending on the distribution and severity of the occlusion or hemorrhage, various subsets of the signs listed would occur.

nervous system (Takahashi and Macdonald, 2004); however, the barrier also prevents certain drugs and protein antibodies from accessing the brain. For example, in the early stages of Parkinson's disease, dopamine delivered to the brain can ameliorate the signs and symptoms. However, dopamine cannot cross the blood-brain barrier. Therefore a metabolic precursor of dopamine, called *l-dopa,* is given to people with Parkinson's disease; l-dopa can cross the blood-brain barrier. Once l-dopa is in the brain, it is converted into dopamine. Currently, the intentional disruption of the blood-brain barrier is an experimental method of delivering some medications to the central nervous system.

The blood-brain barrier is absent in areas of the brain that directly sample the contents of the blood or secrete into the bloodstream. These regions include parts of the hypothalamus and other specialized areas around the third and fourth ventricles. Specialized ependymal cells (tanycytes) separate the leaky regions from the rest of the brain; these special cells may prevent proteins, viruses, and some drugs from entering the brain via the leaky regions.

Cerebral Blood Flow

Because the brain cannot store glucose or oxygen effectively, a consistent blood supply is essential. Oxygen consumption increases from brainstem to cerebral cortex, leaving the cerebral cortex more vulnerable to hypoxia than vital centers in the lower brainstem (Wilson et al., 2003). This differential oxygen requirement explains some incidents of persistent vegetative state. In some cases of persistent vegetative state, severe head trauma or anoxia destroys the cerebral and cerebellar cortices, yet the person survives because the brainstem and spinal cord functions continue (Wilson et al., 2003).

Cerebral arteries **autoregulate** local blood flow, depending primarily on two factors: blood pressure and metabolites. The arteries dilate if blood pressure, oxygen, or pH levels are inadequate, or if carbon dioxide or lactic acid are excessive. Conversely, when blood pressure, oxygen, or pH levels are excessive, or carbon dioxide or lactic acid levels are below functional levels, the arteries constrict. A minor role in regulating arterial diameter is played by autonomic and other neuron systems within the brain; these mechanisms are currently not well understood. Autoregulation is vitally important to ensure adequate blood flow and to prevent brain edema.

Cerebral Edema

Cerebral edema is the accumulation of excess tissue fluid in the brain. Concussion frequently causes cerebral edema because trauma allows fluid to leak from the damaged capillaries. Cardiac arrest and high altitude may also cause cerebral edema. High Altitude Cerebral Edema (HACE) is a frequently fatal form of altitude sickness (Hackett and Roach, 2004). Signs and symptoms include headache, weakness, disorientation, memory loss, hallucinations, psychotic behavior, coma, and less frequently, ataxia. Edema is often progressive because the fluid pressure results in ischemia, causing arterioles to dilate, increasing the capillary pressure, and producing more edema. Also, lack of oxygen to a region of the brain makes the capillaries more permeable, and thus more fluid escapes into the extracellular compartment. Edema can be alleviated by shunts or medications or, in the case of HACE, by moving to a lower altitude.

INCREASES IN INTRACRANIAL PRESSURE

Cerebral edema, hydrocephalus, tumors, and other lesions that occupy space in the brain can cause an increase in intracranial pressure. Symptoms include vomiting and nausea (pressure on vagus nerve), headache (increased capillary pressure), drowsiness, frontal lobe gait ataxia,

and visual and eye movement problems (pressure on optic and oculomotor nerves).

Space-occupying lesions may produce herniation (protrusion) of part of the brain. Pressure from a hemorrhage, edema, or a tumor can cause displacements of brain structures that have grave consequences.

Uncal Herniation

Uncal herniation occurs when a space-occupying lesion in the temporal lobe displaces the uncus medially, forcing the uncus into the opening of the tentorium cerebelli. In turn, this compresses the midbrain, interfering with the function of the oculomotor nerve and consciousness (effect on ascending reticular activating system). Figure 18-14 shows an infarct secondary to uncal herniation.

Central Herniation

Central herniation occurs when a space-occupying lesion in the cerebrum exerts pressure on the diencephalon, moving the diencephalon, midbrain, and pons inferiorly. This movement stretches the branches of the basilar artery, causing brainstem ischemia and edema. Bilateral

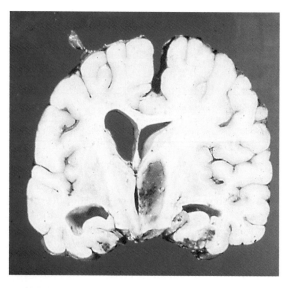

FIGURE 18-14
A large subdural hematoma displaced the right cerebral hemisphere, causing uncal herniation. Note the distortion of the shape of the lateral ventricles and that both lateral ventricles and the third ventricle are to the left of the midline. An infarct of the posterior cerebral artery occurred secondary to the uncal herniation. *(Courtesy Dr. Melvin J. Ball.)*

paralysis ensues (due to damage to upper motor neurons), and consciousness and oculomotor control are impaired.

Tonsillar Herniation

Pressure from an uncal herniation, a tumor in the brainstem/cerebellar region, hemorrhage, or edema may force the cerebellar tonsils (small lobes forming part of the inferior surface of the cerebellum) through the foramen magnum. Tonsillar herniation compresses the brainstem, interfering with vital signs, consciousness, and flow of CSF.

LABORATORY EVALUATION OF CEREBRAL BLOOD FLOW

Blood flow to the brain can be evaluated by **positron emission tomography** (PET) scan or **angiography**. A PET scan is a computer-generated image based on the metabolism of injected radioactively labeled substances (Figure 18-15). A PET scan records local variations in

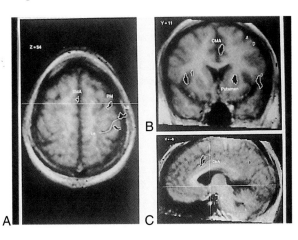

FIGURE 18-15
Positron emission tomography scan. These scans show the cortical areas that have significantly more regional blood flow during self-paced finger flexions than during visually triggered finger flexions or during rest. The colors indicate the level of metabolic activity: red is highest, orange is high, yellow is moderate, green is low, and blue is lowest. SMA, supplemental motor area; PM, premotor area; M1, primary motor cortex; CMA, cingulate motor cortex. The CMA is a region that has not been studied extensively. **A,** Horizontal section. Posterior to the central sulcus (CS), increased activation of the primary somatosensory cortex is visible. **B,** Coronal section. **C,** Midsaggital section. *(From Rapid Science Publishers Ltd. from Larsson J, Bulyas B, et al. (1996). Cortical representation of self-paced finger movement. NeuroReport, 7(2), 466.*

blood flow, reflecting neural activity. Angiography consists of a radiopaque dye injected into a carotid or vertebral artery followed by a sequence of x-rays (Figure 18-16). Typically the end of a plastic catheter inserted into the femoral artery is moved to the origin of the vessel to be visualized, and then the dye is injected. In the first series of x-rays, the arteries are visible; later, as the dye circulates, the veins are seen. Angiography is particularly useful for visualizing aneurysms, occlusions, and malformations of the arteriovenous system; however, thrombosis and embolization are risks with this invasive procedure.

VENOUS SYSTEM

The spinal cord and lower medulla drain into small veins that run longitudinally. These veins drain into radicular veins, which then empty into the epidural venous plexus.

The major venous system of the brain consists of cerebral veins. These veins drain into **dural sinuses** (Figure 18-17) and eventually into the internal jugular vein (Figure 18-18). Cerebral veins interconnect extensively. Two sets of veins drain the cerebrum: superficial and deep. The superficial veins drain cortex and the adjacent white matter, then empty into the superior

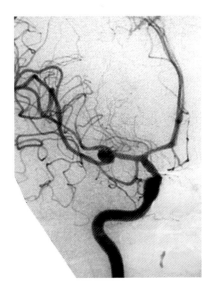

FIGURE 18-16
Angiogram showing an aneurysm arising from the middle cerebral artery.

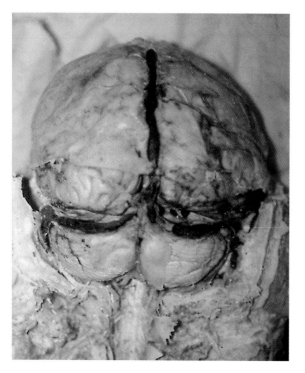

FIGURE 18-17

Posterior view of the dura mater covering the brain, with the dural (venous) sinuses exposed. The superior sagittal sinus (between the superior parts of the cerebral hemispheres) and the transverse sinuses (between the cerebral and cerebellar hemispheres) are visible.

sagittal sinus or one of the sinuses around the inferior cerebrum. The deep cerebral veins drain the basal ganglia, diencephalon, and nearby white matter, then empty into the straight sinus. The superior sagittal and straight sinuses join at the confluence of the sinuses. The transverse sinuses arise from the confluence and connect with the internal jugular veins.

SUMMARY

The CSF is produced in the ventricles as a filtrate of blood. The CSF cushions the brain and spinal cord, provides nutrients and ionic balance in the CNS, and removes waste. CSF flows from the lateral ventricles to the third ventricle via the interventricular foramina then via the cerebral aqueduct into to the fourth ventricle. The fourth ventricle has small openings that allow the flow of CSF into the subarachnoid space. CSF returns to the blood in the dural sinuses. The meninges protect the brain and confine the CSF. Disorders of the CSF system include epidural and subdural hematoma and hydrocephalus.

Blood is supplied to the brain via the vertebral and internal carotid arteries. The two vertebral arteries join to form the basilar artery, and the basilar artery divides to become the posterior cerebral arteries. The internal

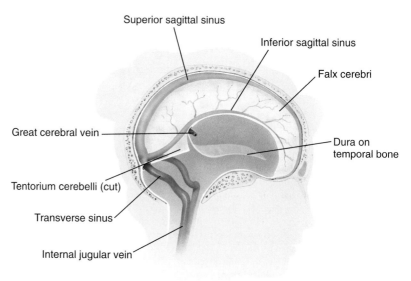

FIGURE 18-18

The venous system of the brain. The venous sinuses eventually drain into the internal jugular vein.

carotid has two large branches, the anterior and middle cerebral arteries. Strokes are classified according to their pattern of progression (transient ischemic attack, completed stroke, or progressive stroke), the etiology (infarction, hemorrhage, subarachnoid hemorrhage), and by arterial location. Developmental disorders of vascular formation include arteriovenous malformations and aneurysms. The blood-brain barrier protects the brain from toxins, pathogens, and specific drugs. Blood flow in local areas is autoregulated by cerebral arteries. Cerebral edema and excessive intracranial pressure interfere with brain function and may be fatal.

CLINICAL NOTES

For each of the following cases, answer the following questions:
1. Which vertical systems are involved?
2. Where is the lesion?
3. What is the likely etiology?

Case 1

BT, a 54-year-old man, reports sudden and complete loss of ability to move his legs. No trauma occurred.

- Pain and temperature sensation have been lost bilaterally below T9. All sensations are intact above T9.
- Localized touch, vibration, and position senses are intact throughout the entire body.
- Motor examination reveals bilateral paralysis below T9. The motor system is normal above T9.

Case 2

LS, a 72-year-old woman, awoke 3 days ago with severe weakness and loss of sensation on the left side of her body and lower face. All sensory and motor functions on the right side are within normal limits.

- Sensory testing reveals responsiveness only to deep pinch on the left side.
- She cannot move any joint on the left side independent of the movement of other joints. When she attempts to reach forward, no flexion occurs at the shoulder; instead, her shoulder elevates, and elbow flexion increases.
- In sitting or assisted standing, she does not bear weight on the left. She cannot walk, even with assistance. She steps forward with the right lower limb, then lurches forward and attempts to continue stepping with the right lower limb, dragging the left lower limb.
- Her gaze tends to be directed toward the right. Even with cuing or loud noises on the left side, she does not turn her head or eyes to the left of midline. She seems unaware of the left side of her body.
- Her ability to converse is normal.

Case 3

KF, a 9-month-old boy, has an enlarged cranium and is being assessed for possible developmental delay.

- Sensation is normal.
- KF cannot sit unsupported. In supported sitting, he is unable to hold his head in neutral for more than 10 seconds. He moves very little. In supine position, his limbs tend to flop out to the sides, and he does not turn from back to side.
- His gaze is directed downward.

Note: Healthy children achieve unsupported sitting between the ages of 4 and 8 months; turning from back to side is usually achieved by 7 months.

REVIEW QUESTIONS

1. What are the functions of the CSF?
2. Where is CSF located?
3. Why is there a difference in pattern of progression between an epidural hematoma and a subdural hematoma?
4. In an infant, an abnormally large head size, inactivity, insufficient feeding, and downward gaze of both eyes may indicate what disorder?
5. Can hydrocephalus occur in adults?
6. What is the watershed area?
7. What is transient ischemic attack?
8. What is a lacuna?
9. A partial occlusion of which artery can result in tetraplegia, loss of sensation, coma, and cranial nerve signs?
10. Hemiplegia and hemisensory loss that are more severe in the lower limb than in the upper limb and face indicate that what part of the brain is affected? What artery supplies this region?
11. Neglect, poor understanding of spatial relationships, and impairment of nonverbal communication are signs of damage to what part of the brain? Which artery supplies this region?
12. If hemiplegia and hemisensory loss affect the upper and lower limbs and the face equally, where is the lesion? Branches of what major artery supply this region?
13. Eye movement paresis with sparing of lateral and inferomedial eye movements combined with contralateral hemiplegia indicates a lesion located where? Which artery supplies this region?
14. What arteries supply the watershed area?
15. What is an arteriovenous malformation?
16. What is an aneurysm?
17. What is an uncal herniation?
18. What is a PET scan?

References

Czosnyka M, Czosnyka Z, et al. (2004). Cerebrospinal fluid dynamics. Physiological Measurement, 25(5), R51-R76.

Ernst E (2002). Manipulation of the cervical spine: A systematic review of case reports of serious adverse events, 1995-2001. Medical Journal of Australia, 176(8), 376-380.

Fisher M (1997). Anterior circulation ischemia. New Horizons, 5(4), 299-304.

Glass TA, Hennessey PM, et al. (2002). Outcome at 30 days in the New England Medical Center posterior circulation registry. Archives of Neurology, 59(3), 369-376.

Graf KJ, Pessin MS, et al. (1997). Proximal intracranial territory posterior circulation infarcts in the New England Medical Center Posterior Circulation Registry. European Neurology, 37(3), 157-168.

Hackett PH, Roach RC (2004). High altitude cerebral edema. High Altitude Medicine & Biology, 5(2), 136-146.

Hankey GJ, Wardlaw JM (2002). Clinical Neurology. (pp. 181-183). New York, Demos Medical Publishing.

Jensen MB, St. Louis EK (2005). Management of acute cerebellar stroke. Archives of Neurology, 62(4), 537-544.

Miklossy J (2003). Cerebral hypoperfusion induces cortical watershed microinfarcts which may further aggravate cognitive decline in Alzheimer's disease. Neurological Research, 25(6), 605-610.

Nguyen-Huynh MN, Johnston SC (2005). Transient ischemic attack: A neurologic emergency. Current Neurology and Neuroscience Reports, 5(1), 13-20.

Rogers JS, Witt PL, et al. (1998). Simultaneous palpation of the craniosacral rate at the head and feet: Intrarater and interrater reliability and rate comparisons. Physical Therapy, 78(11), 1175-1185.

Savitz SI, Caplan LR (2005). Vertebrobasilar disease. New England Journal of Medicine, 352(25), 2618-2626.

Smith E, Delargy M (2005). Locked-in syndrome. British Medical Journal, 330(7488), 406-409.

Takahashi M, Macdonald RL (2004). Vascular aspects of neuroprotection. Neurological Research, 26(8), 862-869.

Tuzun E (1998). Anterior choroidal artery territory infarction: A case report and review. Archives of Medical Research, 29(1), 83-87.

Upledger JE, Vredevoogd JD (1983). Craniosacral Therapy. Seattle: Eastland Press.

Wilson FC, Harpur J, et al. (2003). Adult survivors of severe cerebral hypoxia—Case series survey and comparative analysis. NeuroRehabilitation, 18(4), 291-298.

Wirth-Pattullo V, and Hayes KW (1994). Interrater reliability of craniosacral rate measurements and their relationship with subjects' and examiners' heart and respiratory rate measurements. Physical Therapy, 74, 908-920.

Appendix A

Intracellular Messengers

Neurons frequently use three intracellular messenger molecules:

- Cyclic adenosine monophosphate (cAMP)
- Arachidonic acid
- Inositol triphosphate

Cyclic adenosine monophosphate (cAMP): One example of a G-protein–mediated second-messenger system involves the activation of the enzyme adenylyl cyclase, which converts adenosine triphosphate to cAMP (see Figure 3-10 and Appendix Figure 1-1, A). Increases in cAMP levels modulate membrane receptors or cAMP-dependent cytoplasmic protein enzymes. Membrane channels may be opened, regulating ionic flux into the cell, and a variety of cell regulation and gene expression

pathways may be activated by the cytoplasmic proteins. For example, the transmission of pain information in the peripheral nervous system is thought to involve a cAMP-dependent ion channel. Administering morphine may provide relief of pain when morphine binds to a receptor that activates a G-protein, which then inhibits adenylyl cyclase. Inhibition of adenylyl cyclase and subsequent inhibition of a cAMP-dependent ion channel may inhibit sensory afferents conveying information about tissue damage from the periphery to the central nervous system and thus relieve pain (Ingram and Williams, 1994).

Arachidonic acid: Another second-messenger system that uses G-protein activation targets the enzyme called phospholipase A_2. This system results in the liberation

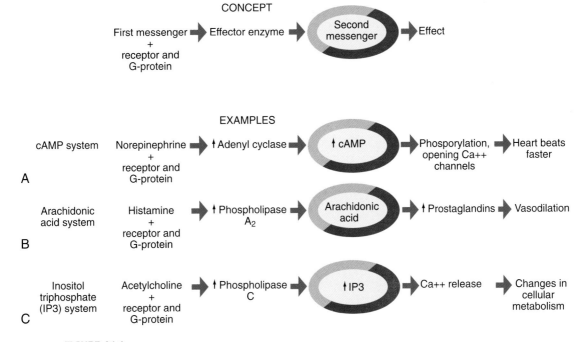

FIGURE A1-1

G-protein-mediated second-messenger systems. All three systems shown involve (1) binding of a neurotransmitter to a G-protein–associated membrane receptor, (2) activation of an effector enzyme, (3) increased levels of a second messenger, and (4) a cellular and physiologic event.

of arachidonic acid as its second messenger and the initiation of a metabolic cascade that leads to the production of prostaglandins (Appendix Figure 1-1, *B*). Prostaglandins are substances that regulate vasodilation and increase inflammation. Histamine is a neurotransmitter that acts through the arachidonic acid pathway. Aspirin and other nonsteroidal anti-inflammatory drugs act to reduce pain by inhibiting one of the enzymes in this G-protein–initiated cascade.

Inositol trisphosphate: In addition to playing a role in the management of pain, G-proteins also play a role in many other nervous system functions. The second-messenger pathway of inositol trisphosphate (IP_3) acts in the release of Ca^{++} from internal stores so that it can be used in a variety of cellular metabolic processes (Stehno-Bittel et al., 1995) (Appendix Figure 1-1, *C*). When a first messenger binds to a receptor, it activates a G-protein, which in turn activates the enzyme phospholipase C. Activation of the enzyme results in the production of the second-messenger IP_3, which diffuses into the cytoplasm to stimulate release of Ca^{++} from the endoplasmic reticulum.

References

Ingram SL, Williams JT (1994). Opioid inhibition of Ih via adenylyl cyclase. Neuron, 13, 179-186.

Stehno-Bittel L, Luckhoff A, et al. (1995). Calcium release from the nucleus by InsP3 receptor channels. Neuron, 14, 163-167.

Appendix B

Neurotransmitters and Neuromodulators

INTRODUCTION

Neurotransmitters and neuromodulators are chemical compounds that convey information among neurons. A neurotransmitter is released by a presynaptic neuron and acts directly on postsynaptic ion channels or activates proteins inside the postsynaptic neuron. The duration of neurotransmitter activity ranges from 1/1,000 of a second to minutes. Neuromodulators are released into extracellular fluid and modulate the activity of many neurons. Typically neuromodulators require seconds before their cellular effects can be observed, and the effects last minutes to days.

Rigid distinctions cannot be made between neurotransmitters and neuromodulators because a single compound may act as a neurotransmitter at some sites in the nervous system and as a neuromodulator at other sites. For example, Substance P acts as a neurotransmitter between the first- and second-order neurons in the nociceptive pathway but as a neuromodulator in the hypothalamus.

ACETYLCHOLINE

Acetylcholine plays the major role in transmitting information in the peripheral nervous system. Acetylcholine is the transmitter released by motor neurons, parasympathetic neurons, and preganglionic sympathetic neurons. In the central nervous system, acetylcholine is involved with the selection of objects of attention and with autonomic regulation. Sources of acetylcholine in the central nervous system include the pedunculopontine nucleus, the basal nucleus of Meynert, and the basal forebrain. Receptors for acetylcholine are nicotinic (brief opening of ion channels) or muscarinic (slow-acting G-protein–mediated effects). Activation of nicotinic receptors initiates skeletal muscle contraction. Activation of muscarinic receptors in cardiac muscle membrane reduces heart rate. An autoimmune disease, myasthenia gravis, causes the destruction of acetylcholine receptors on skeletal muscle membranes.

AMINO ACID TRANSMITTERS

GABA

GABA is a major inhibitory neurotransmitter. Two types of GABA receptors exist: $GABA_A$ and $GABA_B$. When GABA binds with $GABA_A$ receptors, Cl^- channels open, producing hyperpolarization of the postsynaptic membrane. Benzodiazepines (anti-anxiety and anticonvulsant drugs) and barbiturates (tranquilizing drugs) also activate $GABA_A$ receptors and thus hyperpolarize postsynaptic membranes. $GABA_B$ receptors are linked to ion channels via second-messenger systems. Baclofen, a muscle relaxant used to treat excessive muscle activity, increases the presynaptic release of GABA that activates the $GABA_B$ receptors in the spinal cord.

Glycine

Glycine inhibits postsynaptic membranes, primarily in the brainstem and spinal cord. Glycine also prevents desensitization of the N-methyl-D-aspartate (NMDA) receptor.

Glutamate

Glutamate is the excitatory neurotransmitter that activates the NMDA receptor. The NMDA receptor is an excitatory amino acid receptor with six different binding sites. The NMDA receptor has been implicated in long-term potentiation, a possible mechanism of neural plasticity during development and learning. Overactivity of NMDA receptor channels may produce epileptic seizures. Excitotoxicity, the death of neurons from overexcitation, is due to persistent opening of many NMDA receptor channels. The anesthetic ketamine is an NMDA antagonist. Other non-NMDA glutamate receptors are both the direct-action ion-channel type (kainate and AMPA receptors) and the G-protein–mediated receptor type (metabotropic glutamate receptors).

AMINES

The monoamines include the catecholamines dopamine, norepinephrine, and epinephrine, and the indolamine, serotonin. Dopamine, norepinephrine, and serotonin usually have inhibitory effects on postsynaptic membranes, but sometimes are excitatory.

Dopamine

Dopamine has effects on motor activity, motivation, and cognition. Major sources of dopamine are the substantia nigra and the ventral tegmental area. Loss of dopamine from the substantia nigra is the primary deficit in Parkinson's disease. The involvement of dopamine in certain aspects of psychosis is demonstrated by the action of some antipsychotic medications that prevent the binding of dopamine to certain receptor sites. These drugs decrease hallucinations, delusions, and disorganized thinking. However, because these drugs prevent the binding of dopamine, a side effect of many of these medications is tardive dyskinesia. Tardive dyskinesia is a hyperkinetic disorder characterized by involuntary muscle contractions. Clozapine is an antipsychotic drug that binds only to one type of dopamine receptor and does not produce tardive dyskinesia. The motivational aspects of dopamine are evident in addiction to certain drugs. The action of dopamine is potentiated by cocaine, because cocaine interferes with a protein that removes dopamine from its binding site. Amphetamines increase the release of dopamine and block dopamine and norepinephrine reuptake. Finally, although some people with schizophrenia have an excess of a subtype of dopamine receptor, current evidence does not rule out effects of drug treatment as the possible cause of the abnormal concentration of dopamine receptors.

Serotonin

Serotonin adjusts the general arousal level and suppresses sensory information. For example, serotonin plays a role as part of the descending pain control system. Highest levels of serotonin are coincident with alertness; levels are low in non–REM sleep and lowest during REM sleep. Low levels of serotonin are associated with depression and suicidal behavior. The antidepressant Prozac (fluoxetine) is a selective inhibitor of serotonin reuptake.

Norepinephrine

Norepinephrine plays a vital role in active surveillance of surroundings by increasing attention to sensory information. Highest levels of norepinephrine are associated with vigilance, and lowest levels of norepinephrine occur during sleep. Norepinephrine binds to alpha and beta receptors. Norepinephrine is essential in producing the "fight or flight" reaction to stress.

Overactivity of the norepinephrine system produces fear, and in extreme cases panic, by action on cortical and limbic regions. Panic disorder is the abrupt onset of intense terror, a sense of loss of personal identity, the perception that familiar things are strange or unreal, combined with the signs of increased sympathetic nervous system activity. Panic disorder is produced by excessive levels of norepinephrine.

Adrenergic antagonists, such as propranolol, prevent the activation of beta receptors. This action prevents the sweating, rapid heartbeat, and other signs of sympathetic activation that may otherwise occur in stressful situations. Musicians and actors often take propranolol before a performance.

Post-traumatic stress disorder also involves excessive norepinephrine activity. This has been demonstrated by intravenous administration of a drug, yohimbine, that stimulates norepinephrine activity. Veterans with post-traumatic stress disorder experienced flashbacks to the traumatic event, panic, grief, intrusive thoughts about the traumatic event, and emotional numbness when given yohimbine. Control subjects experienced little effect of yohimbine.

Drugs Used to Treat Depression

Drugs effective in treating depression include mono-amine oxidase (MAO) inhibitors, tricyclic antidepressants, and selective serotonin reuptake inhibitors (SSRIs). MAO degrades catecholamines, so inhibiting MAO raises levels of norepinephrine, serotonin, and epinephrine. The main effect of tricyclic antidepressants seems to be increased activity of serotonin and alpha$_1$ (norepinephrine) receptors, and decreased activity of central beta receptors (norepinephrine). The SSRIs include Prozac (fluoxetine).

PEPTIDES

Neuroactive peptides include Substance P and endorphins.

Substance P

Substance P is found in the dorsal horn of the spinal cord, substantia nigra, amygdala, hypothalamus, and cerebral cortex. Within the spinal cord, Substance P acts as a

Table A-1 NEUROCHEMICALS AND THEIR RECEPTORS

Neurochemical	Receptors	Agonists	Antagonists
Acetylcholine	Nicotinic, muscarinic	Nicotine, muscarine	Curare, atropine
GABA	$GABA_A$, $GABA_B$	Benzodiazepines (e.g., Valium), barbiturates, Baclofen	
Glycine	Glycine		
Glutamate	NMDA, non-NMDA		
Dopamine	D_1, D_2, D_3	Cocaine, amphetamines	Antipsychotics that decrease hallucinations, delusions, and disorganized thinking (e.g., clozapine) act on D_2 receptors.
Serotonin	$5\text{-}HT_1$, $5\text{-}HT_2$, $5\text{-}HT_3$	Antidepressants, e.g., fluoxetine (Prozac)	
Norepinephrine	$\alpha 1$, $\alpha 2$ $\beta 1$, $\beta 2$		Propranolol
Substance P	NK 1 (neurokinin l)		
Endorphins	μ_1, μ_2, δ, κ_1, κ_2 (opiate)	Opioids: morphine, heroin, oxycodone	

neurotransmitter in the nociceptive pathway. At the other sites, Substance P acts as a neuromodulator, usually producing long-duration excitation of postsynaptic membranes.

Endorphins

Endorphins are found in areas with opiate receptors, including the substantia gelatinosa, hypothalamus, periventricular gray, and periaqueductal gray. Their primary action is the inhibition of slow nociceptive information.

The receptors for the various neurotransmitters and neuromodulators are summarized in Table A-1.

Suggested Readings

Bremner JD, Innis RB, et al. (1997). Positron emission tomography measurement of cerebral metabolic correlates of yohimbine administration in combat-related posttraumatic stress disorder. Archives of General Psychiatry, 54(3), 246-254.

Brunton LL, Lazo JS, et al. (2006). Goodman and Gilman's The Pharmacological Basis of Therapeutics. (11th ed.). New York: McGraw-Hill.

Cooper JR, Bloom FE, et al. (2003). The biochemical basis of neuropharmacology. (8th ed.). New York: Oxford University Press.

Mosby's Drug Consult 2006. (16th ed.). (2006). St. Louis, Missouri: Elsevier Publishing.

Preston JD, O'Neal JH, et al. (2005). Handbook of Clinical Psychopharmacology for Therapists (4th ed.). Oakland, CA: New Harbinger Publications.

Answers

CHAPTER 2

Case 1

1. The loss of myelin in the peripheral nervous system involves destruction of Schwann cells.
2. The loss of myelin lowers the membrane resistance and allows the leakage of ions across the membrane. The loss of myelin decreases the speed or blocks the propagation of action potentials.
3. The propagation of action potentials is impaired because of the leakage of ions across the membrane. Receptor potentials are not impaired, since the nerve endings of the sensory neurons are not damaged.

Case 2

1. Destruction of oligodendrocytes causes demyelination of axons within the central nervous system.
2. Increases in body temperature may alter the activity of the voltage-gated Na^+ channels, preventing the generation of an action potential.

Review Questions

1. Dendritic projections are input units for the neuron.
2. The sensory neurons that convey information from the body to the spinal cord are pseudounipolar cells. They appear to have one process; however, one axon connects the periphery to the cell body and a second axon connects the cell body to the spinal cord.
3. Multipolar cells are specialized to receive and accommodate huge amounts of synaptic input to their many dendrites.
4. Sodium (Na^+), potassium (K^+), and chloride (Cl^-) contribute to the resting potential of the cell membrane.
5. Depolarization occurs when the membrane potential becomes less negative with respect to the resting membrane potential. Hyperpolarization occurs when the membrane potential becomes more negative with respect to the resting membrane potential.
6. A membrane channel that opens when it is bound by a neurotransmitter is a ligand-gated channel.
7. The term *graded* means that both the amplitude and the duration of the electrical potential can vary depending on the stimulus, and that it is not an all-or-none event.
8. The resting membrane potential is maintained by the unequal distribution of specific ions and charged molecules across the membrane. The unequal distribution is produced by the presence of negatively charged molecules inside the neuron that are too large to diffuse through membrane channels, by the passive diffusion of ions through membrane channels, and by the Na+-K+ pump.
9. Hyperpolarization of a neuronal membrane is considered inhibitory because hyperpolarization makes the neuron less likely to generate an electrical signal.
10. Peripheral receptors have modality-gated channels.
11. Temporal summation and spatial summation of local potentials can bring the membrane to the threshold level.
12. The generation of an action potential requires the influx of Na^+. This influx is mediated by a voltage-gated channel.
13. Large-diameter axons promote faster conduction velocity of an action potential.
14. The nodes of Ranvier have a high density of voltage-gated Na^+ channels, which promotes the generation of an action potential.
15. The spinothalamic tract originates in the spinal cord and terminates in the thalamus.
16. Networks composed of interneuronal convergence and divergence are found throughout the central nervous system.
17. Glial cells have no dendrites or axons, and glial cells cannot conduct an electrical potential.
18. Astrocytes increase or decrease signaling between neurons, clean up ions and transmitters in the extracellular space and synapses, supply nutrition, and protect the central nervous system by serving as part of the blood-brain barrier.
19. Oligodendrocytes and Schwann cells form the myelin sheath around axons to promote the propagation of an action potential.

20. Oligodendrocytes are located in the central nervous system and their processes completely wrap several axons from different neurons. Schwann cells partially or completely wrap a single axon in the peripheral nervous system. In addition to insulation, Schwann cells clean up the cellular environment and provide structural support to neurons.

21. Both Guillain-Barré syndrome (acute idiopathic polyneuritis) and multiple sclerosis are autoimmune disorders that cause demyelination. Guillain-Barré syndrome is a peripheral neuropathy that affects sensory and motor function and, in severe cases, peripheral autonomic function. Most people recover completely from a single bout of Guillain-Barré syndrome. In multiple sclerosis, demyelination in the central nervous system produces plaques in the white matter. Because multiple sclerosis attacks the central nervous system, a greater variety of symptoms occur, including weakness, lack of coordination, visual problems, impaired sensation, slurred speech, memory problems, and abnormal emotional affect. Multiple sclerosis is progressive. Its course is characterized by exacerbations and remissions.

CHAPTER 3

Case 1

1. The influx of Ca^{++} into the axon terminal promotes the release of neurotransmitters. If there are fewer than normal Ca^{++} channels, then intracellular levels of Ca^{++} cannot be elevated sufficiently to cause release of the transmitter ACh.

2. Physical therapy will not be beneficial for increasing strength, since the antibodies are preventing the release of neurotransmitter necessary for muscle contraction.

Case 2

1. Small amounts of botulinum toxin A reduce involuntary muscle activity by decreasing the amount of ACh released at the neuromuscular junction.

2. No, the action of ACh on a nicotinic, ligand-gated receptor is different from the action on the muscarinic, G-protein–mediated receptor. An EPSP is initiated via direct opening of an ion channel associated with the ligand-gated receptor, whereas either an EPSP or an IPSP may be initiated by the action of an intracellular G protein associated with the G-protein–mediated receptor.

Review Questions

1. Postsynaptic inhibition involves the flux of K^+ and/or Cl^- through the membrane of a receiving, postsynaptic cell. This prevents the cell from generating an action potential. Presynaptic inhibition involves the inhibition of an axon terminal by preventing an influx of Ca^{++}. With decreases in Ca^{++} influx associated with presynaptic inhibition, less neurotransmitter is released from the terminal, resulting in decreased stimulation of the postsynaptic cell.

2. The release of neurotransmitter is dependent on Ca^{++}.

3. An EPSP is an excitatory postsynaptic potential, a local depolarization of the neuron's cell membrane. Summation of EPSPs can lead to the generation of an action potential.

4. Direct activation of a membrane channel by a neurotransmitter results in the faster generation of a synaptic potential.

5. The action of a neurotransmitter lasts less than 1/10 of a second. The action of a neuromodulator persist for minutes or days.

6. The binding of the neurotransmitter causes a change in the shape of the membrane ion channel, resulting in its opening.

7. G-proteins function as shuttles that move through the cytoplasm of the neuron to activate an effector molecule that causes cellular events.

8. The effects of a neurotransmitter depend on the action of the receptor.

9. When glutamate binds to a ligand-gated receptor, the associated membrane channel opens quickly, ions that produce membrane depolarization diffuse through the channel, and the channel quickly closes.

10. Dopamine has effects on both motor activity and thinking ability.

11. Substance P serves as a neurotransmitter conveying information interpreted as pain between the peripheral and spinal cord neurons. Substance P also serves as a neuromodulator in pain syndromes.

12. Endogenous opioid peptides inhibit neurons that convey signals interpreted as painful.

13. Glutamate and NMDA receptors are essential for long-term potentiation.

14. No, the number of receptors on a neuron's cell membrane changes according to the amount of activity at the synapses. Thus, changes in neurotransmitter or in neuromodulator activity modify the number of receptors.

CHAPTER 4

Case 1

1. Yes, it is possible for peripheral nerve axons to regenerate and recover following injury.
2. Yes, most likely with recovery of the nerve, the normal sensation should return.

Case 2

1. Damage often is not confined to the oxygen-deprived neurons. As these neurons die, they may cause death of adjacent neurons via the processes of excitotoxicity.
2. Glutamate is the principal excitatory neurotransmitter involved in excitotoxicity.

Review Questions

1. Neuroplasticity is the ability of neurons to change their function, chemical profile (amount and types of neurotransmitters produced), or structure for more than a few seconds.
2. The intent of provoking unwanted reactions in a person with tactile defensiveness is to decrease the neural response by the process of habituation.
3. The mechanism of long-term potentiation is the conversion of silent synapses into active synapses via the action of glutamate on NMDA receptors. Following NMDA activity, AMPA receptors are phosphorylated and inserted into the neuronal membrane, producing active synapses.
4. Wallerian degeneration is the process by which an axon, isolated from the cell body, undergoes a process of degeneration, followed by death of the entire distal segment.
5. The results of axonal sprouts innervating inappropriate targets are confusion of sensory modalities and/or synkinesis.
6. Yes, cortical motor and sensory maps can change, even in the adult mammal.
7. Excitotoxicity is the process by which overexcitation of a neuron leads to cell death.
8. Lactic acid is an end product of glycolysis that contributes to cell death.
9. Excessive levels of intracellular calcium promote cell death by activating calcium-dependent proteases and by activating pathways that produce oxygen free radicals.
10. Yes, some brain damage can potentially be reduced with the administration of pharmaceutical agents.
11. Constraint-induced movement following brain lesions may be harmful or beneficial, depending on how soon after the stroke the intensive therapy begins. Animal studies indicate that vigorous rehabilitation begun immediately after a brain lesion produces enlargement of the lesion. Constraint-induced movement initiated later has been shown to be beneficial in humans post-stroke.

CHAPTER 5

Case 1

1. All three systems are involved. Lack of response to stimulation indicates involvement of the sensory system, inability to voluntarily control the bladder and bowels is an autonomic nervous system problem, and inability to voluntarily move his legs is a motor deficit.
2. The lesion is in the spinal region of the nervous system. The surgery was to move nervous tissue protruding through the bony defect (meningomyelocele) into the vertebral column as much as possible to protect the nervous tissue from infection and injury. Spinal lesions interrupt ascending and descending pathways within the cord, preventing sensory information from being conveyed to the brain and motor information from traveling from the brain to motor neurons. Peripheral lesions are usually not bilateral. Unimpaired sensation and movement of the upper limbs and torso indicate that the brain connections with the upper spinal cord are functionally and anatomically intact.

Case 2

1. The motor system is involved as indicated by the excessive muscle stiffness in the lower limbs, the lower limb muscle weakness, and the motor development delay. The delayed toilet training indicates impaired voluntary control of the autonomic bladder and bowel. In this case, the somatosensory system is normal.
2. The lesion is in the cerebral region, interfering with descending motor signals from the cerebral cortex.
3. The most likely diagnosis is diplegic spastic cerebral palsy.

Review Questions

1. During the embryo stage, from the second to the end of the eighth week, the organs are formed.
2. a. A thickening of the ectoderm becomes the neural plate.
   b. The edges of the plate move toward each other, forming the neural groove.
   c. The folds touch in the dorsal midline, first in the future cervical region.

d. The folds fuse together, forming a tube that detaches from the neural crest cells and from the ectoderm that will become skin.

3. In early development, a myotome is the part of the somite that will become muscle. After the embryo stage, a myotome is a group of muscles innervated by a segmental spinal nerve.

4. After the superior neuropore closes, the region of the neural tube that will become the brain expands to form three enlargements: the hindbrain, midbrain, and forebrain. Next, the hindbrain divides into the myelencephalon and metencephalon, while the forebrain divides into the diencephalon and telencephalon. The myelencephalon and metencephalon further differentiate to become the medulla, pons, and cerebellum. The telencephalon becomes the cerebral hemispheres.

5. The progressive developmental processes are cellular proliferation, migration, and growth; extension of axons to target cells; formation of synapses; and myelination of axons.

6. The regressive developmental processes are neuronal death and axon retraction.

7. "Growing into deficit" is the appearance of signs of nervous system damage during infancy and childhood due to nervous system damage that occurred earlier. The signs are not evident until the infant or child reaches the age when the damaged system(s) would normally have become functional.

8. Anencephaly is the development of only a rudimentary brainstem, without cerebral and cerebellar hemispheres. The Arnold-Chiari deformity is a developmental malformation of the hindbrain, with an elongated inferior cerebellum and medulla that protrude into the vertebral canal. The next four are all due to incomplete closure of the caudal neural tube: in spina bifida occulta, neural tissue does not protrude through the bony defect; in meningocele, the meninges protrude through the bony defect; in meningomyelocele, neural tissue and meninges protrude outside the body; and in myeloschisis, a malformed spinal cord is open to the surface of the body.

9. The Arnold-Chiari malformation is a developmental deformity of the hindbrain. In Type I, the cerebellar tonsils protrude through the foramen magnum into the vertebral canal, and the medulla and pons are small and malformed. Frequently there are no symptoms, or symptoms are delayed until adolescence or adulthood. Headaches, sensory and motor disorders, facial and tongue weakness, hearing loss, dizziness, weakness of lateral eye movements, impaired coordination, and visual disturbances are the most common signs and symptoms. In Type II, the signs are visible during infancy. The brainstem and cerebellum protrude into the vertebral canal. Signs include paralysis of the sternocleidomastoid muscles, deafness, bilateral paresis of lateral eye movements, and facial weakness. Type II is usually associated with meningomyelocele.

10. Severe mental retardation is associated with defects in the structure of dendrites and dendritic spines.

11. Cerebral palsy is a disorder of movement and postural control due to permanent, nonprogressive damage of a developing brain. The major types of cerebral palsy are spastic, athetoid, and mixed. Causes of cerebral palsy include abnormal development in utero, metabolic abnormalities, disorders of the immune system, coagulation disorders, infections, trauma, and hypoxia.

12. Critical periods are the time when neuronal projections compete for synaptic sites. Normal function of neural systems is dependent on appropriate experience during the critical period.

CHAPTER 6

Review Questions

1. The three types of somatosensory receptors are mechanical, chemical, and temperature.

2. Nociceptors are receptors that respond to stimuli that damage or threaten to damage tissue.

3. Primary endings respond to stretch of muscle and to the rate of muscle stretch. Secondary endings respond only to stretch.

4. Firing of the gamma motor neurons causes contraction of the ends of the intrafusal fibers. The contraction maintains the stretch of the central region of the intrafusal fibers so that the sensory endings are able to respond to stretch of the muscle.

5. Muscle stretch information from primary endings in muscle spindles, tension in tendons from Golgi tendon organs, and tension in ligaments from ligament receptors are transmitted by large-diameter Ia and Ib axons.

6. Aδ and C axons convey nociceptive and temperature information.

7. The types of pathways that convey information to the brain are conscious relay, divergent, and unconscious relay.

8. High-fidelity, somatotopically arranged information is conveyed to the primary sensory cortex, located in the postcentral gyrus.

9. Neural signals that are interpreted as dull, aching pain travel in the spinolimbic tract; spinomesencephalic and spinoreticular tract information does not reach conscious awareness.

10. The unconscious relay tracts end in the cerebellum.

11. Synapses between neurons conveying discriminative touch information occur in the left nucleus gracilis in the medulla, right VPL nucleus in the thalamus, and primary somatosensory cortex.

12. Synapses between neurons conveying discriminative pain information occur in the left dorsal horn of spinal cord, right VPL nucleus in the thalamus, and primary somatosensory cortex.

13. Posterior spinocerebellar and cuneocerebellar tracts convey unconscious proprioceptive information. The anterior spinocerebellar and rostrospinocerebellar tracts convey information about activity in spinal interneurons and about descending motor commands.

CHAPTER 7

Case 1

The left lower extremity has lost discriminative touch and conscious proprioception. The tracts for these senses ascend in the ipsilateral cord. The right lower extremity loss is fast pain and discriminative temperature sense. The tracts for these sensations ascend in the contralateral cord. This pattern of sensory loss plus paralysis on the same side as loss of the dorsal column information indicates a hemisection of the cord. The left half of the cord is interrupted at about L2; the right half of the cord is intact. These signs together (paralysis and dorsal column signs on one side, spinothalamic signs on the opposite side) indicate Brown-Séquard syndrome.

Case 2

The sensory and motor signs are both found on only one side of the body, there are no vertical tract signs, and reflexes are intact. Proximal strength and sensation are within normal limits. All these factors indicate that the spinal cord is not involved. Because there are no brainstem or cerebral signs, the most likely location for the lesion is peripheral. The pattern of sensory and motor loss corresponds to the median nerve distribution in the hand, not to a dermatomal distribution. The most likely etiology is carpal tunnel syndrome.

Case 3

Motor and sensory deficits are entirely on the left side of the body. The lower half of the face, trunk, and both limbs are involved, indicating damage to vertical tract neurons. The facial signs indicate a lesion above the lower midbrain, because a spinal cord lesion would not affect the face and a lesion in most areas of the brainstem would have facial signs contralateral to the limb signs. The most likely location is cerebral. The abrupt onset indicates a vascular etiology.

Case 4

The 2 weeks when she was pain free and the recurrence of symptoms with high levels of stress indicate that there may be no current physical lesion. Instead, postural changes secondary to avoiding painful positions after the accident and anxiety may be contributing to muscle guarding, abnormal movement patterns, and disuse.

Case 5

1. The history of minor trauma, constant burning sensation, sharp pain, trophic changes in the fourth and fifth fingers, and unwillingness to move the limb indicate complex regional pain syndrome as a likely diagnosis.

2. The diagnosis was confirmed when a pharmacologic block of sympathetic transmission eliminated the symptoms.

Review Questions

1. For a quick screening, proprioception and vibration are tested in the fingers and toes, and pinprick sensation is tested on the limbs, trunk, and face.

2. Somatosensory evaluations require conscious awareness and cognition and thus do not evaluate how somatosensation is used in movements.

3. Complaints of abnormal sensations or sensory loss, skin lesions that are not painful, and/or localized weakness or atrophy indicate that thorough sensory testing is required.

4. The subject must be prevented from seeing the stimuli during testing, the subject must understand the testing and its purpose, and prediction about stimuli must be prevented by irregular timing of stimuli and by varying the stimuli (for example, randomly presenting dull versus sharp stimuli).

5. An electrical current delivered to a surface electrode stimulates the distal distribution of a peripheral nerve. Surface electrodes placed along the course of the peripheral nerve record the electrical potential evoked in the nerve.

6. Spontaneous tingling and prickling indicate paresthesia.

7. In sensory ataxia, conscious proprioception and vibratory sensation are impaired, and balance when standing with the feet together is worse with the eyes closed than when the eyes are open. In cerebellar ataxia, conscious proprioception and vibratory sensation are normal, and balance is poor when standing regardless of whether the eyes are open or closed.

8. Conscious proprioception and vibratory sense are typically most impaired by demyelination, because the information travels in large-diameter axons that require heavy myelination.

9. A left hemisection of the spinal cord causes loss of voluntary motor control combined with loss of position, vibration, and discriminative touch sensation below the level of the lesion on the left side of the body. Pain and temperature information is lost from the right side of the body, one or two dermatomes below the level of the lesion, because collaterals of the first-order proximal axons ascend and descend a few levels in the dorsolateral column (zone of Lissauer). This combination of signs indicates Brown-Séquard syndrome.

10. Varicella-zoster is a viral infection of the dorsal root ganglion that causes inflammation of the sensory nerves and painful eruptions on the skin. It is usually limited to a single dermatome.

11. A lesion in the left posterolateral lower pons would cause loss of pain and temperature information from the left face and the right side of the body. This pattern arises because the nociceptive information from the left face travels in the left posterolateral pons, while the nociceptive information from the body has crossed midline in the spinal cord.

12. Sensory extinction is a lack of awareness of the stimulus presented on one side of the body when stimuli are provided simultaneously to both sides of the body. If a stimulus is presented only on the affected side, the person is aware of the stimulus.

13. According to the counterirritant theory, pressure on an injured finger stimulates mechanoreceptor afferents that facilitate enkephalin interneurons. The enkephalin released by the interneurons activates

receptors on primary nociceptive afferents and interneurons that decrease the release of substance P by the primary afferents and hyperpolarize interneurons in the nociceptive pathway. Both of these actions decrease the transmission of nociceptive information.

14. The inability to sleep is part of the motivational/affective aspect of the pain experience. Nociception increases arousal, and thus inhibits sleep.

15. The three supraspinal antinociceptive systems originate in the raphe nuclei, periaqueductal gray, and locus ceruleus.

16. Narcotics activate opiate receptors in the raphe nuclei, periaqueductal gray, and dorsal horn of the spinal cord. This activation inhibits nociceptive information by direct and interneuronal inhibition of neurons in the nociceptive pathways, , decreasing transmission of nociceptive information.

17. The levels of the antinociception model are:
   I. Peripheral
   II. Dorsal horn
   III. Neuronal descending
   IV. Hormonal
   V. Cortical

18. Referred pain is pain perceived as arising in a site different from the actual site of origin.

19. Nociceptive chronic pain is due to continued stimulation of nociceptive receptors. Neuropathic chronic pain is due to abnormal activity within the nervous system.

20. Central sensitization is a condition of abnormal, excessive excitability of central nociceptive neurons, produced by depolarization of NMDA receptors and by increased intracellular Ca^{++}.

21. When novel synapses form between A_β afferents and central nociceptive neurons, activity in the A_β fibers produces signals that are perceived as painful.

22. Examples of neuropathic chronic pain include nerve compression, deafferentation pain, phantom pain, and complex regional pain syndrome.

23. Paresthesia is an abnormal, nonpainful sensation. Dysesthesia is an abnormal painful sensation.

24. Ectopic foci are sites along an injured nerve that are abnormally sensitive to mechanical stimulation.

25. Phantom limb pain is pain that seems to originate from a missing limb.

26. Waddell et al. (1993) postulate that chronic low back pain frequently results from muscle guarding, abnormal movements, and disuse syndrome.

CHAPTER 8

Case 1

RD fainted. The most likely cause was excitement, so the diagnosis was vasodepressor syncope.

Case 2

1. Activation of β-adrenergic receptors accelerates heart rate, increases heart contractility, and vasodilates arteries in the heart and in skeletal muscle. Blocking β-adrenergic receptors benefits the heart by decreasing myocardial oxygen demand, allowing BH to accomplish more physiologic work without compromising cardiac function.
2. Because β-blockers decrease heart rate, age-adjusted normal values for heart rate cannot be used as guidelines for exercise prescription. The following guidelines can be used to establish target heart rate. An exercise stress test, monitoring heart rate and blood pressure during treadmill or stationary bicycle exercise, must be administered to determine the heart rate at which symptoms occur, and a percentage (60%-90%) of that heart rate can be used as a guideline for aerobic exercise. If an exercise stress test cannot be performed, a prescription of an exercise heart rate 20 beats per minute above resting heart rate, with instructions to decrease or stop exercise if symptoms occur, is appropriate.

Review Questions

1.

Receptor(s)	Respond to
Pressure receptors	Increased blood pressure secondary to increased heart rate, stroke volume, and the increased venous return by the muscle pump
Stretch receptors in the lungs	Dilation of the bronchi and bronchioles
Chemoreceptors in the carotid and aortic bodies	Concentration of blood oxygen
Chemoreceptors in the medulla	Blood levels of H and carbon dioxide
Chemoreceptors in the hypothalamus	Blood glucose levels and blood osmolality
Hypothalamic thermoreceptors	Increased blood temperature secondary to an increase in metabolic rate

2. Visceral afferents convey information from the internal organs and blood vessels into the central nervous system.
3. Neurons in the medulla and pons, and hormones from the pituitary gland directly control autonomic functions. Parts of the hypothalamus, thalamus, and limbic system modulate the brainstem control.
4. Autonomic regulation is primarily unconscious and can be orchestrated by hormones, functions of the organs regulated can be adjusted by local factors independent of the central nervous system, and the autonomic efferent pathways typically use two neurons as opposed to the single neuron of the somatic efferent pathways.
5. Sympathetic trunks are a series of interconnected paravertebral ganglia. Postganglionic neurons leaving the paravertebral ganglia join either the ventral or dorsal ramus and travel in a peripheral nerve to reach the vasculature in skeletal muscles or skin.
6. Splanchnic nerves are composed of preganglionic axons that innervate abdominal and pelvic viscera.
7. The sympathetic system optimizes blood supply according to the requirements of various organs. Sympathetic activation can elicit vasodilation and, at other times, vasoconstriction because different effects are elicited by activation of subtypes of receptors on the postsynaptic membrane.
8. Capacitance vessels are veins and venules that can hold large quantities of blood when their walls are relaxed. Vasoconstriction of their walls prevents fainting when a person is standing. Blood flow in skeletal muscle arterioles is controlled by α- and β_2-adrenergic receptors, muscarinic cholinergic receptors, and local blood chemistry.
9. Interference with the sympathetic innervation to the muscle that elevates the eyelid and to the pupil of the eye would result in a drooping eyelid and a constricted pupil.
10. The sympathetic system regulates body temperature; blood flow in internal organs, skeletal muscle, and skin; and metabolism.
11. Parasympathetic activity tends to promote energy conservation and storage. In addition, parasympathetic neurons innervate the lacrimal gland, the pupil and lens of the eye, and the bowels, bladder, and external genitalia.
12. The patient with CRPS has very recently had a successful injection of a drug to block the stellate ganglion, producing the signs of decreased sympathetic activity ipsilateral to the block. The purpose of the

block is to reduce pain so that the patient's ability to tolerate active exercise improves temporarily.

CHAPTER 9

Case 1

The corticospinal and corticobulbar fibers have been interrupted, interfering with voluntary control of the left face and body. The sensory information from the left body and face is not reaching consciousness. Therefore, the lesion is in the cerebrum. The lesion is nonprogressive. The abrupt onset indicates a vascular etiology.

Case 2

The loss of voluntary movement and sensation is unilateral and in the ulnar nerve distribution. The lesion is not spinal, because no vertical tract signs are present. The lack of vertical tract signs also excludes the cerebral hemispheres and brainstem as locations of the lesion. The lesion is focal and nonprogressive. Therefore the damage is to a peripheral nerve, probably secondary to the humeral fracture.

Case 3

Bilateral loss of voluntary movement and sensation indicates a central nervous system lesion. Given that her motor and sensory functions are intact above the L1 spinal cord level (corresponding the T10 vertebra), the injury is to the spinal cord. The lesion is focal, nonprogressive, and traumatic.

Case 4

The only system affected is the motor system. The bilateral Babinski's sign and the velocity-dependent hypertonia indicate upper motor neuron involvement. Muscle fibrillation is a sign of motor system pathology, but does not indicate whether upper or lower motor neurons are involved. Because no common disorder only affects upper motor neurons bilaterally, the most likely etiology is amyotrophic lateral sclerosis, which damages both upper and lower motor neurons. The lower motor neuron involvement could be confirmed by motor nerve conduction velocity studies.

Review Questions

1. After Ca^{++} binds to troponin, a change in shape of troponin moves the tropomyosin to uncover active sites on actin. Myosin heads attach to the active sites on actin, then swivel, pulling the actin toward the center of the sarcomere. This shortens the sarcomere, producing contraction of the muscle.

2. In a shortened sarcomere, actin filaments from one side of the sarcomere intrude into the space of the actin filaments from the other side of the sarcomere, interfering with the binding of myosin to active sites on actin.

3. In an intact nervous system, descending motor commands, reflexes, weak crossbridge binding, and titin produce muscle stiffness.

4. After sitting for several hours, many weak bonds have formed between actin and myosin, producing muscle stiffness.

5. Anxiety produces increased activity in the raphespinal and ceruleospinal pathways, which facilitates lower motor neuron firing. This produces muscle contraction and adds a neural contribution to muscle stiffness.

6. A lower motor neuron directly innervates muscle. When a lower motor neuron fires, the muscle fibers it innervates contract. The cell body of a lower motor neuron is in the spinal cord or brainstem, and its axon is in a peripheral nerve. Upper motor neurons synapse with lower motor neurons and thus affect the activity of lower motor neurons. Upper motor neurons are entirely within the central nervous system. Cell bodies of upper motor neurons are in the cerebral cortex or brainstem. The axons of upper motor neurons form the descending motor tracts; examples include the corticospinal, corticobulbar, and reticulospinal tracts.

7. The general function of control circuits is to adjust the activity in descending motor pathways.

8. Slow twitch muscle fibers are usually activated before fast twitch muscle fibers because the alpha motor neurons innervating slow twitch muscle fibers have smaller cell bodies that depolarize earlier than the larger cell bodies of the alpha motor neurons innervating fast twitch muscle fibers.

9. The activity of a motor unit is determined by sensory information from peripheral receptors, by spinal connections, and by activity in descending pathways.

10. Alpha-gamma coactivation is the simultaneous firing of alpha and gamma motor neurons to a muscle so that the extrafusal and intrafusal muscle fibers contract simultaneously.

11. The phasic stretch reflex is elicited by a quick stretch, the afferent is a type Ia fiber, and the connection in the spinal cord between the afferent and efferent is monosynaptic. The tonic stretch reflex is elicited by slow or sustained stretch. The afferents are both type Ia and II fibers, and

the connections within the spinal cord are multisynaptic.

12. Information from the Golgi tendon organ adjusts muscle activity, in concert with information from muscle spindles, cutaneous and joint afferents, and upper motor neurons. GTO signals may facilitate or inhibit the lower motor neuron to the muscle of origin. Signals from Golgi tendon organs do not prevent injury by inhibiting excessive muscle contraction.

13. Changing a person's arousal level alters the response to a quadriceps tendon tap by changing the amount of upper motor neuron input to the lower motor neurons.

14. An H-reflex is produced by electrically stimulating the type Ia afferents in a peripheral nerve. This produces signals that are transmitted into the spinal cord, where alpha motor neurons are activated monosynaptically. Then the alpha motor neurons transmit signals to the skeletal muscles to elicit muscle contraction. Electrodes on the skin surface over the muscle record the depolarization of the muscle membrane. The H-reflex quantifies the level of excitation or inhibition of alpha motor neurons.

15. Reciprocal inhibition prevents antagonist opposition to movements.

16. To motor control researchers, the term *synergy* refers to coordinated activity of muscles that are often activated together by a normal nervous system. Clinicians often use the term *synergy* to indicate pathologic synergies, as when a person with an upper motor neuron lesion cannot flex the knee without simultaneous obligatory flexion of the hip.

17. A stepping pattern generator is a flexible network of spinal interneurons that activates lower motor neurons to produce a muscle activation pattern that approximates gait.

18. The stepping pattern generator is normally activated by descending signals from the brain when the person decides to walk.

19. The medial UMN tracts and their functions are as follows:

Pathway	*Function*
Medial corticospinal	Assist in control of neck, shoulder, and trunk muscles
Medial reticulospinal	Facilitate lower motor neurons to ipsilateral postural muscles and limb extensors
Medial vestibulospinal	Assist in control of neck and upper back muscles
Lateral vestibulospinal	Facilitate lower motor neurons to extensor muscles and inhibit flexor muscles
Tectospinal	Facilitate lower motor neurons that control neck muscles

20. The lateral UMN tracts and their functions are as follows:

Pathway	*Function*
Lateral corticospinal	Influences lower motor neurons that innervate muscles of the hand; fractionation of movement
Corticobulbar	Influences lower motor neurons that innervate facial, tongue, laryngeal, and pharyngeal muscles
Rubrospinal	Influences lower motor neurons that innervate upper limb muscles
Lateral reticulospinal	Facilitates lower motor neurons to flexor muscles and inhibits lower motor neurons to extensor muscles (this action may be reversed in some circumstances)

21. The nonspecific UMN tracts and their functions are as follows:

Pathway	*Function*
Ceruleospinal	Facilitates the activity of interneurons and motor neurons in the spinal cord
Raphespinal	Facilitates the activity of interneurons and motor neurons in the spinal cord

22. Hemiplegia is weakness or paralysis affecting one side of the body.

23. Fibrillations and abnormal movements always indicate pathology. Benign muscle spasms, cramps, and fasciculations may occur following excessive exercise.

24. Hypertonia is unusually strong resistance to passive movement. The difference between the two types of

hypertonia, spasticity and rigidity, is that the resistance in spasticity is velocity dependent and the resistance in rigidity is velocity independent. This means that if spastic muscles are being passively stretched, faster stretch will elicit more resistance than slower stretch. If rigid muscles are being passively stretched, the resistance will remain the same regardless of the speed of stretch. Spasticity is the result of hyperreflexia of the tonic stretch reflex following upper motor neuron lesions. Rigidity is due to a direct upper motor neuron facilitation of alpha motor neurons, producing excess firing of lower motor neurons. Rigidity, in contrast to spasticity, is not associated with clonus or the clasp-knife response.

25. Spinal shock is a temporary condition following injury to the spinal cord during which stretch reflexes cannot be elicited and the muscles are hypotonic owing to edema.

26. Loss of reflexes, muscle atrophy, flaccid paralysis, and fibrillations indicate a lower motor neuron lesion. In contrast, upper motor neuron lesions produce paresis or paralysis and may or may not produce hyperactive reflexes. The muscle atrophy subsequent to upper motor neuron lesions is less severe. Fibrillations may occur in upper motor neuron lesions.

27. Babinski's sign in an adult indicates damage to the corticospinal tract(s).

28. A lesion that produces abnormal cutaneous reflexes, abnormal timing of muscle activation, paresis, and muscle hyperstiffness interrupts upper motor neurons.

29. After a stroke, the factors that contribute to muscle hyperstiffness include weak crossbridge binding, contracture (loss of sarcomeres), and selective atrophy of fast twitch muscle fibers.

30. Changes within the muscle must be producing the excessive force, because if there were activity in the lower motor neuron due to either descending motor commands or to activity in reflexive pathways, the EMG would register muscle membrane depolarization. Weak crossbridge binding, contracture, and selective atrophy of muscle fibers are producing the excessive force.

31. Clonus is involuntary rhythmic muscle contractions elicited by maintained passive dorsiflexion of the ankle or wrist.

32. After a stroke, muscle hyperstiffness is not usually produced by hyperactive stretch reflexes. Post stroke hyperstiffness is typically due to intrinsic changes in muscles and is not reflex based. In the paretic lower limb of adults with chronic hemiplegia, lower motor neurons are less active than in the nonparetic lower limb. If hyperactive stretch reflexes produced hyperstiffness, lower motor neurons to the stiff muscles would be more active than lower motor neurons to muscles in the nonparetic lower limb.

33. Surface EMG can be used to quantify myoplastic hyperstiffness, cocontraction, and hyperreflexia. Myoplastic hyperstiffness is decreased passive range of motion without increased EMG activity. Cocontraction is temporal overlap of EMG activity in antagonist muscles. Hyperreflexia is defined as EMG activity during muscle stretch, with a positive correlation between EMG amplitude and velocity of muscle stretch.

34. In a complete spinal cord injury, there is a total absence of upper motor neuron influence on lower motor neurons. In the typical middle cerebral artery stroke, upper motor neuron influences are abnormal because the corticospinal tracts are interrupted on one side and the activity of some upper motor neurons that originate in the brainstem is altered. However, contralateral corticospinal tracts and all of the upper motor neurons that originate in the brainstem are intact.

35. In spastic cerebral palsy, reflex irradiation and abnormal cocontraction are observed. These motor signs do not occur in adult-onset upper motor neuron disorders.

36. Repetitive movement against resistance and body-weight-support gait training have been shown to improve function in people who have sustained a stroke. These techniques involve forceful movements actively generated by the patient.

37. One week of forced use immediately following a cortical lesion produces greater extent of the lesion and increased behavioral deficits in rats.

38. Amyotrophic lateral sclerosis destroys upper and lower motor neurons only. Amyotrophic lateral sclerosis spares sensory, autonomic, cognitive, language, and all other nonmotor nervous system functions.

CHAPTER 10

Case 1

The resting tremor, difficulty with initiating movements, and muscle rigidity indicate involvement of the basal ganglia. The lesion involves loss of cell bodies in the substantia nigra and pedunculopontine nucleus. The pathology is progressive. This is Parkinson's disease or parkinsonism.

Case 2

The difficulty with initiating movements, postural instability, and rigidity indicate parkinsonism, because the autonomic dysfunctions, Babinski's sign, and ataxia indicate more systems are involved than in pure Parkinson's disease. The lesions are located in basal ganglia, cerebellar, and autonomic systems and the cerebral cortex. The diagnosis is multiple system atrophy.

Case 3

Normal active range of motion in the right upper limb and impaired proprioception and stereognosis combined with muscle cramping during a specific motor activity indicate focal hand dystonia, also known as writer's cramp. The lesion is in the basal ganglia.

Case 4

The coordination problems indicate a cerebellar lesion. Because the cerebellum controls the ipsilateral body, the lesion is located in the right cerebellum. The gradual onset makes a tumor a likely diagnosis.

Review Questions

1. One route for information from the basal ganglia output nuclei to the lower motor neurons is output nuclei → motor thalamus → motor areas of the cerebral cortex → corticospinal and corticobulbar neurons → lower motor neurons. A second route is from the pedunculopontine nucleus → reticulospinal and vestibulospinal tracts → lower motor neurons.

2. The nuclei that comprise the basal ganglia are the caudate, putamen, globus pallidus, subthalamic nucleus, and substantia nigra.

3. The basal ganglia compare proprioceptive information and movement commands, assist in the sequencing of movements, and adjust muscle tone and muscle force.

4. Rigidity, hypokinesia, resting tremor, and visuoperceptive impairments characterize Parkinson's disease. In Parkinson's disease, neurons in the substantia nigra compacta and pedunculopontine nucleus die off.

5. Multiple system atrophy produces the combination of parkinsonism, cerebellar signs, and autonomic dysfunction.

6. Huntington's disease, dystonia, and choreoathetotic cerebral palsy produce hyperkinesia.

7. Involuntary abnormal postures and repetitive twisting movements are signs of dystonia.

8. The major function of the cerebellum is comparing actual to intended motor activity.

9. The major sources of input to the cerebellum are the cerebral cortex, via connections in the pons; internal feedback about spinal cord interneuron activity; and proprioceptor and skin mechanoreceptors.

10. The cerebrocerebellum coordinates finger movements, the spinocerebellum coordinates gross limb movements, and the vestibulocerebellum coordinates postural adjustments.

11. Ataxic gait may indicate damage to the spinocerebellum.

12. Movement decomposition refers to impaired coordination with isolated movements of individual joints instead of coordinated, simultaneous movements of joints. Movement decomposition occurs in cerebellar lesions.

13. The signs of cerebrocerebellar lesions include dysdiadochokinesia, or inability to rapidly alternate movements; dysmetria, or inability to accurately move an intended distance; and action tremor, or shaking of the limb during voluntary movement.

14. The long loop response is the second response of a contracting muscle to stretch. The long loop response is visible on EMG. In the biceps brachii, the long loop response occurs 50-80 milliseconds after the muscle stretch.

15. The asymmetrical tonic neck reflex is the extension of the limbs on the nose side and flexion of the limbs on the skull side when the head is turned toward the right or left. This reflex is frequently observed in normal infants. However, obligatory assumption of this position every time the head is turned to the side indicates that the nervous system has been damaged. An asymmetrical tonic neck reflex in an older child or an adult is a sign of nervous system abnormality.

16. Posturography can reveal the type of sensory information a person typically relies on and the pattern of muscle activity the person uses to maintain equilibrium.

17. Preparatory postural adjustments occur before stepping: the weight is shifted forward and also onto the stance limb.

18. Two identical stimuli may elicit different responses, depending on the instructions a person is given. For example, if a person is asked to maintain 90 degrees

of flexion at the elbow when a weight is placed in the hand, three responses occur in the biceps: stretch reflex, long loop response, and a voluntary response. If the person is asked to let the hand drop when the weight is placed in the hand, only the stretch reflex occurs.

19. For a person with hemiplegia who is having difficulty initiating gait, placing the foot of the swing limb 10-15 cm behind the stance foot may facilitate gait initiation.

20. The two phases of reaching are fast approach and homing in.

21. Diagnostic EMG is used to distinguish between denervated muscle and myopathy.

22. Motor nerve conduction studies are used to differentiate among dysfunctions in nerve, neuromuscular junction, and muscle. Surface EMG for analysis of movement is used to determine which of the following factors contribute to impaired movement: paresis, myoplastic hyperstiffness, cocontraction, and/or hyperreflexia.

CHAPTER 11

Case 1

Rapid onset, motor system more involved than sensory, cranial nerve involvement, and respiratory paresis indicate Guillain-Barré syndrome. Nerve conduction velocity results indicate that the lesions affect the peripheral nerves, specifically the myelin. See Chapter 2 for a review of this disorder.

Case 2

1. Sensory and motor signs with the specific history of trauma indicate crushing injury (axonopathy) of the ulnar nerve.

2. Nerve conduction velocity tests can isolate the location of the lesion prior to Wallerian degeneration of the axon distal to the injury, and the probable rate of recovery of function can be calculated by assuming regrowth of the distal axon of about 1 mm/day.

Case 3

Lack of sensory and coordination deficits, combined with weakness and normal nerve conduction velocity, indicates a primary disease of muscle. The small-amplitude potentials recorded from muscle confirm the diagnosis of myopathy.

Review Questions

1. Peripheral nerves are able to be stretched and shortened without injury due to the following mechanisms: axons wrinkle within the endoneurium when the nerve is not stretched, the endoneurium, perineurium, and external epineurium act as extensible tubes, the fascicles glide relative to each other, fascicular plexuses share the loading, and the entire nerve slides relative to surrounding tissues.

2. Complete severance of a peripheral nerve causes loss of sensation, abnormal sensations, lack of sweating, inability to control smooth muscle in arterial walls, and paralysis of muscles in the area supplied by the portion of the nerve distal to the lesion.

3. The trophic changes that occur in denervated tissues include muscle atrophy, shininess of the skin, brittle nails, and thickening of subcutaneous tissues.

4. Carpal tunnel syndrome is an example of a myelinopathy. The myelin is damaged by repeated mechanical stimuli: focal compression due to pressure, excessive stretch, vibration, and/or friction. Compression of a peripheral nerve decreases epineurial blood flow and axonal transport, causing edema of the endoneurium and epineurium. The edema further restricts blood and axoplasmic flow. The external epineurium and perineurium thicken, causing myelin damage, leading to the development of ectopic foci and decreased nerve conduction velocity. Mechanical or chemical stimulation of ectopic foci generates neuropathic pain in the peripheral nerve distribution. The decreased nerve conduction velocity results in impaired discriminative touch, proprioception, and movements.

5. Axonopathy is typically the result of crushing a nerve, which disrupts all sizes of axons. Reflexes are decreased or absent. Following the injury, Wallerian degeneration and then muscle atrophy occur. Prognosis is good because regenerating axons are confined to intact connective tissue and myelin sheaths and are able to reinnervate appropriate targets.

6. Because the axons and connective tissues are completely severed, regenerating axons are not guided by intact sheaths to the appropriate target organ. The lack of guidance and the presence of tissues that physically interfere with the optimal direction of regrowth lead to inappropriate innervation and neuroma formation.

7. Multiple mononeuropathy is focal damage randomly affecting more than one peripheral nerve. The presentation of signs and symptoms is asymmetrical.

8. Polyneuropathy is most frequently the result of diabetes, nutritional deficiencies secondary to alcohol abuse, and autoimmune disorders.

9. Polyneuropathy usually presents with distal involvement first because the longest axons are most sus-

ceptible to inadequate axonal transport and to the random process of demyelination.

10. Myelinopathy can be distinguished from axonopathy by nerve conduction velocity studies. Myelinopathies produce severe slowing of NCV, and axonopathies primarily produce decreased amplitude of the evoked potential.

11. Electromyography can be used to distinguish neuropathy from myopathy. Myopathy will have small-amplitude compound muscle action potentials (see Chapter 10).

12. Neuronal hyperactivity produces muscle spasms, muscle fasciculations, and cyanosis of the skin. Neuronal hypoactivity produces absent reflexes, lack of sweating, and muscle paralysis.

13. The signs and symptoms listed are characteristic of central nervous system lesions.

CHAPTER 12

Case 1

1. The lesion is in the spinal cord and not in a root because the loss of sensation and motor control throughout the medial upper limb and the entire trunk and lower limb indicates that vertical tracts must be interrupted.

2. The signs include loss of sensation below the C6 dermatome and complete loss of motor control below C6. These signs indicate a complete lesion of the spinal cord at the C6 level.

Case 2

1. BD has anterior cord syndrome at C6. Anterior cord syndrome interrupts descending motor pathways, lower motor neurons, and the spinothalamic tracts. Because some neurons in the spinothalamic tract are intact, pain and temperature sensation is partially preserved. In this case, the incomplete injury slightly damaged anteriorly located tracts on the right side and moderately damaged the same tracts on the left side, leaving parts of the vertical tracts intact.

2. This patient's outcome is very different from the complete lesion of the cord in Case 1 because many axons in vertical tracts were spared.

Case 3

1. Vertical tracts conveying pain and temperature information are not impaired because the spinothalamic tracts are anterior to the lesion.

2. The dermatomal and myotomal patterns of loss indicate a lesion in the right posterolateral cord at the L2 spinal segment. Although the lesion does interfere with transmission of pain information from the dermatome that projects to the right L2 segment, no deficit is evident clinically because of the overlap of adjacent sensory fields in the periphery.

3. The earlier incident of weakness in the left leg, with full resolution, plus the current signs, indicate multiple sclerosis as a possible diagnosis.

Case 4

1. Complete loss of sensation begins at the S1 level on the left. Because the L5 level contributes to ankle kinesthesia, ankle position sense is partially retained. Preserved sensation at the left S4 and S5 levels and intact sensation in the right lower limb indicate that vertical tracts are not damaged. Thus the lesion is likely to be outside the spinal cord.

2. Given the S1-S3 dermatomal distribution of symptoms, a lesion compressing the dorsal roots can be suspected. In this case, the lesion is a small tumor compressing the left S1-S3 dorsal roots.

3. Touch and proprioceptive sensations are more affected than pain and temperature sensations because compression affects large axons more than small axons. A lesion in the dorsolateral cord would have interfered with ascending dorsal column information from the left lower limb and descending lateral corticospinal information to the left lower limb.

Case 5

1. The pain radiating down the posterior right leg indicates impingement of the S1 and S2 sensory nerve roots, and the impaired sensation in the saddle region indicates impingement of the S2-S5 sensory nerve roots. No dermatomal or myotomal signs of lumbar root involvement are present. The bowel and bladder signs indicate involvement of the S2-S4 nerve roots. Because skeletal muscle power in the lower limbs is preserved, the lesion does not involve most anterior nerve roots. However, the weak contraction of the anal sphincter indicates that the lower motor neurons to the anus are affected by the lesion. This case appears to be a cauda equina lesion, primarily affecting sacral sensory nerve roots. Recall that the entire sacral spinal cord is located at the L1 vertebral level. The lesion is most likely at the L5-S1 vertebral level, because the spinal cord ends at L1-L2 vertebral level , no signs of lumbar spinal nerve impingement are present, L5-S1 vertebral level is often the site of disk herniations, and only the sacral roots are present at L5-S1.

2. Because cauda equina syndrome is usually caused by a herniated nucleus pulposis, that is the most likely etiology.

3. The next step is emergency medical referral, because without treatment cauda equina syndrome can cause paraplegia and/or permanent problems with sensory loss and with bowel and bladder control.

Review Questions

1. A spinal nerve is the brief union of the dorsal and ventral roots of a single spinal segment within the intervertebral foramen. The spinal nerve divides into the anterior and posterior rami.
2. A ventral root is a collection of motor and autonomic efferent axons from one segment of the spinal cord. The ventral primary ramus is a branch of the spinal nerve and provides innervation to the anterior and lateral trunk and the limbs.
3. A spinal segment is a section of the spinal cord that is connected with a specific dermatome, myotome, and sclerotome by a spinal nerve, its roots, and its rootlets.
4. The dorsal horn processes sensory information.
5. Lamina II is also known as the substantia gelatinosa.
6. Reflexes and voluntary motor control are not separate because afferent and descending voluntary information converges on the same spinal interneurons. This convergence allows descending voluntary signals to modify reflexive actions and allows afferent input to adjust movements elicited by descending commands.
7. Reciprocal inhibition prevents or decreases activation of an antagonist when an agonist is firing. This prevents opposing muscle forces from being activated when an agonist contracts.
8. Voluntary voiding of urine requires that information regarding fullness of the bladder is conveyed to the sacral spinal cord by afferents, then to the cerebral cortex, where a decision is made. Then the brain initiates voiding by corticospinal inhibition of lower motor neurons that innervate the external sphincter and by brainstem pathways to the autonomic efferents that stimulate contraction of the bladder wall.
9. The differences between segmental and vertical tract signs are as follows: Segmental signs are limited to a dermatomal and/or myotomal distribution. The sensory signs include lost or abnormal sensation, and the motor signs include lower motor neuron signs: flaccid weakness, atrophy, fibrillations, and fasciculations. Vertical tract signs occur at all levels below the lesion and include decreased or lost sensation, decreased or lost voluntary control of pelvic organs, and upper motor neuron signs: muscle hyperstiffness, paresis, phasic stretch hyperreflexia, and Babinski's sign. Signs of interruption of the sympathetic tracts above the T6 level include autonomic dysreflexia, poor thermoregulation, and orthostatic hypotension.

10. The four adult-onset spinal region syndromes are anterior cord syndrome, central cord syndrome, Brown-Séquard syndrome, and cauda equina syndrome. See Figure 12-18 for illustrations of the location of the lesion in each syndrome.
11. Spinal cord functions are depressed or lost immediately below the lesion after a spinal cord injury because descending tracts that supply tonic facilitation to the spinal cord neurons are interrupted by the lesion.
12. Some people with spinal cord injuries have exaggerated withdrawal reflexes because the normal descending reticulospinal inhibition on the neurons within the withdrawal reflex circuit has been removed.
13. An incomplete spinal cord injury is damage to the spinal cord in which sensory and/or motor function is preserved in the lowest sacral segment. Anterior cord, Brown-Séquard, or central cord syndrome can produce incomplete spinal cord injury. Cauda equina syndrome is damage to the cauda equina, not the cord, so cauda equina damage does not produce incomplete spinal cord injury.
14. Autonomic dysreflexia, poor thermoregulation, and orthostatic hypotension arise when the spinal cord below the T6 level is deprived of descending sympathetic innervation.

CHAPTER 13

Case 1

The most likely location of the lesion is the trochlear nerve, damaged or severed by the skull fracture, because the trochlear nerve innervates the superior oblique muscle that moves the eye to look down and in. The intact pupillary and accommodation reflexes and the normal movements of the eyes up, down, in, and up and in indicate that the oculomotor nerve is undamaged. The ability to look laterally indicates that the abducens nerve is also intact.

Case 2

1. This is not an upper motor neuron lesion because an upper motor neuron lesion would spare the pupillary reflexes. In an upper motor neuron lesion, the afferent limb by the optic nerve would be intact, the connections in the brainstem would be intact, and the efferent limb via the oculomotor nerve would be intact.

2. The absence of any cognitive or consciousness disorders and the absence of vertical tract signs, such as paresis elsewhere in the body and/or a loss of sensation, indicate that the lesion is probably in the peripheral nervous system. The oculomotor nerve supplies the extraocular muscles that move the pupil up, down, in, and up and in, as well as the papillary reflexes. The two muscles innervated by the trochlear and abducens nerves are intact. Therefore the lesion involves the oculomotor nerve.

Case 3

There are no signs of vertical tract involvement because the absence of signs below the face indicates that the connections between the brain and the spinal cord are normal. The lesion spares facial sensation, the muscles of mastication, and the tongue, so the trigeminal nerve and hypoglossal nerves are intact. The facial nerve controls the muscles of facial expression, including the orbicularis oculi, so the lesion involves the facial nerve. The disorder affects either the nucleus of cranial nerve VII or its axons. If the axons are affected, the disorder is Bell's palsy.

Review Questions

1. Contraction of the lateral rectus muscle, innervated by the abducens nerve, moves the right eye toward the right. Next, contraction of the superior rectus muscle, innervated by the oculomotor nerve, moves the right eye upward. Contraction of the medial rectus muscle, innervated by the oculomotor nerve, moves the left eye toward the right. Contraction of the inferior oblique muscle, innervated by the oculomotor nerve, moves the left eye upward.
2. The oculomotor nerve provides the efferents for the pupillary reflex.
3. The hypoglossal nerve provides efferents to the tongue muscles.
4. The glossopharyngeal nerve provides afferents for the gag reflex.
5. The facial nerve provides control of the muscles of facial expression.
6. The trigeminal nerve provides somatosensation from the face.
7. See Figure 13-7 for an illustration of the accommodation reflex.
8. The organ of Corti converts mechanical displacement information into neural signals for the perception of sounds.
9. Different brain areas produce authentic and inauthentic smiles. The limbic system is the source of authentic smiles, and voluntary signals from the cerebral cortex produce inauthentic smiles.
10. Cranial nerves V, VII, IX, X, and XII are all involved in swallowing.
11. Double vision can result from lesions of cranial nerves III, IV, or VI or their nuclei, or from lesions of the medial longitudinal fasciculus.

CHAPTER 14

Case 1

1.

Functional losses	Structures involved
Lack of pain and temperature sensation from the right side of the body	Spinothalamic tract
Lack of somatosensation from the left side of the face	Spinal tract and nucleus of cranial nerve V
Ataxia on the left side of the body	Middle cerebellar peduncle
Paralysis of muscles of facial expression on the left side	Facial nerve
Nystagmus, vertigo, nausea, vomiting	Vestibular nuclei
Loss of corneal reflex on the left side	Nucleus of cranial nerve V

2. The cranial nerve signs indicate that the lesion must be in the brainstem. The lesion affects the left side of the brainstem because the loss of pain and temperature sensation is from the right side of the body (the axons conveying pain and temperature information from the body cross the midline in the spinal cord) and the cranial nerve signs involve the left side of the head. All of the structures involved are located in the lateral pons; thus the lesion is in the lateral pons.

Case 2

Normal voluntary control of both sides of the upper face, including the orbicularis oculi, plus the movement of the right lower face when she frowns in response to frustration, indicates that the facial nerve, cranial nerve VII, is intact. Thus the lesion is an upper motor neuron lesion that prevents corticobulbar information from the left cerebral cortex from reaching the right facial nerve nucleus, resulting in paralysis of voluntary movements of the right lower face. The lesion is in the corticobulbar tract that influences cranial nerve VII.

Case 3

1. MZ's ability to respond appropriately to requests for eye movements indicates he is not in a vegetative state. In the vegetative state, the person is not conscious. MZ's responses to the requests demonstrate that he is conscious.

2. Because he is unable to move any part of his body other than his eyes, the condition is locked-in syndrome.

Case 4

1.

Functional losses	*Structures involved*
Decreased control of trunk and proximal limb muscles and paralysis of distal limb muscles on the right side of the body	Upper motor neurons, including corticospinal tracts
Unable to voluntarily move the right lower face	Corticobulbar tracts
Inability to move the left eye medially, downward, or upward; drooping of left upper eyelid; dilated left pupil that is nonresponsive to light	Oculomotor nerve

2. The combination of cranial nerve signs on the left side (oculomotor nerve) and loss of voluntary motor control of the right lower face and right body indicate a brainstem lesion on the left side. Because the oculomotor nuclei are in the midbrain, the lesion must affect the midbrain. The corticospinal and corticobulbar tracts cross the midline below the midbrain, therefore a lesion in the left midbrain produces contralateral paresis of the body and the lower face.

Review Questions

1. The dorsal column/medial lemniscus, spinocerebellar, some parasympathetic, corticobulbar, corticopontine, and corticoreticular tracts are modified in the brainstem.

2. The reticular formation integrates sensory and cortical information, regulates somatic motor activity, autonomic function, and consciousness, and modulates nociceptive/pain information.

3. The major reticular nuclei and the neuromodulators they produce are the ventral tegmental area: dopamine; pedunculopontine nucleus: acetylcholine; raphe nuclei: serotonin; and locus ceruleus and medial reticular area: norepinephrine.

4. Dopamine from the ventral tegmental area is involved in activating cerebral areas essential for motivation and decision making.

5. The pedunculopontine nucleus affects movement by its connections with the globus pallidus, subthalamic nucleus, and reticular formation areas that are the source of the reticulospinal tracts.

6. The raphe nuclei in the medulla are part of the descending pain control system. Other structures that are part of the descending pain control system are the locus ceruleus and the periaqueductal gray, located in the pons and midbrain, respectively.

7. Ascending fibers from the locus ceruleus direct attention.

8. For each function, the nucleus required and its brainstem location are as follows:

Function	*Nucleus*	*Brainstem location*
Control voluntary muscles in the pharynx and larynx	Ambiguus	Upper medulla
Integrate and transmit pain information from the face	Spinal nucleus of the trigeminal nerve	Lower medulla
Control tongue muscles	Hypoglossal	Upper medulla
Process information about sounds	Cochlear	Junction of medulla and pons
Perception of time	Inferior olivary nucleus	Upper medulla
Control muscles of mastication	Trigeminal motor nucleus	Pons
Contract the papillary sphincter, and change curvature of the lens to focus on near objects	Parasympathetic oculomotor	Midbrain

9. The substantia nigra and pedunculopontine nucleus in the midbrain are part of the basal ganglia circuit.

10. The functions of the cerebellum include coordination of movements, motor planning, and cognitive functions, including rapid shifts of attention.

11. Brainstem lesions above the inferior medulla cause contralateral loss of discriminative touch information from the body because the second-order neuron in the dorsal column/medial lemniscus pathway crosses the midline in the inferior medulla.

12. The periaqueductal gray coordinates somatic and autonomic reactions to pain, threats, and emotions.

13. Corticobulbar tracts convey motor signals from the cerebral cortex to cranial nerve motor nuclei.

14. A complete facial nerve lesion produces paralysis of the ipsilateral muscles of facial expression, and the person cannot close the ipsilateral eye. Eye closure is intact with a corticobulbar lesion because cortical control of muscles in the upper face is bilateral.

15. A person with a complete left facial nerve lesion would not be able to smile on the left side of the face because there is no neural connection between the brainstem and the muscles of facial expression on the left side.

16. In the brainstem, damage to the reticular formation or the ascending reticular activating system can cause disorders of consciousness.

17. A person with complete loss of consciousness and normal vital functions is in a vegetative state.

18. Because the brainstem is tightly confined within the bone and dura, space-occupying lesions compress the brainstem and thus interfere with its function.

CHAPTER 15

Case 1

1. AJ has deficient input from both the cochlear and vestibular branches of cranial nerve VIII on the right side.

2. The nerve damage secondary to the fracture interferes with hearing and disrupts the reciprocal relationship between signals from the semicircular canals. Alteration in the pattern of vestibular signals is misinterpreted as signifying movement, resulting in illusions of changes in head position and movement. The nervous system attempts to maintain equilibrium by responding to the illusory changes, resulting in inappropriate muscle activity and nystagmus. Over time, with movement and practice, the central nervous system will adapt to the altered signals, and balance will improve. However, if AJ continues to restrict his movements to prevent provoking the dizziness and nausea, the signs and symptoms will remain unchanged or worsen.

Case 2

1. The cranial nerve signs—loss of sensation and movement of the face, inability to move the right eye toward the right, and deafness—are all on the right side. Ataxia of the limbs, a cerebellar sign, is also on the right side. Cerebellar signs are ipsilateral, on the same side as the lesion (see Chapter 10). The vertigo, nystagmus, oscillopsia, and vomiting indicate a lesion involving the vestibular system. BF also has loss of pain and temperature sensations on the left side of the body. The mix of cranial nerve signs on the right side of the head with vertical tract signs on the left side of the body indicate a brainstem lesion. The cranial nerve nuclei involved are trigeminal, abducens, facial, and vestibulocochlear. All of these cranial nerve nuclei are in the lateral pons, and their axons supply ipsilateral structures. Thus the lesion is in the lateral pons on the right side.

2. The localized loss of function and the slow onset indicate a neoplastic etiology.

Case 3

1. Conscious awareness of visual information occurs only in the cerebral region, so the lesion must be in the cerebrum. The visual loss is restricted to the right visual field of both eyes. This means that the information from the left half of each retina is not being conveyed to or processed in the left visual cortex. To interrupt the fibers from the left half of the retina of both eyes, the lesion must be posterior to the optic chiasm. So the lesion could be affecting the left optic tract, left lateral geniculate, left optic radiation, or left visual cortex.

2. Neural connections of the left motor and somatosensory cortex have been interrupted. The axons connecting motor and somatosensory cortex with subcortical areas travel through the internal capsule, and the initial section of the optic radiations travels in the internal capsule, so the internal capsule is the most likely location for the lesion.

Review Questions

1. Inertia of fluid in the semicircular canals causes bending of hairs in the crista during rotational acceleration of the head. Bending of the hairs stimulates or inhibits the hair cells, eliciting excitation or inhibition of vestibular nerve endings, depending on the direction of bend. Head position relative to

gravity is signaled by bending of hairs in the macula when the weight of otoconia displaces the gelatinous mass. The bending of the hairs stimulates or inhibits the hair cells, which in turn facilitate or inhibit vestibular nerve endings.

2. "Each pair of semicircular canals produces reciprocal signals" means that increased frequency of signals from one canal occurs simultaneously with decreased signals from its partner.

3. The tracts that use vestibular information to control posture include the medial corticospinal, reticulospinal, tectospinal, and vestibulospinal.

4. Signals conveyed by the medial longitudinal fasciculus coordinate eye and head movements.

5. Nystagmus is involuntary back-and-forth movements of the eyes. Physiologic nystagmus is a normal response of an intact nervous system to moving visual objects, head rotation, caloric stimulation of the semicircular canals, or extreme positions of the eyes. Pathologic nystagmus is abnormal oscillating eye movements that are caused by a nervous system disorder.

6. Information from the left visual field reaches the right visual cortex via the following pathways: Light from the left visual field strikes the right half of each retina. From the left eye, signals travel in the left optic nerve, cross the midline in the optic chiasm, travel in the optic tract to the right lateral geniculate body, and from the geniculate body to the right optic cortex. Visual information from the right eye travels in the right optic nerve, stays ipsilateral in the optic chiasm, and then follows the same route as visual information from the nasal half of the left eye.

7. The ability to see yet not recognize an object in the left visual field would result from a lesion in the right perceptual stream for visual information. Information in this stream flows from visual areas of the cortex to recognition areas in the temporal lobe.

8. Eye movements are directed by information from the vestibular, visual, proprioceptive, limbic, and voluntary eye movement systems.

9. The objectives of eye movements are to stabilize gaze and to direct gaze toward visual targets.

10. The vestibulo-ocular reflex stabilizes the visual world when the head moves during walking.

11. The optokinetic reflex is an involuntary eye movement reaction elicited by moving visual stimuli. The eyes reflexively follow large objects in the visual field.

12. When the head is moving rapidly and the visual object is stationary, the vestibulo-ocular reflex compensates for the head movements using feed-forward, producing a clear, stable visual image. When the object is moving rapidly and the head is stationary, the loss of the target and the new position of the target must be recognized, and movements generated to move the eyes to the new position. However, if the object is moving rapidly, the position of the object changes before the eye movements are completed. Thus, when this feedback process is used, the object cannot be seen clearly.

13. Normally, detailed visual information is suppressed when the head is turned rapidly.

14. Vertigo is the most common symptom in peripheral vestibular disorders.

15. A lesion that produces hearing loss, tinnitus, vertigo, and nystagmus is most likely to be located in the inner ear.

16. BPPV is benign paroxysmal positional vertigo, a syndrome of a brief (less than 2 minutes) sensation of whirling movement evoked by a rapid change in head position.

17. The abrupt onset of dysequilibrium, spontaneous nystagmus, nausea, and severe vertigo characterizes vestibular neuritis.

18. Oscillopsia is the visual sensation of movement of nonmoving objects. The objects appear to jump or bounce.

19. Peripheral vestibular disorders always produce nystagmus, which is never vertical; may be associated with hearing loss or tinnitus, but never with signs of a brainstem region lesion; are associated with severe nausea and vomiting; and do not produce oscillopsia unless there are bilateral peripheral lesions. In contrast, central vestibular disorders may produce nystagmus, which may be vertical; are not associated with hearing loss or tinnitus; are accompanied by brainstem region signs; cause only mild nausea and vomiting; and oscillopsia is often present.

20. The ocular tilt reaction is a triad of signs produced by a unilateral lesion of the otoliths or of the vestibular nuclei. The signs include lateral head tilt, rotation of the eyes toward the downward side of the head, and skew deviation of the eyes with one eye looking upward while the other eye looks downward.

21. A left homonymous hemianopia is produced by a complete lesion of the visual pathway anywhere posterior to the optic chiasm on the right side: in the

optic tract, lateral geniculate, optic radiations, or primary visual cortex. Any of these lesions produce a loss of information from the contralateral visual field.

22. Phoria is a tendency for one eye to deviate from looking straight ahead when binocular vision is unavailable. When a person is attempting to look straight ahead at a target with both eyes, the deviation of one eye from forward gaze is a tropia.

23. Cerebellar ataxia is unaffected by whether the person is standing, sitting, or lying down, and in standing, vision does not improve balance. Vestibular ataxia is gravity dependent; when the person is lying down, coordination is normal. Cerebellar and vestibular ataxia both may be associated with vertigo and nystagmus. Sensory ataxia is characterized by decreased or lost proprioceptive and vibratory senses and ankle reflexes. No vertigo or nystagmus occurs with sensory ataxia.

CHAPTER 16

Review Questions

1. Damage to the ventral anterior nucleus would interrupt fibers from the globus pallidus to the premotor areas; damage to the ventral lateral nucleus would interrupt circuits from the dentate nucleus to primary motor cortex and premotor areas; damage to the ventral posterolateral nucleus would prevent relay of somatic information from the body to the somatosensory cortex; damage to the ventral posteromedial nucleus would stop somatic sensation from the face from reaching the somatosensory cortex; and lesions of the medial and lateral geniculates would interrupt axons transmitting auditory and visual information to the cerebral cortex.

2. The hypothalamic regulation of body temperature, metabolic rate, and blood pressure are essential for survival.

3. A lesion of the genu of the internal capsule would cause contralateral loss of corticobulbar control, resulting in inability to voluntarily control the cranial nerves that receive cortical input: oculomotor, trochlear, trigeminal, abducens, facial, glossopharyngeal, accessory, and hypoglossal. Thus the person would be unable to voluntarily control the muscles that move the eyes, chew, form facial expressions, swallow, produce speech, elevate the shoulders, and turn the head. Cortical control of reticular activity would be decreased because corti-

coreticular fibers travel through the genu and then project bilaterally to the reticular formation.

4. The functional categories of the cerebral cortex are primary sensory, sensory association, association, motor planning, and primary motor.

5.

Primary auditory cortex → Auditory association cortex → Parieto-temporal association areas → Visual cortex

↓

Sensorimotor cortex ← Premotor area ← Visual cortex ← Cortical eye fields

↓

Spinal cord

6. The stress response is produced by activity of the voluntary, autonomic, and neuroendocrine systems.

7. Excessive, prolonged cortisol secretion may contribute to the development of stress-related diseases, including colitis, adult-onset diabetes, cardiovascular disorders, and emotional and cognitive disorders.

8. The hippocampus consolidates declarative short-term memory into long-term memory, although the hippocampus does not store the long-term memories.

9. Motor and parietal cortex and striatum are involved in learning procedural memories. Supplementary motor area and the putamen/globus pallidus are involved in storing procedural memories.

10. Visual information in the ventral stream is used to identify objects and people.

11. The right frontal and parietal lobes contribute to the maintenance of attention, the right parietal lobe disengages attention, and the midbrain shifts attention to a new focus.

CHAPTER 17

Case 1

1. Thalamic activity determines the level of cortical activity, so severe bilateral thalamic damage prevents consciousness.

2. The reticular formation of the brainstem, the reticular activating system, the thalamus, thalamic projections to the cerebral cortex, and the cerebral cortex are all required for consciousness.

Case 2

1. External temperature control is being substituted for the patient's impaired ability to adjust her own body temperature.

2. Pressure from edema following surgery is compressing the hypothalamus, compromising blood flow and thus hypothalamic function. Despite lack of direct damage, the hypothalamus cannot currently regulate temperature. As the fluid is reabsorbed, the hypothalamus will gradually regain its ability to regulate body temperature.

Case 3

The primary motor and somatosensory cortices are damaged. Primary motor cortex neurons control fractionation of movement, particularly of distal muscles, so the lesion interferes with fine-motor control of the hand. The primary somatosensory cortex is necessary for localization of tactile stimuli and conscious proprioception. The lesion does not affect the somatosensory association area because the ability to distinguish sharp from dull is intact.

Case 4

1. RB demonstrated a form of agnosia called **astereognosis,** the inability to identify objects by touch and manipulation despite intact discriminative somatosensation. Astereognosis results from lesions in the somatosensory association area.
2. The disuse of a hand with normal strength may occur as a result of perceptual loss if information from the other hand is processed normally.

Case 5

This patient's apathy and lack of goal-directed behavior are typical of patients with lesions in the prefrontal area. Patients with damage to this region have difficulty choosing goals, planning, executing plans, and monitoring the execution of a plan.

Case 6

Despite intact intellectual ability, BG demonstrated the poor judgment and inability to conform to social conventions often seen in patients with orbitofrontal brain injury. In addition, his left premotor and primary motor areas were also damaged, resulting in decreased voluntary movement on the right side.

Case 7

The disorder is apraxia, the inability to correctly perform purposeful movements despite intact sensation, comprehension, and physical ability to perform the movement. In this case, the errors were entirely sequencing errors, and discrete movements within the sequence were performed correctly.

Case 8

1. **Spastic dysarthria,** characterized by harsh, awkward speech, occurs when upper motor neurons are damaged.
2. In this case, the upper motor neurons could be damaged at their origin in the primary motor cortex, adjacent white matter, or in the internal capsule. The lesion also damaged neurons that control the arm and hand and somewhat affected control of the trunk and lower limb; again, the lesion is in the primary motor cortex, adjacent white matter, or internal capsule, disrupting corticospinal control of lower motor neurons in the cord.

Case 9

1. The lesion is in the left hemisphere because the sensory and motor losses are contralateral to cerebral lesions.
2. The language dysfunction is **Broca's aphasia,** characterized by grammatical omissions and errors, short phrases, and effortful speech. Interference with the programming of language output is consistent with a left hemisphere lesion because Broca's area usually is in the left hemisphere.

Case 10

1. The communication disorder is Wernicke's aphasia.
2. The lesion is probably in the left hemisphere, in Wernicke's area, disrupting the ability to comprehend language.

Case 11

1. The disorder is neglect.
2. AG shows signs of both personal and spatial neglect because he seems unaware of his own left side, he becomes lost easily, and his drawings omit features that should be included on the left side.

Case 12

1. The condition is optic ataxia.
2. The damage is to both parietal lobes.

Case 13

HL has focal contusions of the inferior frontal and anterior temporal and medial lobes, impairing judgment, self-control, and declarative memory. He also has diffuse axonal injury to the superior cerebellar peduncle, which impairs cerebellar projections to the motor areas of the cerebral cortex via the ventrolateral nucleus of the thalamus.

Review Questions

1. The most probable location of the lesion is the right posterior limb of the internal capsule.
2. Astereognosis: inability to recognize an object by touch and manipulation; lesion is in the somatosensory association area. Visual agnosia: inability to recognize objects by vision, despite intact vision; lesion is in the visual association area. Apraxia: inability to perform voluntary movement in spite of preserved sensation, muscular power, and coordination; lesion is in the premotor area. Spastic dysarthria: speech disorder is due to upper motor neuron damage. The damage can cause paralysis, spasticity, and/or uncoordinated activity of the speech muscles; lesion is in the primary motor and primary somatosensory cortex.
3. The lesion is in the area analogous to Wernicke's area in the right hemisphere.
4. Broca's aphasia is not an upper motor neuron disorder. Broca's area provides grammatical function words and planning of speech movements. Information from Broca's area projects to the adjacent sensorimotor cortex, which is the source of most upper motor neurons that control cranial nerves involved in producing speech.
5. Dysarthria interferes with the motor production of sounds. Thus dysarthria can be a lower or upper motor neuron disorder. The lower motor neuron form of dysarthria produces flaccidity of the muscles of speech, causing soft, imprecise speech. The upper motor neuron form of dysarthria is characterized by harsh, awkward speech. Unlike dysarthria, a disorder of speech, aphasia interferes with language. Broca's aphasia interferes with the language output, whereas Wernicke's aphasia interferes with understanding language.
6. The left inferior frontal cortex and adjacent parietal cortex are the most probable sites of the lesion.
7. Nonverbal communication, using gestures and demonstration, is most effective in conveying information to people who cannot understand language.
8. JH has spatial neglect.

CHAPTER 18

Case 1

Because the anterior spinal artery supplies the anterior two-thirds of the cord, occluding this artery interrupts upper motor neurons and spinal tract neurons conveying nociceptive and temperature information, resulting in the deficits seen. The posterior spinal arteries supply the dorsal columns, so vibration and position senses are unaffected.

Case 2

Vertical tracts: all sensations and voluntary movement are affected on one side of the body. Lack of attention to the left side of the body (neglect of the left limbs, lack of response to stimuli on the left side) indicates a cortical lesion. Because at the cortical level all vertical systems project contralaterally, the lesion is in the right cortex. The sudden onset suggests a vascular etiology. The artery supplying the lateral part of the sensorimotor cortex is the middle cerebral artery. Because the lower limb is affected, the lesion involves the deep branches of the middle cerebral artery.

Case 3

The vertical tract sign is the motor deficits; the sensory system is unaffected. In conjunction with the enlarged cranium and eye position, the motor signs indicate hydrocephalus.

Review Questions

1. The cerebrospinal fluid provides water, some amino acids, and ions to the extracellular fluid and protects the central nervous system by absorbing some of the impact when the head receives a blow. Cerebrospinal fluid may also remove metabolites from the extracellular fluid.
2. Cerebrospinal fluid is located in the ventricles and the subarachnoid space.
3. An epidural hematoma arises from arterial bleeding. Because arteries bleed quickly, the signs and symptoms develop rapidly. In contrast, a subdural hematoma is produced by venous bleeding. Veins bleed slowly, causing slow progression of the signs and symptoms.
4. An enlarged head, difficult feeding, downward looking eyes, and inactivity in an infant may indicate hydrocephalus.
5. Hydrocephalus can occur in adults, but the head does not enlarge because bone growth has stopped, and thus the signs and symptoms differ from hydrocephalus in infants.
6. The watershed area is the region on the surface of the lateral cerebral hemisphere that receives blood from small anastomoses linking the ends of the cerebral arteries. The watershed area is susceptible to insufficient blood flow.

7. A transient ischemic attack is a brief, focal loss of brain function that lasts less than 24 hours. The neurologic deficits must be completely resolved within 24 hours.

8. A lacuna is a small cavity that remains after the necrotic tissue is cleared following an infarct in a small artery.

9. A partial occlusion of the basilar artery may result in tetraplegia, loss of sensation, coma, and cranial nerve signs because the basilar artery supplies both the left and right sides of the medulla and pons; thus interference with its blood flow deprives the descending upper motor neuron axons and the ascending sensory axons, as well as the reticular formation, cranial nerve nuclei, and cranial nerves of adequate perfusion.

10. More severe hemiplegia and hemisensory loss in the lower limb indicate that the lesion is in the medial sensorimotor cortex and adjacent subcortical white matter. This region is supplied by the anterior cerebral artery.

11. Neglect, problems comprehending space, and impaired nonverbal communication occur with damage to the area analogous to Wernicke's area in the hemisphere that is nondominant for language (usually the right hemisphere). This area is supplied by the middle cerebral artery.

12. Hemisensory loss and hemiplegia affecting the limbs and face equally indicate a lesion in the internal capsule, supplied by deep branches of the middle cerebral artery.

13. The loss of eye movements combined with contralateral hemiplegia indicates a lesion of the anterior midbrain, supplied by branches of the posterior cerebral artery.

14. Distal branches of the anterior, middle, and posterior cerebral arteries supply the watershed area.

15. An arteriovenous malformation is an abnormal connection between arteries and veins, with thin-walled vessels larger than capillaries connecting the vessels. Arteriovenous malformations are developmental defects.

16. An aneurysm is a dilation of the wall of an artery or vein. Aneurysms are prone to rupture because their walls are thinner than normal vessel walls.

17. An uncal herniation is displacement of the uncus medially, so that the uncus protrudes through the tentorium cerebelli and compresses the midbrain.

18. A positron emission tomography (PET) scan is a computer-generated image reflecting the metabolic activity throughout biological tissues. PET scans of the central nervous system record the relative activity and inactivity of areas in the brain or spinal cord.

Glossary

accommodation   Adjustments of the eyes to view a near object: the pupils constrict, the eyes converge (adduct), and the lens becomes more convex. The optic nerve is the afferent (sensory) limb of the reflex, while the oculomotor nerve provides the efferent (motor) limb.

acetylcholine   A neurotransmitter released by axons from the pedunculopontine nucleus and nucleus basalis of Meynert, by lower motor neurons, by preganglionic autonomic axons, by postganglionic parasympathetic axons, and by postganglionic sympathetic axons that innervate sweat glands. Binds with nicotinic or muscarinic receptors. Action on postsynaptic membranes is usually excitatory.

adrenergic   (1) Referring to neurons that secrete norepinephrine or epinephrine. (2) referring to drugs that bind with and activate the same receptors as norepinephrine or epinephrine. (3) referring to receptors that bind norepinephrine, epinephrine, or agonist drugs.

agnosia   General term for the inability to recognize objects when using a specific sense, even though discriminative ability with that sense is intact. Specific types of agnosia include astereognosis, visual agnosia, and auditory agnosia.

agnosia, visual   Inability to visually recognize objects despite intact vision.

agraphia   Diminished or lost ability to produce written language.

alexia   Diminished or lost ability to comprehend written language.

allodynia   Sensation of pain in response to normally nonpainful stimuli.

all-or-none   Term applied to the generation of an action potential, indicating that every time even minimally sufficient stimuli are provided to generate an action potential, an action potential will be produced. Stimuli that are stronger than the minimally sufficient stimuli produce action potentials of the same voltage and duration as the minimally sufficient stimuli.

γ-aminobutyric acid (GABA)   neurotransmitter released by the caudate nucleus and putamen and by cerebellar Purkinje's cells and spinal interneurons. Action on postsynaptic membranes is inhibitory.

amygdala   Nuclei that interpret facial expressions and social signals. Together the amygdala, orbitofrontal cortex, and anterior cingulate gyrus regulate emotional behaviors and motivation. The amygdala consists of an almond-shaped collection of nuclei deep to the uncus in the temporal lobe.

analgesia   Absence of pain in response to stimuli that would normally be painful.

anencephaly   Developmental defect characterized by development of a rudimentary brainstem without cerebral and cerebellar hemispheres.

aneurysm   Saclike dilation of the wall of an artery or vein. These swellings have thin walls that are prone to rupture.

angiography   Radiopaque dye injected into a carotid or vertebral artery, followed by a sequence of x-rays.

antinociception   Top-down inhibition of pain signals.

antinociception, stress-induced   Absent or reduced perception of pain due to activation of the pain inhibition systems during an emergency or in competitive situations.

aphasia   Disorder of language expression or comprehension. Deficit in the ability to produce understandable speech and writing, or the ability to understand written and spoken language.

aphasia, Broca's   Difficulty expressing oneself by language or symbols. A person with Broca's aphasia has deficits in both speaking and writing. Syn.: motor aphasia, expressive aphasia.

aphasia, conduction   Language disorder resulting from damage to the neurons that connect Wernicke's and Broca's areas. The ability to understand written and spoken language is normal. In mild cases, only paraphrasias occur. In the most severe form, speech and writing produced are meaningless.

aphasia, global   Inability to use language in any form. People with global aphasia cannot produce understandable speech, comprehend spoken language, speak fluently, read, or write.

aphasia, Wernicke's   Impairment of language comprehension. People with Wernicke's aphasia easily produce spoken sounds, but the output is often meaningless. Listening to other people speak is equally meaningless, despite the ability to hear normally. Syn.: receptive aphasia, sensory aphasia.

apparatus, vestibular   The part of the inner ear that detects position and movement of the head. Consists of the semicircular canals, the saccule, and the utricle.

apraxia   Inability to perform a movement or sequence of movements despite intact sensation, automatic motor output, and understanding of the task.

apraxia, constructional   Inability to comprehend the relationship of parts to the whole.

arachnoid   Middle layer of the membranes surrounding the central nervous system.

area, Broca's   Region of cortex that provides instructions for language output, including planning the movements to produce speech and providing grammatical function words, such as the articles *a, an,* and *the.* Located inferior to the premotor area and anterior to the face and throat region of the primary motor cortex, usually in the left hemisphere.

area, corresponding to Broca's area   Region of the cerebral cortex inferior to the premotor area and anterior to the face and throat region of the primary motor cortex. Usually in the right hemisphere. Plans nonverbal communication, including emotional gestures and adjusting the tone of voice.

area, corresponding to Wernicke's area   Subregion of the parietotemporal cortex where interpretation of the nonverbal signals from other people and understanding of spatial relationships occur. Usually located on the right side.

area, lateral premotor   A region of the cerebral cortex involved in preparing for movement and controlling trunk and girdle muscles via the medial upper motor neurons. Located anterior to the upper body region of the primary motor cortex, on the lateral surface of the hemisphere.

area, limbic association   Part of the cerebral cortex involved in regulating mood (subjective feelings), affect (observable demeanor), and processing of some types of memory. Located in the anterior temporal lobe and in the orbitofrontal cortex (above the eyes).

area, preoptic   Part of the limbic system, located anterior to the septal area.

area, septal   Part of the limbic system in the basal forebrain region, anterior to the anterior commissure.

area, somatosensory association   A region of cerebral cortex that analyzes information from the primary somatosensory cortex and from the thalamus. Provides stereognosis and memory of the tactile and spatial environment. Located posterior to the primary somatosensory cortex.

area, supplementary motor   A region of the cerebral cortex involved in preparing for movement, orientation of the eyes and head, and planning bimanual and sequential movements. Located anterior to the lower body region of the primary motor cortex, on the superior and medial surface of the hemisphere.

area, ventral tegmental   A region in the midbrain that provides dopamine to cerebral areas important in motivation and in decision making.

area, watershed   Area of marginal blood flow on the surface of the lateral hemispheres, where small anastomoses link the ends of the cerebral arteries.

area, Wernicke's   Subregion of the parietotemporal cortex where comprehension of language occurs. Usually located on the left side.

areas, association   Regions of the cerebral cortex that are not directly involved with sensation or movement. Involved with personality, integration and interpretation of sensations, processing of memory, and generation of emotions. The three association areas are prefrontal, parietotemporal, and limbic.

areas, Brodmann's   Histologic regions of the cerebral cortex mapped by Brodmann. Often used to designate functional areas.

areas, motor planning   Regions of the cerebral cortex involved in organizing movement. Motor planning areas include supplementary motor area, premotor area, Broca's area, and the area corresponding to Broca's area.

areas, parietotemporal association   Part of the cerebral cortex devoted to intelligence, problem solving, and comprehension of communication and spatial relationships. Located at the junction of the parietal, occipital, and temporal lobes.

areas, primary sensory Areas of the cerebral cortex that receive sensory information directly from the ventral tier of thalamic nuclei. Each primary sensory area discriminates among different intensities and qualities of one type of sensory input. Separate primary sensory areas are devoted to somatosensory, auditory, visual, and vestibular information.

areas, sensory association Areas of the cerebral cortex that analyze sensory input from both the thalamus and the primary sensory cortex. Sensory association areas contribute to the analysis of one type of sensory information.

artery, anterior cerebral Vessel that provides blood to the medial surface of the frontal and parietal lobes and the anterior head of the caudate. A branch of the internal carotid artery.

artery, anterior choroidal A branch of the internal carotid artery that provides blood to the optic tract, choroid plexus in the lateral ventricles, and parts of the optic radiations, putamen, thalamus, internal capsule, and hippocampus.

artery, basilar Vessel that provides blood to the pons and most of the cerebellum. Formed near the pontomedullary junction by the union of the vertebral arteries. Divides to become the posterior cerebral arteries.

artery, internal carotid Vessel that provides blood to the anterior, superior, and lateral cerebral hemispheres via its branches, the anterior and middle cerebral and the anterior choroidal arteries.

artery, middle cerebral Vessel whose branches fan out to provide blood to most of the lateral hemisphere. A branch of the internal carotid artery.

artery, posterior cerebral Vessel that provides blood to the midbrain, occipital lobe, and parts of the medial and inferior temporal lobes. A branch of the basilar artery.

artery, posterior choroidal A branch of the posterior cerebral artery that provides blood to the choroid plexus of the third ventricle and parts of the thalamus and hippocampus.

artery, striate Any of several arteries arising from the proximal part of either the anterior or middle cerebral arteries to supply the basal ganglia and parts of the thalamus and internal capsule.

artery, vertebral Vessel that provides blood to the brainstem, cerebellum, and the posteroinferior cerebrum. Branch of the subclavian artery.

ascending reticular activating system Part of the brainstem reticular formation that projects to areas of the thalamus that project to the cerebral cortex. Involved in arousal.

astereognosis Inability to identify objects by touch and manipulation despite intact discriminative somatosensation.

astrocytes Macroglia that play a critical role in nutritive and cleanup functions within the central nervous system.

ataxia Abnormal voluntary movements that are of normal strength but jerky and inaccurate.

ataxia, cerebellar limb Uncoordinated voluntary movements of the limbs.

ataxia, sensory Uncoordinated movement caused by a lesion along peripheral or central proprioceptive pathways.

ataxia, vestibular Gravity-dependent uncoordinated movement. Limb movements are normal when the person is lying down but are ataxic during walking.

athetosis Involuntary slow, writhing, purposeless movements.

atrophy Loss of muscle bulk.

atrophy, disuse Loss of muscle bulk resulting from lack of use.

atrophy, multiple system Progressive degenerative disease affecting the basal ganglia, cerebellar, and autonomic systems, the peripheral nervous system, and the cerebral cortex.

atrophy, neurogenic Loss of muscle bulk resulting from damage to the nervous system.

atrophy, olivopontocerebellar Multiple system atrophy presenting initially with incoordination, dysarthria, and balance deficits.

attack, transient ischemic A brief, focal loss of brain function, with full recovery from neurologic deficits within 24 hours. Transient ischemic attacks are believed to be due to inadequate blood supply.

attention Ability to maintain focus on a particular input or activity.

autoregulation Adjustment of local blood flow to the demands of the surrounding tissues.

axon Process that extends from the cell body of a neuron. Most axons conduct signals away from the cell body. The only axons that conduct information toward the cell body are the distal axons of primary afferent neurons, which conduct signals to the dorsal root ganglion or cranial nerve ganglion.

axon hillock Specialized region of a neuron cell body that gives rise to the axon. The axon hillock is densely populated with voltage-gated Na^+ channels.

axons, myelinated Axons that are completely enveloped by a myelin sheath.

axons, unmyelinated Axons that are only partially enveloped by myelin.

basal ganglia Interconnected group of nuclei involved in comparing proprioceptive information and movement commands, sequencing movements, and regulating muscle tone and muscle force. May select and inhibit muscle synergies. Consist of the caudate, putamen, globus pallidus, subthalamic nucleus, substantia nigra, and pedunculopontine nucleus.

basal of Meynert Part of the limbic system in the basal forebrain region, inferior to the preoptic area.

bundle, medial forebrain Axons connecting anterior structures (septal area, nucleus accumbens, amygdala, anterior cingulate gyrus), the hypothalamus, and the midbrain reticular formation.

calcitonin gene-related peptide A neuromodulator that activates second messengers. The end result is decreasing the likelihood that acetylcholine (ACh) will activate its own receptor when bound. Also involved in long-term neural changes in response to pain stimuli.

canals, semicircular Three hollow rings in the inner ear, oriented at right angles to each other. Each canal has an enlargement called the *ampulla,* which contains the receptor mechanism for detecting rotational acceleration or deceleration of the head.

cell body The metabolic center of any cell that contains the nucleus and the energy-producing/storing apparatus. The cell body of neurons also includes neurotransmitter-synthesizing mechanisms.

cells, bipolar Neurons having two primary processes, a dendritic root,

and an axon, which extend from the cell body.

cells, multipolar Neurons having multiple dendrites arising from many regions of the cell body and possessing a single axon.

cells, pseudounipolar Neurons that have one projection from the cell body that later divides into two axonal roots. A pseudounipolar cell has no true dendrites.

cells, Renshaw Interneurons that produce recurrent inhibition in the spinal cord. Act to focus motor activity.

cells, Schwann Macroglia that form myelin sheaths enveloping only a single neuron's axon or partially surrounding several axons. Found in the peripheral nervous system.

cells, stem Immature and undifferentiated cells that give rise to both neurons and glial cells.

cells, tract Cells with long axons that connect the spinal cord with the brain.

cerebellum Part of the brain posterior to the brainstem. Involved in coordination of movement and postural control, motor planning, and rapid shifting of attention.

cerebral hemispheres The right and left halves of the cerebrum.

cerebral palsy, choreoathetoid Motor disorder that develops in utero or during infancy. Characterized by involuntary movements that are jerky and rapid or slow and writhing.

cerebral palsy, spastic Motor disorder that develops in utero or during infancy. Characterized by muscle hyperstiffness.

cerebrocerebellum Part of the cerebellum that coordinates voluntary movements via influence on corticofugal pathways, plans

movements, judges time intervals, and produces accurate rhythms. Located in the lateral cerebellar hemispheres.

channels, G-protein–mediated Ion neuronal membrane channels that open in response to the activation of a G-protein or its second messenger.

channels, ligand-gated Neuronal membrane ion channels that open in response to the binding of a chemical neurotransmitter.

channels, modality-gated Membrane ion channels, specific to sensory neurons, which open in response to mechanical forces (i.e., stretch, touch, pressure) or thermal or chemical changes.

channels, voltage-gated Membrane ion channels that open in response to changes in electrical potential across a neuron's cell membrane.

chemoreceptor Receptor that responds to chemical change. Found in the carotid body, brainstem respiratory centers, specialized sensory cells for taste and smell, and the skin, muscles, and viscera.

chiasm, optic Site where the optic nerve fibers from the nasal half of the retina cross the midline.

cholinergic (1) Referring to a neuron that secretes acetylcholine. (2) referring to drugs that bind with and activate the same receptors as acetylcholine. (3) referring to receptors that bind acetylcholine or agonist drugs.

chorea Involuntary, jerky, rapid movements.

choreoathetosis A combination of involuntary, jerky, rapid movements and slow, writhing, purposeless movements.

choroid plexus A network of capillaries embedded in connective tissue and epithelial cells that produce cerebrospinal fluid.

circle of Willis   Anastomotic ring of nine arteries, supplying all of the blood to the cerebral hemispheres. Consists of two anterior cerebral arteries, two internal carotid arteries, two posterior cerebral arteries, one anterior communicating artery, and two posterior communicating arteries.

circuits, control   Neural connections that adjust activity in the upper motor neurons, resulting in excitation or inhibition of the lower motor neurons. Consist of the basal ganglia and cerebellum.

cleft, synaptic   The space between the presynaptic and postsynaptic neuron terminals.

clonus   Involuntary rhythmic muscle contractions elicited by passive dorsiflexion of the foot or passive extension of the wrist. Occurs in upper motor neuron lesions, secondary to the loss or alteration of descending motor control.

coactivation, alpha-gamma   Simultaneous firing of alpha and gamma motor neurons. Ensures that the muscle spindle maintains its sensitivity even when the extrafusal fibers surrounding the spindle contract.

cochlea   Snail-shell–shaped organ, formed by a spiraling, fluid-filled tube. The cochlea contains a mechanism, the organ of Corti, which converts mechanical vibrations into the neural impulses that produce hearing.

cochlear duct   Membranous tube within the inner ear that contains the organ of hearing (the organ of Corti).

cocontraction   Simultaneous contraction of agonist and antagonist muscles. May occur in an intact nervous system when

learning a new movement, or may be a sign of neural dysfunction.

colliculus, superior   Part of the tectum of the midbrain, the superior colliculus integrates various sensory inputs and influences eye movement, head and body orientation, and postural adjustments.

columns, anterolateral   White matter in the anterior and lateral spinal cord that contains spinothalamic and motor axons.

coma   Condition of being unarousable; no response to strong stimuli such as strong pinching of the Achilles tendon.

complex regional pain syndrome (CRPS)   Chronic syndrome of pain, vascular changes, and atrophy in a regional distribution. Syn.: causalgia, Sudeck's atrophy, sympathetically maintained pain, reflex sympathetic dystrophy.

concussion   Mild traumatic brain injury.

conduction, saltatory   Rapid propagation of an action potential by jumping from one node of Ranvier to the next along a myelinated axon.

contracture, muscle   Adaptive shortening of muscle, caused by the muscle remaining in a shortened position for prolonged periods of time. The decrease in length is caused by loss of sarcomeres.

convergence   (1) Multiple inputs from a variety of different cells terminating on a single neuron. (2) movement that directs the eyes toward the midline.

corpus callosum   Large fiber bundle connecting the right and left cerebral cortices.

cortex, cerebral   Gray matter covering the cerebral hemispheres.

cortex, limbic   Part of the limbic system. A *C*-shaped region of cortex located on the medial

hemisphere, consisting of the cingulate gyrus, parahippocampal gyrus, and uncus (a medial protrusion of the parahippocampal gyrus).

cortex, prefrontal   Anterior part of the frontal cortex, responsible for self-awareness and executive functions (also called *goal-oriented behavior*). Executive functions include deciding on a goal, planning how to accomplish the goal, executing the plan, and monitoring the outcome of the action.

cortex, primary motor   Part of the cerebral cortex. Origin of many cortical upper motor neurons that influence contralateral voluntary movements, particularly the fine, fractionated movements of the hand and face. Located in the precentral gyrus, anterior to the central sulcus.

cortex, primary sensory (primary somatosensory)   Cerebral cortex that receives somatosensory information from the body and face. Located posterior to the central sulcus.

cortically blind   Person has no awareness of any visual information yet is able to orient his or her head position to objects.

cortisol   Steroid hormone that mobilizes energy (glucose), suppresses immune responses, and serves as an anti-inflammatory agent. Secreted by the adrenal glands. Syn.: hydrocortisone.

cramp   Severe and painful muscle spasm associated with fatigue or local ionic imbalances.

crest, neural   During development, the part of the ectoderm that will become the peripheral sensory neurons, myelin cells, autonomic neurons, and endocrine organs (adrenal medulla and pancreatic islets).

deafferentation   Interruption of sensory information from part of the body, usually caused by a lesion affecting first-order somatosensory neurons.

deafness, conductive   Hearing defect due to inability to transmit vibrations in the outer or middle ear.

deafness, sensorineural   Hearing defect due to damage of the receptor cells or the cochlear nerve.

deformity, Arnold-Chiari Developmental malformation of the hindbrain, with elongation of the inferior cerebellum and medulla. The inferior cerebellum and medulla protrude into the vertebral canal.

degeneration, Wallerian Degeneration and death of the distal segment of a severed axon.

delirium   Reduced attention, orientation, and perception, associated with confused ideas and agitation.

dementia   Severe impairment or loss of intellectual capacity and personality integration, due to the loss of or damage to neurons in the brain.

dementia, Parkinson's   Cognitive deficit that interferes with the ability to plan, to maintain goal orientation, and to make decisions.

dementia, with Lewy bodies Type of parkinsonism with cognitive decline and visual hallucinations.

dendrite   Process that extends from the cell body of a neuron. Dendrites conduct information toward the cell body.

depolarization   Process whereby a neuron's cell membrane potential becomes less negative than its resting potential.

depolarized   The electrical state of a neuron's cell membrane when the membrane potential becomes less negative than the resting potential.

depression   Syndrome of hopelessness and a sense of worthlessness, with aberrant thoughts and behavior.

dermatome   The part of the somite that becomes dermis, or after the embryo stage, the dermis innervated by a single spinal nerve.

diencephalon   Centrally located part of the cerebrum, consisting of the thalamus, hypothalamus, epithalamus, and subthalamus.

diffuse axonal injury   Stretch injury to the membrane of an axon initiating changes that cause the axon to rupture.

diplopia   Double vision. Perceiving a single object as two objects.

disease, Charcot-Marie-Tooth   An inherited peripheral neuropathy that causes distal paresis and decreased ability to sense heat, cold, and pain Syn.: hereditary motor and sensory neuropathy.

disease, diffuse Lewy body Progressive cognitive decline, memory impairments, deficits in attention, executive function, and visuospatial ability secondary to abnormal protein aggregates in the cerebral cortex, brainstem nuclei, and limbic areas.

disease, Huntington's   Autosomal dominant hereditary disorder that causes degeneration in many areas of the brain, primarily in the striatum and cerebral cortex. Characterized by hyperkinesia.

disease, Ménière's   Sensation of fullness in the ear, tinnitus (ringing in the ear), severe acute vertigo, nausea, vomiting, and hearing loss. Cause is unknown.

disease, Parkinson's   The most common disorder of the basal ganglia, resulting from death of dopamine-producing cells in the substantia nigra compacta and

acetylcholine-producing cells in the pedunculopontine nucleus. Characterized by muscular rigidity, slowness of movement, shuffling gait, droopy posture, resting tremors, diminished facial expression, and visuoperceptive impairments.

disorder, attention deficit Difficulty sustaining attention, with onset during childhood.

disorder, panic   Abrupt onset of intense terror, a sense of loss of personal identity, and the perception that familiar things are strange or unreal, combined with signs of increased sympathetic nervous system activity.

divergence   The branching of a single neuronal axon to synapse with a multitude of neurons.

dopamine   Neurotransmitter released by axons from the substantia nigra and the ventral tegmental area. Action on postsynaptic membranes is usually inhibitory.

dorsal root   The afferent (sensory) root of a spinal nerve.

dysarthria   Speech disorder resulting from paralysis, incoordination, or hyperstiffness of muscles used for speaking. Due to upper or lower motor neuron lesions or muscle dysfunction. Comprehension of spoken language, writing, and reading are not affected by dysarthria. Two types of dysarthria may be distinguished: spastic, due to damage of upper motor neurons, and flaccid, resulting from damage to lower motor neurons.

dysarthria, flaccid   Breathy, soft, imprecise speech caused by damage to lower motor neurons in cranial nerve IX, X, and/or XII.

dysarthria, spastic   Harsh, awkward speech caused by an upper motor neuron lesion.

dysdiadochokinesis Inability to rapidly alternate movements. For example, inability to rapidly pronate and supinate the forearm, or inability to rapidly alternate toe tapping. Syn.: dysdiadochokinesia.

dysesthesia Painful abnormal sensation, including burning and aching sensations.

dyskinesia Involuntary movement that resembles chorea (brisk, jerky movements) and/or dystonia (involuntary sustained postures or repetitive movements).

dysmetria Inability to accurately move an intended distance.

dysreflexia, autonomic Excessive activity of the sympathetic nervous system, usually elicited by noxious stimuli below the level of a spinal cord lesion.

dystonia Hereditary movement disorder, usually nonprogressive, characterized by involuntary sustained muscle contractions causing abnormal postures or twisting, repetitive movements.

ectopic foci Site on neural membrane that is abnormally sensitive to mechanical stimulation.

edema, cerebral Accumulation of excess tissue fluid in the brain.

effectiveness, synaptic Functional activation of postsynaptic receptors in response to the release of a neurotransmitter from a presynaptic terminal.

electromyography Recording of electrical activity produced by contracting muscle.

embolus Blood clot that formed elsewhere and has been transported to a new location before occluding a vessel.

emotional lability Abnormal, uncontrolled expression of emotions.

ending, primary Sensory ending of a type Ia axon that responds phasically to stretch of the central region of intrafusal fibers in the muscle spindle.

ending, secondary Sensory ending of a type II axon that responds tonically to stretch of the central region of intrafusal fibers (primarily nuclear chain fibers) in the muscle spindle.

endogenous opioid peptides Peptides that bind to the same receptors that opium binds to and inhibit the transmission of nociceptive signals. Includes endorphins, enkephalins, and dynorphins.

endoneurium Connective tissue that separates individual axons.

endorphins Endogenous, or naturally occurring, substances that activate analgesic mechanisms. Endorphins include enkephalins, dynorphin, and β-endorphin.

enkephalin A neurotransmitter that, when bound to receptor sites, depresses the release of Substance P and hyperpolarizes interneurons in the nociceptive pathway, thus inhibiting the transmission of nociceptive signals.

epilepsy Sudden attacks of excessive neuronal discharge interfering with brain function.

epineurium Connective tissue that surrounds an entire nerve trunk.

epithalamus The major structure of the epithalamus is the pineal gland, an endocrine gland innervated by sympathetic fibers. The pineal gland is believed to help regulate circadian (daily) rhythms and influence the secretions of the pituitary gland, adrenals, and parathyroids.

equation, Nernst Mathematical equation used to determine the equilibrium potential for a diffusible ion.

Erb's paralysis Loss of shoulder abduction, external rotation, and elbow flexion (waiter's tip position) caused by a lesion of the upper trunk of the brachial plexus or the fifth and sixth cervical nerve roots.

executive functions Goal-oriented behavior.

excitotoxicity Overexcitation of a neuron, leading to cell death.

extinction, sensory A form of unilateral neglect. Loss of sensation is evident only when symmetrical body parts are tested bilaterally.

eye movements, conjugate Both eyes move in the same direction.

eye movements, vergence Eyes move toward the midline or away from the midline.

facilitation, presynaptic At an axoaxonic synapse, the excitatory process by which transmitter released by one axon terminal causes the second axon terminal to release a greater than normal amount of neurotransmitter.

fasciculation A quick twitch of muscle fibers in a single motor unit, which is visible on the surface of the skin.

fasciculus cuneatus Axons that transmit discriminative touch and conscious proprioceptive information from the upper half of the body to the brain. Located in the lateral section of the dorsal column of the spinal cord.

fasciculus gracilis Axons that transmit discriminative touch and conscious proprioceptive information from the lower half of the body to the brain. Located in the medial section of the dorsal column of the spinal cord.

fasciculus, medial longitudinal (MLF) Brainstem tract that coordinates head and eye movements by providing bilateral connections among vestibular, oculomotor, and accessory nerve nuclei and the superior colliculus.

feedback Information resulting from a movement. For example, when a person flexes the elbow, feedback consists of information from sensory receptors in muscles, tendons, and skin.

feed-forward Neural preparation for anticipated movement, based on instruction, previous experience, and the ability to predict the movement requirements and/or outcome.

fiber, intrafusal Specialized muscle fiber inside the muscle spindle.

fibers, association Axons connecting cortical regions within one hemisphere.

fibers, commissural Axons connecting homologous areas of the nervous system.

fibers, corticobulbar Axons that influence the activity of lower motor neurons innervating the muscles of the face, tongue, pharynx, and larynx. Corticobulbar fibers arise in motor planning areas of the cerebral cortex and the primary motor cortex, then project to cranial nerve nuclei in the brainstem.

fibers, extrafusal Contractile skeletal muscle fibers outside of the muscle spindle.

fibers, projection Axons connecting subcortical structures to the cerebral cortex, and axons connecting the cerebral cortex with the subcortical structures.

fibrillation Brief contraction of a single muscle fiber, not visible on the surface of the skin.

fibromyalgia Tenderness of muscles and adjacent soft tissues, stiffness of muscles, and aching pain. The painful area shows a regional rather than dermatomal or peripheral nerve distribution.

flat affect Lack of emotional facial expressions and gestures.

forebrain Anterior part of the developing brain; becomes the cerebrum.

formation, reticular Complex neural network in the brainstem, including the reticular nuclei and their connections. Source of ascending and descending reticular tracts.

fornix Arch-shaped fiber bundle connecting the hippocampus with the mamillary body and anterior nucleus of the thalamus.

fractionation Ability to activate individual muscles independently of other muscles.

freezing Episodes when movements abruptly cease. Characteristic of Parkinson's disease.

functional electrical stimulation (FES) Use of electrical currents to activate nerves.

ganglion, dorsal root Collection of primary somatosensory neuron cell bodies located in the dorsal root.

ganglion, stellate A sympathetic ganglion located at the level of the seventh cervical vertebra. Site of local anesthetic injection for upper limb complex regional pain syndrome. Syn.: cervicothoracic ganglion.

gate theory of pain Theory that transmission of pain information can be blocked in the dorsal horn by stimulation of large-fiber primary afferent neurons.

generator, stepping pattern Flexible network of interneurons that activate repetitive, rhythmical, reciprocal movement in the lower limbs, similar to stepping during walking.

geniculate, lateral Site of synapse between axons from the retina and neurons that project to the visual cortex. Part of the thalamus, located inferiorly and posteriorly.

geniculate, medial Site of synapse in the auditory pathway. Part of the thalamus, located inferiorly and posteriorly.

genu Most medial part of the internal capsule, containing cortical fibers that project to cranial nerve motor nuclei, to the reticular formation, and to the red nucleus.

glia Support cells of the nervous system, including oligodendrocytes, Schwann cells, astrocytes, and microglia.

globus pallidus internus Part of the globus pallidus specialized for output to the motor thalamus and pedunculopontine nuclei.

glutamate Excitatory amino acid neurotransmitter. Excessive amounts can be toxic to neurons.

glycine Neurotransmitter released by axons from spinal cord interneurons.

gray, periaqueductal Area around the cerebral aqueduct in the midbrain. Involved in somatic and autonomic reactions to pain, threats, and emotions. Activity of the periaqueductal gray results in the fight-or-flight reaction and in vocalization during laughing and crying.

groove, neural During development, the depression formed by the infolding of the neural plate; becomes the neural tube.

growing into deficit Signs and symptoms of nervous system damage that do not become evident until the systems damaged would have become functional.

growth cone The moving tip of a growing axon.

gyrus, cingulate Gyrus on the medial cerebral hemisphere, superior to the corpus callosum. Contributes to processing of memory and emotions.

gyrus, parahippocampal Most medial gyrus of the inferior temporal lobe. Contributes to memory processing.

habituation A form of short-term plasticity. Repeated stimuli result in a decreased response, owing to a decrease in the amount of neurotransmitter released from the presynaptic terminal of a sensory neuron.

Hallpike maneuver Rapid inversion of the posterior semicircular canal. Tests for benign paroxysmal positional vertigo; vertigo and nystagmus indicate a positive test.

hematoma, epidural Collection of blood between the skull and the dura mater.

hematoma, subdural Collection of blood between the dura mater and the arachnoid.

hemianopia, bitemporal Loss of information from both temporal visual fields. Produced by damage to fibers in the center of the optic chiasm, interrupting the axons from the nasal half of each retina. Also called *bitemporal hemianopsia.*

hemianopia, homonymous Loss of visual information from one hemifield. A complete lesion of the visual pathway anywhere posterior to the optic chiasm, in the optic tract, lateral geniculate, or optic radiations, results in loss of information from the contralateral visual field. Also called *homonymous hemianopsia.*

hemiplegia Weakness or paralysis affecting one side of the body.

hemisphere, lateral Part of the cerebellar hemisphere lateral to the paravermis. Involved in coordination of voluntary movements, planning of movements, and the ability to judge time intervals and produce accurate rhythms.

Henneman's size principle Order of recruitment from smaller to larger alpha motor neurons.

herniation, central Movement of the diencephalon, midbrain, and pons inferiorly, caused by a lesion in the cerebrum exerting pressure on the diencephalon. This movement stretches the branches of the basilar artery, causing brainstem ischemia and edema.

herniation, tonsillar Protrusion of the cerebellar tonsils (small lobes forming part of the inferior surface of the cerebellum) through the foramen magnum.

herniation, uncal Protrusion of the uncus into the opening of the tentorium cerebelli, causing compression of the midbrain.

hindbrain Posterior part of the developing brain; becomes the pons, medulla, and cerebellum.

hippocampus Part of the limbic system. Important in processing, but not storage of, declarative memories. Formed by the gray and white matter of two gyri rolled together in the medial temporal lobe.

homunculus Figure representing the parts of the body controlled by or transmitting sensory information to a specific part of the cerebral cortex.

horn, dorsal Posterior section of gray matter in the spinal cord. Primarily sensory in function, the dorsal horn contains endings and collaterals of first-order sensory neurons, interneurons, and dendrites and somas of tract cells.

horn, lateral Lateral section of gray matter in the spinal cord. Contains the cell bodies of preganglionic sympathetic neurons.

horn, ventral Anterior section of gray matter in the spinal cord. Contains endings of upper motor neurons, interneurons, and dendrites and cell bodies of lower motor neurons.

hydrocephalus Accumulation of an excessive amount of cerebrospinal fluid in the ventricles.

hyperalgesia Excessive sensitivity to painful stimuli.

hyperalgesia, primary Excessive sensitivity to stimuli that are normally mildly painful in the injured tissue.

hyperalgesia, secondary Excessive sensitivity to stimuli that are normally mildly painful in uninjured tissue.

hypereffectiveness, synaptic Increased response to a neurotransmitter because damage to some branches of a presynaptic axon results in larger than normal amounts of transmitter being released by the remaining axons onto postsynaptic receptors.

hyperkinetic Characterized by abnormal involuntary movements. Includes dystonic, choreic, athetotic, and choreoathetotic movements.

hyperpolarization Process whereby a neuron's cell membrane potential becomes more negative than its resting potential.

hyperpolarized The electrical state of a neuron's cell membrane when the membrane potential becomes more negative than its resting potential.

hyperreflexia Excessive phasic and/or tonic stretch reflex response. Hyperreflexia often contributes to movement disorders post spinal cord injury and in spastic cerebral palsy. Hyperreflexia usually does not interfere with active movement post stroke.

hypersensitivity, denervation Increased response to a neurotransmitter because new receptor sites have developed on the postsynaptic membrane.

hyperstiffness, muscle Excessive resistance to muscle stretch, regardless of whether the stretch is active or passive. Produced by neutral input to muscles (active muscle contraction) and/or by changes within the muscle (myoplastic hyperstiffness: contracture, selective atrophy of specific muscle fiber types, and weak actin-myosin bonding).

hyperstiffness, myoplastic Excessive resistance to muscle stretch due to changes within the muscle secondary to upper motor neuron lesion. Produced by contracture and increased weak actin-myosin bonding. Post stroke, selective atrophy of type II muscle fibers also contributes to the excessive resistance.

hypertonia Abnormally strong resistance to passive stretch. Occurs in chronic upper motor neuron disorders and in some basal ganglia disorders. Two types are (1) spastic (resistance is dependent on velocity of stretch) and (2) rigid (resistance is independent of velocity of muscle stretch).

hypotension, orthostatic Decrease of 20 mm Hg or more in systolic blood pressure when moving from prone or supine to sitting or standing.

hypothalamus The ventromedial part of the diencephalon. Plays a major role in regulation of the autonomic and endocrine systems, and contributes to emotional and motivational states.

hypotonia Abnormally low muscular resistance to passive stretch. Occurs in lower motor neuron, and primary afferent neuron disorders. Also occurs temporarily following upper motor

neuron lesions owing to a period of neural shock (electrical silence) post injury. Syn.: flaccidity.

incidence Rate of new disease or disorder in a population. Usually expressed as the number of new cases in a year in a population.

infarct, lacunar Obstruction of blood flow in a small, deep artery. Lacunae are small cavities that remain after the necrotic tissue is cleared away.

inhibition, presynaptic At an axoaxonic synapse, the inhibitory process by which transmitter released by one axon terminal causes the second terminal to release a lower than normal amount of neurotransmitter.

inhibition, reciprocal Decreased activity in an antagonist when an agonist is active.

inhibition, recurrent Inhibition of agonists and synergists, combined with disinhibition of antagonists.

insula Cortex located in the lateral fissure of the cerebrum.

internal capsule Axons connecting the cerebral cortex with subcortical structures. The internal capsule is white matter bordered by the caudate and thalamus medially and lenticular nucleus laterally. The internal capsule has three parts: anterior limb, genu, and posterior limb. Anterior limb: located lateral to the head of the caudate, contains corticopontine fibers and fibers interconnecting thalamic and cortical limbic areas. Genu: most medial part of the internal capsule, containing cortical fibers that project to cranial nerve motor nuclei and to the red nucleus. Posterior limb: located between the thalamus and lenticular nucleus, with additional fibers traveling posterior and inferior to the lenticular nucleus

(retrolenticular and sublenticular fibers). The posterior limb contains corticobulbar, corticospinal, and thalamocortical projections.

interneurons Neurons that either process information locally or convey information short distances from one site in the nervous system to another.

internuclear ophthalmoplegia Loss of adduction of one eye during horizontal gaze due to a lesion of the medial longitudinal fasciculus. Convergence is preserved.

junction, neuromuscular Synapse between a nerve terminal and the membrane of a muscle fiber. Acetylcholine is the neurotransmitter released at the neuromuscular junction.

Klumpke's paralysis Paralysis and atrophy of the hand intrinsic muscles and the long flexors and extensors of the fingers caused by avulsion of the motor roots of C8 and T1.

labyrinth The inner ear, consisting of the cochlea and the vestibular apparatus.

laminae, Rexed's Histologic divisions of the spinal cord gray matter.

layer, mantle During development, the inner wall of the neural tube.

layer, marginal During development, the outer wall of the neural tube.

lemniscus, medial Axons of second-order neurons conveying sensory information related to discriminative touch and conscious proprioception from the body to the cerebral cortex. Begins in the nucleus cuneatus and nucleus gracilis and ends in the ventral posterolateral nucleus of the thalamus.

lesion An area of damage or dysfunction; a pathologic change that may be structural or functional.

level, cortical   Areas of cerebral cortex that induce antinociception.

level, neurologic   Describing spinal cord injury, neurologic level is the most caudal level with normal sensory and motor function bilaterally.

limb, anterior   Part of the internal capsule located lateral to the head of the caudate; contains corticopontine fibers and fibers interconnecting thalamic and cortical limbic areas.

limb, posterior   Part of the internal capsule located between the thalamus and lenticular nucleus, with additional fibers traveling posterior and inferior to the lenticular nucleus (retrolenticular and sublenticular fibers). Contains corticobulbar, corticospinal, and thalamocortical projections.

locus ceruleus   Nucleus in the upper pons involved in direction of attention, nonspecific activation of interneurons and lower motor neurons in the spinal cord, and inhibition of pain information in the dorsal horn. Transmitter produced is norepinephrine.

M1   The shortest latency response after stretch of a muscle, produced by the monosynaptic phasic stretch reflex.

M2   The second response after stretch of a muscle, probably involving neural circuits in the brainstem. Also called the *long loop response.*

macroglia   Large support cells of the nervous system, including oligodendrocytes, Schwann cells, and astrocytes.

malformations, arteriovenous Developmental abnormalities with arteries connected to veins by abnormal, thin-walled vessels larger than capillaries. Arteriovenous malformations usually do not cause signs or symptoms unless they rupture.

marginal layer   Most dorsal part of the spinal gray matter. Involved in processing nociceptive information. Syn.: lamina 1.

mater, dura   Tough, outer membrane surrounding the central nervous system.

mater, pia   Inner layer of the membranes surrounding the central nervous system.

medial geniculate body   Thalamic relay station for auditory information to the primary auditory cortex.

mechanoreceptor   Receptor that responds to mechanical stimulation (e.g., stretch or pressure). For example, receptors in the muscle spindle, touch receptors in skin, and stretch receptors in viscera.

medulla   Inferior part of the brainstem. Contributes to the control of eye and head movements, coordinates swallowing, and helps regulate cardiovascular, respiratory, and visceral activity.

memory, declarative   Recollections that can be easily verbalized. Declarative memory is also called *conscious, explicit,* or *cognitive memory.*

memory, procedural   Recall of skills and habits. This type of memory is also called *skill, habit,* or *nonconscious* or *implicit memory.*

meninges   Membranes that enclose the brain and spinal cord. Include the dura mater, arachnoid, and pia mater.

meningitis   Inflammation of the membranes that surround the central nervous system.

meningocele   Congenital defect in which the meninges protrude through a deficiency in the vertebral column or skull.

meningomyelocele   Developmental defect in which the inferior part of the neural tube remains open.

mesencephalic nucleus of the trigeminal nerve   Collection of cell bodies that process proprioceptive information from the face.

messenger, second   Molecule that diffuses through the intracellular environment of a neuron and initiates cellular events including opening or closing of membrane ion channels, activation of genes, or modulation of calcium concentrations inside the cell.

microglia   Small support cells of the nervous system.

midbrain   The uppermost part of the brainstem.

migraine   Syndrome including headache, nausea, vomiting, extreme sensitivity to light and sound, dizziness, and cognitive disturbances. Caused by inherited abnormalities in genes that control activity of certain brainstem neurons. Some migraines do not include headache. Some migraines are preceded by an aura; some are not.

modulation   Long-lasting changes in the electrical potential of a neuron's cell membrane that alter the flow of ions across the cell membrane.

mononeuropathy   Dysfunction of a single peripheral nerve.

mononeuropathy, multiple Dysfunction of several separate peripheral nerves. Signs and symptoms show an asymmetrical distribution.

motor neurons, alpha   Lower motor neurons that innervate extrafusal fibers in skeletal muscle. When these neurons fire, skeletal muscle fibers contract.

motor neurons, gamma   Lower motor neurons that innervate intrafusal fibers in skeletal muscle.

When these neurons fire, the ends of intrafusal fibers contract, stretching the central region of muscle fibers within the muscle spindle.

motor neurons, lower Neurons with their cell bodies in the spinal cord or brainstem whose axons directly innervate skeletal muscle fibers. Two types are alpha motor neurons that innervate extrafusal muscle fibers, and gamma motor neurons that innervate intrafusal muscle fibers.

motor neurons, upper Neurons that transmit information from the brain to lower motor neurons and movement-related interneurons in the spinal cord or brainstem. Although upper motor neurons do not directly innervate skeletal muscle, they contribute to the control of movement by influencing the activity of lower motor neurons.

motor plate Ventral section of the neural tube that becomes the ventral horn in the mature spinal cord.

motor perseveration Uncontrollable repetition of a movement.

muscle synergy Muscle contraction that produces coordinated action.

myasthenia gravis Immune disorder in which antibodies attack acetylcholine receptors on muscle membranes, producing weakness that worsens with repetitive or continuous use of the muscles.

myelin Sheath of proteins and fats formed by oligodendrocytes and Schwann cells to envelop the axons of nerve cells. Provides physical support and insulation for conduction of electrical signals by neurons.

myelination Process of acquiring a myelin sheath.

myeloschisis Congenital defect in which the malformed spinal cord is open to the surface of the body.

myoclonus Brief, involuntary contractions of a muscle or group of muscles.

myofibrils Individual muscles fibers composed of proteins arranged in sarcomeres.

myopathy Abnormality or disease intrinsic to muscle tissue.

myotome During development, the part of a somite that becomes muscle, or after the embryo stage, a group of muscles innervated by a segmental spinal nerve.

neglect Tendency to behave as if one side of the body and/or one side of space does not exist.

nerve, abducens Cranial nerve VI. Controls the lateral rectus muscle that moves the eye laterally.

nerve, accessory Cranial nerve XI. Motor nerve innervating the trapezius and sternocleidomastoid muscles.

nerve, facial Cranial nerve VII. Mixed nerve containing both sensory and motor fibers. The sensory fibers transmit touch, pain, and pressure information from the tongue and pharynx and information from taste buds of the anterior tongue to the solitary nucleus. Motor innervation by the facial nerve includes the muscles that close the eyes, move the lips, and produce facial expressions. The facial nerve provides the efferent limb of the corneal reflex and also innervates salivary, nasal, and lacrimal (tear-producing) glands.

nerve, glossopharyngeal Cranial nerve IX. Mixed nerve containing both sensory and motor fibers. The sensory fibers transmit somatosensation from the soft palate and pharynx and taste information from the posterior tongue. The motor component innervates a pharyngeal muscle and the parotid salivary gland.

nerve, hypoglossal Cranial nerve XII. Motor nerve providing innervation to the intrinsic and extrinsic muscles of the ipsilateral tongue.

nerve, oculomotor Cranial nerve III. Controls the superior, inferior, and medial rectus, the inferior oblique, and the levator palpebrae superioris muscles. These muscles move the eye upward, downward, and medially; rotate the eye around the axis of the pupil; and assist in elevating the upper eyelid. Parasympathetic efferent fibers in the oculomotor nerve innervate the ciliary muscle and the sphincter pupillae, controlling reflexive constriction of the pupil and the thickness of the lens of the eye.

nerve, olfactory Cranial nerve I. Transmits information about odors.

nerve, optic Cranial nerve II. Transmits visual information from the retina to the lateral geniculate body of the thalamus and to nuclei in the midbrain.

nerve, spinal Nerve located in the intervertebral foramen, formed by the dorsal and ventral roots, which contains both afferent and efferent axons. Spinal nerves branch to form dorsal and ventral rami.

nerve, trigeminal Cranial nerve V. Mixed nerve containing both sensory and motor fibers. The sensory fibers transmit information from the face and temporomandibular joint. The motor fibers innervate the muscles of mastication. Three branches: ophthalmic, maxillary, and mandibular.

nerve, trochlear Cranial nerve IV. Controls the superior oblique muscle, which rotates the eye or, if the eye is adducted, depresses the eye.

nerve, vagus Cranial nerve X. Provides sensory and motor innervation of the larynx, pharynx, and bidirectional communication with the viscera.

nerve, vestibulocochlear Cranial nerve VIII. Sensory nerve with two distinct branches. The vestibular branch transmits information related to head position and head movement. The cochlear branch transmits information related to hearing.

neuralgia, post herpetic Severe pain that persists more than 1 month after an infection with Varicella zoster virus. Occurs along the distribution of a peripheral nerve or branch of a peripheral nerve.

neuralgia, trigeminal Dysfunction of the trigeminal nerve, producing severe, sharp, stabbing pain in the distribution of one or more branches of the trigeminal nerve.

neuritis, vestibular Inflammation of the vestibular nerve, usually caused by a virus. Dysequilibrium, spontaneous nystagmus, nausea, and severe vertigo persist up to 3 days.

neuroma Tumor composed of axons and Schwann cells.

neuromodulator Chemical released into the extracellular fluid at a distance from the synaptic cleft. The effects manifest more slowly and usually act longer than effects at a synapse. Typically neuromodulators require seconds before their effects are manifest. The same molecule can act as both a neurotransmitter and a neuromodulator, depending upon whether it is released at a synapse or extrasynaptic site.

neuron The electrically excitable nerve cell of the nervous system.

neuron, afferent (1) Neuron that brings information into the central nervous system. (2) neuron that transmits information toward a structure.

neuron, efferent (1) Neuron that relays commands from the central nervous system to the smooth and skeletal muscles and glands of the body. (2) neuron that transmits information away from a structure.

neuron, postganglionic Autonomic neuron with its cell body in an autonomic ganglion and its termination in an effector organ.

neuron, preganglionic Autonomic neuron with its cell body in the brainstem or spinal cord and its termination in an autonomic ganglion.

neuropathy Dysfunction or pathology of one or more peripheral nerves.

neuroplasticity Ability of neurons to change their function, chemical profile (amount and types of neurotransmitters produced), or structure.

neurotransmitters Chemicals contained in the presynaptic terminal that are released into the synaptic cleft to transmit information between neurons.

nociceptive Able to receive or transmit information about stimuli that damage or threaten to damage tissue.

nociceptors Receptors that are sensitive to information about tissue damage or potential tissue damage.

nodes of Ranvier Interruptions in the myelin sheath that leave small patches of axon unmyelinated. These unmyelinated patches contain a high density of voltage-gated Na^+ channels that contribute to the generation of action potentials.

norepinephrine A neurotransmitter released by axons from the locus ceruleus and medial reticular zone and by postganglionic sympathetic axons except those innervating sweat glands. Binds with α- and β-adrenergic receptors.

nuclei, association Thalamic nuclei that connect reciprocally with large areas of cerebral cortex. Association nuclei are found in the anterior thalamus, medial thalamus, and dorsal tier of the lateral thalamus.

nuclei, cochlear Site of synapse between first- and second-order neurons involved in hearing. Located laterally at the pontomedullary junction.

nuclei, nonspecific Thalamic nuclei that receive multiple types of input and project to widespread areas of cortex. This functional group includes the reticular, midline, and intralaminar nuclei, important in consciousness and arousal.

nuclei, raphe Brainstem nuclei that modulate activity throughout the central nervous system. Major source of serotonin. The midbrain raphe nuclei are important in mood regulation and onset of sleep. Pontine raphe nuclei modulate activity in the brainstem and cerebellum. Medullary raphe nuclei modulate activity in the spinal cord via raphespinal tracts. Projections to the spinal cord inhibit transmission of nociceptive information, adjust levels of interneuron activity, and produce nonspecific activation of lower motor neurons.

nuclei, relay Thalamic nuclei that receive specific information and serve as relay stations by sending the information directly to localized areas of cerebral cortex. All relay nuclei are found in the ventral tier of the lateral nuclear group.

nuclei, vestibular   Site of synapse between first- and second-order neurons involved in detecting head movement and head position. Located laterally at the pontomedullary junction.

nucleus   Collection of nerve cell bodies in the central nervous system.

nucleus accumbens   Group of neurons located at the junction of the head of the caudate and the anterior part of the putamen. Involved in reward, pleasure, and addiction.

nucleus, Clarke's   Site of synapse between first- and second-order neurons that convey unconscious proprioceptive information to the cerebellum. The second-order axon is in the posterior spinocerebellar tract. Clarke's nucleus is located in the medial dorsal horn of the spinal cord, from T1 to L2 spinal segments. Syn.: nucleus dorsalis.

nucleus cuneatus   Site of synapse between fasciculus cuneatus and medial lemniscus neurons. Relays discriminative touch and conscious proprioceptive information. Located in the dorsal part of the lower medulla.

nucleus dorsalis   Site of synapse between first- and second-order neurons that convey unconscious proprioceptive information to the cerebellum. The second-order axon is in the posterior spinocerebellar tract. The nucleus dorsalis is located in the medial dorsal horn of the spinal cord, from T1 to L2 spinal segments. Syn.: Clarke's nucleus.

nucleus gracilis   Site of synapse between fasciculus gracilis and medial lemniscus neurons. Relays discriminative touch and conscious proprioceptive information.

Located in the dorsal part of the lower medulla.

nucleus, inferior olivary   Nucleus in the upper medulla that receives input from most motor areas of the brain and spinal cord. Axons from the inferior olivary nucleus project to the contralateral cerebellar hemisphere. May be involved in the perception of time.

nucleus, lateral cuneate   Nucleus that receives proprioceptive information from the upper body. Relays unconscious proprioceptive information to the cerebellum, via the cuneocerebellar tract. Located in the dorsolateral medulla.

nucleus, lentiform   Globus pallidus and putamen.

nucleus, main sensory of trigeminal   Site of synapse between first- and second-order discriminative touch neurons in the trigeminothalamic pathway.

nucleus, mesencephalic of the trigeminal nerve   Location of cell bodies of primary afferents conveying proprioceptive information from the muscles of mastication and extraocular muscles.

nucleus, pedunculopontine   Nucleus within the caudal midbrain that influences movement via connections with the globus pallidus, subthalamic nucleus, and reticular areas. The neurons produce acetylcholine.

nucleus proprius   Part of the dorsal gray matter in the spinal cord. Processes proprioceptive and two-point discrimination information. Syn.: laminae III and IV.

nucleus, red   Sphere of gray matter that receives information from the cerebellum and cerebral cortex and projects to the cerebellum, spinal cord (via rubrospinal tract), and

reticular formation. Activity in the rubrospinal tract contributes to upper limb flexion.

nucleus, solitary   Main visceral sensory nucleus. Receives information from the oral cavity and thoracic and abdominal viscera via the vagus, glossopharyngeal, and facial nerves. Involved in regulation of visceral function. Located in the dorsal medulla.

nucleus, spinal trigeminal   Site of synapse between first- and second-order neurons conveying nociceptive information from the face. Located in the lower pons and medulla.

nucleus, subthalamic   Collection of cell bodies located inferior to the thalamus and superior to the substantia nigra. Part of the basal ganglia.

nucleus, trigeminal main sensory   Nucleus that receives touch information from the face. The information is transmitted to the ventral posteromedial nucleus of the thalamus, then to the cerebral cortex.

nucleus, ventral posterolateral of the thalamus   Site of synapse between neurons that convey somatosensory information from the body to the cerebral cortex. The spinothalamic and medial lemniscus axons end in this nucleus.

nucleus, ventral posteromedial   Site of synapse between neurons that convey somatosensory information from the face to the cerebral cortex. Located in the thalamus.

nystagmus   Involuntary back-and-forth movements of the eyes. Physiologic nystagmus is a normal response that can be elicited in an intact nervous system by rotational or temperature stimulation of the semicircular canals or by moving the eyes to the extreme horizontal position. Pathologic nystagmus, a sign of nervous system abnormality, is abnormal oscillating eye movements that occur with or without external stimulation.

nystagmus, pathologic   Abnormal oscillating eye movements that occur with or without external stimulation.

obtunded   Sleeping more than awake; drowsy and confused when awake.

oculomotor complex   Oculomotor nucleus and the oculomotor parasympathetic nucleus. The oculomotor nucleus supplies efferent somatic fibers to the extraocular muscles innervated by the oculomotor nerve. The oculomotor parasympathetic (Edinger-Westphal) nucleus supplies parasympathetic control of the pupillary sphincter and the ciliary muscle (adjusts thickness of the lens in the eye).

oligodendrocytes   Macroglia that form myelin sheaths, enveloping several axons from several neurons. Found within the central nervous system.

olive   Small oval lump on the anterolateral medulla that lies external to the inferior olivary nucleus.

organ of Corti   Organ of hearing, located within the cochlea.

organs, otolithic   The utricle and saccule, part of the inner ear. Contain receptors that respond to head position relative to gravity and to linear acceleration and deceleration of the head.

oscillopsia   Lack of visual stabilization. The world appears to bounce up and down due to failure of the vestibulo-ocular reflex.

outflow, craniosacral   Parasympathetic nervous system.

outflow, thoracolumbar   Sympathetic nervous system.

pain, chronic   Persistent pain. The three major types are (1) nociceptive (continuing tissue damage), (2) chronic neuropathic pain, and (3) chronic pain syndrome. Continuing tissue damage arises from rheumatoid arthritis, cancer, and other physically identifiable causes. Chronic neuropathic pain is due to abnormal neural activity within the central nervous system. An example is phantom limb pain. Chronic pain syndrome is pain that persists more than 6 months after normal healing would have been expected. An example is chronic low back pain syndrome without continuing tissue damage. Disuse syndrome may be a contributing factor to chronic low back pain syndrome.

pain, fast   Discriminative information about stimuli that damage or threaten to damage tissue. Conveyed to cerebral cortex.

pain, myofascial   A controversial diagnosis: pressure on sensitive points (called trigger points) reproduces the person's pattern of referred pain. Advocates contend that the diagnosis is confirmed when stretch or injecting a local anesthetic into the trigger points eliminates the pain.

pain, neuropathic chronic   Persistent pain due to abnormal neural activity in various locations in the nervous system.

pain, nociceptive chronic   Persistent pain due to stimulation of nociceptive receptors.

pain, phantom limb   Neuropathic pain that seems to originate from a missing body part, caused by central nervous system overactivity subsequent to an amputation.

pain, referred   Pain that is perceived as arising in a site different from the actual site producing the nociceptive information.

pain, slow   Nonlocalized information about stimuli that damage or threaten to damage tissue. Conveyed by divergent pathways to areas in the midbrain and reticular formation and to the medial and intralaminar nuclei of the thalamus. This information reaches widespread areas of the cerebral cortex.

pain, spinothalamic   Discriminative information about stimuli that damage or threaten to damage tissue. Conveyed to cerebral cortex. Syn.: fast pain.

palsy, Bell's   Paralysis or paresis of the muscles of facial expression on one side of the face, caused by a lesion of the facial nerve.

palsy, cerebral   Movement and postural disorder resulting from permanent, nonprogressive damage to the developing brain.

paralysis   Inability to voluntarily contract muscle(s). Reflexive contraction may be intact if the paralysis is due to an upper motor neuron lesion. Reflexive contraction is absent if paralysis is due to a complete lower motor neuron lesion.

paralysis, flaccid   Loss of voluntary movement and muscle tone.

paraphrasia   Word substitution. Syn.: paraphasia.

paraplegia   Paresis or paralysis of both lower limbs. May also involve part of the trunk.

paravermis   Part of the cerebellar hemisphere adjacent to the vermis; influences the activity of the lateral activation pathways.

paresis   Weakness; decreased ability to generate the amount of force required for a task.

paresthesia   Nonpainful abnormal sensation, often described as pricking and tingling.

parkinsonism A general term for basal ganglia disorders with signs and symptoms characteristic of Parkinson's disease. Includes disorders caused by drugs, infection, or trauma. The term excludes idiopathic Parkinson's disease.

pathway, conscious relay Three-neuron series that transmits somatosensory information about location and type of stimulation to the cerebral cortex.

pathway, cuneocerebellar A two-neuron series that transmits proprioceptive information from the arm and upper half of the body to the cerebellum.

pathway, divergent Series of neurons that transmits somatosensory information to the brainstem and cerebrum.

pathway, posterior spinocerebellar A two-neuron series that transmits proprioceptive information from the legs and the lower half of the body to the cerebellum.

pathway, spinolimbic Axons that convey nonlocalized nociceptive information to the medial and intralaminar nuclei of the thalamus. The information is then transmitted to limbic and other areas of the cerebral cortex. Involved in arousal, withdrawal, and autonomic and affective responses to pain.

pathway, retinogeniculocalcarine Neural connections that convey visual information from the retina to the visual cortex.

pathway, spinomesencephalic Series of neurons that transmits nociceptive information to the superior colliculus and to the periaqueductal gray in the midbrain. Activates parts of the descending pain control system.

pathway, spinoreticular Series of neurons that convey nonlocalized nociceptive information to the reticular formation. The information influences arousal and is transmitted to the medial and intralaminar nuclei of the thalamus.

peduncles, cerebellar Bundles of axons that connect the cerebellum with the brainstem. The superior peduncle connects with the midbrain, the middle peduncle with the pons, and the inferior peduncle with the medulla.

peduncles, cerebral The most anterior part of the midbrain, formed by axons descending from the cerebrum to the pons, medulla, and spinal cord. Specifically the corticospinal, corticobulbar, and corticopontine tracts.

perception Interpretation of sensation into meaningful forms.

perineurium Connective tissue that surrounds bundles of axons.

period, absolute refractory The time period during an action potential when no stimulus, no matter how strong, will elicit another action potential.

period, critical Time period during which neuronal projections are competing for synaptic sites.

period, relative refractory Time period soon after the peak of an action potential when only a stronger than normal stimulus can elicit another action potential.

peripheral nerve distribution Area of skin innervated by a single peripheral nerve.

periphery Parts of the body outside the vertebra and skull.

perseveration, motor Uncontrollable repetition of a movement.

phoria Tendency for one eye to deviate from looking straight ahead when binocular vision is not available.

plaques Patches of demyelination.

plasmapheresis Replacement of blood plasma with a plasma substitute, to remove circulating antibodies.

plate, association Dorsal section of the neural tube that becomes the dorsal horn in the spinal cord.

plate, neural During development, the thickened ectoderm on the surface of an embryo; becomes the neural tube.

polyneuropathy Generalized disorder of peripheral nerves that typically presents distally and symmetrically.

polyneuropathy, diabetic Distal, usually symmetrical impairment of axon and myelin function secondary to diabetes.

positron emission tomography (PET) Computer-generated image based on the metabolism of injected radioactively labeled substances. The image indicates metabolic activity of the central nervous system.

post-ganglionic An axon that originates from a cell body located in an autonomic ganglion.

postural instability Tendency to lose one's balance.

posturography Recording of force plate information and electromyograms from postural muscles during postural tests.

potential, action A large change in the electrical potential of a neuron's cell membrane, resulting in the rapid spread of an electrical signal along the cell membrane.

potential, equilibrium The electrical membrane potential at which any diffusible ion is electrically and chemically distributed equally on the two sides of the membrane.

potential, excitatory postsynaptic (EPSP) Electrical depolarization of a neuron's cell membrane. Initiated by the binding of a neurotransmitter to membrane receptors and produced by the instantaneous flow of Na^+, K^+, or Ca^{++} into the cell.

potential, inhibitory postsynaptic (IPSP) Electrical hyperpolarization of a cell membrane. Initiated by the binding of a neurotransmitter to membrane receptors and produced by the instantaneous flow of Cl^- into the cell and/or K^+ out of the cell.

potential, local A small change in the electrical potential of a neuron's cell membrane that is graded in both amplitude and duration.

potential, resting membrane The difference in electrical potential across the cell membrane of a neuron when the neuron is neither receiving nor transmitting information, i.e., the electrical state of a neuron's cell membrane when the cell is at rest (neither electrically excited nor inhibited).

potentials, auditory evoked A method of testing brainstem function by auditory stimulation combined with recording electrical potentials from the scalp.

potentials, receptor Local potentials generated at the receptor of a sensory neuron.

potentials, postsynaptic Graded, local changes in ion concentration across the postsynaptic membrane. May be excitatory or inhibitory.

potentials, synaptic Local potentials generated at a postsynaptic membrane.

potentiation, long-term (LTP) Cellular mechanism for memory that results from the synthesis and activation of new proteins and the growth of new synaptic connections.

premotor area Controls trunk and girdle muscles via the medial upper motor neurons.

preganglionic Neuron or axon proximal to an autonomic ganglion.

prevalence Number of existing cases of a disease or disorder at a specific time per number of people in a population.

progressive supranuclear palsy (PSP) A type of parkinsonism characterized by depression, psychosis, rage attacks, and impairment of voluntary movement of the eyes.

pronociception Biological amplification of pain signals.

proprioception, conscious Awareness of the movements and relative position of body parts.

propriospinal Within the spinal cord. Usually refers to neurons that are located entirely within the spinal cord.

pyramids Ridges on the anteroinferior medulla, formed by the lateral corticospinal tracts.

radiculopathy Lesion of a dorsal or ventral nerve root. Clinical use of the term may refer to a spinal nerve lesion.

rami, anterior Branch of a spinal nerve that innervates the skeletal, muscular, and cutaneous areas of the limbs and the anterior and lateral trunk.

rami, posterior Branch of a spinal nerve that innervates paravertebral muscles, posterior parts of the vertebrae, and overlying cutaneous areas.

ramus, dorsal primary Branch of a spinal nerve that innervates the paravertebral muscles, posterior parts of the vertebrae, and overlying cutaneous areas.

ramus, ventral primary Branch of a spinal nerve that innervates the skeletal, muscular, and cutaneous areas of the limbs and/or of the anterior and lateral trunk.

receptor, muscarinic Receptor on an organ innervated by a postganglionic parasympathetic neuron. Acetylcholine binding to muscarinic receptors initiates a G-protein–mediated response.

receptor, phasic A sensory nerve ending that adapts to a constant stimulus and stops responding.

receptor, tonic A sensory nerve ending that responds as long as a stimulus is present.

receptors, adrenergic Receptors in the sympathetic nervous system that respond to norepinephrine or epinephrine or to adrenergic drugs. Subtypes are α- and β-adrenergic receptors.

receptors, cholinergic Receptors that respond to acetylcholine. Found in the autonomic and central nervous systems and on the motor end-plate in skeletal muscle membranes. Subtypes include nicotinic and muscarinic.

receptors, nicotinic Receptors on postsynaptic neurons in autonomic ganglia and on the motor end-plate of skeletal muscle. Acetylcholine binding to nicotinic receptors causes a fast excitatory postsynaptic potential in the postsynaptic membrane.

reflex An involuntary response to an external stimulus.

reflex, asymmetrical tonic neck Head rotation to the right or left elicits extension of the limbs on the nose side and flexion of limbs on the skull side.

reflex, consensual Constriction of the pupil in the opposite eye when a bright light is shined into one eye. The optic nerve is the afferent (sensory) limb of the reflex, while the oculomotor nerve provides the efferent (motor) limb.

reflex, crossed extension Extension of the opposite lower limb when one lower limb is moved away from a stimulus.

reflex, H-   Reflexive muscle contraction elicited by electrically stimulating the skin over a peripheral nerve. Used to assess the degree of excitation of alpha motor neurons.

reflex, phasic stretch   Muscle contraction in response to quick stretch. Syn.: myotatic reflex, muscle stretch reflex, deep tendon reflex.

reflex, pupillary   Pupil constriction in the eye directly stimulated by a bright light. The optic nerve is the afferent (sensory) limb of the reflex, while the oculomotor nerve provides the efferent (motor) limb.

reflex, symmetrical tonic neck   Flexion of the upper limbs and extension of the lower limbs when the neck is flexed and the opposite pattern in the limbs when the neck is extended.

reflex, tonic labyrinthine   Tilting the head back causes flexion of the upper limbs and extension of the lower limbs. Tilting the head forward elicits extension of the upper limbs and flexion of the lower limbs.

reflex, tonic stretch   Sustained alpha motor neuron firing and muscle contraction in response to maintained stretch of muscle spindles. At velocities of muscle stretch typically used in clinic, the tonic stretch reflex is only present following upper motor neuron lesions.

reflex, vestibulo-ocular   Automatic movements of the eyes that stabilize visual images during head and body movements.

reflex, withdrawal   Movement of a limb away from a stimulus.

reflexive bladder function   Stretching of the bladder wall initiates bladder emptying.

refractory   The time following an action potential during which another action potential cannot be generated or more stimulation than normal is required to generate an action potential.

reuptake   Process of taking neurotransmitters back into cells for reuse or recycling.

response, clasp-knife   When a spastic muscle is slowly and passively stretched, resistance to stretch is suddenly inhibited at a specific point in the range of motion.

response, long loop   The second response after stretch of a contracting muscle, probably involving neural circuits in the brainstem. Also called M2.

response reversal   Modification of ongoing motor activity to adapt the movement to environmental conditions. For example, if one catches a foot under an object while walking, the foot is moved to clear the object rather than continue to collide with the object.

rhizotomy, dorsal   Surgical severance of selected dorsal roots. Purpose is to decrease pain or to decrease hyperreflexia.

rigidity   Velocity-independent muscle hypertonia.

saccade   High-speed eye movement.

saccule   Part of the inner ear that contains receptors that respond to head position relative to gravity and to linear acceleration and deceleration of the head.

sarcomere   Functional unit of skeletal muscle consisting of the proteins between two adjacent Z-lines.

schizophrenia   Group of disorders consisting of disordered thinking, delusions, hallucinations, and social withdrawal.

sclerosis, amyotrophic lateral   Disease that destroys only the lateral activating pathways and anterior horn cells in the spinal cord, thus producing upper and lower motor neuron signs.

sclerosis, multiple   Disease characterized by random, multifocal demyelination limited to the central nervous system. Signs and symptoms include numbness, paresthesias, Lhermitte's sign, asymmetrical weakness, and/or ataxia.

sclerotome   During development, the part of a somite that becomes the vertebrae and skull.

section, basilar   Anterior part of the brainstem, containing predominantly motor system structures.

segmental organization   Arrangement of spinal cord according to the spinal nerves that connect a section of the cord with a specific region of the body.

sensitivity   Ability to detect a specific stimulus. For example, the ability to detect light touch.

sensitize   To make neurons fire with less stimulation than is usually required.

serotonin   Neurotransmitter released by axons from the raphe nuclei. See *nuclei, raphe* for a summary of functions.

severance   Physically division of a nerve, by excessive stretch or laceration.

sheath, myelin   Covering of fat and protein that surrounds axons.

sign, Babinski's   Reflexive extension of the great toe, often accompanied by fanning of the other toes. The sign is elicited by firm stroking of the lateral sole of the foot, from the heel to the ball of the foot, then across the ball of the foot.

sign, Lhermitte's   Radiation of a sensation like electrical shock down the back or limbs, elicited by neck flexion.

sign, Tinel's   Sensation of pain or tingling in the distal distribution of a peripheral nerve, elicited by tapping on the skin over an injured nerve.

sinus, dural   Spaces between layers of dura mater that collect venous blood.

smooth pursuits   Eye movements that follow a moving object.

soma   Cell body, the metabolic center of a cell.

somatotopic   Information arranged similarly to the anatomical organization of the body.

somatic marker hypothesis   Theory that emotions are crucial for sound judgment. Proposed by Antonio Damasio.

somite   During development, the part of the mesoderm that will become dermis, bone, and muscle.

spasm, muscle   Sudden, involuntary contraction of muscle fibers.

spasticity   (1) Velocity-dependent muscle hypertonia. (2) the entire upper motor neuron syndrome.

spina bifida   A developmental defect resulting from failure of the inferior part of the neural tube to close.

spinal cord injury, complete   Lack of sensory and motor function in the lowest sacral segment (American Spinal Cord Injury Association definition).

spinal cord injury, incomplete   Preservation of sensory and/or motor function in the lowest sacral segment (American Spinal Cord Injury Association definition).

spinal shock   Temporary suppression of spinal cord function at and below the lesion following spinal cord injury. Caused by edema.

spindle, muscle   Sensory organ embedded in muscle that responds to stretch of the muscle.

spinocerebellum   Functional name for the vermis and paravermal region of the cerebellum. Controls ongoing movements.

spondylosis, cervical   Degeneration of the cervical vertebrae and disks that produces narrowing of the vertebral canal and intervertebral foramina.

sprouting   The regrowth of damaged axons.

sprouting, collateral   Reinnervation of a denervated target by branches of intact axons.

sprouting, regenerative   Injured axon sends out side sprouts to a new target.

stage, embryonic   Developmental stage lasting from the second to the end of the eighth week in utero; during this time, the organs are formed.

stage, fetal   Developmental stage lasting from the end of the eighth week in utero until birth; the nervous system continues to develop, and myelination begins.

stage, pre-embryonic   Developmental stage lasting from conception to the second week in utero.

state, vegetative   Complete loss of consciousness, without alteration of vital functions.

stenosis   Narrowing of the vertebral canal.

stepping pattern generators (SPGs)   Adaptable networks of spinal interneurons that activate lower motor neurons to elicit alternating flexion and extension of the lower limbs.

stereognosis   Ability to use manipulation, touch, and proprioceptive information to identify an object.

stream, action   Stream of visual information that flows dorsally and is used to direct movements.

stream, perception   Stream of visual information that flows ventrally and is used to recognize visual objects.

striatum   Caudate and putamen.

striatum, ventral   Inferior junction of the caudate and putamen. Includes the nucleus accumbens.

striatonigral degeneration   Multiple system atrophy presenting initially with rigidity and bradykinesia.

stroke   Sudden onset of neurologic deficits due to disruption of the blood supply in the brain. Syn.: cerebrovascular accident (CVA), brain attack.

stroke, completed   Neurologic deficits, resulting from vascular disorders affecting the brain, which persist more than 1 day and are stable (not progressing or improving).

stroke, progressive   Neurologic deficits, resulting from vascular disorders, which increase intermittently over time. Progressive strokes are believed to be due to repeated emboli or continued formation of a thrombus in the brain.

stupor   Condition of being arousable only by strong stimuli, such as strong pinching of the Achilles tendon.

Substance P   Neurotransmitter produced by primary nociceptive neurons. Also produced in other areas of the central nervous system.

substantia gelatinosa   Part of the dorsal gray matter in the spinal cord. Involved in processing nociceptive information. Syn.: lamina II.

substantia nigra   One of the nuclei in the basal ganglia circuit, located in the midbrain. The compacta part provides dopamine to the caudate nucleus and putamen. The reticularis part serves as one of the output nuclei for the basal ganglia circuit.

substantia nigra reticularis   Part of the substantia nigra specialized for output to the motor thalamus and pedunculopontine nuclei.

subthalamus   Part of the basal ganglia circuit, involved in regulating movement. The subthalamus facilitates the basal ganglia output nuclei. The subthalamus is located superior to the substantia nigra of the midbrain.

summation, spatial   The cumulative effect of either receptor or synaptic potentials occurring simultaneously at different receptor sites of the neuron.

summation, temporal   The cumulative effect of a series of either receptor or synaptic potentials that occur within milliseconds of each other.

supplementary motor cortex   Initiates movement, orients the eyes and head, and plans bimanual and sequential movements.

syncope   Fainting. Loss of consciousness due to an abrupt decrease in blood pressure that deprives the brain of adequate blood supply.

syndrome, anterior cord   Signs and symptoms produced by interruption of ascending spinothalamic tracts, descending motor tracts, and damage to the somas of lower motor neurons. This spinal cord syndrome interferes with pain and temperature sensation and with motor control.

syndrome, Brown-Séquard's   Signs and symptoms produced by a hemisection of the spinal cord. Segmental losses are ipsilateral and include loss of lower motor neurons and all sensations. Below

the level of the lesion, voluntary motor control, conscious proprioception, and discriminative touch are lost ipsilaterally, and temperature and nociceptive information are lost contralaterally.

syndrome, cauda equina   Signs and symptoms produced by damage to the lumbar and/or sacral nerve roots, causing sensory impairment and flaccid paralysis of lower limb muscles, bladder, and bowels.

syndrome, central cord   Signs and symptoms produced by interruption of spinothalamic fibers crossing the midline, producing loss of pain and temperature sensation at the involved segments. Larger lesions also impair upper limb motor function because the lateral corticospinal tracts to the upper limb are located in the medial part of the white matter and because the lesion typically occurs in the cervical region.

syndrome, chronic pain   Physiologic impairment consisting of muscle guarding, abnormal movements, and disuse syndrome.

syndrome, Guillain-Barré   Acute, autoimmune peripheral polyneuropathy characterized by progressive paralysis, burning/tingling sensations, and pain.

syndrome, Horner's   Drooping of the upper eyelid, constriction of the pupil, and vasodilation with absence of sweating on the ipsilateral face and neck. Due to lesions of the cervical sympathetic chain or its central pathways.

syndrome, locked-in   Complete inability to move, despite intact consciousness. Due to damage to upper motor neurons.

syndrome, Ramsay-Hunt   Varicella zoster infection of the facial and vestibular nerves.

syndrome, Shy-Drager   Multiple system atrophy presenting initially with autonomic dysfunction.

syndrome, tethered cord   Abnormal attachment of the sacral spinal cord to surrounding structures. Signs and symptoms include low back and lower limb pain, difficulty walking, excessive lordosis, scoliosis, problems with bowel and/or bladder control, foot deformities, and paresis. If the spinal cord is excessively stretched, may cause upper motor neuron signs.

synkinesis   Unintended movements when lower motor neurons fire. Occurs when severed motor neurons regrow to innervate different muscles than they innervated prior to being severed.

syringomyelia   Rare, progressive disorder. A syrinx, or fluid-filled cavity, develops in the spinal cord, almost always in the cervical region. Segmental signs occur in the upper limbs, including loss of sensitivity to pain and temperature stimuli. Upper motor neuron signs in lower limbs include paresis, muscle hyperstiffness, and phasic stretch hyperreflexia. Often loss of bowel and bladder control also occurs.

system, consciousness   Neural connections governing alertness, sleep, and attention. Includes the reticular formation, the ascending reticular activating system, the basal forebrain (anterior to the hypothalamus), the thalamus, and the cerebral cortex.

system, dorsal column/medial lemniscus   Pathway that transmits information about discriminative touch and conscious proprioception to the cerebral cortex.

system, hormonal   System that provides antinociception by the release of hormones.

system, limbic Group of structures involved in emotions, processing of declarative memories, and autonomic control. Includes parts of the hypothalamus, thalamus, limbic cortex (cingulate gyrus, parahippocampal gyrus, uncus), hippocampus, amygdala, and the basal forebrain (septal area, preoptic area, nucleus accumbens, and the basal nucleus of Meynert).

system, neuronal descending Brainstem areas that contain cell bodies of descending axons involved in antinociception.

tectum Part of the midbrain posterior to the cerebral aqueduct, consisting of the pretectal area and the superior and inferior colliculi. Involved in reflexive movements of the eyes and head.

tegmentum Posterior part of the brainstem, including sensory nuclei and tracts, reticular formation, cranial nerve nuclei, and the medial longitudinal fasciculus.

terminal, postsynaptic The membrane region of a cell containing receptor sites for a neurotransmitter.

terminal, presynaptic The end projection of an axon, specialized for releasing a neurotransmitter into the synaptic cleft.

tetraplegia Impairment of arm, trunk, lower limb, and pelvic organ function, usually due to damage involving the cervical spinal cord.

thalamus Group of nuclei deep in the cerebrum that relays information to and from the cerebral cortex.

theory, counterirritant Theory that inhibition of nociceptive signals by stimulation of non-nociceptive receptors occurs in the dorsal horn of the spinal cord.

thermoreceptor Receptor that responds to changes in temperature.

threshold (1) The least amount of stimulation that can be perceived when testing sensation. (2) the minimum stimulus necessary to produce action potentials in an axon.

thrombus Blood clot within the vascular system.

tinnitus Sensation of ringing in the ear.

tomography, positron emission (PET scan) Computer-generated image based on metabolism of injected radioactively labeled substances. The PET scan records local variations in blood flow, reflecting neural activity.

tone, muscle Amount of resistance to passive stretch exerted by a resting muscle.

touch, discriminative Localization of touch and vibration, and the ability to discriminate between two closely spaced points touching the skin.

tract A bundle of axons with the same origin and a common termination.

tract, anterior spinocerebellar Axons that transmit information about the activity of spinal interneurons and of descending motor signals from the cerebral cortex and brainstem. The neurons arise in the thoracolumbar spinal cord and end in the cerebellar cortex. The information does not reach consciousness and is used to adjust movements.

tract, ceruleospinal Axons originating in the locus ceruleus that 1. enhance activity in spinal interneurons and motor neurons. The effects of ceruleospinal activity are generalized (not related to specific movements). 2. inhibit the nociceptive pathway neurons in the dorsal horn.

tract, cuneocerebellar Axons that transmit high-fidelity, somatotopically arranged tactile and proprioceptive information from the upper half of the body to the cerebellar cortex. The information does not reach consciousness and is used to adjust movements.

tract, dorsolateral White matter dorsal to the dorsal horn in the spinal cord. Axons of first-order nociceptive neurons ascend or descend in this tract before synapsing in the dorsal horn lamina. Syn.: zone of Lissauer.

tract, geniculocalcarine Axons that convey visual information from the lateral geniculate body of the thalamus to the visual cortex.

tract, internal feedback Axons of neurons that monitor the activity of spinal interneurons and of descending motor signals from the cerebral cortex and brainstem. The information is transmitted to the cerebellum. The information does not reach consciousness and is used to adjust movements.

tract, lateral corticospinal Axons that arise in motor planning areas of the cerebral cortex and the primary motor cortex and synapse with lower motor neurons that innervate limb muscles. Essential for fractionated hand movements.

tract, lateral (medullary) reticulospinal Axons originating in the medullary reticular formation that descend bilaterally to facilitate flexor muscle motor neurons and to inhibit extensor muscle motor neurons.

tract, lateral vestibulospinal Axons arising in the lateral vestibular nucleus that project ipsilaterally to facilitate lower motor neurons to extensor muscles and simultaneously inhibit lower motor neurons to flexor muscles via interneurons.

tract, medial corticospinal   Axons that convey information from motor areas of the cerebral cortex to the spinal cord. The axons end in the cervical and thoracic cord and influence the activity of lower motor neurons that innervate neck, shoulder, and trunk muscles.

tract, medial reticulospinal   Axons that project from the pontine reticular formation to the spinal cord. Activation of this tract facilitates ipsilateral lower motor neurons innervating postural muscles and limb extensors.

tract, medial vestibulospinal   Axons arising in the medial vestibular nucleus that project bilaterally to the cervical and thoracic spinal cord. Affect the activity of lower motor neurons controlling neck and upper back muscles.

tract, spinothalamic   Axons of second-order nociceptive specific neurons that convey localized pain information and second-order neurons that convey temperature information from the spinal cord to the ventral posterolateral nucleus of the thalamus. Part of the discriminative pain and temperature conscious relay pathway to the cerebral cortex.

tract, optic   Axons that convey visual information from the optic chiasm to the lateral geniculate body of the thalamus.

tract, posterior (dorsal) spinocerebellar   Axons that transmit high-fidelity somatotopically arranged tactile and proprioceptive information from Clarke's nucleus (information from the lower half of the body) to the cerebellar cortex. The information does not reach

consciousness and is used to adjust movements.

tract, raphespinal   (1) Axons originating in the raphe nuclei that enhance activity in spinal interneurons and motor neurons. The effects of raphespinal activity are generalized (not related to specific movements). (2) axons originating in the raphe nuclei that inhibit the transmission of nociceptive information in the spinal cord.

tract, rostrospinocerebellar   Axons that transmit information about the activity of spinal interneurons and of descending motor signals from the cerebral cortex and brainstem. The neurons arise in the cervical spinal cord and end in the cerebellar cortex. The information does not reach consciousness and is used to adjust movements.

tract, rubrospinal   Axons that originate in the red nucleus of the midbrain, cross to the opposite side, then descend to synapse with lower motor neurons primarily innervating upper limb flexor muscles.

tract, tectospinal   Axons that project from the superior colliculus to synapse with lower motor neurons in the cervical spinal cord. Involved in reflexive movements of the head toward stimuli.

tracts, corticobulbar   Axons that convey motor signals from the cerebral cortex to cranial nerve nuclei in the brainstem.

tracts, descending motor   Axons that convey movement-related information from the brain to lower motor neurons in the spinal cord or brainstem.

tracts, fine movement   Axons involved in the descending control of skilled, voluntary movements.

tracts, high-fidelity   Two groups of axons, the posterior spinocerebellar

and cuneocerebellar, which relay accurate, detailed, somatotopically arranged tactile and proprioceptive information from the spinal cord to the cerebellar cortex. The information does not reach consciousness and is used to adjust movements.

tracts, lateral upper motor neuron   Neurons that influence the activity of lower motor neurons innervating limb muscles. Includes the lateral corticospinal, rubrospinal, and lateral reticulospinal tracts.

tracts, medial upper motor neuron   Neurons that influence the activity of lower motor neurons innervating postural and girdle muscles.

tracts, motor corticofugal   Axons of upper motor neurons whose cell bodies are in the cerebral cortex: the corticospinal, corticopontine, and corticobulbar tracts.

tracts, nonspecific upper motor neurons   Axons of upper motor neurons that influence the general level of activity in lower motor neurons.

tracts, postural/gross movement   Axons of upper motor neurons that synapse with lower motor neurons controlling automatic skeletal muscle activity.

tracts, spinocerebellar   Groups of axons that convey proprioceptive information or information from spinal interneurons to the cerebellum. The information does not reach consciousness and is used to adjust movements.

tracts, unconscious relay   Axons of neurons that convey proprioceptive information from the spinal cord or information from spinal interneurons to the cerebellum. The information does not reach consciousness and is used to adjust movements.

transmission, ephaptic Cross-excitation of axons, due to loss of myelin. Excitation of one axon induces activity in a parallel axon.

transport, anterograde Movement of proteins and neurotransmitters from the soma to the axon.

transport, retrograde Movement of some substances from the axon back to the soma for recycling.

traumatic axonopathy Severance of an axon by injury.

traumatic myelinopathy Loss of myelin limited to the site of injury.

tremor Involuntary, rhythmic shaking movements of the limbs produced by contractions of antagonist muscles.

tremor, action Shaking of a limb during voluntary movement.

tremor, resting Repetitive alternating contraction of the extensor and flexor muscles of the distal extremities during inactivity. The tremor diminishes during voluntary movement. A classic resting tremor is the movement of the hands as if using the thumb to roll a pill along the fingertips (pill-rolling tremor); characteristic of parkinsonism and Parkinson's disease.

tropia Deviation of one eye from forward gaze when both eyes are open.

uncus Most medial part of the parahippocampal gyrus.

unit, motor Alpha motor neuron and the muscle fibers it innervates.

unmasking of silent synapses Disinhibition or reactivation of functional synapses that are unused unless injury to other pathways necessitates their activation.

unmyelinated Refers to axons that are not completely wrapped by Schwann cells. Unmyelinated axons conduct more slowly than myelinated axons.

utricle Part of the inner ear that contains receptors that respond to head position relative to gravity and to linear acceleration and deceleration of the head.

ventral root The efferent (motor) root of a spinal nerve.

ventricle A space in the brain that contains cerebrospinal fluid. The lateral ventricles are within the cerebral hemispheres, the third ventricle is in the midline of the diencephalon, and the fourth ventricle is located between the pons and medulla anteriorly and the cerebellum posteriorly.

ventricle, fourth A fluid-filled space located posterior to the pons and medulla and anterior to the cerebellum.

ventricle, third A fluid-filled space between the two thalami.

ventricles, lateral Fluid-filled spaces within the cerebral hemispheres.

vermis The midline part of the cerebellum, involved in controlling ongoing movements and posture via the brainstem descending pathways.

vertigo An illusion of motion, common in vestibular disorders.

vertigo, benign paroxysmal positional Acute onset of vertigo provoked by change of head position that quickly subsides even if the provoking head position is maintained.

vessels, capacitance Vessel whose relaxed walls expand to contain more blood. Blood pools in these vessels.

vestibulocerebellum Functional name for the flocculonodular lobe of the cerebellum. Influences the activity of eye movements and postural muscles.

zoster, Varicella Infection of a dorsal root ganglion or cranial nerve ganglion with Varicella zoster virus. Syn.: herpes zoster.

Index

Page numbers followed by b indicate box(es); f, figure(s); t, table(s).

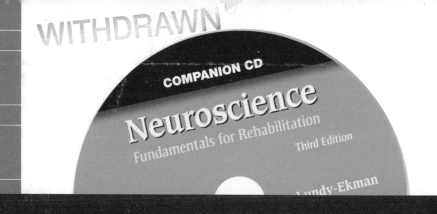

COMPANION CD

Neuroscience
Fundamentals for Rehabilitation
Third Edition

Lundy-Ekman

Better understand important concepts
in the text with this CD!

Designed to enhance your learning, this companion CD provides you with over **30 animations** of concepts offered in *Neuroscience: Fundamentals for Rehabilitation, 3rd Edition*.

You'll find animations of...

▶ motor neuron function and control

▶ the development of the nervous system

▶ the electrical properties of neurons

▶ and more!

TRY IT NOW!